SOFT TISSUE
RHEUMATIC PAIN

RECOGNITION, MANAGEMENT, AND PREVENTION
Third Edition

SOFT TISSUE RHEUMATIC PAIN

RECOGNITION, MANAGEMENT, AND PREVENTION

Third Edition

ROBERT P. SHEON, M.D., F.A.C.P.
Consultant in Musculoskeletal Medicine
Washington, D.C.
Medical Director, ArthritisCare Center of America
Nashville, Tennessee
Emeritus Clinical Professor of Medicine
Medical College of Ohio at Toledo
Toledo, Ohio

ROLAND W. MOSKOWITZ, M.D.
Professor of Medicine
Case Western Reserve University School of Medicine
Director, Division of Rheumatic Diseases
University Hospitals
Cleveland, Ohio

VICTOR M. GOLDBERG, M.D.
Charles H. Herndon Professor and Chairman
Department of Orthopaedics
Case Western Reserve University School of Medicine
Attending Orthopaedist
University Hospitals and Veterans' Administration
Cleveland, Ohio

Illustrations by
Claire B. Kirsner
Roy C. Schneider
Alan Weintraub

Editor: Jonathan W. Pine, Jr.
Managing Editor: Molly L. Mullen
Production Coordinator: Linda Carlson
Copy Editor: John J. Guardiano
Designer: Rita Baker-Schmidt
Illustration Planner: Wayne Hubbell
Cover Designer: Rita Baker-Schmidt
Typesetter: Automated Graphic Systems
Printer: R. R. Donnelley & Sons Co., Inc.

First Edition, 1982
Second Edition, 1987

Library of Congress Cataloging-in-Publication Data

Sheon, Robert P.
    Soft tissue rheumatic pain : recognition, management, and
prevention / Robert P. Sheon, Roland W. Moskowitz, Victor M.
Goldberg ; illustrations by Claire B. Kirsner, Roy C. Schneider,
Alan Weintraub.—3rd ed.
        p.   cm.
    Includes bibliographical references and index.
    ISBN 0-683-07678-7
    1. Nonarticular rheumatism.   2. Pain.   I. Moskowitz, Roland W.
II. Goldberg, Victor M., 1939–   . III. Title.
        [DNLM: 1. Rheumatic Diseases.   2. Muscular Diseases.   3. Pain-
-therapy.   4. Physical Therapy.   WE 544 S546s   1966]
    RC927.5.N65S48   1996
    616.7'23—dc20
    DNLM/DLC
    for Library of Congress   95-44778
                                                                                                        CIP

The publishers have made every effort to trace the copyright holders for borrowed material. If they have inadvertently overlooked any, they will be pleased to make the necessary arrangements at the first opportunity.

96 97 98 99 00
1 2 3 4 5 6 7 8 9 10

Reprints of chapters may be purchased from Williams & Wilkins in quantities of 100 or more. Call Isabella Wise, Special Sales Department, (800) 358-3583.

To Irma, Peta, and Harriet
for their love and support

PREFACE

Musculoskeletal disorders consume a significant portion of health care dollars, are occurring more often, and are of concern to experts in health care planning.

Most musculoskeletal disorders are managed successfully with a skillful blend of the science and art of medicine using medication, physical interventions, and education. With current challenges such as the increase in an aging population, reduction in available health care dollars, and ever-increasing job and family demands, we medical practitioners must learn to deliver care as efficiently and effectively as possible.

This third edition of *Soft Tissue Rheumatic Pain* has reflected these concerns by incorporating the expertise of experienced rheumatology physical therapist clinicians (Patricia A. Hoehing and Barbara Banwell), nursing educators (Janet E. Jeffrey and Patty M. Orr), and the viewpoint of the corporate world in health care (Dr. Orr). Dr. Orr's experience also extends to having provided guidance to the ArthritisCare Center of The Toledo Hospital, a facility that has put the principles of this book into practice. The implementation of these principles has resulted in more efficient delivery of comprehensive care for musculoskeletal disorders with equal or improved patient outcomes. For example, we have observed a reduced number of missed work days for patients with cumulative movement disorders, even with fewer physical and occupational therapy visits. When soft tissue rheumatic disorders occur in patients with concomitant generalized osteoarthritis or inflammatory rheumatic diseases, a team of clinical rheumatology specialists can deliver more efficient and cost-effective care than can nonspecialized clinicians working independently of one another. In the integrated team approach, the need for social service, dietary, or psychological interventions is quickly identified and appropriately addressed.

We hope that this edition will be useful to an even wider range of health care practitioners than in the past. More information about exercises and other physical interventions, as well as patient education, has been included so that the text will be of value to the broadest range of practitioners. Physicians should be able to make direct use of this information in their practices.

Nearly 200 illustrations have been added or changed to reflect advances in the practice of musculoskeletal medicine, using gray tones to yield better photocopies. We are indebted to the staff of The Toledo Hospital Medical Library and of the ArthritisCare Center for the many hours and expertise needed to make these changes. Irma S. Sheon fulfilled many indispensable roles, including research, proofreading, and the assembly and typing of references. Alan Weintraub, medical photographer at The Toledo Hospital, devoted many hours to the illustrations.

Hundreds of readers have provided helpful comments over the years; the authors are grateful to them and have incorporated their ideas and suggestions.

The medical publishing field has undergone considerable consolidation and change. Our new editors at Williams & Wilkins have been most helpful, thoughtful, and encouraging.

Robert P. Sheon, M.D.,   Washington, D.C.
Roland W. Moskowitz, M.D.,   Cleveland, Ohio
Victor M. Goldberg, M.D.,   Cleveland, Ohio

CONTRIBUTORS

BARBARA BANWELL, M.A., B.S., P.T.
Founder and Owner
Joint Approaches to Health
East Lansing, Michigan

PATRICIA A. HOEHING, P.T.
Senior Physical Therapist
ArthritisCare Centers of America
Toledo Hospital
Toledo, Ohio

JANET E. JEFFREY, R.N., Ph.D.
Faculty of Nursing
The University of Western Ontario
London, Ontario

PATTY M. ORR, R.N., Ed.D.
Vice President, Clinical Services
American Healthcorp
Nashville, Tennessee

CONTENTS/SOFT TISSUE RHEUMATIC PAIN:
RECOGNITION, MANAGEMENT, AND PREVENTION
Third Edition

CHAPTER 3: UPPER LIMB DISORDERS

CHAPTER 6: LOWER LIMB DISORDERS

CHAPTER 7: FIBROMYALGIA AND OTHER GENERALIZED SOFT TISSUE RHEUMATIC DISORDERS

CHAPTER 8: PHYSICAL INTERVENTIONS, EXERCISE, AND REHABILITATION
Barbara Banwell and Patricia Hoehing

CHAPTER 9: ROLE OF NURSING IN THE MANAGEMENT OF SOFT TISSUE RHEUMATIC DISEASE
Janet Jeffrey

Introduction: An Overview of Diagnosis and Management

Current trends in health care mandate several important philosophic underpinnings in the diagnosis and management of musculoskeletal symptoms:

1. Reliance on *practical approaches* that can be carried out in cost-effective strategies.
2. Emphasis on *self-management* strategies that enlist patient responsibility and adoption of appropriate healthy behaviors.
3. Reliance on techniques that have demonstrated *efficacy* in controlled studies or have strong anecdotal histories of effectiveness.
4. The development of long-term healthy lifestyle habits that assist in the *prevention* of disease.

Health care is now measured at least in part by its effect on functional outcomes rather than on symptoms. Soft tissue rheumatic diseases are major sources of work-related disability and possible loss of independence. Increasing attention is now being focused on diagnoses such as "cumulative movement disorders" and other task/function-related disorders. These disabilities and their resultant costly impact exist both in home and leisure environments as well as in industrial settings. Earlier management programs for the soft tissue rheumatic diseases cited "decrease in pain" as a main goal of treatment, since pain is often the primary presenting symptom of these syndromes. Today, however, a primary goal of treatment is *return to function* rather than simply decrease in pain.

Pain, spasm, and disability, though they are major features of soft tissue rheumatic diseases, often lack objective measurement. Outcome measurement is frequently based on scales that summarize global musculoskeletal performance. These scales are used as tools for research—none is widely used in the office management of nonarticular rheumatic pain disorders. However, several function scales, such as the Functional Independence Measure, are now being used on a limited scale (see Chapter 8). For these reasons, clinical and basic research are in evolution; much of what is reported is anecdotal, to some extent arbitrary, and often controversial.

Results of expensive and invasive procedures are under scrutiny for relevance; often findings do not change clinical strategy and therefore are a wasteful use of resources. Application of a careful and intelligent history and physical examination may lead to prompt diagnosis and identify probable causation without expensive and invasive procedures. Figure I.1 presents a pyramid of management for rheumatic pain.

Treatment, though often empiric, is in most cases safe and economical. Simple observations of functional improvement, such as degree of difficulty in rising from a chair or dressing, are recommended as measures of treatment outcome. Returning the patient to work armed with principles of energy-saving strategies, joint protection measures, and other behavior modifications will prevent recurrent soft tissue disorders. This book is, to some extent, a "What it is" and "How to treat it" book. Throughout the text, practical approaches are recommended with emphasis on functional outcomes.

This text is a resource for the evaluation and treatment of an increasingly common and expensive major segment of health problems and has been widely used in the United States, Germany, the Scandinavian countries, and Brazil, with translations into German and Portuguese.

The previous edition was selected by the American College of Physicians' Core Library

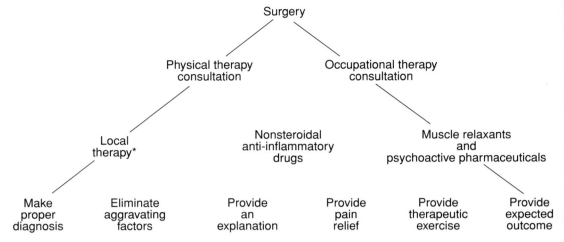

Fig I.1 A pyramid of management for nonarticular soft tissue rheumatic disorders. The pyramid builds from six essential points of management at the base. *Local therapy may be ice or heat; massage; pressure point therapy; spray and stretch; or intralesional injection(s).

for Internists. It was also recommended in *Medical Secrets,* published by the Department of Medicine, Baylor College of Medicine.

TERMINOLOGY

The designation of a regional pain disorder as a tendinitis or as myofascial pain is in common use, yet physical findings often require an examining "finger of faith." Insurers are increasingly accepting a symptom diagnosis such has "neck pain" or "hand pain." For coding purposes in the U.S., the reader may use either an anatomic or a symptom code (see Appendix D).

Cumulative Movement Disorders: Overuse may be defined as a level of repetitive microtrauma sufficient to exceed the tissues' ability to adapt. "Repetitive strain injury" or "cumulative trauma" have been used to describe tendinitis and carpal tunnel syndrome in many instances of "occupational injury." Because specific diagnostic findings and pathology are often lacking, and trauma or injury are pejorative terms to industry, the term *cumulative movement disorders* will be used here.

When a regional soft tissue disturbance results from improper sport or work habits, the condition is considered in terms of its anatomic designation (e.g., "bursitis" or "tendinitis") but categorized from an etiopathologic viewpoint as a cumulative movement disorder.

TABLE I.1 SOFT TISSUE RHEUMATIC PAIN DISORDERS

1. Regional myofascial pain: Regional pain with trigger point (See Anatomic Plates XIV and XV)
2. Tendinitis and bursitis
3. Structural disorders: Examples include short leg, scoliosis, lateral patellar subluxation, flatfeet
4. Neurovascular entrapment: Examples include thoracic outlet syndrome, carpal tunnel syndrome, and tarsal tunnel syndromes
5. Generalized pain disorders: Examples include the fibromyalgia syndrome, chronic benign pain syndrome, reflex sympathetic dystrophy, and psychogenic rheumatism

DIAGNOSIS OF SOFT TISSUE RHEUMATIC PAIN

The disorders described in this book fall into five major groups (summarized in Table I.1)

1. Regional Myofascial Pain Disorder
2. Tendinitis and Bursitis
3. Structural Disorders
4. Neurovascular Entrapment Disorders
5. Generalized Pain Disorders

Regional Myofascial Pain

Regional myofascial pain is defined by Travell and Simons as "hyperirritable spots, usually within a taut band of skeletal muscle or in the muscle's fascia that is painful on compression and can give rise to characteristic referred pain, tenderness, and autonomic phenomena'' (1).

The pain of myofascial pain disorder is of a deep, aching quality, occasionally accompanied by a sensation of burning or stinging. The pain occurs only in one body region. Patients often have restricted active movement of the involved area. One or more *trigger points* or tender points will be found if the examiner gains familiarity with the likely point locations for each body region. These are presented in Anatomic Plates XIV and XV. The trigger points often feel indurated, and palpation reproduces the pain in the ''target zone,'' often some distance away. Palpation of a trigger point may cause a muscle twitch and an electromyographic response (2–4).

Many health care professionals do not accept the concept of trigger points because they occur in normal subjects without pain and disability. Furthermore, in certain regions of the body, interobserver reliability and specificity have been found to be poor. Fibromyalgia *tender points* (discussed below) add semantic confusion. Chapter 1 discusses some of the current research on trigger points and tender points, as well as the similarities and differences between myofascial pain disorder and fibromyalgia.

Nevertheless, points of indurated bands of tissue in which pain—not tenderness—is induced on examination are commonly found in regional pain, and they aid in distinguishing a local musculoskeletal disorder from referred pain; they also imply a treatable disorder.

We have often used the combined term ''tender (trigger) point'' to denote these points in this text, in the hope that the reader will thus worry less about the semantics involved.

First noted by Swedish masseurs and described in the literature of the early 1800s, and popularized along with trigger points by Travell following World War II (6, 7), myofascial pain accounts for a significant proportion of pain complaints. For example, it was the primary complaint in 30% of patients who presented with a pain problem to a UCLA clinic (5). These patients often have a chronic, regional, perplexing pain disorder.

Tender points of fibromyalgia (see below) occur in more widespread locations and may coexist with myofascial pain. Hence, a myofascial pain disorder may bring the patient to the physician, but features of fibromyalgia may be evident in the history and physical examination. Simply palpating the opposite, uninvolved side for tenderness would alert the examiner that myofascial pain may be a presentation for the more generalized fibromyalgia. If myofascial pain disorder is the only disease process present, then palpation at other locations will be normal.

Trigger points may result from acute trauma or from repeated microtrauma of daily living, or from a chronic strain of sedentary work or living habits.

Tendinitis and Bursitis

Tendinitis is a clinical and pathologic disorder with common features of local pain and dysfunction, inflammation, and degeneration, often resulting from overuse. *Triggering* is a unique disturbance associated with tendinitis. Usually a digit will suddenly lock up and must be pulled passively for release. A snapping is perceived as the digit ''unlocks.'' Triggering occurs in 20% of upper limb occurrences of tendinitis.

Tendinitis may result from inflammatory rheumatic diseases or from metabolic disturbances such as calcium apatite deposition; a careful history will often suggest the systemic disorder. Achilles tendinitis may result from use of a fluoroquinolone antibiotic (8). The pathology of tendinitis is described in Chapter 1.

Clinical diagnosis rests on subjective features of local pain, tenderness, and dysfunction. Often local swelling is evident, and sometimes tendinitis crepitans is demonstrable as a rubbery grating sensation noted during palpation while the patient actively moves the involved digit.

Bursitis is an inflammation of the sac-like structures that form in utero to protect the soft tissues from underlying bony prominences. The origin of the term ''bursitis'' as recalled by Bywaters is of interest (9). Monro provided the first atlas of some 40 bursae. At the time (1788), the society that had followed the second bourgeois revolution consisted of princes and their political power, laborers and freemen who

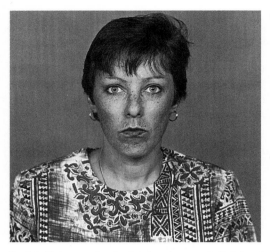

Fig I.2 Note smaller facial structure on left side of face. When one side of the face is smaller, temporomandibular joint dysfunction is more common. Other associated features may include scoliosis and a short leg.

provided the basic work, and the new middle-men—the businessmen and the banks, who ensured that the lubrication of *la bourse* (the purse) made for a frictionless and smoothly running society. Hence the aptly applied term—the bursa!

Clinically, bursitis is a diagnosis based upon exquisite local tenderness at sites where bursae are usually present, pain on motion and at rest, and sometimes regional loss of active movement. When bursitis occurs close to the body surface (e.g., bunion, prepatellar bursitis) swelling is evident.

Structural Disorders

Up to seven different musculoskeletal structural abnormalities were noted in 69% of healthy normal medical students in one study. *Joint laxity* was the most common; next was *restricted joint motion* (muscular tightness) (10). Other common findings were scoliosis, short leg, and lateral patellar subluxation. *Body asymmetry* is a common cause for many regional pain disorders. When one side of the face is smaller, temporomandibular joint dysfunction is more common (Fig. I.2); in addition, the remainder of the ipsilateral body may also be smaller, and the patient may present with a scapulotho-

racic syndrome related to a scoliosis or might suffer back pain in association with a short leg or an underdeveloped buttock.

Clinically, a structural disorder is rarely mentioned in the patient's history, but it must be considered—and searched for. Clinical correlation is necessary.

Neurovascular Entrapment Disorders

Neurovascular entrapment disorders may occur within the spinal canal (spinal stenosis) or along the course of a peripheral nerve. A sensation of *swelling* and *pain,* and *paresthesias* distal to the site of entrapment should suggest the condition. Tapping over the peripheral nerve or compression with an inflated blood pressure cuff proximal to the nerve may reproduce or accentuate symptoms and aid in diagnosis.

Generalized Pain Disorders

Generalized pain disorders include the hypermobility syndrome, fibromyalgia, the clencher syndrome, polymyalgia rheumatica, and somatoform disorders. The *hypermobility syndrome* results from loss of muscle tone in a person with joint laxity. Widespread arthralgia and a sensation of joint swelling lasting for hours, not days, are suggestive. *Fibromyalgia* is a symptomatic disorder with widespread pain and fatigue and the presence of 11 or more tender points in specific locations, with no more than 3 painful control points. *Chronic fatigue syndrome* typically includes widespread pain as well as the additional features of a past history suggestive of a preceding infection, tender lymph nodes, sore throat, and low-grade fever. Fibromyalgia and chronic fatigue syndrome share the symptoms of long-standing and often overwhelming fatigue and problems with memory and recall, but chronic fatigue syndrome is not characterized by the 11 or more tender points of fibromyalgia. Nevertheless, about 30% of patients diagnosed with chronic fatigue syndrome do have 11 or more tender points. The two conditions also have similar neuroendocrine and diminished cerebral blood flow findings. (See Chapters 1 and 7.)

The clencher syndrome occurs when a person under stress or caffeine intoxication uncon-

TABLE I.2 FEATURES OF NONARTICULAR RHEUMATIC PAIN DISORDERS

Inflammatory Rheumatic Diseases	Nonarticular Disorders
Pain during movement	Pain after rest
Palpable joint swelling	Swelling is sensation only
Abnormal laboratory test results	All laboratory tests normal
Aggravating factors possible	Aggravating factors likely
Diagnosis based on clinical examination and test results	Diagnosis based on physical examination maneuvers and outcome

From Sheon RP: Nonarticular rheumatism and nerve entrapment disorders. Resident and Staff Physician 35(12):65–70, 1989.

sciously clenches the jaw, fists, and rectal muscles. This may give rise to head and neck pain, arm and hand pain, and low back pain and coccygodynia, all at the same time.

Other symptom disorders that physicians are familiar with include vertigo, migraine headaches, and angina pectoris. These disorders often lack any pathognomonic feature, but treatment is specific and is associated with a good response in most patients. Relief from pain becomes a corroborative part of the syndrome recognition. A majority of patients with nonarticular rheumatic disorders respond favorably to treatment, which often helps to corroborate or establish the diagnosis in them as well.

CLINICAL FEATURES

Laying on of hands to palpate tender, indurated, trigger points of muscle tissue, to determine passive range of movement of joints, or to elicit joint hypermobility, is particularly important. Careful joint palpation for synovial thickening or synovial effusion is essential in order to detect the subtle manifestations of various connective tissue diseases.

Nonarticular rheumatic pain disorders have clinical features that are also helpful in diagnosis (summarized in Table I.2):

- First, the usual physical findings and tests of inflammation, as well as roentgenographic features of arthritis, are normal or expected for age.
- Second, symptoms often are worse after resting. Whereas intraarticular disease is worse with use and relieved by rest, these conditions often will awaken the patient from sleep or will be accentuated after sitting and relieved with movement. Of course, overuse may aggravate them as well.

- Third, most of these conditions have aggravating factors that lead to recurrences. These include improper resting position, prolonged repetitive movements, lack of respect for pain, and a personality trait characterized by the attitude, "I'm going to finish this even if it kills me!"
- Fourth, physical examination tests and maneuvers can reproduce or exacerbate symptoms.
- Lastly, simple office management can provide relief, and this response to treatment will corroborate the diagnosis.

COST-EFFECTIVE SYNDROME ANALYSIS

Somatic symptoms and fatigue are among the most common reasons for seeking medical care. The average cost for evaluation of a somatic symptom is in the thousands of dollars per patient (11). For example, Kroenke et al. reported that the average workup for back pain in 1986 was $7,263, chest pain $4,354, and fatigue $1,486 (12).

Cost-effective care must begin with a comprehensive appropriate history and physical examination. Only then can efficient further diagnostic studies and care be rendered. We stress the cost-effectiveness of artful diagnoses based on careful observation and a structured history. Appendix A provides a review of the art of the rheumatologic history and physical examination.

Imaging

When pain is persistent and debilitating, imaging is too often ordered on the assumption

HELPFUL HINTS

1. Laying on of the examiner's hands often provides more useful information than do roentgenograms.
2. Osteoarthritis seen on roentgenograms is often unrelated to the pain syndrome.
3. Localized musculoskeletal pain disorders may be layered over another established disease process.
4. When morning stiffness does not *mainly* involve the hands and feet, rheumatoid arthritis is an unlikely diagnosis.
5. Pain so severe that the limbs cannot be touched (the ''touch-me-not'' syndrome), and with no discernible spasm, is usually of psychogenic origin.
6. Pain localized to a body quadrant is seldom due to a psychogenic cause.
7. Observing the patient while seated, while rising from a chair, while standing, and while bending forward can lead to recognition of basic *structural* alterations. ''Misuse'' of the musculoskeletal system may also be observed.
8. Drugs may be the least important part of treatment. Stretching exercises and avoiding aggravating factors often provide more sustained benefit than pills.

that it will provide answers. Yet the information acquired rarely changes the course of treatment. Imaging procedures of the cervical and lumbar spine have high sensitivity but low specificity: findings in normal subjects reveal significant abnormality in 20% of normal 20-year-olds, in 40% of normal 40-to-50-year-olds, and in more than half of normal persons over 60 years of age (13, 14).

Magnetic resonance imaging (MRI), computed tomography (CT), arthrography, ultrasonography, arthroscopy, and electromyography have results that depend on the operator's skill, experience, and technique. The choice and timing of a procedure will depend upon the clini-

cal impression, response to past treatment, potential duration of disability, cost, and availability of an experienced operator of the procedure. The skill of those in the community who perform the procedure will also be a major determinant for use (15).

Do not order imaging if:
• there is no evidence of a critical disease process
• criteria for surgical intervention are not present
• the patient states ''I'd never have surgery, it isn't that bad.'' Too often the physician presents the MRI finding of disc herniation only to be told by the patient ''Oh, no, I'm not ready for that!'' Do not waste this resource. Imaging can be a significant tool for research in soft tissue disease etiology and pathogenesis. Unfortunately, many reports are uncontrolled or lack tests for interobserver reliability.

Thermography remains outside of currently accepted imaging technology, though it has been undergoing refinement and gaining in quality. Infrared emission from the body can be recorded by telethermography, contact thermography, and microwave thermography and may provide a simple, noninvasive, permanent record of sympathetic nervous system change in association with impingement of nerve roots, myofascial pain, and pain referred from cardiac or visceral diseases (16–18).

If no critical features are detected at the initial patient encounter, begin symptomatic treatment and provide the patient with an expected outcome, with the advice that the patient return within a reasonable time and proceed with laboratory or radiologic procedures if symptoms persist. (Table I.3 lists potentially critical features of rheumatic pain.)

TABLE I.3 LIST OF POTENTIALLY CRITICAL FEATURES

Fever, chills, sweats
Weight loss
Pain localized to a single site, and worsening
Skin color change
Raynaud's phenomenon
Bruits or diminished pulse
Lymphadenopathy
Joint swelling and tenderness
Limitation of spinal or joint movement
Asymmetric weakness
Neurologic deficit
Any unexplained laboratory abnormality

SIX POINTS FOR MANAGEMENT OF SOFT TISSUE RHEUMATIC PAIN DISORDERS

Six points of management (summarized in Table I.4) can often be initiated during the patient's *first visit,* even before appropriate laboratory and radiologic findings are available.

1. Exclude Systemic Disease. Satisfy yourself and the patient that serious systemic disease is not present. Systemic inflammatory connective tissue disorders must be excluded, as well as such entities as diabetes mellitus, thyroid dysfunction, occult neoplasm, and drug reactions.

Treatment need not wait for results from such tests in many patients. If roentgenograms are likely to add little information to the findings, they may be deferred until results of the treatment program are evaluated a few weeks later. Expensive, time-consuming, and possibly hazardous procedures (e.g., angiography for a thoracic outlet syndrome) should only be considered if they are clinically justified. More often, such procedures can and should be reserved for patients who fail to benefit from the conservative therapy initiated on the first visit.

A patient with tendinitis or bursitis following a cumulative movement strain would not likely benefit from radiologic or laboratory studies. But for patients presenting with bilateral carpal tunnel syndrome or frozen shoulder or fibromyalgia, we would certainly order appropriate screening tests, including complete blood counts, urinalysis, Westergren sedimentation rate, and appropriate serum chemistry determinations.

- An "arthritis screen" consisting of an antinuclear antibody and rheumatoid factor screening test, a uric acid determination, and a Wintrobe sedimentation rate determination may provide more misinformation than help. None of these tests is pathognomonic; each should be ordered only if the syndrome analysis reveals enough features to consider rheumatoid arthritis, systemic lupus erythematosus, or gout.
- Palpation will often provide more information than roentgenograms. (See "Helpful Hints" above.) If roentgenograms have been taken elsewhere recently, the films may be requested for review.

2. Recognize and Eliminate Aggravating Factors. Events and activities preceding the pain state must be reviewed in an effort to recognize aggravating activities that can cause recurrences. Improper resting, sitting, or working positions are common precipitating factors (Figs. I.3–I.6). Strain resulting from job performance, a new hobby, or repetitive, tiring tasks should be recognized and altered. Strain resulting from structural features, such as flatfoot or heavy, pendulous breasts, can also be altered with appropriate instructions. Too often, a job is blamed for symptoms that really resulted from a combination of factors in and outside of the workplace. Joint protection advice is detailed in the chapters covering each body region and in Appendix B.

- Chronic pain causes anxiety, depression, physical tension, and disturbed sleep. Let the patient know that emotional stress can be an aggravating factor, and that it may not only play a primary role in the pain syndrome, but may also lower a patient's pain threshold and compound the pain-spasm-pain cycle. Similarly, secondary pain resulting in dependent interpersonal relationships can prolong treatment. Frank discussion usually leads to a satisfactory solution.

Chapter 9 contains a wealth of information on both assessment strategies and psychosocial interventions. Readers who lack familiarity with any of the techniques can find recommended further reading in the references list of that chapter.

- Somatic delusions that accompany certain psychoses may at first confound the clinician, though the need for psychiatric care in such patients soon becomes obvious.

3. Provide an Explanation to the Patient. The physician should provide the patient with a suspected cause for his or her symptoms. For

TABLE I.4 SIX POINTS FOR MANAGEMENT

1. Exclude systemic disease
2. Recognize and eliminate aggravating factors
3. Provide an explanation to the patient
4. Provide instruction in self-help exercises
5. Provide relief from pain
6. Project an expected outcome

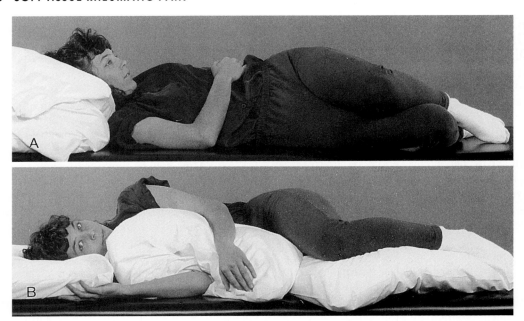

Fig I.3 A. Improper resting position: 1) poorly placed pillows; 2) neck in excessive flexion; 3) unsupported shoulder and upper arm; 4) twisted spine; and 5) unsupported knee and foot. **B.** Pillows strategically placed to support body in good alignment.

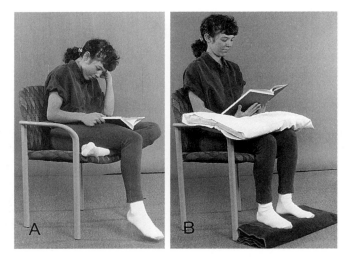

Fig I.4 A. Improper sitting position: 1) forward tilted head; 2) reading material at wrong angle and distance; 3) rounded shoulders; 4) foot tucked under knee; and 5) foot dangling free. **B.** Proper sitting position: 1) good cervical alignment; 2) support at elbows, forearms, and feet; and 3) correct positioning of reading material relieves neck strain.

example, if after the examination a benign hypermobility syndrome (see Chapter 7) is considered to be the cause of the patient's symptoms, this may be explained to the patient and he or she may be reassured immediately. Hypermobility syndrome is a more welcome diagnosis than systemic lupus erythematosus or rheumatoid arthritis. When a myofascial pain syndrome, such as gluteal fasciitis or trochanteric bursitis, is superimposed upon another disorder, such as osteoarthritis of the hip, the patient's comprehension of the findings is vital to future

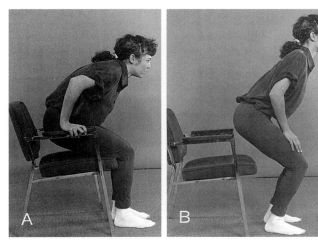

Fig I.5 A. This sit-to-stand technique demonstrates poor joint protection: 1) hands and wrists are strained to push off from chair arms; 2) hips too far back as subject attempts to stand; 3) excessive use of head and neck muscles; and 4) minimal use of thigh muscles. **B.** Incorporating joint protection principles, the subject moves to front of chair before rising, aligns head and neck, and pushes up to standing using thigh (quadriceps) muscles. This relieves strain on arms and strengthens quadriceps.

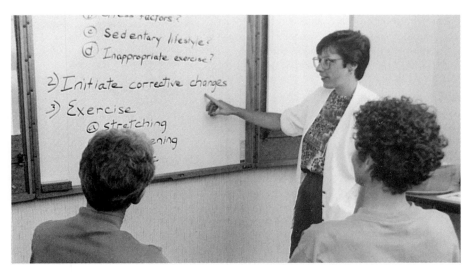

Fig I.6 It is imperative that the patient understand the role of exercise and other self-help techniques in the management of myofascial pain syndromes.

care. The myofascial or bursitis pain may cause more suffering than the coexisting arthritis. Alternatively, nonarticular rheumatic pain may disrupt a physical therapy program that is essential for treatment of the accompanying arthritis. Treatment of the bursitis or fasciitis provides relief from pain, which in turn allows the patient to follow conservative care necessary for the arthritis. If a myofascial pain syndrome has been found and trigger points identified, the patient can be informed that the pain is real, that a pain-spasm-pain cycle may be prolonging the condition, and that the persistence of pain may be due to an ongoing aggravating movement.

4. Provide Instruction in Self-Help Strategies. A prescription program of home physical therapy and exercises should be outlined on the first visit, if appropriate. Myofascial pain syndromes appear to respond best to a twice-daily stretching regimen performed first thing in the morning and last thing at night (Figs. I.6 and I.7). Even if pain has subsided, twice-daily stretching exercises should be continued until the involved region no longer tightens up during sleep. The ease or flexibility of morning stretching should be comparable to the ease of stretching the preceding evening. The exercises should be continued until the morning and evening exercise regimens can be performed with equal flexibility. Exercise strategies are described throughout the text for each body region (see also Chapter 8).

5. *Provide Relief from Pain.* Throughout history people have sought pain relief (Figs. I.8 and I.9). As mentioned, when pain is present, it may stimulate a vicious cycle, promoting greater muscular spasm. When the clinician fails to address the patients' pain needs, they will often turn to the use of alternative strategies, some of which may be unhelpful and costly. The self-help therapy program can be more effective and results obtained more quickly when pain is relieved. If spasm is minimal, pain relief may be obtained by such time-honored therapy as heat or cold applications and aspirin prior to performing the exercises (Figs. I.10 and I.11.). Acetaminophen use at the beginning of a more active day may be helpful for the patient with fibromyalgia.

- Intense muscle spasm can usually be relieved by local application of ice followed by stretching. If spasm is prolonged, injecting the "trigger point" with a long-acting corticosteroid–local anesthetic mixture can be curative. Similarly, if local application of ice and the use of nonsteroidal antiinflammatory drugs (NSAIDs) has failed, local injection for treatment of a suspected bursitis, tendinitis, or carpal tunnel syndrome can provide prompt pain relief and may help to establish a nonarticular rheumatic disease diagnosis. The technique is fully described in each chapter and in Appendix C.

There continues to be some disagreement on the decision to inject, and then whether to use

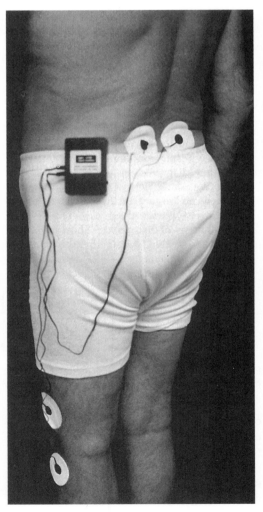

Fig I.8 One of several types of transcutaneous electrical nerve stimulator (TENS), with electrodes in place for sciatica.

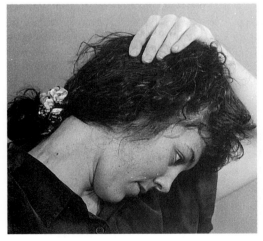

Fig I.7 A twice-daily stretching program to painful tight areas can be an effective relief strategy.

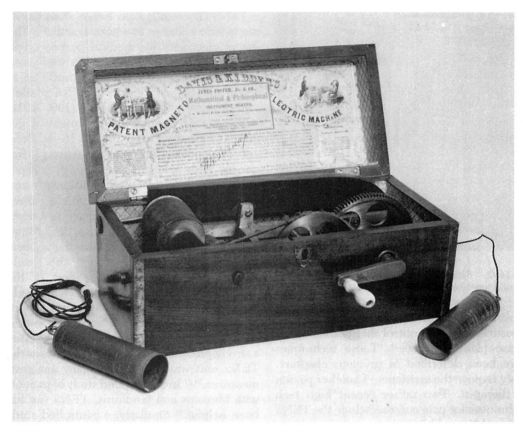

Fig I.9 A hand-cranked electrical nerve stimulater, 1856. The use of electricity for pain management dates to antiquity; after its beginnings with the use of electric eels, modern devices such as this one were devised.

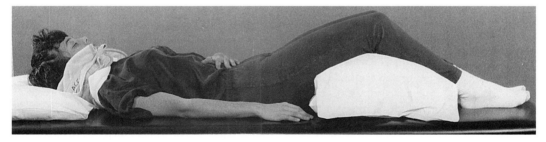

Fig I.10 Moist heat to a painful area can relieve myofascial pain and tension as well as emotional stress related to the pain. Apply heat for 15 to 20 minutes while relaxing in a comfortable, well-aligned position.

a local anesthetic agent alone, or a mixture of a steroid and a local anesthetic agent. Physiatrists tend to use anesthetic agents alone combined with physical therapy; orthopaedists and rheumatologists tend to use the combination without physical therapy; many soft tissue problems can also be alleviated by manipulation by a skilled manipulator. Where data are available to compare these techniques, the results are presented throughout the chapters of this text.

- NSAIDs are often helpful but may require a trial-and-error routine to determine efficacy and tolerability. Toxicity increases with age and in those with impaired renal or hepatic function. Persons older than 70 years of age may be given salsalate in low dosages, or acetaminophen.

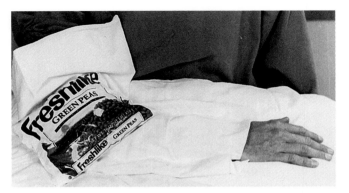

Fig I.11 Ice often provides adequate relief to tender points. A package of frozen peas conforms nicely to small areas. Freezing a mixture of 1 part rubbing alcohol and 2 parts water in doubled zipper bags also provides a reusable cold "slush." Commercial ice packs are also available. Apply ice for 7–10 minutes.

- If pain chronicity suggests a pain-spasm-pain cycle, tricyclic antidepressant agents, such as amitriptyline, may be helpful even in patients without apparent depression. Used at night, in ascending dosage, amitriptyline or other tricyclics may help to diminish pain as well as to provide more restful sleep (19–24). Patients who find a "morning hangover" effect with tricyclics taken at bedtime may find them more helpful if taken with the evening meal. A low dose of amitriptyline is often used, beginning with 10 mg and increasing by 5 or 10 mg every few days to weeks. Complaints of a dry mouth may be treated with increased fluid intake, sucking on sourball candy, or sipping water to which a few drops of oil of peppermint are added. Patients taking tricyclics should be warned not to drink alcoholic beverages or to increase caffeine ingestion.

Some muscle relaxants, such as cyclobenzaprine, carisoprodol, or meprobamate, may be helpful, particularly in patients with an acute regional pain disorder overlaid upon fibromyalgia. More information on medication can be found in Chapter 7.

Pain management must be approached from many perspectives. Gradual return to normal activity and beginning daily exercise should be accompanied by taking medication and by using other pain management strategies as well as stress management. Learning to think differently about pain is equally important. The whole person must be considered, and a program of pain management may require tailoring to the needs of the individual.

Too often the patient focuses on "I feel. . ." instead of focusing on goals. "How can I. . ." changes the attitude to one of self-efficacy. Patients need to have achievable goals, such as ways to reduce stressful confrontations, rest injured joints and yet continue employment, and make time for an exercise program.

6. Project an Expected Outcome. The physician should be familiar enough with soft tissue rheumatic pain disorders that the expected outcome and time required for benefits to become evident can be projected. Relief from carpal tunnel syndrome, bursitis, or tendinitis may require only a few days, whereas symptoms due to hypermobility syndrome or disorders of other structural deficits may require several months before moderate or great improvement is seen. This should be explained to the patient at the outset. The patient should also understand that the physician's diagnosis may depend upon the patient's achieving symptomatic relief; this in turn often depends upon the patient's performing the self-help program. The patient must work with the physician and other health care team members. Goals can be obtained, but their achievement will take time.

WORK-RELATED INJURIES

Many facets of work-related injuries must be considered:

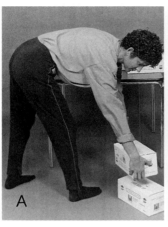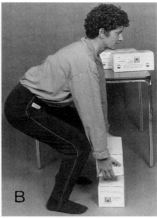

Fig I.12 A. Improper lifting techniques contribute to the high incidence of back injuries in the workplace. Note that keeping the knees straight while reaching out to pick up this heavy object significantly increases the forces on this subject's spine. **B.** To lift an object properly, one should use good body mechanics to protect the spine. Squat and keep the weight close to the body during the lifting process. Use the thigh muscles for power.

1. The work effort: Does the worker have to perform a repetitive task, remain in a fixed position for long periods of time, lift above or below a height that may cause strain (Fig. I.12*A,B*), or perform a tedious and monotonous task? What number of workers performing the same job have been disabled?
2. The workplace environment: Are lighting and temperature adequate? Are tools and machines adaptable to the physical features of the worker? Is the workplace safe? When the workplace is in the home, consider additionally the height of the work surface and its location, urgency of interruptions that promote tripping injuries, and frequent need to climb steps.
3. Does the worker have a good relationship with coworkers and management? Is the milieu conducive to good work habits? How does the company manage the injured worker? How quickly is proper care given?
4. What personal characteristics, habits, and attitudes does the worker bring to the workplace? What is the worker's past history in regard to time lost from work? Are the physical characteristics of the worker important to satisfactory job placement? Are there off-site aggravating factors

such as sports participation or a second job or hobby that contribute to the so-called work-related injury?

The "clencher syndrome" is a good example. The patient, Henry C., drives a long distance to work, has a boss he cannot tolerate, and he perceives his job environment as stressful. Each morning, the patient unconsciously clutches the steering wheel with excessive force, grits his teeth, and tightly clenches the muscles of the pelvic floor (levator ani, coccygeus muscles) all the way to work. By the time he gets there, he is exhausted! He soon has the features of carpal tunnel syndrome, coccygodynia, and a headache.

Workers under stress who develop myofascial pain disorders have diminished skin conductance and higher electromyographic response than those under stress but without symptoms (25). Also, they have evidence of autonomic nervous system dysfunction generally (26).

Long-lasting disability is not necessarily related to the seriousness of the injury, but rather to the age of the worker, lack of work skills, inadequate treatment, compensation neurosis, and worker motivation; these factors are difficult to measure (27). Yet, in everyday practice, the clinician can consider the impact that these factors might have on the patient and provide appropriate advice in an effort to improve the worker's health and productivity and to prevent recurrences. It is noteworthy, too, that delay in referral to specialists is correlated with longer periods of disability (28, 29).

Psychologic tests demonstrate that higher scores for anxiety and depression may precede disability in workers. Such workers are more likely to develop a cumulative movement disorder disability or to ask for medical consultation than workers with normal preemployment psychological test results (30).

Both medical and social factors are involved in disability (31). The interest in unconscious harmful motivation toward injury was stimulated by Hirschfeld and Behan in their research on what they called *the accident process.* From their study of the causes of accidents and injuries in the workplace (300 cases), the authors hypothesize that the accident process (recognized in seven cases) consisted of a state of conflict and anxiety within the patient; the worker then finds a self-destructive, injury-producing act which causes the "death" of the person as a worker. Instead of presenting with a classical psychiatric syndrome, the patient presents with physical symptoms that defy medical solution (32). This physical disturbance provides a solution to the original conflict. Others have found similar important psychologic factors in prolonged disability; they stress the importance of psychologic counseling and behavioral modification in treatment (33–37).

Malingering

Some characteristics of the consciously motivated (or malingering) patient include extensive "documentation" of the problem, a defensive attitude, demands for surgery, anger, withholding of information, inconsistent behavior, the "importance" of litigation to patient, and a relentless search for pain relief provided by someone else (38). They seldom perform self-help exercises. Isokinetic measurement often demonstrates significant variation in patient effort. Motivation may be directed toward secondary gain.

Newer treatment methods utilize symptom control, stimulus control, and social system modification. Symptom control is sometimes obtained by relaxation training, biofeedback, and autohypnosis. Data on outcome are meager. Simply introducing an interview with questions concerning job stress, ambiguity of the worker's role, overwork, and job suitability, was found to result in a marked decrease in worker absenteeism in one controlled study (39).

Neustadt (40) suggests consideration of the four R's when a patient develops increasing disability despite apparently adequate management:

1. *Roles*—the ability to carry on relationships as parent, spouse, student, or breadwinner. Look for loss of self-esteem.
2. *Reactions*—the patient's emotional response to the disorder, including anger, hostility, anxiety, discouragement, or defeat. Patient education is needed here.
3. *Relationships*—look for insurmountable problems at work, in the family, in school, or with friends. The patient may be beating his head against such "brick walls."
4. *Resources*—has the patient tapped community programs, counselors, minister, or used simple joint protection methods that reduce stress?

Disabled persons who keep pain in order to control others must be guided by the health professional to weigh the benefits of the pain against the risk of ultimately losing these persons with time. Holding onto pain as a means of avoiding work or home activities must be addressed by the health care professional, but only when trust has been established. Most patients want to "get better" even if unable to resume all former activities.

Much more work is required in prevention. Repetitive tasks that are not evaluated, boring tasks that not examined for ways to reduce the boredom and the risk of cumulative movement disorders, result in either "injury," errors, and ultimately lost work time. Recognition of a psychological motivation toward injury and disability may help to prevent accidents in the workplace. Employees remain active and fulfill job requirements and are less likely to use injury and pain to "get off" work when they feel appreciated and valued in the organization. Occupational health and safety are equally important, and, given the spiraling costs of disability to society, both are the responsibility of industry.

Chapter 8 may be helpful to the occupational health care professions as well as others concerned with patient attitude or motivation. Resources within the community, including agencies and public and private health care practitioners, are helpful and are also discussed in Chapters 8 and 9. Solutions to ergonomic problems in the workplace may be found in each chapter, or in consultation with an occupational therapist, or by using the following resources and literature for occupational problems:

- CTD News
  Center for Workplace Health
  Haverford, PA 19041
  Tel: (800) 554-4283

- Human Factors and Ergonomics Society
  Box 1369
  Santa Monica, CA 90406

- Applied Ergonomics
  Elsevier Science Ltd.
  Langford Lane
  Kidlington
  Oxford
  OX5 1GB
  UK

- U.S. Department of Health and Human
  Services

4676 Columbia Pkwy
Cincinnati, OH 45226
Ergonomics in Manufacturing, by C. Drury and S. Czaja (Philadelphia: Taylor & Francis, 1987).

OUTCOME APPRAISAL TECHNIQUES

Few studies have been conducted to evaluate the therapeutic interventions in nonarticular and soft tissue disorders because few valid and reliable measures of outcomes exist. What endpoints should be used? Pain intensity is the most common outcome measure of research and clinical assessment. Among the simplest tools for pain measurement are a 100-mm visual analog scale or a simple pain rating scale (Table I.5). This subjective self-report of pain is the most straightforward method available to measure pain. Reduction in pain intensity indicates, at least, that something is working.

Other measures that are as important as pain intensity include the impact of pain on daily life as well as the impact of other symptoms or problems, including fatigue and sleep disorder. Other outcomes might include onset to fatigue and the ability to perform tasks without pain.

Functional assessment can include determination of walking time, ease of putting on clothing or rising from a chair, or independence in bathing. Sleep patterns also reflect clinical

TABLE I.5 SCALES FOR MEASURING DEGREE OF PAIN

Visual Analogue Scale
A visual analogue scale by definition is a 100-mm line:

No Pain _____ Pain as
    0   1   2   3   4   5   6   7   8   9   10 bad as it
    could be

Verbal Rating Scale
_____ No pain
_____ Some pain
_____ Considerable pain
_____ Pain that could not be more severe

Numerical Rating Scale
Choose the number that best represents your pain, with 0 as ''no pain'' and 100 as ''pain as bad as it could be.''

After Whitaker OC, Warfield CA: The measurement of pain. Hospital Practice (15 Feb):155–161, 1988.

improvement. These simple functions are good indicators of the effectiveness of treatment and management strategies.

Clinimetrics, the study of the use of self-rating questionnaires to collect and analyze comparative clinical data, may provide a quantitative measurement of patient care (41). The measurement of functional ability, disability, quality of life, and coping with pain can all be performed with the use of valid and reliable questionnaires. Many of these measures have been used in studies of persons with soft tissue rheumatic disease. Unfortunately, these measures may not detect the patient's sense that quality of life is more than health status. Gill and Feinstein believe that quality of life can be measured only by determining the opinions of patients, which are not measured in current instruments (42). Lawrence et al. point out that the burden of illness is inaccurately measured, that little is known about such factors as provider and patient compliance, and that the economics of therapy can guide us when no therapy is clearly superior. Return to work and patient self-management programs should be considered as well as other therapeutic options (43).

A seven-point scale for a Functional Independence Measure, under study at the State University of New York at Buffalo and at Vanderbilt University, may be adapted for regional soft tissue disorders.

Psychometric studies are extremely important and correlate well with perceived disability. Some investigators believe that for every person with a disability from a rheumatic disease, there are five persons working who have just as much disease, but suffer less. Suffering should not be confused with severity of disease. It is hoped that the measures described in each section of this text will help to reduce suffering, reverse disability, and provide for more cost-effective care.

Involving workers in decision making provides the employer with other points of view and provides the worker with a greater sense of personal esteem. Having the workforce working smarter is better than working harder.

REFERENCES

1. Travell JG, Simons DG: Myofascial pain and dysfunction: the trigger point manual. Baltimore: Williams & Wilkins, 1983.
2. Simons DG: Electrogenic nature of palpable bands and ''jump sign'' associated with myofascial trigger points. In: Bonica JJ, Albe-Fessard DG, eds. Advances in pain research and therapy. Vol 1. New York: Raven Press, 1976:913–918.
3. Cobb CR, deVries HA, Urban RT, et al.: Electrical activity in muscle pain. Am J Phys Med 54: 80–87, 1975.
4. Fricton JR, Auvinen MD, Dykstra D, et al.: Myofascial pain syndrome: electromyographic changes associated with local twitch response. Arch Phys Med Rehabil 66:314–317, 1986.
5. Skootsky SA, Jaeger B, Oye RK: Prevalence of myofascial pain in general internal medicine practice. Western J Med 151:157–160, 1989.
6. Travell J, Rinzler SH: The myofascial genesis of pain. Postgrad Med 11:425–434, 1952.
7. Travell J: Conferences on therapy: management of pain due to muscle spasm. New York State J Med 45:2085–2097, 1945.
8. Ribard P, Audisio F, Kahn, et al.: Seven Achilles tendinitis including 3 complicated by rupture during fluoroquinolone therapy. J Rheumatol 19:1479–1481, 1992.
9. Bywaters EGL: Lesions of bursae, tendons, and tendon sheaths. Clin Rheum Dis 5:883–918, 1979.
10. Raskin RJ, Lawless OJ: Articular and soft tissue abnormalities in a ''normal'' population. J Rheumatol 9:284–288, 1981.
11. Kroenke K: Symptoms in medical patients: an untended field. Am J Med 92(Suppl 1A):1A-3S–1A-6S, 1992.
12. Kroenke K, Mangelsdorff AD: Common symptoms in ambulatory care: incidence, evaluation, therapy, and outcome. Am J Med 86:262–266, 1989.
13. Teresi LM, Lufkin RB, Reicher MA, et al.: Asymptomatic degenerative disk disease and spondylosis of the cervical spine: MR imaging. Radiology 164:83–88, 1987.
14. Boden SD, Davis DO, Dina TS, et al.: Abnormal magnetic-resonance scans of the lumbar spine in asymptomatic subjects. J Bone Joint Surg 72A(3):403–408, 1990.
15. Halbrecht JL, Wolf EM: Office arthroscopy of the shoulder: a diagnostic alternative. Orthop Clin North Am 24(1):193–200, 1993.
16. Hobbins WB: Thermography and pain. Progr Clin Biol Res 107:361–375, 1982.
17. Fischer AA: Thermography and pain. Arch Phys Med Rehabil 62:542–543, 1981.

18. Abraham EA: Thermography: uses and abuses. Contemp Orthop 8:95–99, 1984.
19. Raskin NH, Prusiner S: Carotidynia. Neurology 27:43–46, 1977.
20. Gomersall JD, Stuart A: Amitriptyline in migraine prophylaxis. J Neurol Neurosurg Psychiatry 36:684–690, 1973.
21. Halpern LM: Analgesic drugs in the management of pain. Arch Surg 112:861–869, 1977.
22. Duthie AM: The use of phenothiazines and tricyclic antidepressants in the treatment of intractable pain. S Afr Med J 51:246–247, 1977.
23. Beaumont G: The use of psychotropic drugs in other painful conditions. J Int Med Res 4(Suppl 2):56–57, 1976.
24. DeJong RH: Central pain mechanisms. JAMA 239:2784, 1978.
25. Kapel L, Glaros AG, McGlynn FD: Psychophysiological responses to stress in patients with myofascial pain-dysfunction syndrome. J Behavioral Med 12:397–406, 1989.
26. Perry F, Heller PH, Kamiya J, et al.: Altered autonomic function in patients with arthritis or with chronic myofascial pain. Pain 39:77–84, 1989.
27. Woodyard JE: Injury, compensation claims, and prognosis: Part II. J Soc Occup Med 30:57–60, 1980.
28. Lehmann TR, Brand RA: Disability in the patient with low back pain. Orthop Clin North Am 13:559–568, 1982.
29. Lehmann TR: Compensable back injuries and their management. J Iowa Med Soc 71: 527–530, 1981.
30. Helliwell PS, Mumford DB, Smeathers JE, et al.: Work-related upper limb disorder: the relationship between pain, cumulative load, disability, and psychological factors. Ann Rheum Dis 51: 1325–1329, 1992.
31. Jeune B, Mikkelsen S, Olsen J, Sabroe S: Epidemiological research in disability pensioning. Scand J Social Med 16:5–7, 1980.
32. Hirschfeld AH, Behan RC: The accident process. I. Etiological considerations of industrial injuries. JAMA 186:193–199, 1963.
33. Phillips AM, Weirton W: A study of prolonged absenteeism in industry. J Occup Med 575–578, 1961.
34. Maltbie AA, Cavenar JO Jr, Hammett EB, et al.: A diagnostic approach to pain. Psychosomatics 19:359–366, 1978.
35. Khatami M, Rush AJ: A pilot study of the treatment of outpatients with chronic pain: symptom control, stimulus control, and social system intervention. Pain 5:163–172, 1978.
36. Diamond MD, Weiss AJ, Grynbaum B: The unmotivated patient. Arch Phys Med Rehabil 49:281–284, 1968.
37. Cinciripini PM, Floreen A: An evaluation of a behavioral program for chronic pain. J Behav Med 5:375–389, 1982.
38. Florence DW, Miller TC: Functional overlay in work-related injury: a system for differentiating conscious from subconscious motivation of persisting symptoms. Postgrad Med 77(8):97–108, 1985.
39. Seamonds BC: Extension of research into stress factors and their effect on illness absenteeism. J Occup Med 25:821–822, 1983.
40. Neustadt DH: Commentary. Psychosocial factors in rheumatic disease. Orthop Rev 13:114–115, 1984.
41. Feinstein AR: An additional basic science for clinical medicine. IV. The development of clinimetrics. Ann Intern Med 99:843–848, 1983.
42. Gill TM, Feinstein AR: A critical appraisal of the quality of Quality of Life measurements. JAMA 272:619–626, 1994.
43. Lawrence VA, Tugwell P, Gafni A, et al.: Acute low back pain and economics of therapy: the iterative loop approach. J Clin Epidemiol 45(3): 301–311, 1992.

ANATOMIC PLATES
and
TRIGGER POINT MAP

Plates I to XIII are from *Gray's Anatomy,* 30th American Edition, 1985, Lea & Febiger, Media, Pennsylvania. Used with permission.

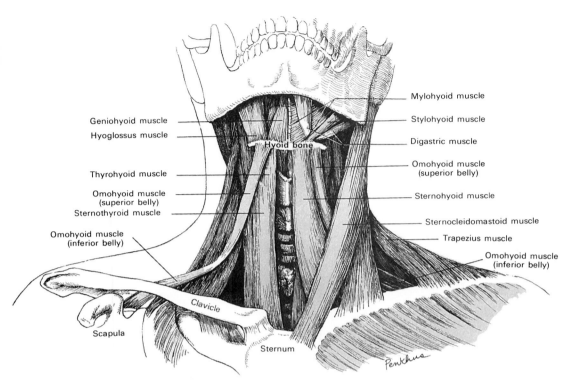

Geniohyoid muscle

Hyoglossus muscle

Thyrohyoid muscle

Omohyoid muscle
(superior belly)

Sternothyroid muscle

Omohyoid muscle
(inferior belly)

Hyoid bone

Clavicle

Scapula

Sternum

Penthus

Mylohyoid muscle

Stylohyoid muscle

Digastric muscle

Omohyoid muscle
(superior belly)

Sternohyoid muscle

Sternocleidomastoid muscle

Trapezius muscle

Omohyoid muscle
(inferior belly)

Plate I.   Muscles of the neck, anterior view

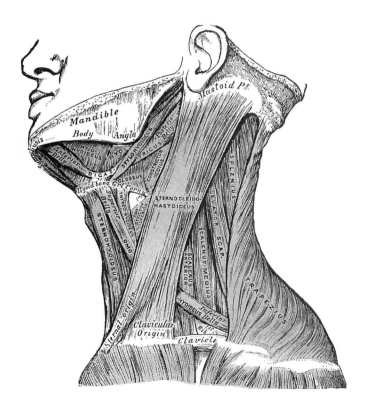

Plate II.   Muscles of the neck, lateral view.

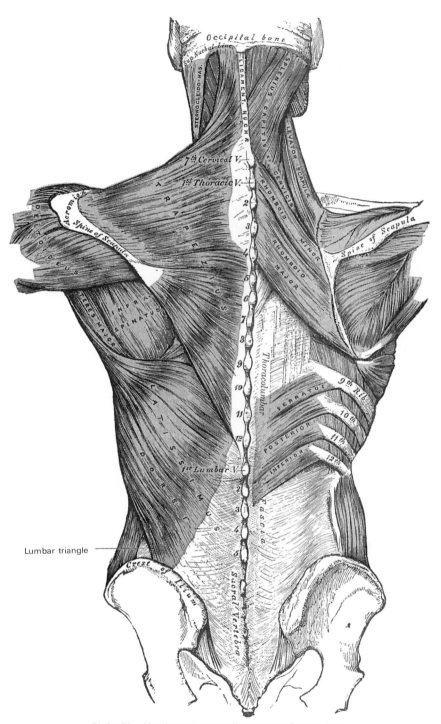

Lumbar triangle

Plate III.   Neck and upper thorax, posterior view.

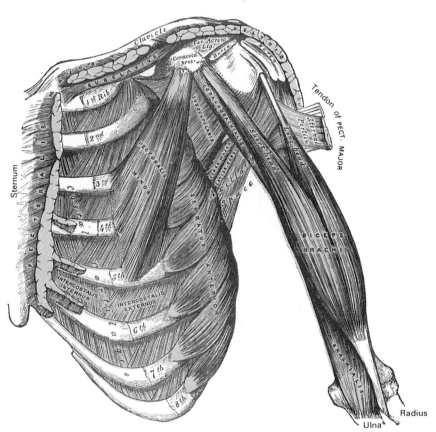

Plate IV. Shoulder, anterior view.

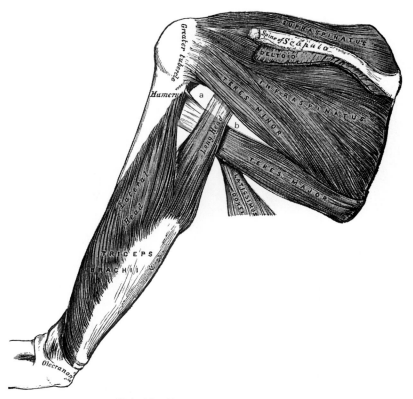

Plate V.   Shoulder, posterior view.

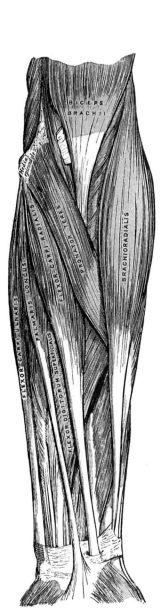

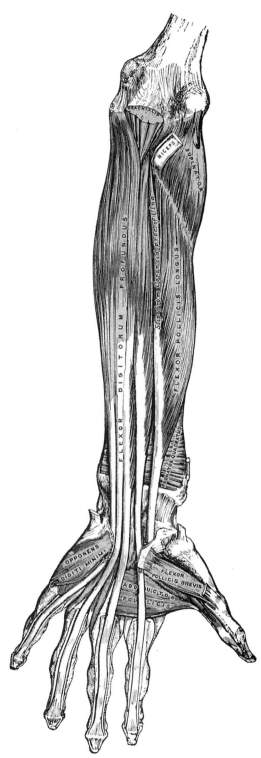

Plate VI. Forearm, superficial muscles.

Plate VII. Forearm, deep muscles.

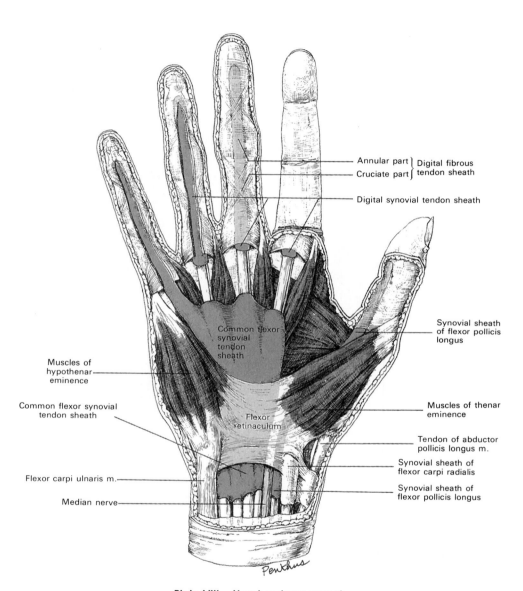

Annular part ⎱ Digital fibrous
Cruciate part ⎰ tendon sheath

Digital synovial tendon sheath

Synovial sheath
of flexor pollicis
longus

Common flexor
synovial
tendon
sheath

Muscles of
hypothenar
eminence

Muscles of thenar
eminence

Common flexor synovial
tendon sheath

Flexor
retinaculum

Tendon of abductor
pollicis longus m.

Synovial sheath of
flexor carpi radialis

Flexor carpi ulnaris m.

Median nerve

Synovial sheath of
flexor pollicis longus

Penthus

Plate VIII.   Hand, palmar aspect.

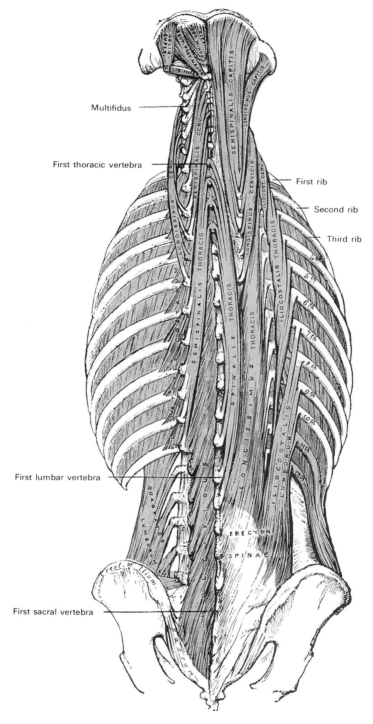

Multifidus

First thoracic vertebra

First rib

Second rib

Third rib

First lumbar vertebra

First sacral vertebra

Plate IX. Low back, deep muscles.

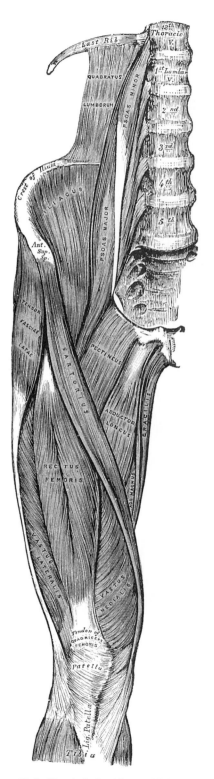

Plate X.   Anterior hip and thigh.

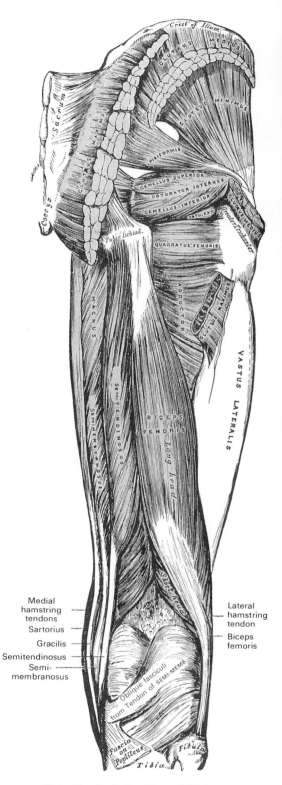

Plate XI.   Posterior hip and thigh.

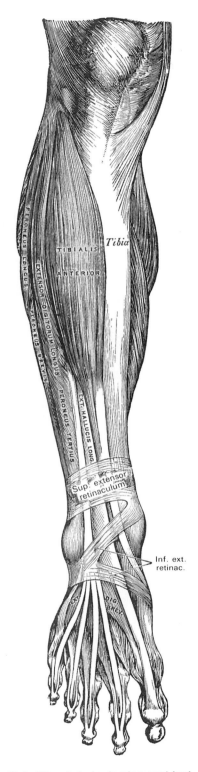

Plate XII.   Anterior foreleg and foot.

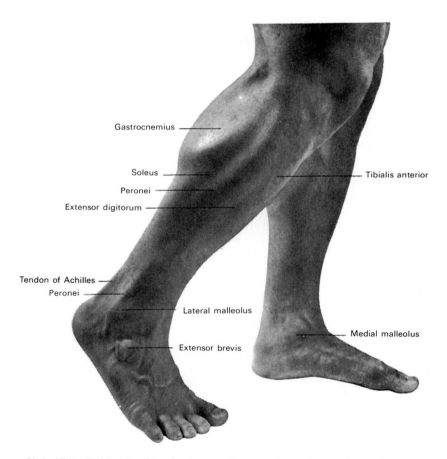

Gastrocnemius

Soleus

Peronei

Extensor digitorum

Tibialis anterior

Tendon of Achilles

Peronei

Lateral malleolus

Medial malleolus

Extensor brevis

Plate XIII.   Right side of leg to show surface contours of muscles and bones.

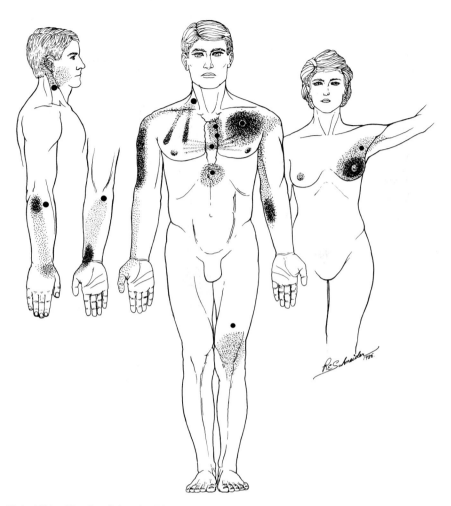

Plate XIV.   Myofascial pain (trigger) points and zones of pain referral, anterior view.

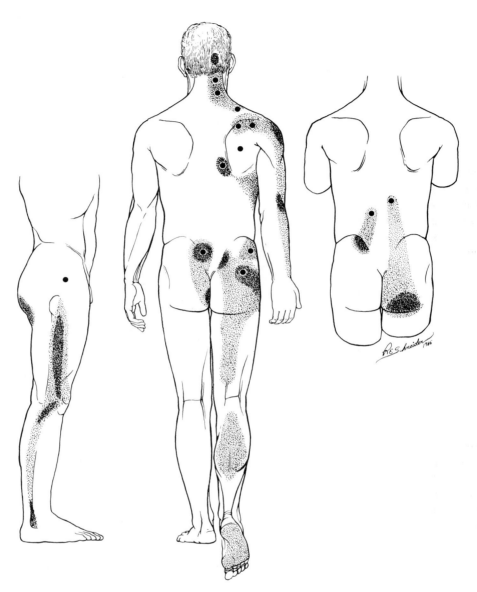

Plate XV.   Myofascial pain (trigger) points and zones of pain referral, posterior view.

1: Pathology and Pathogenesis

Etiopathologic aspects of soft tissue rheumatic pain conditions to be discussed in this section include those pertaining to myofascial pain and fibromyalgia (formerly referred to as fibrositis), bursitis, tendinitis, and nerve entrapment disorders. Often, the etiology is microtrauma or macrotrauma, but a number of factors may predispose the soft tissues to injury. Deconditioning, joint laxity, diabetes, and dietary factors may play a role in soft tissue injury (1).

CUMULATIVE MOVEMENT DISORDERS

Overuse may be defined as a level of repetitive microtrauma sufficient to exceed the tissues' ability to adapt. Tissues thought to be affected include muscle, tendons, and neurovascular structures as they pass through the extremities. The clinical disorders often are symptomatic regional problems such as carpal tunnel syndrome, epicondylitis, myofascial pain disorders, bursitis, and stenosing tenosynovitis.

Pathologic Studies

Structural and biochemical changes in the affected tissues have been described by several authors. In the hand, Dennett and Fry (2) performed open biopsy of the affected first dorsal interosseous muscle in 29 patients with upper extremity cumulative movement strain disorder and in eight volunteer controls. Affected and unaffected limbs were compared, and the histopathologic findings were categorized according to the severity (grade) of overuse described by Fry (3):

Grade 1: Pain in one site on repetitive activity.
Grade 2: Pain in multiple sites on repetitive activity.

Grade 3: Pain with some other uses of the hand, tender structures demonstrable, may show pain at rest or loss of muscle function.
Grade 4: Pain with all uses of the hand, postactivity pain with minor uses, pain at rest and at night, marked physical signs of tenderness, loss of motor function, weakness.
Grade 5: Loss of capacity for use because of continuous pain; loss of muscle function, particularly weakness; gross physical signs.

Findings demonstrated structural differences in affected muscles including increased type 1 fibers, decreased type 2 fibers, type 2 fiber hypertrophy, increased internal nuclear count, mitochondrial changes, and other ultrastructural changes. In Grade 3 complainants little difference in histology was noted from controls. But the findings were much more significantly abnormal in patients in Grades 4 and 5 compared to controls and to those in Grade 3 (2).

In an in vitro study Almekinders et al. used human tendon fibroblasts that were repetitively stretched with a cyclical computer-controlled device providing various levels of strain, after which the results were compared to control fibroblasts. Prostaglandin (PGE_2) and leukotriene (LTB_4) were significantly elevated, and lactic dehydrogenase was unchanged from normal compared to controls (4).

Larsson et al. report pathologic changes in open biopsies from painful areas of the upper trapezius in 17 patients with localized pain attributed to static load during repetitive assembly work. Findings, though not controlled, include pathologic ragged red fibers (Type 1 fibers only). Prior to biopsy, blood flow to the involved muscle was assessed using a laser-Doppler flowmeter with comparison to the less affected side. The authors noted a greater reduction in blood flow directly in correlation with the greater pain. Mitochondrial changes were also described (5). In another study muscle fiber changes were found not to be correlated with duration of symptoms (6).

These findings support the view that *some individuals can have tissue alterations that result from repetitive movement*. Chronic injury is followed by inflammation and repair with fibroblast proliferation, collagen deposition and regeneration, and tissue contraction may lead to swelling, pain, and some loss of motion and strength. Injury often arises from inappropriate personal work and play habits. Persistent pain rarely follows an isolated single injury. Cumulative injury from inappropriate use often arises at home as well as at the work site.

Tendinitis and Fasciitis

Tendon sheaths, like bursae, develop in response to motion as tendons pull and transmit power. Some tendons are short and without sheaths. They are supplied with blood from their muscular origin and from the investing paratenon. Where there is excessive motion, the tendon is enveloped in a synovial sheath. The visceral sheath has a flat synovial lining, and the parietal layer has vesicular and granular patches; there is no basement membrane, only a fatty or collagenous connective tissue (7). Tendon healing is facilitated by an intact tendon sheath. Tendinitis was first described in 1763 (8).

Connective tissue sheets called fasciae hold in place and separate individual muscles and groups of muscles. Other fasciae exist, also. Superficial fascia, a loose, fat-filled layer, intervenes between the skin and the deep fascia. The deep fascia invests and penetrates between the various structures that form the body wall and the limbs. The subserous fascia lies within the body cavities.

Tendon function can be impaired by local trauma, systemic disease, inflammation, fibrosis, impaired blood supply, atrophy, or degeneration (7, 9, 10). Recently, Achilles tendinitis has been linked to use of fluoroquinolone antibiotics (11). In most cases of chronic nonspecific tendinitis the upper limb is involved, and in 20% ''triggering'' occurs (12). Snap-

ping or triggering of joint movement can be due to nodular enlargement of the tendon, stenosis of the sheath, or both. Triggering—a momentary locking up of joint motion—can result from diverse etiologies, the most common of which is excessive repetitive hand use. Other causes include anomalous muscles (13), stenosing tenosynovitis at the wrist (14), and as a familial disorder (15). In most cases a stenosing tenosynovitis is found. Impingement of tendons between bone or ligamentous structures, most common at the shoulder, can result from repetitive motion of bone and a constricting second bone or ligamentous band (16, 17).

Inflammatory tendinitis may precede or accompany many systemic disorders ranging from tuberculosis, gonorrhea, and other infectious causes; rheumatic fever, rheumatoid arthritis, and other connective tissue diseases; gout, pseudogout, apatite deposition disease, lipemias, ochronosis and other metabolic disorders; giant cell tumors of tendon sheaths, and pigmented villonodular synovitis (7, 9, 17).

Dystrophic calcareous deposits in tendons and bursae that develop after injury or inflammation are of uncertain pathogenesis (7). Amorphous calcium or urate do not provoke inflammation whereas crystals do. Calcific tendinitis may result from apatite or calcium pyrophosphate (pseudogout) deposition disease after the calcific deposits erupt out of the tendon into the tendon sheath or bursa. Attacks of calcific tendinitis have a predilection for the shoulder, wrist, and ankle. Other types of crystals deposited in soft tissues include monosodium urate, xanthine, hypoxanthine, calcium oxalate, and various other calcium and lipid crystals (18). Hydroxyapatite, the most common type of calcification, is thought to precipitate as a result of a preceding degenerative process.

The enthesis, the site of attachment of a ligament or muscle into bone, is involved in a wide variety of diseases. Thirty-nine such sites have been described (10). They have specialized nerve endings, and the bone is not covered by periosteum. The tendon fibers pass directly into perforating (Sharpey's) fibers of bone. The tendon widens and attaches in a fanlike zone of attachment and hyaline cartilage is interposed at this site. The peritenon, perichondrium, and periosteum are connected to one another and contain much of the blood supply. This site is vulnerable to inflammation and is the typical site of involvement in patients with HLA-B27 associated spondyloarthropathies. Osteoarthritis has a predilection for this site as does ochronosis, calcium apatite deposition disease, hypoparathyroidism, osteomalacia, fluorosis, and acromegaly. Ischemia also plays an important role in degenerative lesions at these attachment sites (10).

Injury at these sites frequently is the result of conditioning and sport activities. A large gap exists between physiologic loads and the stress needed to cause tendon failure. Following a stress of as much as 17 times the body weight, a tendon can recover if given adequate time (19). Reapplying the force before recovery may lead to tendon rupture. Tendons are most vulnerable when tension is applied quickly, when tension is applied obliquely, when the tendon is tensed before trauma, when the attached muscle is maximally innervated, when the muscle group is stretched by external stimuli, or when the tendon is weak in comparison to muscle. With increasing strains that elongate a tendon, some of the cross links between neighboring tropocollagen molecules break, and, as more links break, the weakest fibers rupture. The load is then increased on the remaining fibers. Initial lesions are probably molecular, and with shearing force, the microvasculature is probably injured (20). This may lead to decreased oxygen, nutrition, and rupture of the cross-links between tropocollagen molecules. Chronic strain results in marked degenerative changes with focal necrosis and hemorrhage into the tendinous and cartilaginous tissues, followed by reparative tissue changes. The amount of acid mucopolysaccharides in small ''lake-like accumulations'' between fibers is distinctly greater than that found in the aging process (21, 22). Vascular proliferation is a regular feature in these tendon lesions, and signifies reparative processes (21, 23).

Acute overuse tenosynovitis may be serous or fibrinous, the latter sometimes referred to as ''peritendinitis crepitans'' (17). The basic feature is an inflammation due to changes in permeability of the cell membranes. Release of mediators of inflammation is followed by pain and edema, leading to impaired circulation.

Fibrin deposits then become organized, followed by adhesions (24).

Prolonged overstrain and inflammation result in similar pathologic changes. Pathologic changes resulting from repetitive strain disorder were described earlier. Electron microscopic findings suggest simultaneous degeneration and repair in chronic tendinitis (23). In summary, the pathologic findings of tendinitis are variable and may include features of degeneration, fibrin deposition, increased vascularity, edema, and occasionally inflammation. The pathologic condition in typical lesions is presented in Figures 1.1 to 1.3. However, if the tenosynovitis is secondary to a systemic disease, then features characteristic of that disease are found.

Fascia lata fasciitis, plantar fasciitis, and gluteal fasciitis are clinical diagnoses in which pathologic changes may be minimal or absent. This tissue has rarely been excised, examined by biopsy, or studied. The relation of fasciitis to myofascial pain phenomena is unclear. The etiology is thought to be of traumatic origin. The pathogenesis of fasciitis may include, in addition to traumatic factors, other biochemical, metabolic, inflammatory, neurogenic, aging, and central nervous system contributions. Plantar fasciitis can be objectively assessed with scintigraphy (25).

Bursitis

An atlas of the bursae was published by Monro in 1788 (26). Bursae are formed in response to movement. They are lined by synovial cells that secrete collagen and proteoglycans as well as collagenases and other enzymes. Subcutaneous bursae, such as at the olecranon, are formed after birth and develop in response to friction. Deep bursae develop in utero (7, 27). ''Adventitious'' bursae (superficial cutaneous bursae) form in response to shearing stress at the first metatarsophalangeal joint (forming a bunion), over exostoses, and over prominent spinous processes (7).

The normal bursa consists of a thin layer of sparse synovial cells supported by an adipose, a reticular, and a fibrous layer. Synovianalysis of normal bursal fluid, which consists of a thin fluid film, has not been reported. Traumatic

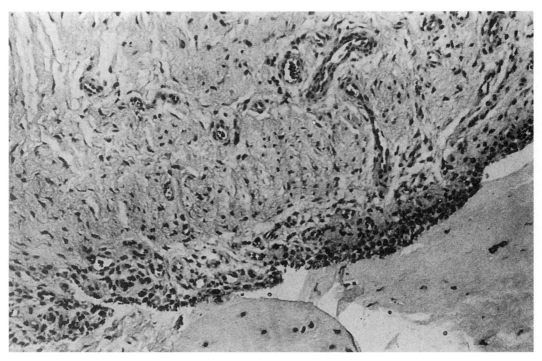

Figure 1.1. de Quervain's disease. Tenosynovium with slight synoviocyte hyperplasia and inflammation.

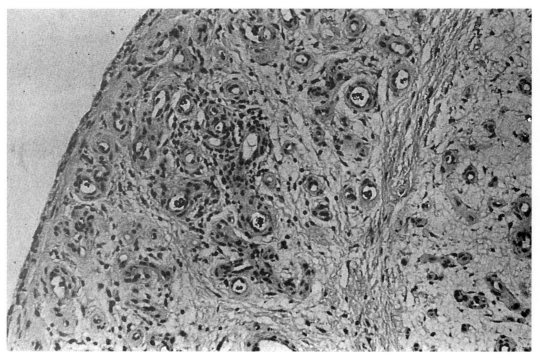

Figure 1.2. de Quervain's disease. Increased vascularity and slight perivascular cuffing by lymphocytes. (H&E × 100)

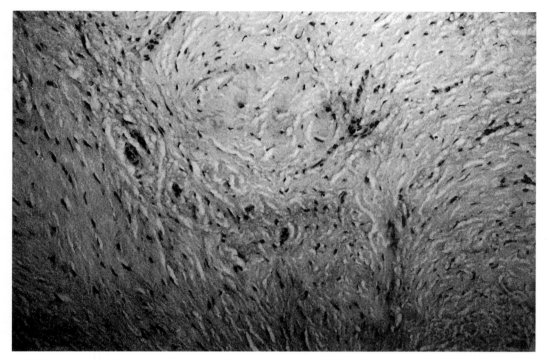

Figure 1.3. Trigger thumb. Tenosynovium with marked collagenized fibrosis. Note lack of vascularity, inflammation, or edema. (H&E × 100)

fluid is hemorrhagic or xanthochromic, with fair to poor mucin clot. Glucose content may be 80% of serum levels. Mononuclear cells predominate (27). Traumatic inflammation of the deep bursae results in the synovial cell lining becoming denuded in places, with fibrin deposits developing and the bursal walls becoming thickened. In some cases of metatarsal bursitis, the bursal wall shows fibrinoid necrosis (28).

In addition to trauma or friction, other causes of inflammation of the bursae include septic, metabolic, hematologic, and inflammatory connective tissue diseases. Also, villonodular synovial lesions may develop in bursae. Septic bursitis most often arises in the subcutaneous bursae (olecranon, bunion area, and prepatellar bursae); the inflammatory response in septic bursitis is less intense than that of joints. The septic bursal fluid white blood count may range from only 1200 cells upward and the bursal sugar content may not be as depressed as that of septic joint synovial fluid (29, 30). This is thought to be due to the lesser vascularity of bursae as compared to synovial membranes (27).

Gout, pseudogout, and calcium apatite deposition disease frequently cause bursitis. Intense inflammation follows, resulting in local warmth, redness, and exquisite tenderness. Calcium apatite deposition disease may affect tendons, tendon sheaths, joint synovium, and bursae. Roentgenographic evidence of calcification is noted. Involvement of the shoulder, elbow, wrist, hip, knee, and ankle are well known (31, 32). The pathogenesis involves a number of inflammatory pathways. Severe destruction of the shoulder cuff in association with calcium apatite deposition, the "Milwaukee shoulder," results from collagenase and neutral protease activity. Enzymatic release of hydroxyapatite crystals from the synovium and endocytosis by synovial macrophage-like cells with subsequent crystal-stimulated release of the enzymes complete a pathogenetic cycle (33). Hydroxyapatite crystal deposition also occurs in patients with hyperlipidemia, gout, diabetes, and in association with HLA-Bw35 and HLA-A2 genes (18).

Villonodular synovitis and, rarely, Gaucher's disease, may result in a hemorrhagic bursitis (34). Thus, in addition to trauma, the bursae may be afflicted by all the diseases that affect synovial joints, but the synovial fluid response is usually less intense.

MYOFASCIAL PAIN DISORDER AND FIBROMYALGIA

The findings and definitions of *trigger points* and myofascial pain, and of *tender points* and fibromyalgia, are controversial. Myofascial pain disorders are usually defined as prolonged regional pain at rest and with movement, without discernable disease. Myofascial pain is a local disorder of muscle that usually occurs in one body region. Perhaps the first reference to this subject was that of William Balfour in 1816 (35). An extensive literature followed the popularity of massage therapy in Europe in the early 1800s, and has been extensively reviewed by Reynolds, Simons, and Travell (36–41). Trigger points were mapped out and popularized during the 1940s by Travell (40). Trigger points can be eliminated with local modalities including ice massage, stretching, dry needling or local injections of an anesthetic agent alone, or combined with a corticosteroid agent. Tender points, however, cannot be eliminated by these methods but may be rendered less painful.

In one study designed to assess the interobserver reliability of trigger point identification, four experts on fibromyalgia and four experts on trigger points examined subjects divided into three groups: seven patients with fibromyalgia, eight patients with myofascial pain disorder (MFD), and eight healthy persons. Local tenderness was elicited in a greater proportion of MFD experts' manual examinations. Active trigger points were found in 18% of examinations of patients with fibromyalgia and MFD, but were not as common as the examiners would have expected. Taut muscle bands and muscle twitches were common to all groups (42). Thus there is need for more objective determinants.

The distinctions between trigger points and tender points of fibromyalgia may be artificial but are presented in an effort to provide a clear separation between myofascial pain and fibromyalgia (Table 1.1). Tender points, characteristic of fibromyalgia, occur not only in

muscle, but also in fascia, fat, or periosteal locations; they are seldom indurated; and they are considered secondary phenomena at the site of referred pain. Trigger points completely disappear with treatment; tender points do not (43).

Trigger Points of Myofascial Pain

The trigger point is the "lesion" of myofascial pain and is the result of injury. Trigger points are palpable bands within muscle.

The trigger point may represent sensitive areas over the site of innervation of the underlying muscle, where it is most accessible to percutaneous electrical stimulation. Needle electromyographic evaluation does not distinguish between fibromyalgia points and trigger points (44). Transcutaneous electrical nerve stimulation (TENS) of trigger points, compared with a sham TENS procedure, demonstrated reduced pain sensation generally, but not trigger point sensitivity when measured with a pressure algometer (45).

Trigger points presumably involve a circular or reflex pain-spasm-pain cycle, likely involving the autonomic nervous system. Although trigger points, when indurated, do not disappear with general anesthesia (46), they are abolished with a sympathetic nerve block (47).

Fine et al. demonstrated involvement of the endogenous opioid system. Following intravenous naloxone and trigger point injection with bupivacaine, the expected decrease in pain and the expected improvement in range of motion was abolished when compared to controls given intravenous saline (48). This study suggests that trigger points create high levels of muscle tension that is abolished with an injection.

Hendler et al. used electromyogram recording and noted a 7-fold increased muscle tension reading in trigger points that was then reduced to 1.5 times normal after bupivacaine injection (49).

Skin resistance is lower in the vicinity of a trigger point than in the surrounding tissue (50) and this can be reversed with treatment.

Most studies of the histopathologic changes reported in myofascial pain lack controls or do not distinguish between fibromyalgia and localized myofascial pain disorder. Two con-

TABLE 1.1 FEATURES OF TRIGGER POINTS AND TENDER POINTS

Feature	Trigger Point	Tender Point
	MYOFASCIAL PAIN	FIBROSITIS/FIBROMYALGIA
Tenderness and pain location	Local tenderness variable but pain zone always distant	Tenderness and pain at same site
Local twitch after stroking	Fiber twitch response	None
Aggravating factors	Mechanical injury such as strain overuse, direct injury	Dampness, cold, fatigue, overuse
Local pathology	None evident; local ischemia, or neurogenic factors suspected	Electron microscopic abnormalities; motheaten appearance; fiber atrophy, glycogen and fat deposition
Electrodiagnostic findings	Measurable during twitch response	None reported

trolled studies in fibromyalgia also were not definitive (51–53). However, fibromyalgia biopsy specimens show fewer capillaries per square millimeter than controls (54).

The "fasciitis" of myofascial pain has seldom been described histologically. The investing fascia of myofascial points was examined by Simon, Ringel, and Sufit (55) who reported normal findings in eight of nine patients who underwent biopsy examination. The one positive biopsy analysis revealed marked lymphocytic and plasma cell infiltrates in the fascia with extension deep into the dermis. Skin and muscle were otherwise normal. In ten noninflammatory neuromuscular disease control patients, the investing fascia was histologically normal.

Specific metabolic or chemical etiologies for regional myofascial pain are often lacking but must be considered. For example, Mills and Edwards found endocrine and enzymatic myopathies as a cause of muscle pain in 22 of 109 patients, inflammatory rheumatic disease in eight cases, and neurogenic causes in seven instances; in 72 patients they were unable to find any histologic diagnosis (56). Whether these patients had myofascial pain is unclear.

Local ischemia may play a role in persistent muscle induration and tenderness. The swollen muscle bundles may constrict the muscle's own blood supply. Ischemia as a cause for muscular pain has been suggested by findings of degenerated mitochondria and increased glycogen deposits in muscle fibers obtained from trapezius muscle biopsy specimens and examined by electron microscopy (57). However, in one controlled study with 12 patients and matched

controls using a xenon-133 clearance method to measure muscle blood flow in the involved trigger points, no difference in blood flow was found (58).

Muscle fiber injury as a cause for the induration and abnormality of trigger points is also supported by the report of Danneskiold-Samsoe et al. They measured plasma myoglobin (by radioimmunoassay) before and after 45 minutes of massage to tender muscle areas and to control areas. A tenfold increase in plasma myoglobin was found after tender point massage compared to the control area (quadriceps muscle) massage. Furthermore, as the measured area of tenderness receded with successive treatments, the plasma myoglobin "leakage" diminished (59). These findings suggest inherent brittleness of muscle fibers at tender point locations. Muscle injury may heal more slowly due to depressed levels of somatomedin C (60). Inasmuch as growth hormone is secreted during sleep, and sleep is of poor quality in patients with fibromyalgia, it is likely that sleep and healing are related. Sleep disorder is similar among patients with myofascial pain and fibromyalgia (61).

The American College of Rheumatology criteria for the classification of fibromyalgia has allowed investigation of a more homogeneous group of patients with a reasonably identifiable disorder (62). Speculation on the etiology of fibromyalgia has varied from a suspected peripheral lesion (fibrositis "nodule") to neuroendocrine dysfunction. Both local and central nervous system factors may operate together to create a chronic pain disorder with sensations of stiffness, tightness, and fatigue.

Mean maximum workload capacity of fibromyalgia patients was lower than that of controls (63) and lower than that of patients with myofascial pain disorder (64). Using an orthostatic test, a deep breathing test, Valsalva maneuver, and a hand grip test, 17 young men with fibromyalgia demonstrated greater cardiovascular functional variability when compared to normal age-matched controls (65). Muscle fatigue measurement using electrically stimulated tetanic forces failed to demonstrate central fatigue, and the relaxation rate of the muscle became gradually faster than noted in normal subjects (66). Thus, from a number of directions, there is accumulating evidence for a central nervous system disorder in fibromyalgia.

Histopathologic features of fibromyalgia reveal no consistent abnormality. Singular reported findings include interstitial inflammatory changes (67–69), necrosis and fibrosis, papillary projections of sarcolemmal membrane (36, 66–69, 51), and a metachromatic substance in interfibrillar spaces (51, 53, 59, 60, 69–84). Muscle ischemia, energy metabolism, and other functional abnormalities have been hypothesized but not universally accepted (64, 85–88).

For many years researchers have tried to identify serologic markers for fibromyalgia, including substance P and enkephalins and endorphins. Then, in 1982, Terenius presented findings of low levels of endorphins in cerebrospinal fluid (CSF) using a receptor assay in patients with chronic headache or back pain (89). Cleeland et al. confirmed and extended this finding in 1984 using a radioimmunoassay test (90). More recently, Vaeroy et al. found normal levels of CSF endorphin in fibromyalgia (91).

Substance P, one of the somatostatins, is generated in peripheral nerves and the spinal cord and is a modulator or transmitter of afferent pain stimuli. Vaeroy et al., using a radioimmunoassay test, have demonstrated increased activity of substance P in the CSF of fibromyalgia patients, sometimes as much as three times normal (92). However, the highest levels are not correlated with severity of pain.

Studies also reveal biogenic amine abnormality in fibromyalgia. Findings suggest decreased brain serotonin levels (93) and low levels of CSF metabolites of serotonin, norepi-nephrine, and dopamine (94). Deficiency of serotonin is thought to account for many of the features of fibromyalgia as well as for the improvement provided by medications directed at this deficiency. However, not all patients with fibromyalgia are deficient in CSF serotonin.

MYOPATHIES

Trigger points and tender points are absent in most cases of myopathy. Thus careful assessment for generalized myopathic disease states must be considered if trigger points are not detected. Disorders to be differentiated include polymyalgia rheumatica and other inflammatory rheumatic diseases, alcoholism, metabolic bone diseases, defects in muscle energy metabolism, myoadenylate deaminase deficiency (95, 96), idiopathic paroxysmal myoglobinurias, muscle pain syndromes of unknown etiology, and drug-induced myopathies. Myoadenylate deaminase deficiency may cause myalgia complaints, weakness, and exercise intolerance. Drugs to be considered as pathogenic factors in myopathies include anticonvulsants, heroin, amphetamines, clofibrate, ϵ-aminocaproic acid, vincristine, emetine, cimetidine, diuretics, laxatives, and licorice. Muscle cramp and fasciculation may further result from use of clofibrate, lithium, and cytotoxic drugs (97). Thus the requirement for a careful history and examination is stressed. The distinction between myofascial pain with trigger points and myopathies is usually not difficult.

NERVE ENTRAPMENT DISORDERS

Entrapment neuropathies (98) occur at many locations where neurovascular compression causes localized nerve damage. Entrapment may result from direct external nerve compression or contusion from work, hobby, or sport activities including such entities as harp player's thumb, bowler's thumb, or by a constricting watch or belt (99). Structural abnormalities such as a cervical rib, anomalous nerves, muscles, or bands may constrict adjacent nerves (100, 101). Stenosis of the cervical spinal canal (102) or lumbar spinal canal (103) results in both neurologic and vascular impairment. A peripheral neuropathy may coexist and create significant diagnostic confusion.

The more common sites for nerve entrapment are the thoracic outlet, the cervical and lumbar spine, the coracoacromial arch, the elbow, the wrist and hand, the pelvic region, the popliteal region, and the ankle and foot (104, 105). Imaging studies of normal subjects have raised questions concerning the relevance of spinal stenosis to symptoms, as a significant proportion of middle-aged and aged asymptomatic subjects have moderate stenoses.

The carpal tunnel syndrome is the most common entrapment neuropathy and was first reported in 1913 (106). Median nerve impingement may result from diseases that invade the carpal tunnel, from swelling of tendon sheaths within the tunnel, from stenosis of the tunnel by bone enlargement, or from thickening and degeneration of the volar carpal ligament. The elliptically shaped space enclosed by the inelastic flexor retinaculum ventrally and the carpal bones dorsally contains eight deep and superficial flexor tendons and their sheaths, the flexor pollicis longus tendon and sheath, and the median nerve. Occasionally, the space also contains the radial and ulnar palmar bursae, or the median artery (107). The application of computed tomography to the carpal canal has suggested that the bony canal may become stenosed. Normal and affected women in a study had significantly smaller carpal canals than healthy males, and carpal size was inversely proportional to age. Hand size alone did not correlate with the development of a carpal tunnel syndrome (108). When compared to normal controls, CT scan of symptomatic patients demonstrated significant stenosis of the proximal part but not the distal part of the carpal canal (109). A genetic propensity toward carpal tunnel stenosis has been suggested (110).

The nerve compression may result from externally applied trauma or from factors within the canal such as tenosynovitis due to systemic rheumatic disorders, thickening of the retinaculum, hypertrophy of muscles, infiltrative diseases of the canal such as amyloid, myeloma, or myxedema, or bone involvement by disease or tumor. Nerve compression can result from synovitis of the long flexor tendons due to overuse (111), fluid retention states, and systemic inflammation. Aberrant or hypertrophied muscles may also be found as contributing factors (104). Overuse is thought to be a precipitating event rather than a primary etiologic factor in carpal tunnel syndrome (112).

In cases of carpal tunnel syndrome, histologic examination reveals an increase in perineurial and endoneurial connective tissue and a marked reduction in the caliber of the nerve fibers (112). Pathologic findings are so variable that they provide few clues as to the mechanism responsible for impaired nerve conduction.

One mechanism may be the complex pressure system which operates within the canal (112). Pressure within the carpal canal rises threefold during flexion or extension (113). Once the carpal canal pressure rises, progressive nerve involvement occurs with edema of nerve tissue. Anoxia, caused by venous congestion and stasis, may be the result (111).

REFERENCES

1. Jacobsson L, Lindgarde F, Manthorpe R, et al.: Fatty acid composition of adipose tissue and serum micronutrients in relation to common rheumatic complaints in Swedish adults 50–70 years old. Scand J Rheumatol 21:171–177, 1992.
2. Dennett X, Fry HJH: Overuse syndrome: a muscle biopsy study. Lancet 1:905–908, 1988.
3. Fry HJH: Overuse syndrome in musicians: prevention and management. Lancet 2:728–731, 1986.
4. Almekinders LC, Banes AJ, Ballenger CA: Effects of repetitive motion on human fibroblasts. Med Sci Sports Exer 25:603–607, 1993.
5. Larsson SE, Bodegard L, Henriksson JG, et al.: Chronic trapezius myalgia: morphology and blood flow studied in 17 patients. Acta Orthop Scand 61:394–398, 1990.
6. Uhlig Y, Weber BR, Grob D, Muntener M: Fiber composition and fiber transformations in neck muscles of patients with dysfunction of the cervical spine. J Orthop Res 13(2):240–249, 1995.
7. Bywaters EGL: Lesions of bursae, tendons, and tendon sheaths. Clin Rheum Dis 5:883–926, 1979.
8. DeSauvages de la Croix FB: Nosologia Methodica Sistens Morborum Classes, Genera et Species

Juxta Sydenhami Mentum et Botanicorum Ordinem. Amsterdam, 1763.

9. Borgsmiller WK, Whiteside LA: Tuberculous tenosynovitis of the hand (''compound palmar ganglion''): literature review and case report. Orthopedics 3:1093–1096, 1980.

10. Niepel GA, Sit'aj S: Enthesopathy. Clin Rheum Dis 5:857–863, 1979.

11. Ribard P, Audisio F, Kahn, et al.: Seven Achilles tendinitis including 3 complicated by rupture during fluoroquinolone therapy. J Rheumatol 19:1479–1481, 1992.

12. Lipscomb PR: Chronic nonspecific tenosynovitis and peritendinitis. Surg Clin North Am 24: 780–797, 1944.

13. Aghasi MK, Rzetelny V, Axer A: The flexor digitorum superficialis as a cause of bilateral carpal-tunnel syndrome and trigger wrist. J Bone Joint Surg 62A:134–135, 1980.

14. Parker HG: Dupuytren's contracture as a cause of stenosing tenosynovitis. J Maine Med Assoc 70:147–148, 1979.

15. Weber PC: Trigger thumb in successive generations of a family. Clin Orthop 143:167, 1979.

16. Hawkins RJ, Hobeika P: Physical examination of the shoulder. Orthopedics 6:1270–1278, 1983.

17. Moritz AR: The pathology of trauma. 2nd Ed. Philadelphia: Lea & Febiger, 1954.

18. Dieppe PA, Huskisson EC, Crocker P, Willoughby DA: Apatite deposition disease: a new arthropathy. Lancet 1:266–268, 1976.

19. Curwin S, Stanish WD: Tendinitis: its etiology and treatment. Lexington, Mass.: The Collamore Press, 1984.

20. Kalyan-Raman UP, Kalyan-Raman K, Yunus MB, Masi AT: Muscle pathology in primary fibromyalgia syndrome: a light microscopic histochemical and ultrastructural study. J Rheumatol 11: 808–813, 1984.

21. Merkel KHH, Hess H, Kunz M: Insertional tendopathy. Pathol Res Pract 173:303–309, 1982.

22. Riley GP, Harrall RL, Constant CR, et al.: Glycosaminoglycans of human rotator cuff tendons: changes with age and in chronic rotator cuff tendinitis. Ann Rheum Dis 53(6):367–376, 1994.

23. Sarkar K, Uhthoff HK: Ultrastructure of the common extensor tendon in tennis elbow. Virchows Arch A Pathol Anat Histopathol 386:317–330, 1980.

24. Kvist M, Jarvinen M: Clinical, histochemical, and biomechanical features in repair of muscle and tendon injuries. Int J Sports Med 3:12–14, 1982.

25. Dasqupta B, Bowles J: Use of technetium scintigraphy to locate the steroid injection site in plantar fasciitis. (Abstract #581) Arthritis Rheum 38(9 [Suppl.]):S250, 1995.

26. Monro A (Secundus): A description of all the bursae mucosae of the human body. Edinburgh: Elliot, 1788.

27. Canoso JJ, Yood RA: Reaction of superficial bursae in response to specific disease stimuli. Arthritis Rheum 22:1361–1364, 1979.

28. Bossley CJ, Cairney PC: The intermetatarsophalangeal bursa: its significance in Morton's metatarsalgia. J Bone Joint Surg 62B:184–187, 1980.

29. Thompson GR, Manshady BM, Weiss JJ: Septic bursitis. JAMA 240:2280–2281, 1978.

30. Ho G Jr, Tice AD: Comparison of nonseptic and septic bursitis: further observations on the treatment of septic bursitis. Arch Intern Med 139: 1269–1273, 1979.

31. Pinals RS, Short CL: Calcific periarthritis involving multiple sites. Arthritis Rheum 9:566–574, 1966.

32. Fam AG, Pritzker KPH, Stein JL, Houpt JB, Little AH: Apatite-associated arthropathy: a clinical study of 14 cases, 2 with calcific bursitis. J Rheumatol 6:461–470, 1979.

33. Halverson PB, Cheung HS, McCarty DJ, et al.: ''Milwaukee shoulder'': association of microspheroids containing hydroxyapatite crystals with rotator cuff defects. II. Synovial fluid studies. Arthritis Rheum 24:474–476, 1981.

34. Gelfand G, Bienenstock H: Hemorrhagic bursitis and bone crises in chronic adult Gaucher's disease: a case report. Arthritis Rheum 25: 1369–1373, 1982.

35. Balfour W: Illustrations of the efficacy of compression and percussion in the cure of rheumatism and sprains, scrofulous affections of the joints and spine, chronic pains arising from a scrofulous taint in the constitution, lameness, and loss of power in the hands from gout, paralytic debility of the extremities, general derangement of the nervous system; and in promoting digestion, with all the secretions and excretions. Lon Med Phys J 51:446–462; 52:104–115, 200–208, 284–291, 1824.

36. Reynolds MD: The development of the concept of fibrositis. J Hist Med & Allied Sci 38:5–35, 1983.

37. Simons DG: Muscle pain syndromes—part I. Am J Phys Med 54:289–311, 1975.

38. Simons DG: Muscle pain syndromes—part II. Am J Phys Med 55:15–42, 1976.

39. Travell J, Rinzler SH: The myofascial genesis of pain. Postgrad Med 11:425–434, 1952.

40. Travell J: Conferences on therapy: management of pain due to muscle spasm. New York State J Med 45:2085–2097, 1945.

41. Travell JG, Simons DG: Myofascial pain and dysfunction: the trigger point manual. Baltimore: Williams & Wilkins, 1983.

42. Wolfe F, Simons DG, Fricton J, et al.: The fibromyalgia and myofascial pain syndromes: a preliminary study of tender points and trigger points in persons with fibromyalgia, myofascial pain syndrome, and no disease. J Rheumatol 19: 944–951, 1992.

43. Sheon RP: Regional myofascial pain and the fibrositis syndrome (fibromyalgia). Compr Ther 12:42–52, 1986.

44. Durette MR, Rodriquez AA, Agre JC, et al.: Needle electromyographic evaluation of patients with myofascial or fibromyalgic pain. Am J Phys Med Rehabil 70:154–156, 1991.

45. Graff-Radford SB, Reeves JL, Baker RL, et al.: Effects of transcutaneous electrical nerve stimulation on myofascial pain and trigger point sensitivity. Pain 37:1–5, 1989.

46. Reynolds MD: The development of the concept of fibrositis. J Hist Med Allied Sci 38:5–35, 1983.

47. Procacci P, Francini F, Zoppo M, et al.: Role of the sympathetic system in reflex dystrophy. Adv Pain Res Ther 1:953–957, 1976.

48. Fine PG, Milano R, Hare BD: The effects of myofascial trigger point injections are naloxone reversible. Pain 32:15–20, 1988.

49. Hendler N, Fink H, Long D: Myofascial syndrome: response to trigger-point injections. Psychosomatics 24:990–999, 1983.

50. Hyvarinen J, Karlsson M: Low resistance points that may coincide with acupuncture loci. Med Biol 55:88–94, 1977.

51. Kalyan-Raman UP, Kalyan-Raman K, Yunus MB, Masi AT: Muscle pathology in primary fibromyalgia syndrome: a light microscopic histochemical and ultrastructural study. J Rheumatol 11:808, 1984.

52. Yunus MB, Kalyan-Raman UP, Masi AT, et al.: Electron microscopic studies of muscle biopsy in primary fibromyalgia syndrome: a controlled and blinded study. J Rheumatol 16:97–101, 1989.

53. Bengtsson A, Henriksson KG, Larsson J: Muscle biopsy in primary fibromyalgia. Light-microscopal and histochemical findings. Scand J Rheumatol 15:1–6, 1986.

54. Lindh M, Johansson G, Hedberg M, et al.: Muscle fiber characteristics, capillaries, and enzymes in patients with fibromyalgia and controls. Scand J Rheumatol 24(1):34–37, 1995.

55. Simon DB, Ringel SP, Sufit RL: Clinical spectrum of fascial inflammation. Muscle Nerve (Sept): 535–537, 1982.

56. Mills KR, Edwards RHT: Investigative strategies for muscle pain. J Neuro Sci 58:73–88, 1983.

57. Fassbender HG, Wegner K: Morphologie und Pathogenese des Weichteilrheumatismus. Z Rheumaforsch 32:355, 1973.

58. Klemp P, Nielsen HV, Korsgard J: Blood flow in fibromyotic muscles. Scand J Rehabil Med 14:81–82, 1982.

59. Danneskiold-Samsoe B, Christiansen E, Lund B, Andersen RB: Regional muscle tension and pain (fibrositis). Scand J Rehabil Med 15:17–20, 1982.

60. Bennett RM, Clark SR, Campbell SM, et al.: Low levels of somatomedin C in patients with the fibromyalgia syndrome. Arthritis Rheum 35: 1113–1116, 1992.

61. Scudds, RA, Trachsel LC, Luckhurst BJ, et al.: A comparative study of pain, sleep quality, and pain responsiveness in fibrositis and myofascial pain syndrome. J Rheumatol Suppl 19(Nov): 120–126, 1989.

62. Wolfe F, Smythe HA, Yunus MB, et al.: The American College Of Rheumatology 1990 criteria for the classification of fibromyalgia. Arthritis Rheum 33:160–172, 1990.

63. Van Denderen JC, Boersma JW, Zeinstra P, et al.: Physiological effects of exhaustive physical exercise in primary fibromyalgia syndrome (PFS): is PFS a disorder of neuroendocrine reactivity? Scand J Rheumatol 21:35–37, 1992.

64. Jacobsen S, Danneskiold-Samsoe B: Dynamic muscular endurance in primary fibromyalgia compared with chronic myofascial pain syndrome. Arch Phys Med Rehabil 73:170–173, 1992.

65. Visuri MB, Lindholm H, Lindqvist A, et al.: Cardiovascular function disorder in primary fibromyalgia. Arthritis Care Res 5:210–215, 1992.

66. Mengshoel AM, Saugen E, Forre O, et al.: Muscle fatigue in early fibromyalgia. J Rheumatol 22:143–150, 1995.

67. Abel O, Siebert WJ, Earp R: Fibrositis. J Missouri Med Assn 36:435, 1939.

68. Awad EA: Interstitial myofibrositis: hypotheses of the mechanism. Arch Phys Med Rehabil 54: 449–453, 1973.

69. Brendstrup P, Jespersen K, Asboe-Hansen G: Morphological and chemical connective tissue changes in fibrositic muscles. Ann Rheum Dis 16:438–440, 1957.

70. Bengtsson A, Henriksson KG: The muscle in fibromyalgia: a review of Swedish studies. J Rheumatol Suppl 19:144, 1989.

71. Backman E, Bengtsson A, Bengtsson M, et al.: Skeletal muscle function in primary fibromyalgia: effect of regional sympathetic blockade with guanethidine. Acta Neurol Scand 77:187, 1988.

72. Bartels EM, Danneskiold-Samsoe B: Histological abnormalities in muscle from patients with certain types of fibrositis. Lancet 1:755, 1986.

73. Danneskiold-Samsoe B, Christiansen E, Andersen RB: Myofascial pain and the role of myoglobin. Scan J Rheumatol 15:174, 1986.

74. Elert JE, Rantapaadahlqvist SB, Henriksson-Larsen K, et al.: Muscle performance, electromyography, and fibre type composition in fibromyalgia and work-related myalgia. Scand J Rheumatol 21:28, 1992.

75. Elert JE, Dahlqvist SBR, Henriksson-Larsen K, Gerdle B: Increased EMG activity during short pauses in patients with primary fibromyalgia Scand J Rheumatol 18:321, 1989.

76. Bennett, RM: Beyond fibromyalgia: ideas on etiology and treatment. J Rheumatol Suppl 19: 185, 1989.

77. Bennett RM: Muscle physiology and cold reactivity in the fibromyalgia syndrome. Rheum Dis Clin North Am 15:135, 1989.

78. Bennett RM: Physical fitness and muscle metabolism in the fibromyalgia syndrome: an overview. J Rheumatol Suppl 19:28, 1989.

79. Bennett RM, Clark SR, Goldberg L, et al.: Aerobic fitness in patients with fibrositis: a controlled study of respiratory gas exchange and 133xenon clearance from exercising muscle. Arthritis Rheum 32:454–460, 1989.

80. Elam M, Johansson G, Wallin BG: Do patients with primary fibromyalgia have an altered muscle sympathetic nerve activity? Pain 48:371, 1992.

81. Yunus MB, Kalyan-Raman UP, Masi AT, Alday JC: Electron microscopic studies of muscle biopsy in primary fibromyalgia syndrome: a controlled and blinded study. J Rheumatol 16:97, 1989.

82. Yunus MB, Kalyan-Raman UP: Muscle biopsy findings in primary fibromyalgia and other forms of nonarticular rheumatism. Rheum Dis Clin North Am 15:115, 1989.

83. Yunus MB, Kalyan-Raman UP, Kalyan-Raman K, Masi AT: Pathologic changes in muscle in primary fibromyalgia syndrome. Am J Med 81:38, 1986.

84. Drewes AM, Andreasen A, Schroder HD, et al.: Pathology of skeletal muscle in fibromyalgia: a histo-immuno-chemical and ultrastructural study. Br J Rheumatol 32:479–483, 1993.

85. Simms RW, Roy SG, Hrovat M, et al.: Lack of association between fibromyalgia syndrome and abnormalities in muscle energy metabolism. Arthritis Rheum 37:794–800, 1994.

86. De Blecourt AC, Wolf RF, van Rijswijk MH, et al.: In vivo 30P-MR spectroscopy of tender points in patients with fibromyalgia. (Abstract) Scand J Rheumatol Suppl 21:24, 1992.

87. Wigers SH, Aasly J: 31 phosphorus magnetic resonance spectroscopy of leg muscle of patients with fibromyalgia. (Abstract) Scand J Rheumatol Suppl 21:26, 1992.

88. Jacobsen S, Jensen KE, Thomsen C, et al.: 31P magnetic resonance spectroscopy of skeletal muscle in patients with fibromyalgia. J Rheumatol 19:1600–1603, 1992.

89. Terenius L: Endorphins and modulation of pain. Adv Neurol 33:59–64, 1982.

90. Cleeland C, Schacham S, Dahl J, et al.: CSF B-endorphin and the severity of pain. Neurology 34:378–380, 1984.

91. Vaeroy H, Nyberg F, Terenius L: No evidence for endorphin deficiency in fibromyalgia following investigation of cerebrospinal fluid (CSF) dynorphin A and Met-enkephalin-Arg6-Phe7. Pain 46:139–143, 1991.

92. Vaeroy H, Helle R, Forre O, et al.: Elevated CSF levels of substance P and high incidence of Raynaud phenomenon in patients with fibromyalgia: new features for diagnosis. Pain 32:21–26, 1988.

93. Yunus MB, Dailey JW, Aldag JC, et al.: Plasma and urinary catecholamines in primary fibromyalgia: a controlled study. J Rheumatol 19:95–97, 1992.

94. Russell IJ, Vaeroy H, Javors, M, et al.: Cerebrospinal fluid biogenic amine metabolites in fibromyalgia/fibrositis syndrome and rheumatoid arthritis. Arthritis Rheum 35:550–556, 1992.

95. Valen PA, Nakayama DA, Veum JA, Wortmann RL: Myoadenylate deaminase deficiency: diagnosis by forearm ischemic exercise testing and oxypurine. (Abstract #A26) Arthritis Rheum 27:(4 [Suppl]):546, 1984.

96. Gertler PA, Jacobs RP: Myoadenylate deaminase deficiency in a patient with progressive systemic sclerosis. Arthritis Rheum 27: 586–590, 1984.

97. Morgan-Hughes JA: Painful disorders of muscle. Br J Hosp Med 22:360–365, 1979.

98. Kopell HP, Thompson WAL: Peripheral entrapment neuropathies. Huntington NY: RE Krieger, 1976.

99. Goldner JL: Symposium: upper extremity nerve entrapment syndrome. Contemp Orthop 6: 89–112, 1983.

100. Levy M, Goldberg I: Four unusual causes of carpal tunnel syndrome. Orthop Rev 11: 67–73, 1982.

101. Moss SH, Switzer HE: Radial tunnel syndrome: a spectrum of clinical presentations. J Hand Surg 8:414–420, 1983.

102. Hashimoto I, Tak YK: The true sagittal diameter of the cervical spinal canal and its diagnostic significance in cervical myelopathy. J Neurosurg 47:912–916, 1977.

103. Choudhury AR, Taylor JC: Occult lumbar spinal stenosis. J Neurol Neurosurg Psychiatry 40: 506–510, 1977.

104. Wakefield G: Entrapment neuropathies. Clin Rheum Dis 5:941–956, 1979.

105. Sunderland S: The nerve lesion in the carpal tunnel syndrome. J Neurol Neurosurg Psychiatry 39:615–626, 1976.

106. Marie, Pierre, et Foix: Atrophie isolée de l'éminence thénar d'origine névritique: rôle du ligament annulaire antérieur du carpe dans la pathogénie de la lésion. Rev Neurol 26:647–649, 1913.

107. Zucker-Pinchoff B, Hermann G, et al.: Computed tomography of the carpal tunnel: radioanatomical study. J Comput Assist Tomography 5:525–528, 1981.

108. Armstrong TJ, Chaffin DB: Carpal tunnel syndrome and selected personal attributes. J Occup Med 21:481–486, 1979.

109. Papaioannou T, Rushworth G, Atar D., et al.: Carpal canal stenosis in men with idiopathic carpal tunnel syndrome. Clin Orthop 285: 210–213, 1992.

110. Dekel S, Papaioannou T, Rushworth G, Coates R: Idiopathic carpal tunnel syndrome caused by carpal stenosis. Br Med J 120:1297–1303, 1980.

111. Phalen GS: Soft tissue affections of the hand and wrist. Hosp Med 7:47–59, 1971.

112. Sunderland S: Nerve and nerve injuries. New York: Churchill Livingstone, 1978.

113. Werner CO, Elmqvist D, Ohlin P: Pressure and nerve lesion in the carpal tunnel. Acta Orthop Scand 54:312–314, 1983.

2: The Head and Neck

INTRODUCTION

The past decade has witnessed significant advances in our knowledge of the anatomy and aging changes of the cervical spine. Meticulous neck dissection and imaging studies demonstrate moderate and sometimes severe degenerative or developmental changes in the cervical spine in asymptomatic subjects. Aging is normally associated with bone and ligament hypertrophy (1). Teresi et al., in a study of patients having magnetic resonance imaging (MRI) of the larynx, reported protrusions of the cervical disc in 20% to 57% (stratified by age ranging from 45 to 82 years) in these normal subjects. Cord compression was evident in 7% (2). In another MRI study of 63 normal subjects (age 20 to 73 years), cervical spinal stenosis was seen in 20% of asymptomatic subjects over the age of 40 (3). Furthermore, wide interobserver variation exists in the interpretation of roentgenography and imaging of the spine. Therefore, when addressing the question "Where does the pain arise?" the clinician must first and foremost apply good clinical skills in history-taking and physical examination.

History and Physical Examination

The cervical spine is remarkably mobile because of its 37 separate joints and 6 intervertebral discs. When the head is held upright for very long, however, the muscles are subject to rapid fatigue. This is even more evident if the head is deviated from its normal alignment with the trunk. When the patient with skeletal disease also subjects the neck to prolonged or repetitive motion, pain of muscle origin may be more important than the known skeletal disease. Prolonged neck flexion and arm elevation significantly contributes to neck and shoulder symptoms (3a). If the improper pos-

ture is not identified and corrected, repeated bouts of pain can lead to exorbitant costs associated with unnecessary treatment.

John H., a 44-year-old professor, changed occupations and was spending 4 or more hours a day at his computer terminal. He complained of painful clicking in the posterior neck during head turning. Results of roentgenography were normal for his age. He had diffuse soft tissue tenderness. Physical therapy provided little relief. Fortunately, after reviewing postures that might contribute to his problem, he recognized forward neck thrust, also called "birdwatcher's neck": the head and neck are jutted forward as if birdwatching through a pair of binoculars (4). He did this while driving, not when working. After he corrected this habit, he recovered.

The disorders included in this chapter result from inappropriate use and from injury (myofascial pain disturbances, tendinitis, and bursitis); structural disorders such as body asymmetry or an elongated styloid process; neurovascular entrapment disorders; and discogenic cervical pain. Table 2.1 presents potential sources for cervical spine symptoms.

Key points in the history and physical examination include immediate recognition of potentially critical signs as shown in Table 2.2, and the following:

- Are symptoms worse when at rest or asleep than at other times?
- Does the patient use proper or improper neck positions at home or at work? (Refer to Table 2.5 below for joint protection measures.)
- Does patient report bruxism (grinding and clenching the teeth) at night, or jaw complaints after sleep?
- Has the patient had a personal or family history of migraine? This can be related to carotodynia and can be overlooked.

TABLE 2.1 SOURCES OF NECK PAIN

Soft Tissue
  Pharynx—pharyngitis, Ludwig's angina,
    inflamed pharyngeal cyst (branchial cleft
    remnants)
  Tonsils—tonsillitis, neoplasm
  Tongue—ulcers, neoplasm
  Esophagus—inflamed diverticulum, peptic
    esophagitis, radiation esophagitis
  Skin and subcutaneous tissues—furuncle,
    carbuncle, erysipelas, soft tissue calcemia
    of C1 and C2
Glands
  Thyroid gland—acute suppurative thyroiditis,
    subacute thyroiditis with pain radiating to
    the ear, hemorrhage
  Salivary gland—mumps, suppurative parotitis,
    calculus in duct
  Lymph node—acute adenitis, chronic
    conditions (e.g., Hodgkin's disease,
    scrofula, gummas, actinomycosis,
    carcinomatous metastases)
Blood Vessels
  Carotodynia—carotid body tumor, subclavian
    artery aneurysm
Bones
  Mandible—fracture, osteomyelitis, periodontitis
  Cervical vertebrae—whiplash, subluxation,
    acute or subacute fracture, spondylosis,
    primary metastatic neoplasm, osteomyelitis,
    tuberculosis
Joints
  Temporomandibular joint—associated with
    myofascial pain syndrome in neck
  Facet joint—facet joint syndrome and
    dislocation
  Infectious arthritis
  Occipital neuralgia with C1, C2 arthrosis
    syndrome
Discs
  Herniated intervertebral disc
Muscles and Ligaments
  Myofascial pain disorders
  Eagle's syndrome
  Cervical intervertebral bursitis
  Sternocleidomastoid—acquired or congenital
    torticollis
Compression Syndromes
  Anterior scalenus syndrome, costoclavicular
    syndrome, pectoralis minor
    (hyperabduction) syndrome
Nerves
  Cervical herpes zoster, spinal cord tumor,
    epidural abscess or hematoma,
    poliomyelitis, occipital neuralgia,
    suprascapular neuralgia, reflex sympathetic
    dystrophy
Referred Pain
  Bronchial tumor, Pancoast tumor, angina from
    the sixth cervical dermatomal band,
    spontaneous pneumomediastinum

Reprinted with permission from Gilbert R, Warfield CA:
Evaluating and treating the patient with neck pain. Hosp
Pract (Off Ed) 22(8):223–232, 1987.

TABLE 2.2 POTENTIALLY CRITICAL SIGNS IN THE HEAD AND NECK

1. Fever and chills
2. Intense headache or spasmodic stabbing
   pains
3. Mental dullness
4. Visible swelling
5. Swollen lymph glands
6. Blood in the ear, nose, or mouth
7. Disturbed vision, smell, or taste
8. Numbness or weakness
9. Horner's syndrome
10. Axillary pain
11. Ischemic upper limb appearance
12. Absent pulses in upper limb
13. Arm claudication
14. Upper limb atrophy

- Does the patient have any sensory impairment, especially of the vision or hearing, that can cause unconscious head tilting?
- What job tasks, activities of daily living, or hobbies are performed for longer than an hour that can give rise to neck muscle fatigue?
- Has the patient had previous trauma or neck problems that required medical attention?
- If involved in a motor vehicle accident, what occurred? What external trauma was evident? Was the patient seat-belted? Was the headrest in place? How much damage to the car occurred? Were roentgenograms obtained?
- When the patient claims an occupation-related disorder, what other tasks, daily activities, or hobbies could be related? Were there previous neck problems? How long does it take the patient to drive to work? Does the patient unconsciously jut the head forward when driving, or unconsciously clench jaw or hands? The clencher syndrome is not rare.
- What changes have recently occurred in daily activity patterns? Too often, workplace stress is just added to many accumulating neck aggravations. (Refer to Table 2.5 below for joint protection measures.)

Physical examination should begin with immediate impressions of posture and structure, quality of movement and physical features:

Skeletal disorders such as body asymmetry (for example, the left side of the face and cheekbone are smaller than the right side—see Figure I.2); the head held immobile when you entered the examination room (suggesting ankylosing spondylitis or severe osteoarthritis); dowager hump; forward inclination and droop of the neck and shoulders.

Quality of movement including the features of Parkinsonism such as loss of facial movement or arm tremor; gait; arm and hand use during gesturing.

Physical features such as hair and eyebrow appearance (sparse lateral brows suggest hypothyroidism); prominence of temporal arteries; proptosis; muscle atrophy.

Then proceed to the remainder of the physical examination:

- Active and passive range and tone of cervical motion.
- Palpation of scalp (tenderness can suggest temporal arteritis); muscles for tenderness and induration; fibromyalgia tender points; medial (internal) pterygoid muscles for silent temporomandibular joint dysfunction; and for nodes, masses, and trigger points. Inspection of ears, eyes, nose, and mouth.
- Maneuvers, when symptoms warrant, including the Spurling maneuver, Adson's test; tests for carpal tunnel syndrome (retrograde nerve irritation can sometimes cause neck and shoulder pain).
- General examination and neurologic examination as clinical features warrant.

In this chapter disorders of the head and neck are presented beginning with those generating frontal region symptoms, then those affecting the side of the face and neck, and finally, those affecting the posterior elements of the head and neck.

CRANIOMANDIBULAR JOINT DISORDERS

In recent years the TMJ has been approached with tomograms, arthrograms, arthroscopic examination, and magnetic resonance imaging (MRI). As in other joint regions, a wide discrepancy occurs between objective findings and clinical relevance. Furthermore, the cost-effectiveness and functional efficacy of these more recent methods have not been established. TMJ disorders may be categorized as either intracapsular or extracapsular.

The American Academy of Craniomandibular Disorders states that the vast majority of symptomatic patients have an extraarticular *myofascial pain disorder* that is unrelated to intrinsic disease of the TMJ (5). Studies of craniomandibular disorders in the population at large demonstrate that a majority of people have derangements: 23% have a muscle disorder, 19% have a joint disorder, 27% have both, and only 31% were normal (6). Only 5% of involved persons seek medical attention.

Studies of school children in Japan (7), in Saudi Arabia (8), and in western nations demonstrate that malocclusion is very common, and jaw noise is common, but only 2% have TMJ complaints. Therefore, it is difficult to attribute symptoms to malocclusion. Certainly, the experienced dentist will be helpful when malocclusion is present, but when symptoms are out of proportion with malocclusion, then myofascial pain disorder should be considered. Hyperplasia of the coronoid process of the mandible is another cause for restricted jaw mobility that can be overlooked.

Craniomandibular disorders include a number of clinical problems that involve the masticatory musculature, the temporomandibular joint, or both (5).

Intracapsular disorders include rheumatoid arthritis, osteoarthritis, and articular disc displacements. Osteoarthritis with erosions may be secondary to myofascial pain disorder with overloading of the masticatory system during bruxism and jaw clenching.

Diagnostic criteria for articular disc displacement include (5):

1. Pain, when present, precipitated by joint movement and caused by inflammation.
2. Reproducible joint noise at different positions during opening and closing mandibular movements; closing noise (click) usually located close to intercuspal position.
3. Soft tissue imaging reveals displaced disc that usually reduces on opening.
4. No coarse crepitus.
5. Range of motion usually normal.

Many patients with articular disc displacement have generalized joint laxity (9). MRI findings of articular disc displacement occur in a minority of symptomatic patients.

Occlusal disharmony and meniscus changes, when present, may not be relevant to symptoms. Clicks and grinding sounds are usually present only when an articular disc displacement is present (10). One-fifth of asymptomatic individuals have clinical signs of TMJ articular disc displacement, and cadaver studies demonstrate a 40 to 60% incidence of articular disc displacement.

Temporomandibular Joint (TMJ) Disorders

Extracapsular disorders are far more common and are collectively known as myofascial pain of the masticatory muscles (11).

TMJ MYOFASCIAL PAIN SYNDROME OR TMJ DYSFUNCTION SYNDROME (TMJDS)

TMJDS may present as pain in the jaw, face, ear, neck, or with headache and is often associated with a stressful life event. The term ''myofascial pain'' refers to pain that is assumed to occur when regional muscle tightness and associated symptoms result from persistent, unconscious, repetitive use of the involved muscles. Not infrequently, the jaw is not recognized as contributing to the problem, although characteristic localized tenderness in taut muscle bands within the muscles of mastication establishes the nature of the pain disorder (11). However, in one study, use of occlusal adjustment and splint therapy did not significantly alter headache when compared to a control group treated with mock adjustment (12).

Usually seen in young women, symptoms of TMJDS include chronic pain in the muscles of mastication, sometimes with pain radiating to the ear and neck. Other common features are jaw noise, irregular mandibular movements, and limitation of jaw movement or opening. Many patients present with occipital headache. Lip and mouth biting that can occur as a result of jaw clenching may contribute to facial pain (12a).

Physical Examination: TMJ examination begins with inspection from the front. Ask the patient to open and close the mouth so that any jaw deviation may be noted. Then palpate over the joint as the mouth is opened and closed. To elicit joint tenderness, place the tips of the

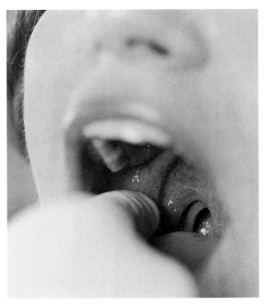

Figure 2.1. Using a gloved finger, the examiner palpates the internal (medial) pterygoid muscle on the inner aspect of the ramus of the mandible between the tonsillar pillars. Each side is compared for pain reproduction. Tenderness is elicited on the symptomatic side.

forefingers behind the tragi at each external acoustic meatus and pull forward while the patient opens the mouth.

Next, using gloves, palpate the medial pterygoid muscles located at the back of the mouth on the inner aspect of the ramus of the mandible, between the tonsillar pillars. Introduce a finger into the mouth and gently palpate the muscle; this causes mild to exquisite pain in the patient with TMJ dysfunction (Fig. 2.1). Before attempting the examination, the clinician should warn the patient not to bite!

Etiology: In addition to stress and personal habits, the temporomandibular joint dysfunction syndrome is often associated with malocclusion, which may be a cause for, may be independent of, or may result from, the chronic muscle tension compressing the joint (13). Costen's syndrome (temporomandibular joint pain, limited joint excursion, hearing deficits, and headaches) has been reassessed in the light of myofascial pain mechanisms and this eponym has been abandoned (14).

The temporomandibular joint dysfunction syndrome may result from the use of cervical traction, dental manipulation, trauma or, most often, from muscle fatigue due to jaw clenching.

In a controlled study in which direct measurements of nocturnal tooth contact were taken by continuous computer monitoring, Trenouth demonstrated that most patients with TMJDS had bruxism at night, whether they were aware of it or not. Tooth contact occurred an average of 360 times per night in ten normal volunteers, 1325 times in nine patients with known bruxism, and 999 times in six patients without known bruxism. In addition, the duration of tooth contact was 5.4 minutes per night for the control group, 38.7 minutes in the bruxism group, and 11.5 minutes in those without bruxism. Overall, evidence for tooth grinding was found in 78% of patients (15).

Jaw clenching, in turn, is often due to anxiety and leads to a myofascial syndrome with a trigger point in the medial pterygoid muscles. Psychologic investigation has yielded conflicting information (16, 17). Although these patients usually suffer from anxiety, the psychoneurosis apparently does not interfere with the response to treatment. However, those with a severely disturbed capacity for interpersonal relationships were found least likely to gain from therapy (18).

Radiographic changes, including erosions of the mandibular condyle or degenerative arthritis, are difficult to relate to symptoms. Toller found no correlation of erosions to symptoms (19). The most severe degenerative joint changes were found in those patients who had the poorest results from therapy (19). Persistent joint compression by the temporomandibular joint dysfunction syndrome may lead to degenerative arthritis (13).

Myofascial TMJ dysfunction occurs in persons with other musculoskeletal problems including articular disc displacement, joint laxity, body asymmetry, increased cervical and lumbar lordosis, scoliosis, poor positioning of the head or tongue, and other posture problems (11). Migraine headaches are also more common in these patients.

Radiologic, Imaging, and Laboratory Studies: As has been stated, only a minority of patients will have significant articular disc displacement. When disabling pain or locking occurs, MRI is the procedure of choice but must be interpreted by an experienced radiologist or dental surgeon. Indications for MRI include severe symptoms, palpable abnormality, and failure with conservative treatment.

Panoramic roentgenograms with open and closed views should be obtained for evaluation of bony architecture. False positive diagnoses of erosive osteoarthritis of the temporal components can occur.

Arthrography is an excellent means for evaluating the articular disc, but the procedure is painful, invasive, and largely replaced by MRI.

MRI is very expensive and the findings may not be relevant to symptoms. The procedure should be reserved for patients who have significant functional impairment despite good attempts at conservative care including behavior change, use of night splinting, stress management, and proper dental evaluation. Too often, articular disc derangement is found and treated without discernable benefit.

Laboratory studies should be considered, depending upon the findings of a careful history and physical examination, the age of the patient, and features listed in Table 2.2. Results of a complete blood count and erythrocyte sedimentation rate may point toward infection in the young or temporal arteritis in the elderly.

Differential Diagnosis: Organic diseases, as a cause for symptoms, include the inflammatory rheumatic diseases such as rheumatoid arthritis or ankylosing spondylitis. Regional infection and disease of the neck, teeth, tonsils, and cervical lymph nodes should be excluded. Table 2.3 presents a decision chart for head and neck pain.

Management: Management of TMJDS is summarized in Table 2.4. Treatment requires exclusion of mechanical abnormalities and inflammatory diseases. Dental evaluation by an experienced practitioner is often required for evaluation and possible correction of occlusive abnormalities.

- Basic treatment consists of the correction of improper movement patterns and posture habits, behavior changes, stress management, and physical and occupational therapy principles as detailed in Tables 2.5 and 2.6; then, if necessary, occlusal bite appliance, TMJ local corticosteroid injection, and consideration for surgical intervention.

TABLE 2.3 DECISION CHART: THE HEAD AND NECK

Problem	Action	Other Actions	Further Actions
A. Chronic Neck Pain Trigger points present No limitation of motion No neurologic signs B. Subacute Neck Pain Minor injury Limitation of movement No neurologic signs C. Acute Neck Injury Soft tissue tenderness No swelling No neurologic signs Normal passive motion Normal roentgenograms	CONSERVATIVE CARE Correct aggravating factors (joint protection) → Provide pain relief; NSAIDS, ice, trigger point injections, TENS, anti- depressants, relaxants, mild analgesics, ultrasound Prescribe exercises	*Tests for inflammation* *Radiologic studies* *Bone Scan* *MRI* → *Electrodiagnostic tests* *Review exercises and* *joint protection* *measures*	*Repeat physical* *examination* *Consultation with:* *Orthopaedist/* *Neurosurgeon* *Physiatrist* *Rheumatologist*
D. Danger List Present Neurologic findings present Bleeding from any orifice Fever, chills, swelling Meningismus	URGENT CONSULTATION Orthopaedist/ Neurosurgeon Emergency medicine specialist, traumatologist Oral examination Lumbar puncture		

TABLE 2.4 MANAGEMENT OF TEMPOROMANDIBULAR JOINT DYSFUNCTION SYNDROME

1. Exclude infections and inflammatory diseases
2. Recognize aggravating factors (e.g., spasm, jaw muscle fatigue, dental malocclusion, anxiety, or stress)
3. Eliminate nocturnal jaw clenching with an acrylic bite plate appliance
4. Provide dental care if indicated
5. Provide jaw exercises
6. Provide muscle relaxants, sedatives, and amitriptyline or similar tricyclic compounds at bedtime
7. Perform local anesthetic–corticosteroid joint injections for persistent symptoms

- An occlusal joint splint is helpful when used during sleep to gently stretch the medial pterygoid muscles and to prevent jaw clenching during sleep (20) (Fig. 2.2). Its use should be continued for months. Although some dentists think these retainers are nothing more than placebos, others believe they prevent dam-

age to the joint (15). In one study, the use of occlusal splints provided relief from clicking in 40% of patients, from pain in 85% of patients, and from other muscular complaints in 88% of patients (21). Jaw relaxation during the day may be provided by the occlusal bite splint, if necessary. Using electromyographic voltage tension curves to quantitate the effect of splinting, Kotani et al. noted that symptom improvement preceded objective electromyogram improvement in 15 patients (22).

- Sleep instructions include the use of a neck contour or soft tubular pillow that holds the neck in a neutral position. The head should not drop off the end of the pillow.
- Isometric jaw exercises are helpful. Refer to Table 2.6 to locate appropriate exercises.
- Nocturnal sedation is helpful during the first few weeks. If fibromyalgia is a coexisting problem, the use of amitriptyline

TABLE 2.5 JOINT PROTECTION FOR THE HEAD AND NECK

General

Avoid sitting or standing for more than 30 minutes. It can induce more neck strain than lifting heavy objects.

Take frequent breaks during tasks in which the body does not move (e.g., knitting). Includes tasks that allow the body greater movement (e.g., sweeping).

Align the head, neck, and trunk during rest and activities.

Avoid stressful head positions (e.g., lying on a sofa with the head propped up; falling asleep in a chair and allowing the head to drop forward; using more than one thin pillow).

Align the entire trunk, chest, and head on a slanted wedge or a very large pillow if you must watch television or read in a reclining position.

If required to sleep with the head high, elevate the entire mattress or the head of the bed.

Sleep on the side or the back, keeping the arms below chest level.

Clenching the jaw can cause muscle spasms in the neck; use relaxation techniques or a bite spacer.

Store heavy items that are used daily no higher than shoulder height and no lower than knee height.

Use a step stool when lifting heavy items from shelves higher than the shoulders.

Avoid the ``birdwatcher's neck'' (jutting the head forward as if watching birds through field glasses) (also called video display terminal or VDT neck).

Be conscious of stressful head positions when concentrating, when driving, or when tense.

Use headsets or a speaker phone for prolonged or frequent telephone calls.

Place a computer screen at eye level and use a ``draft holder'' to place work at eye level next to the screen.

Use an adjustable chair and vary the height of the seat frequently during prolonged sitting.

Maintain the proper hand-to-eye work or reading distance of 16 inches.

Position the body and work materials in such a way that the neck remains straight during activities.

Sports

Use plastic goggles or eyeglasses with plastic lenses.

Wear a safety helmet when cycling.

Vary swim strokes and head position during swimming and water exercise. When diving, be certain that pools are of proper depth.

and/or a muscle relaxant such as cyclobenzaprine or carisoprodol may be useful at night in small doses.

- If the above measures are not helpful, a single injection of a corticosteroid–local anesthetic mixture into the temporomandibular joint may provide pain relief with subsequent relaxation of the pterygoid muscles and allow the rest of the treatment program to take hold. *Technique:* Strict attention to injection principles is essential (Appendix C). Palpate the involved joint just in front of the ear while the patient opens and closes the mouth. Note the depression as the joint opens. This site can be marked with pressure from the end of a ballpoint pen. After preparation with surgical soap or povidone-iodine and alcohol, apply gloves, and in a 3 mL syringe draw up a maximum of 20 mg methylprednisolone or equivalent steroid mixed with 1% lidocaine hydrochloride. A macroscopic flocculate occurs with the use of methylprednisolone, thus further impeding absorption from the injection site. For the temporomandibular joint, a 1-inch No. 25 or No. 27 needle can be used (Fig. 2.3).

Outcome and Additional Suggestions: The outcome is satisfactory with relief from pain, headache, and bruxism in most cases (18, 23, 24). In one study, after 5 years of follow-up, 52% of patients with temporomandibular joint pain and erosions had relief from pain and radiographic improvement. This radiographic improvement of the erosion followed treatment that included a single corticosteroid injection of the temporomandibular joint (19). The relief from chronic joint compression may have allowed healing to occur.

Another study reported long-term outcome (3–15 years) in 190 patients with clicking and with myofascial pain dysfunction treated without mandibular reposition or irreversible surgical procedures. Of those in college at the time of treatment, 73% reported either cessation of symptoms or improvement and 15% were symptomatically improved but still noted clicking. Of older patients seen, 54% were either free of clicking or improved. Thus status of clicking carries no worse prognosis (10). The occlusal splint should be used for some period of time after symptoms are relieved.

- Biofeedback has been advocated for patients with less than 2 or 3 years' duration of symptoms (25).
- For the few patients who fail to benefit after these measures, reassessment is indicated, both from a mechanical and a

TABLE 2.6 HEAD AND NECK EXERCISES

Condition	Exercise(s)	Exercise Number
Temporomandibular joint dysfunction	Axial Extension	2.A
	Jaw Balancing (Isometric)	2.B(a–c)
	Neck Flexion	2.C(a)
Cervical syndrome (sprain ``whiplash'') (myofascial neck pain)	Axial Extension	2.A
	Head/Neck Isometric Strengthening	2.C(a–c)
	Neck Erector Strengthening	2.D(a,b)
	Resisted Strengthening	2.E(a,b)
	Active Range of Motion (Flexibility)	2.F(a–d)
	Assisted Stretches	2.G(a,b)
	Shoulder Shrugs	2.H
	Cervical Traction	2.J
Torticollis (traumatic)	Appropriate stretching, range of motion, and strengthening exercises would be determined by existing head posture	
	Assisted Stretches	2.G(a,b)
	Active Range of Motion (Flexibility)	2.F(a–d)
	Head/Neck Isometric Strengthening	2.C(a–c)
	Corner Stretch	2.I
	Cervical Traction	2.J
Cervical nerve root syndrome	Axial Extension	2.A
	Head/Neck Isometric Strengthening	2.C(a–c)
	Neck Erector Strengthening	2.D(a,b)
	Active Range of Motion (Flexibility)	2.F(a–d)
	Cervical Traction	2.J
Thoracic outlet syndrome	Axial Extension	2.A
	Head/Neck Isometric Strengthening	2.C(a–c)
	Neck Erector Strengthening	2.D(a–b)
	Corner Stretch	2.I
	Shoulder Shrugs	2.H

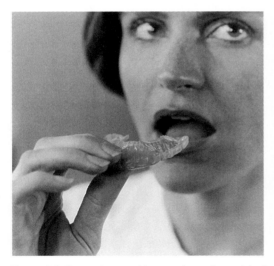

Figure 2.2. One of several types of acrylic molded bite plate appliances used to prevent jaw clenching and to provide gentle stretching of the pterygoid muscles.

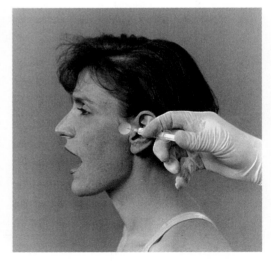

Figure 2.3. After sterile preparation, with the mouth open, the temporomandibular joint may be injected using a No. 25 or No. 27 short needle with 1 mL of a mixture of 20 mg methylprednisolone (or equivalent) and lidocaine hydrochloride 1%.

psychological standpoint. Often, the addition of a tricyclic antidepressant is helpful.

- When temporomandibular joint pain occurs in a patient with concomitant rheumatoid arthritis, the arthritis may produce constant muscle spasm, and the patient cannot fully open the jaw. The joint should be injected with a steroid–local anesthetic mixture if symptoms require it. The patient should be instructed to obtain three or four corks, ranging in size up to $1\frac{1}{2}$ inches in diameter. Several times a day the patient should insert the series of corks between the front teeth, beginning with the smallest cork. Each is held in place for 1 minute. Relief from pain and return to normal function is expected within 10 days.

OTHER FACE AND NECK DISORDERS

Carotodynia

Young and middle-aged men and women with carotodynia, often with a past history or family history of migraine, present with persistent or intermittent aching pain over one temporomandibular joint, radiating forward along the mandible, up to the temple, and into the ear (26). The pain is described either as a dull ache or as an intermittent throbbing. Often, these patients have seen a dentist and otolaryngologist to no avail. Muscle contraction headache may coexist. Visual abnormalities do not occur, and jaw motion is normal.

Physical examination reveals tenderness and sometimes palpable swelling of the external carotid artery (27). Gentle pressure upon the external carotid artery often reproduces and intensifies the neck and facial pain (Fig. 2.4). Examination and comparison of the carotid vessels on each side of the neck may reveal unilateral swelling and/or tenderness of the involved vessel. Pain points within the trapezius and posterior neck muscles commonly coexist. Tenderness and fullness within the temporal and masseter muscles may be found (28, 29).

Etiology: Most current opinion suggests that carotodynia is a migraine equivalent (27, 28). Often, drugs useful in migraine prophylaxis (e.g., amitriptyline) appear effective in caroto-

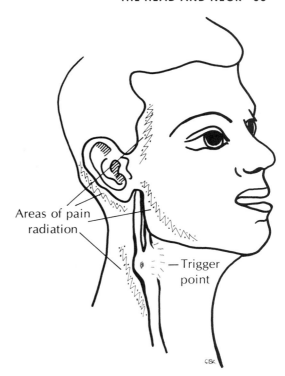

Areas of pain radiation

—Trigger point

Figure 2.4. Palpation of the carotid artery just below the bifurcation accentuates pain referral forward along the mandible, up toward the temple, and occasionally into the ear.

dynia. An elongated styloid process probably is not a cause for this syndrome.

Radiologic, Imaging, and Laboratory Studies: Laboratory and roentgenographic findings are not revealing. The normal Westergren sedimentation rate should exclude underlying sepsis or polymyalgia rheumatica, or giant cell arteritis in the elderly. Radiographic evidence of cervical degenerative arthritis is not related to this syndrome and should be considered a coincidental abnormality.

MRI and arteriography may be used if symptoms suggest ischemia resulting from vasculitis or dissection.

Differential Diagnosis: Differential diagnosis includes occult infection within the oropharyngeal structures, giant cell arteritis (to be considered in the elderly), neoplasm, carotid body tumors, dissection, and the temporomandibular joint dysfunction syndrome.

Management: Treatment begins with explaining the origin of pain to the patient. Once a patient realizes that the pain originates from the carotid artery, there is a tendency to stroke

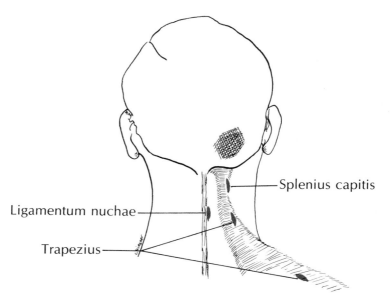

Splenius capitis

Ligamentum nuchae

Trapezius

Figure 2.5. Myofascial pain (trigger) points in the cervical region.

the area, thus exacerbating the condition. Advise the patient not to stroke the neck. Search for coexisting myofascial trigger points in the trapezius and posterior neck muscles (Fig. 2.5). In patients who have such trigger points, relaxing the trapezius muscle with heat or cold applications, exercises (Table 2.6) including shoulder shrugging (Exercise 2.H) and axial extension (Exercise 2.A), and the use of a tricyclic antidepressant (amitriptyline) have been helpful (27, 28). Manual techniques such as massage applied by a therapist or in a self-management program can be helpful in relieving tender/trigger points. A steroid–local anesthetic injection (Fig. 2.6) into the points may be performed as an alternative. Restoring strength and flexibility to all cervical muscles may be important. Occasionally ergot preparations or propranolol useful in the treatment of migraine are helpful (27–31).

Outcome and Additional Suggestions: Most patients will be greatly improved following this treatment regimen. Therapy is continued for at least 3 months, and the exercises should be continued twice daily for several months. Patients should be instructed to avoid sleeping on their stomachs because neck hyperextension may intensify distress. Patients should avoid extreme neck positions and be aware of neck posture during work, when on the phone, or when at rest. Calcium channel blocking agents,

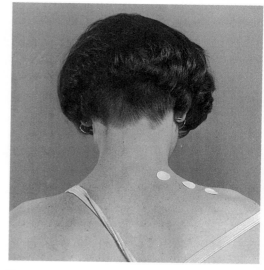

Figure 2.6. Sites of injection for trapezius pain (trigger) points (see text for details).

such as verapamil and nifedipine, may be of value for patients with resistant pain (32).

Eagle's Syndrome (Stylohyoid Syndrome)

An elongated styloid process (normal length is 2.5 cm) can compress the carotid vessels; this results in dysphagia, pharyngeal pain, and referred otalgia (33). Abnormalities of the stylohyoid ligament with resulting stretching of muscles that attach to the hyoid bone may cause similar pain. Sometimes pain occurs just below the angle of the jaw, and is aggravated when talking. Panoramic radiography may show calcification of the stylohyoid ligament (34).

The trigger point may be palpated within the tonsillar crypt. Intralesional injection with a local anesthetic will provide immediate temporary relief. Only those familiar with this technique should attempt it.

Another source for the pain may be tendinitis adjacent to muscular attachments to the hyoid bone. This ''hyoid syndrome'' can be alleviated with intralesional corticosteroid–local anesthetic injection (10 mg methylprednisolone plus 1 mL 1% procaine) near the cornua of the hyoid bone in the lateral anterior neck between the mandible and the larynx (35). Only those familiar with this technique should attempt it.

In children, following tonsillectomy, a chronic sore throat may be the presenting symptom; the syndrome is thought to result from scar tissue within the tonsillar fossa.

Myofascial Face Pain

Travell (36) describes a number of potential myofascial sources for head and face pain. Trigger points in the orbicularis oculi, temporalis, masseter, medial and lateral pterygoid, and trapezius muscles may refer pain to facial areas and present as atypical neuralgia. Palpation of the involved muscles will discern the trigger points; treatment of the points with either ice massage and stretching or intralesional injections is usually helpful (36). Exercise should be included during all phases of treatment and continued after pain is relieved to restore flexibility and strength. Exercises should include isometric head and neck strengthening (Exercise 2.C) and range of motion in straight and diagonal planes (Exercise 2.F).

Omohyoid Syndrome

A trigger point in the inferior belly of the omohyoid muscle located adjacent to the sternal division of the sternocleidomastoid muscle has been described as a cause for pain in the shoulder, neck, arm, and mandible (37). The etiology may be trauma, intense vomiting, or inflammation from regional or systemic disease. Local injection can be helpful.

Pterygoid Hamulus Bursitis

A pricking and burning sensation in the soft palate and oropharynx accompanied by tenderness within the whole mouth and throat may result from a bursitis adjacent to the area inferior to the pterygoid hamulus. Injection of 1 mL dexamethasone (4 mg/mL) into the area of tenderness corresponding to the hamular notch was reported to provide cure (38). Other steroid agents would likely work as well.

Neuralgias

Glossopharyngeal neuralgia presents with a cluster of lancinating, burning, stabbing pains in the region of the tonsil and radiates to the ear, neck, or anterior jaw. Swallowing may trigger the attack. The attacks may provoke cardiac arrhythmias due to irritation of the carotid sinus.

Superior laryngeal neuralgia is characterized by similar paroxysms of unilateral pain above the lateral thyroid cartilage with radiation to the angle of the jaw and the ear. Lesions of the larynx may involve the nerve, so careful examination is important to exclude other causes of the syndrome. Use of phenytoin (Dilantin) or carbamazepine (Tegretol) is often helpful. When performed by an experienced physician, direct nerve block into the pyriform sinus can provide diagnostic relief. Surgical intervention may require posterior cranial fossa root sections as last resort therapy (31).

Other conditions to be considered include trigeminal neuralgia, postherpetic neuralgia, and temporal arteritis. A careful neurologic examination, tests of inflammation, and consultation with an otolaryngologist may be needed (39).

OCCUPATION-RELATED HEAD AND NECK PAIN

Workplace ergonomic factors as a cause of head and neck pain are difficult to analyze because they are hard to segregate from all other possible causes. A meta-analysis revealed that only two of 54 relevant studies met the stringent criteria required to demonstrate causality (40). Head and neck positions are only slightly relevant to neck disorders and better methods of measurement are needed.

Use of video display terminals and head and neck symptoms were studied among Massachusetts clerical workers. Dose-dependent symptomatology was noted, but workers in data processing, public utilities, and those working for the Commonwealth complained more than those working in banking, communications, and hospitals (41).

Executives and others who rush through airports carrying heavy luggage may develop a cervical traction radiculopathy involving C6 and C7 nerve roots. Pain and paresthesia should alert the physician to the need to advise such persons to use a folding wheeled baggage cart (42).

If the patient considers the job as a cause, and if review of joint protection principles (Table 2.5) has not been of value, then referral to an occupational therapist should be considered for functional analysis and individual guidance. More often than not, factors outside of the workplace can be significantly aggravating and the job is only a corollary to the problem.

THE CERVICAL SYNDROME: SPRAIN (WHIPLASH)

Whiplash, a lay term, signifies a flexion-extension injury to the neck. Because such injuries may range from mild muscle tears to vertebral fractures and dislocations, the term should not be used for diagnosis. This chapter considers the conditions that can be managed by the personal physician (refer to Table 2.3 for diagnostic considerations). (See Anatomic Plates II and III.)

Obviously, neurologic deficits demand immediate expert attention. For patients without danger signs MRI should be reserved for those with persistent spasm, reversal of the cervical curve, paresthesias into the hands, or persistent interscapular pain.

Management: According to McKinney, rest, heat, and home mobilization exercises (Table 2.6, Exercises 2.A, 2.D, 2.E, 2.F, 2.G, and 2.H) will usually suffice (43). Others suggest the use of ice, isometric exercise (Exercise 2.C), cervical traction exercise (Exercise 2.J), and breathing and relaxation exercises. Patients may benefit from intermittent use of a soft collar. Comfort may be aided by sleeping with the neck and shoulders raised. For longer-term management, refer to the treatment measures for Cervical Myofascial Pain, below. One study showed that when symptoms persisted beyond 2 years, follow-up after 10 years showed persistence of those symptoms (44).

Partial tear of the sternocleidomastoid muscle may occur as a result of or accompany a hyperextension injury. A fibrotic band with torticollis may occur. The band is hard, indurated, and tender. After proper and sterile preparation, injection with lidocaine hydrochloride mixed with methylprednisolone, 1 mL each, is often helpful; inject the band throughout its length using multiple injections with a No. 25 needle. Resection of the band has been helpful in resistant cases (45).

Posttraumatic torticollis is a cervical dystonia following a blow to the neck, a sudden forced postural neck strain in falling down, or a flexion-extension motor vehicle injury (46). Onset begins within 1–4 days following the trauma. Two features that differ from idiopathic torticollis are the inability to actively turn the neck further in the direction of the torticollis, and the torticollis persists during sleep. The torticollis does not worsen with activity in most patients. They simply cannot perform tasks that require changing neck position. The disorder generally does not respond to local treatment measures (47). We have not found treatment to be helpful in restoring cervical motion; however, pain relief can be managed with physical therapy and exercise (refer to Table 2.6 and appropriate listed exercises). A trial of botulinum toxin has been recommended (47a). The disorder is long lasting. (One of us (RPS) has followed several patients for longer than 10 years with striking persistence of the torticollis.)

CERVICAL MYOFASCIAL PAIN

Cervical myofascial pain is characterized by neck pain and tenderness, accompanied by stiffness and weather sensitivity; it is often caused by postural strain or repetitive head movements. Most patients have an aching and irritating discomfort in the lower posterior neck region, worse after rest, or while sitting. Clicking noise is common. Paresthesia in the neck and parascapular area may occur. When the process occurs after trauma, several weeks often elapse before the onset of chronic diffuse neck pain.

Physical Findings: Active and passive neck motion may be restricted. Palpation of trigger points, often with bands of indurated muscle, reproduces or accentuates the pain. Sometimes a tight, tender ligamentum nuchae is noted during neck flexion (Fig. 2.5).

To palpate trigger points, use a consistent firmness: use enough pressure that the fingernail begins to blanche. However, proceed slowly. If pain in a target zone occurs, no further pressure is needed.

Cervical myofascial pain often is associated with either temporomandibular joint dysfunction (myofascial pain disorder) or fibromyalgia. Whenever examining the patient with neck region pain, the examiner should also palpate the medial pterygoid muscles for tenderness (Fig. 2.1) and for fibromyalgia tender points located at 18 locations as described in Chapter 7.

When subjective findings do not match physical findings, compensation or reimbursement issues may have influenced the perception of pain. In such cases, neurologic motor examination is normal; objective signs of injury are absent; imaging reveals no significant abnormality; indurated trigger points are usually not present; and exaggerated tenderness may occur at control areas, such as the styloid process or forehead. Symptoms may include burning, throbbing, numbness, tingling, weakness, and disability.

Etiology: The cause is often an improper head position during sedentary activity such as:

- Allowing the head and neck to jut forward (birdwatcher's neck (4)—as if birdwatching through field glasses).
- Falling asleep in a chair with the chin drooped onto the chest.
- Watching television with the head malaligned to one side. The screen should be directly in front of the viewer.

- Lying with the head propped up on the arm of a sofa or reading propped up in bed.
- Maintaining improper posture while using a computer, engaging in prolonged hand work, and the like.

Differential Diagnosis: Neck pain and stiffness that follow rest and improve during movement seldom result from more serious disease. However, a careful history and physical examination are necessary, including the exclusion of referred pain from the temporomandibular joint, diaphragm, and a hiatus hernia, and with consideration of neurologic or cardiovascular disease. The cervical zygapophyseal joints are not a usual cause for myofascial pain. Barnsley et al. found no benefit from using nerve blocks and intraarticular injections of these joints (48). Sometimes spinal enthesopathies can cause chronic neck discomfort and stiffness. They can affect the paraspinal ligaments with degeneration and calcification. Involvement of the anterior longitudinal ligament (Forestier's disease) also involves other segments of the spine. Characteristic flowing ossifications are usual roentgenographic findings. (See also the discussion below on ossification of the posterior longitudinal ligament.)

Polymyalgia rheumatica and giant cell arteritis should be considered if morning stiffness, restricted shoulder motion, scalp tenderness, headache, or jaw claudication is noted.

Stress-related (psychogenic) neck pain tends to occur episodically and does not improve with activity; pain is out of proportion to the physical findings, and palpation during the physical examination often reveals tenderness in excess of usual trigger point tenderness. Treatment of psychogenic pain requires that the patient learn to deal with stress.

Laboratory and Radiologic Examination: If pain is mild and not disabling and is of recent onset, treatment should precede laboratory and radiologic examination. Patients with any danger signs, those older than 50, and those with restricted range of motion should be studied promptly. Upright anteroposterior and lateral neck roentgenograms in the neutral, flexion, and extension positions, and open-mouth odontoid views, should be obtained to exclude cervical spine disease. Oblique views of the cervical spine are obtained for evaluation of the neuroforamina. Muscle spasm may lead to loss of the normal forward curve; skeletal injuries can be identified. Osteoporosis, neoplasm, and other diseases can also be ruled out.

Radiologic examination of the neck may reveal degenerative changes expected for age, but abnormalities are often unrelated. A Westergren sedimentation rate should be performed in elderly patients to exclude giant cell arteritis.

MRI should be considered if objective findings or potentially critical signs (Table 2.2) suggest intraspinal disease; if pain persists despite conservative treatment; or following significant head or neck trauma. Unfortunately, MRI often reveals significant unrelated abnormality in normal subjects.

Tests for metabolic disorders, inflammatory disease, or neoplasia should be performed depending upon clinical signs. Note also the decision chart presented in Table 2.3.

Management for Cervical Myofascial Pain Syndromes

Treatment begins with excluding ominous findings by careful history and physical examination. The history should also be directed to searching for unrecognized aggravating habits.

- Tasks requiring sitting or standing should be interrupted frequently. Lying on a sofa with the head propped up on the sofa arm induces neck strain and should be avoided. Sleep position with the head preferably in a neutral position (lying on the back with the legs elevated) is helpful.
- Joint protection will help patients with structural abnormalities such as adult round back or scoliosis, and patients with unilateral loss of vision or hearing who have alterations in head and neck motion.
- If work requires that both hands be free when on the phone, then the use of a headphone or speaker phone is helpful.
- Users of computer video display terminals may develop musculoskeletal complaints resulting from such factors as surface screen glare, poor screen and keyboard heights relative to the user, inappropriate seating, and the type of tasks being performed.
- Tasks consisting of high volume work, those under rigid control and continuous performance, can produce significant job stress and health complaints (49).
- The birdwatcher's neck is a frequent strain. The neck is unconsciously jutted forward during certain activities or during times of stress (4). Being aware of the possibility and then changing the behavior can be helpful.
- Neck mobilizing and strengthening exercises have been helpful in our experience. Exercises are selected for posture control, body alignment, flexibility, and strengthening. They must be performed gradually and repeated twice daily. Refer to Table 2.6 and the appropriate listed exercises. If pain is severe, assisted exercise with a physical therapist might be appropriate, or various combinations may be tried, but these should lead up to active, isometric, and resisted strengthening exercise.
- Stress management may require referral to a psychologist or other counselor skilled in dealing with psychophysiological problems and who is expert in teaching behavioral modification.
- Ice and stretching may be carried out using ice held in a sandwich bag, stroked gently along the length of the involved muscle while the patient stretches the involved area. Two slow strokes with the ice are sufficient (4).
- Two additional local treatment measures include topical capsaicin (50) and microcurrent electrical nerve stimulation (MENS) (51). Topical capsaicin (0.025% and 0.075%) depletes substance P. Originally recommended for relieving the pain of herpes zoster, capsaicin is recommended in many superficial pain disorders including myofascial pain. Derived from hot peppers, the product is available without prescription, with easily followed instructions. Some brands are in applicator tubes so that fingers are not contaminated, making eye contact less likely.
- Overhead cervical traction is useful when lateral rotation remains limited either from muscle tightness or from osteoarthritis (Exercise 2.J). Cervical traction should not be prescribed without first obtaining roentgenograms of the cervical spine if significant disease is suspected.

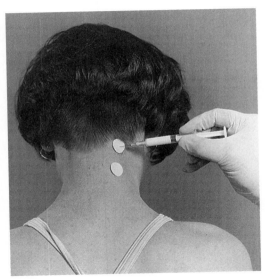

Figure 2.7. Injection of cervical myofascial pain (trigger) points in the splenius capitis and upper cervical muscles (see text for details).

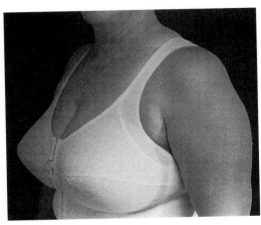

Figure 2.8. One example of a proper brassiere with wide elastic straps and good support.

We use up to 25 or 30 pounds of traction to distract the vertebrae. Cervical traction should be performed at least twice daily (morning and evening) if possible, for 5 to 10 minutes. Beginning with 8 to 10 pounds, the weight is increased gradually until benefit results. Home traction of up to 20 pounds is usually well tolerated. Traction is followed by range of motion and neck strengthening exercises (Table 2.6, Exercises 2.A, 2.C, 2.D, 2.E, and 2.F).

- Injection of a steroid-anesthetic combination into pain (trigger) points in the trapezius (Fig. 2.6) and neck erector muscles (Fig. 2.7) may be performed on the first visit. *Technique:* After sterile preparation, use a No. 23 or No. 25 ¾-inch needle to probe for tenderness. Trigger or pain points may be injected with 1% lidocaine hydrochloride mixed with 10–20 mg methylprednisolone or equivalent corticosteroid. A macroaggregation flocculate occurs when methylprednisolone is used. Inject the mixture instilling about 0.5 mL per lesion, not to exceed 60 mg of methylprednisolone in total. Ice application following the injection reduces crystal-induced local pain. The injections rarely have to be repeated.

- If patient has heavy pendulous breasts with shoulders drooping forward, suggest use of a proper brassiere (Fig. 2.8).

Outcome and Additional Suggestions: After these therapeutic measures, relief from cervical myofascial pain should begin within a week or two in the majority of patients. Exercises are done on a long-term basis. Whenever cervical traction is prescribed, the patient may have to continue the twice daily traction therapy for a prolonged period. Initial and periodic supervision by a physical therapist is desirable.

A tricyclic antidepressant (such as amitriptyline) or muscle relaxant (such as carisoprodol), given at bedtime to relieve a pain-spasm-pain cycle, may be helpful. Biofeedback relaxation has also been advocated (52, 53).

Related syndromes include the sternomastoid myofascial syndrome, muscle contraction headache (tension headache), occipital neuralgia, and interspinous bursitis.

Sternomastoid Myofascial Syndrome

Trigger points in the sternocleidomastoid muscle may refer pain widely to the forehead, face, orbit, occiput, throat, ear, or sternum. To find the trigger points, have the patient turn the head away from the painful side, then palpate the tensed sternomastoid muscle. Often the trigger point is palpably indurated. Pain radiation into the jaw, temple, or ipsilateral arm may be noted. The offending repetitious head turning, or improper sleep position must be identified and changed (Table 2.5).

Muscle Contraction Headache

This common headache involves the base of the neck, with a tight band sensation around the head. Pain may radiate into the retroorbital area. The headache often is noted after sleep. Similar headache may result from intense bearing down during prolonged labor (postpartum headache) (54).

Physical examination reveals a normal range of passive neck motion (when the examiner moves the patient's head laterally, forward, and backward, with the patient relaxed). Trigger or painful points within the trapezius as well as the neck erector muscles are uniformly present. The upper posterior neck region and the splenius capitis are sometimes associated with C2 neuralgia. Palpation produces local tenderness but rarely the headache. Occasionally, inflammation of the posterior ligamentum nuchae is felt as a thickened, indurated, tender band. Other physical findings and tests for inflammation are normal.

Etiology: The cause of muscle contraction headache is usually improper head position during the previous evening. Sitting over a puzzle or bingo cards with the head dropped forward, falling asleep in a chair with the head dropped forward, or lying with the head propped up on the arm of a sofa results in overstretching of the muscles and ligaments.

Differential Diagnosis: Musculoskeletal symptoms consisting of pain in the neck and at the back of head, with a sensation of tightness and pressure, can usually be differentiated from headache of intracranial origin (55). Attributes of pain, as determined by history, can follow the PQRST questioning (56):

Provocative factors: head position, coughing, straining, emotion

Quality: burning, aching, throbbing, continuous, superficial

Region: location of pain

Severity: on a scale from none to terrible

Timing: duration and periodicity

Potentially critical signs, as detailed in Table 2.2, should be sought in the examination of any patient with significant headache complaints.

Management: Muscle contraction headache responds well to treatment as described for cervical myofascial pain. Correcting rest and sitting positions is essential in order to prevent recurrences. Biofeedback, relaxation training, and the use of a simple relaxation audio tape were compared (57). The audio tape did just as well—and at the least expense!

Cervical epidural nerve blocks for persistent neck pain and headache have been described in very well-selected patients; these are not without risk, however, and should be undertaken only by those with expertise (58). The complication of dural puncture may require cervical epidural blood patch (59).

Occipital Neuralgia

Pain at the base of the skull posteriorly, with occasional burst of pain and paresthesia traveling up the occiput, sometimes to the entire scalp, can be due to irritation of the greater occipital nerve. Neck strain, from working with the head hyperextended, may have precipitated the pain. Occipital neuralgia may occur as a result of trauma, often in association with degenerative disease of the atlantoaxial joint. Palpation at the base of the skull may reproduce or exacerbate the sensation.

Applications of ice or heat, injection of splenius capitis trigger points with a steroid–local anesthetic mixture, instructions in sleep position (head and neck in line with trunk), and axial extension exercises (Table 2.6, Exercises 2.A and 2.D) should provide prompt relief. Wearing a soft cervical collar to sleep can be helpful if symptoms persist. Proper imaging assessment of the upper neck region should be obtained if these measures fail. Lateral flexion and extension roentgenographic views and open-mouth odontoid views can identify underlying abnormalities, which may rarely require C1-C2 fusion. Unfortunately, most patients are very elderly and surgery is not feasible; symptoms may at times spontaneously improve but often only after months or years have elapsed.

CERVICAL SPINAL STENOSIS

Spinal stenosis with bilateral neurologic impairment (cervical myelopathy) may be a devastating result of osteoarthritis and spur formation. Upper limb weakness and impairment and limitation of neck notion are the usual presenting features. Long tract signs are usually present. Careful diagnostic assessment with imaging and, if required, myelography should be performed when surgical decompression is considered. Only a surgeon with wide experience and conservative judgment should be involved.

CERVICOTHORACIC INTERSPINOUS BURSITIS

Midline posterior cervical pain may result from formation of a bursa between the posterior spinous processes (60, 61). The pain is dull, usually constant, and localized in the region between the posterior processes of C7 and T1. The patient usually has a dorsal kyphosis with a forward inclination of the neck in relation to the shoulders. The pain is worse with resting or sitting, but improves during movement. Often, the provoking cause is an activity requiring hyperextension of the neck and head, such as cleaning the upper shelves of a cupboard.

Physical examination reveals point tenderness directly at the midline of the lower cervical or upper thoracic spine. Rubbery swelling of the soft tissues may be palpated. Passive range of motion is normal. Roentgenograms to exclude osteoporosis and an erythrocyte sedimentation rate to exclude sepsis should be obtained.

Treatment includes injection of the interspinous space, approached from a lateral point of entry about ½ inch from the midline. A long-acting steroid–local anesthetic mixture is injected into each side of the bursa (Fig. 2.9). Proper sleep position, with the neck in a neutral position, is advised, and neck erector strengthening and shoulder shrugging exercises are provided (Table 2.6, Exercises 2.A, 2.C, 2.D, 2.E, and 2.H). The patient should choose the single most comfortable strengthening exercise among Exercises 2.C, 2.D, and 2.E. Only one of the three is necessary for a continued, twice daily exercise regimen along with Exercises 2.A and 2.H. The patient is instructed to avoid hyperextension of the neck.

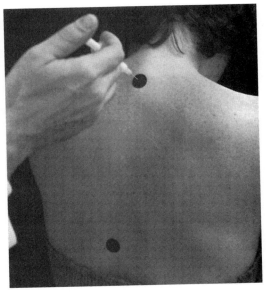

Figure 2.9. Injection of interspinous bursitis: a 1-inch No. 25 or No. 23 needle is used with a 45-degree angulated approach. Up to 2 mL volume is used.

FLOPPY HEAD SYNDROME

The floppy head syndrome has features of severe neck weakness. The weakness seems to be limited to the neck, and is often associated with generalized fatigue. These patients often have either hypothyroidism or polymyositis (62).

NECK PAIN OF LIGAMENTOUS ORIGIN

Ossification of the posterior longitudinal ligament may result in a cervical myelopathy with added complaints of altered sensation and motor function in the upper and lower limbs. Most cases occur among Japanese persons (63, 64). Similar findings can occur in association with diffuse idiopathic skeletal hyperostosis (Forestier's disease), spondylosis, and ankylosing spondylitis (65). Treatment of the spinal stenosis and myelopathy is surgical, with decompression.

Calcific tendinitis of the longus colli muscle tendon can result in a self-limited condition with neck and throat pain and dysphagia of several months' duration. Pain is aggravated by neck motion, and neck motion is severely restricted (66–68).

The crowned dens syndrome is due to ligamentous calcification posterior to the odontoid process. Radiopaque densities surround the top and sides of the odontoid process like a crown. Calcium apatite deposition or calcium pyrophosphate deposits can give rise to severe acute pain in the upper cervical region and may occur in association with acute attacks of pseudogout in peripheral joints. Treatment with nonsteroidal antiinflammatory agents is helpful (69).

TORTICOLLIS

Posttraumatic torticollis was presented earlier.

Acute wryneck of nontraumatic origin is usually a self-limited spasm of the sternocleidomastoid muscle in a child, and often follows an upper respiratory infection. The head is tilted with the chin directed away from the involved sternomastoid muscle. Treatment may be achieved with use of a tilt board. The patient is gently strapped supine with a head-down tilt of about 20 degrees. The dependent head provides traction, and after 5 or 10 minutes the spasm of the involved neck muscles may be relieved (70).

Inflammatory torticollis in children with the occiput rotated to the affected side and the chin rotated to the contralateral side may be severe, with resulting subluxation of the atlantoaxial joint. Search for overt or occult otolaryngologic infection, which may require imaging (71).

Spasmodic torticollis (focal cervical dystonia) tends to be chronic and disabling. Clonic or tonic contractions of the neck muscles with rotation of the head can result from organic disease of the nervous system or hysteria. The condition is thought to arise from neurovascular compression (72). Remission is rare after the first year (73).

Palliative treatment includes trigger point injections, neck stretching, and biofeedback. More radical measures include botulinum toxin (40–56) (47a, 74–76) or neurosurgical procedures including denervation of the involved muscles (77).

CERVICAL NERVE ROOT IMPINGEMENT

Presentation of cervical nerve root impingement will depend upon the nerve root involved

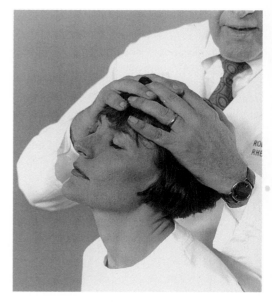

Figure 2.10. The Spurling maneuver. Downward force for 10 seconds' duration is used to reproduce symptoms resulting from cervical nerve impingement.

and the mode of onset. Pain aggravated by coughing or with bowel movement is suggestive of nerve compression. Neurologic history, combined with assessment of strength, reflexes, and tests for neurocompression aids diagnosis and suggests the site of compression. Sensory nerve testing has poor interobserver reliability.

The neck compression test (Spurling maneuver), the shoulder abduction test, and the axial traction test are helpful, although they have low sensitivity (78).

The *Spurling maneuver* is an attempt to reproduce the pain by direct compression of the nerve. With hands placed on the seated patient's head, the examiner rotates the head slightly to the painful shoulder. Pressure is then exerted downward with approximately 20 pounds of force for 10 seconds. Nerve root compression is strongly suggested if shoulder pain occurs or is increased (Fig. 2.10).

The *axial manual traction test* is performed with the patient supine. The patient's head is pulled with a traction force corresponding to 20 to 35 pounds; a positive test is the decrease or disappearance of radicular symptoms.

The *shoulder abduction test* is performed with the patient in the sitting position. When the patient lifts a hand above his or her head, the decrease or disappearance of the radicular symptoms represents a positive result.

Differential diagnosis includes other disorders that can cause radicular type of pain including herpes zoster, polyradiculitis (Landry-Guillain-Barré syndrome), Lyme disease, syringomyelia, rheumatoid arthritis involving the cervical spine, and acute brachial radiculitis.

Radiologic study and MRI should be considered if neurologic abnormality is noted. Electrodiagnostic studies may be normal during the first month of symptoms.

Management: Treatment begins with instructing the patient in proper sleep and sitting positions and avoidance of hyperextension of the neck (79). A helpful sleep position is to have the patient lie flat on his or her back with the thighs elevated on pillows, thus flattening the long spinal muscles. A rolled-up towel under the neck may be used. Some patients prefer the use of a soft neck collar or neck pillow. Reducing cervical erector muscle spasm is imperative. Measures to do this include the application of local moist heat or cold, the injection of cervical muscle trigger points with a local anesthetic–corticosteroid mixture, and the use of neck erector strengthening exercises (Table 2.6, Exercises 2.A, 2.C, 2.D, and 2.F). Manual techniques to relieve muscle spasm and trigger points can also be effective in therapy or self-management regimes. Cervical traction performed several times a day with a motorized intermittent traction machine or with a home traction kit is helpful (Table 2.6, Exercise 2.J) (80). Use of a mild muscle relaxant–analgesic preparation is most beneficial when used in conjunction with physical therapy measures; if cervical traction is necessary, the patient may need to use it daily for several months.

Isometric and strengthening neck exercises following each traction treatment can be helpful (Table 2.6, Exercise 2.A, 2.C, 2.D, and 2.E). Cervical collars are of value for protecting the neck from further injury especially while driving.

Most patients respond quickly and do not require electrodiagnostic studies or consideration for a surgical procedure. As a rule, we treat patients initially with local heat and exercises, and if no benefit occurs in the first few weeks, we then add cervical traction. A cervical spine radiologic examination to exclude malalignment or fractures should be considered before instituting cervical traction. If traction fails, we then proceed to EMG and surgical consultation. In our experience, fewer than 1% of these patients require surgical intervention; young women with nontraumatic herniated cervical disc lesions are more likely to require surgery than are older patients.

THORACIC OUTLET SYNDROME

The triangular space between the scalene muscles, the costoclavicular space, and the pectoralis minor space under the pectoralis minor muscle are frequent sites for congenital and acquired lesions that can lead to obstruction of the neurovascular bundle serving the arm (Fig. 2.11). Sir Ashley Cooper may have provided the first description in 1821.

Because multiple sites of obstruction in individual patients are commonly found at surgery, older terms based upon a presumed site of obstruction, such as the scalenus anticus (or anterior) syndrome, the cervical rib syndrome, the costoclavicular syndrome, and the hyperabduction or Wright's syndrome, are no longer used as the diagnosis. Many authors, particularly in the neurologic literature, have expressed skepticism regarding the diagnosis of thoracic outlet syndrome. However, the purely vascular types with objective change and the purely neurologic types with objective change are clearly accepted but are rarely seen. Much more common is the disputed form of neurologic presentation without objective features.

We stress how important it is to avoid unnecessary invasive measures when objective abnormality is not present. Many congenital deformities of this region occur in normal uncomplaining persons; therefore causality is uncertain without objective evidence. Clinical tests with poor discrimination include the elevated arm stress test, Adson's maneuver, plethysmography, and electrodiagnostic study. Clinical presentation depends upon whether the obstruction is predominantly vascular or neurogenic.

Purely vascular obstruction can be either venous or arterial; both are rare. Color change

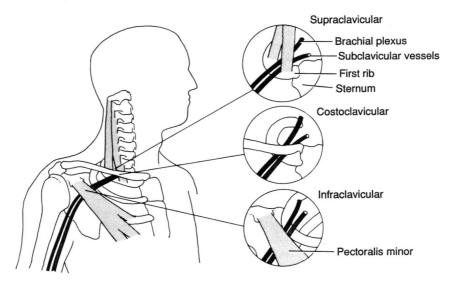

Figure 2.11. The thoracic outlet. The neurovascular bundle passes through three potential spaces: the triangular space between the scalene muscles; the costoclavicular space; and a space beneath the pectoralis minor muscle. (From Steinberg GG et al., eds. Ramamurti's orthopaedics in primary care. 2nd ed. Baltimore: Williams & Wilkins, 1992.)

and/or ischemic symptoms are evident. Patients may note swelling, venous dilatation, and diffuse arm, forearm, and hand pain. Purely neurologic presentation, also rare, includes evidence of neurogenic compression, usually with loss of sensation and intrinsic muscle atrophy. Much more common is the disputed neurogenic type with overlapping vascular symptoms and without objective findings.

A triad of numbness, weakness, and a sensation of swelling of the upper limbs is strongly suggestive of thoracic outlet syndrome.

Presentation: Paresthesia, pain, and often a sensation of swelling of the arm and hand on one or both sides occur. Occasional complaints include weakness of the hands, chest wall pain (81), and less often, discomfort of the entire shoulder girdle. Intermittent pain and paresthesia occur in nearly all patients, and usually follow the ulnar nerve distribution or involve the entire hand and lower arm (82, 83). Vascular disturbances, which accompany neurologic symptoms, include a sensation of coldness, congestion of the entire hand (rings feel tight in the morning), and distension of the veins of the hand.

Of 149 patients reviewed by Dale and Lewis (83), all had reported painful upper extremities; 58% suffered intermittent paresthesia, 23% reported motor incoordination, and only 16% had edema of the upper extremities. In two large series, over 80% of patients had

neurologic complaints of intermittent paresthesia or motor incoordination; less than 20% had vascular symptoms or edema (83, 84).

A carpal tunnel syndrome may coexist (83, 85), and retrograde neurologic symptoms from a carpal tunnel syndrome are common and may be confusing diagnostically. Patients may complain of hand congestion, arm weakness, shoulder pain, and nocturnal paresthesia relieved only by elevating and hyperabducting the arm—all due to a carpal tunnel syndrome (85). Positive tests for median nerve compression at the wrist, or relief following a corticosteroid injection into the carpal tunnel, will help to resolve the cause of symptoms in most patients. Thus, the carpal tunnel syndrome can accompany a thoracic outlet syndrome, or can cause similar symptomatology.

Chest pain often results from thoracic outlet syndrome but this syndrome may be overlaid upon coronary artery disease or reflux esophagitis. In fact, it is not uncommon for all three conditions to be present at the same time.

Etiology: By far the most common cause of thoracic outlet syndrome is sagging musculature related to aging, obesity, or heavy breasts and arms. Swift and Nichols have aptly designated this condition "the droopy shoulder syndrome" (86).

Occupational and other aggravating causes should be elicited. Painters, welders, mail carriers, and auto mechanics who frequently work with their arms overhead may acquire the syndrome during hyperabduction. Poor sleep position, with the arms hyperabducted, leads to neurovascular compression. Sedentary activities that allow the shoulders to drop down and forward may provoke symptoms.

Anatomic anomalies include cervical ribs with or without radiolucent cervical bands, first rib anomalies, elongation of a cervical transverse process, hypertrophy of the omohyoid or the scalenus anterior muscles, and post-stenotic aneurysms of the subclavian artery (87).

Roos described surgical findings in 232 patients who required surgical decompression (88). Of these, 27 cases were associated with cervical ribs or clavicle anomalies; other anatomic anomalies found included cervical bands (22 cases) and hyperplastic first ribs (three cases). Roos found no anatomic anomalies in the remaining 81% of his cases.

Cervical ribs are common, and may or may not contribute to thoracic outlet syndrome. Often, the cause is a functional change in the thoracic outlet due to aging (sagging muscles from sedentary activities) with no significant anatomic fault (83, 89).

Makhoul and Machleder (90) describe developmental anomalies found at surgery: among 200 consecutive cases, 86 scalene and 39 subclavius muscles had developmental abnormality, often at their insertions. But the scalene muscles vary considerably in their attachments and arrangement of their fibers. Again, causality is often difficult to establish in the individual patient.

Neurography of the brachial plexus, instillation of contrast media (meglumine iothalamate) into peripheral nerves, has been described by Takeshita, et al. in 180 patients with features of thoracic outlet syndrome, and in 30 patients with cervical symptoms without brachial plexus involvement. Abnormalities were noted in 85% of the patients; only an insignificant compression was observed in one of the control subjects. Narrowing was seen in the scalene triangle (30%), in the costoclavicular space (75%) and at the subcoracoid level (6%). When performed postoperatively, the compression was no longer evident except in the single patient with persistent postoperative complaints (91).

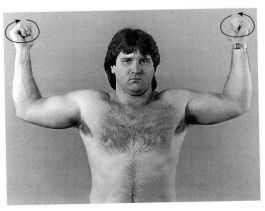

Figure 2.12. Roos Test. The patient repeatedly clenches and unclenches the fists while keeping the arms abducted and externally rotated (palms forward and upward). The elbows are braced slightly behind the frontal plane. When symptoms are reproduced, the test is positive.

Subluxation of the first rib at the costotransverse joint can lead to restricted cervical rotation and lateral flexion. This can be demonstrated during physical examination and relieved with exercise (see below).

Physical Examination: A careful history and physical examination are essential. The most important factor in the physical examination is to *look at the patient.* Is there a postural problem? In the female with heavy pendulous breasts, a tight brassiere, deep strap marks, and drooping shoulders will often be evident. Is the patient's thorax unusually narrow at the apex? Does the patient have poor muscle tone with drooping clavicles? Palpation and auscultation of the costoclavicular space for the presence of a cervical rib, tumor, aneurysm, or malformation of the body structures are quick, simple, and necessary procedures (83). The scalene muscles and brachial plexus may be tender to palpation or percussion, and if the condition is unilateral, the tenderness of the involved side should be compared with the uninvolved side (92).

A clinical test described by Roos (93) is very suggestive and easily performed. The patient repeatedly clenches and unclenches the fists while keeping the arms abducted and externally rotated (palms forward and upward) (Fig. 2.12). The elbows are braced slightly behind the frontal plane. When symptoms are reproduced, the test is positive. The test was validated

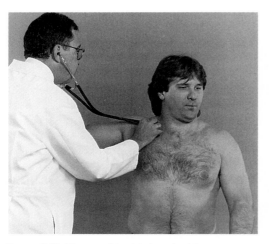

Figure 2.13. The modified Adson test for neurovascular compression by the scalenus anterior muscle. A positive test includes reproduction of symptoms, diminution of the pulse at the wrist, and the development of a bruit over the axillary vessels.

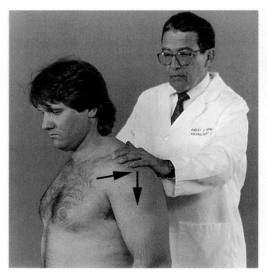

Figure 2.14. The costoclavicular maneuver (*arrows*) reproduces symptoms and decreases the pulse amplitude at the costoclavicular space. Backpacking is a common cause for the costoclavicular syndrome.

in an industrial setting and was predictive of neck, shoulder, and carpal tunnel distress among workers regardless of line of work (94).

The cervical rotation–lateral flexion test for obstruction of the thoracic outlet due to subluxation of the first rib is performed as follows. The neutrally positioned cervical spine is first rotated, passively and maximally, away from the side being tested. Then, while still in this position, the neck is gently flexed as far as possible, moving the ear toward the chest. The test is repeated on and compared with the uninvolved side. A positive test occurs if lateral flexion is totally blocked by bony restriction (95).

Other tests and maneuvers that can be helpful are the modified Adson test, the costoclavicular maneuver, and the hyperabduction maneuver.

The modified *Adson test or maneuver* is performed with the patient seated, arms at the sides. The pulse is palpated at the wrist and is auscultated for a bruit in the supraclavicular space (84). During the Adson test, the patient performs a Valsalva maneuver with the neck fully extended, arm elevated and the chin turned both toward and away from the involved side (87) (Fig. 2.13). The purpose of this test is to tense the scalenus anterior muscle. A positive test results in diminished pulsation of the radial artery and a bruit over the axillary vessels; the patient becomes aware of increased paresthesia.

The *costoclavicular maneuver* is performed by having the patient's shoulder rotated backward and downward; neurovascular features similar to those of Adson's test become evident as a positive result (Fig. 2.14). Yet another technique entails having the patient stand with elbows flexed at 90 degrees; in the coronal plane of the body (arms abducted 90 degrees), the arms are placed in three positions: at 45 degrees, 90 degrees, and 135 degrees (arms on top of the head): at each position the radial pulses are palpated and the examiner auscultates inferior to the midpoint of the clavicle for a bruit. Pulse diminution and bruit occur in cases of obstruction by the first rib (56).

The *hyperabduction maneuver* reproduces symptoms when the patient laterally circumducts the arms and clasps the hands over the head (Fig. 2.15). This results in compression of the neurovascular bundle beneath the insertion of the tendon of the pectoralis minor muscle at the coracoid process.

Of normal asymptomatic persons, 38% have a positive Adson's test, 68% have a positive costoclavicular maneuver, and 54% have a positive hyperabduction maneuver (85). But used in conjunction with other findings and history, these tests serve to bolster the benign nature of the symptoms.

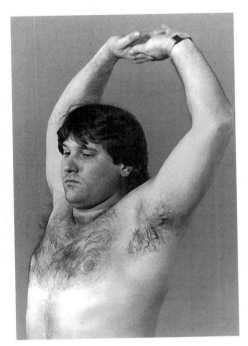

Figure 2.15. The hyperabduction maneuver reproduces symptoms when compression occurs beneath the insertion of the pectoralis minor tendon into the coracoid process.

Taking a complete history, observing for neurovascular compression, reproducing symptoms with one or another of the test maneuvers, and determining any occupational or positional aggravating causes for thoracic outlet compression certainly helps the clinician (83). A good response to therapy is excellent support for the diagnosis.

Laboratory and Radiologic Examination: Roentgenograms of the chest and cervical spine are necessary to exclude the presence of tumors, cervical ribs, or other skeletal anomalies. An erythrocyte sedimentation rate should be performed to exclude inflammatory and neoplastic conditions. Special tests, including nerve conduction or invasive vascular studies, can be withheld as long as vascular signs are not objectively present at the time of the first visit. Stress electrocardiograms may be necessary to exclude other causes if chest pain is a prominent feature (83). If the patient does not respond to initial therapy, nerve conduction velocities can sometimes provide diagnostic information.

The value of electrodiagnostic study was reevaluated in several studies (96, 97); elec-trodiagnostic testing was found to be useful only in order to exclude cervical nerve root compression or a carpal tunnel syndrome (83, 84). The cost-benefit ratio of the test is poor in our experience as well as that of others (92). Vascular studies, including arteriography and venography, are indicated when physical findings suggest a vascular disorder, such as an aneurysm or venous thrombosis (85), but otherwise help little in making the diagnosis.

Magnetic resonance angiography and intravascular ultrasound are undergoing evaluation for patients with a predominantly vascular presentation (98). Neurography may provide the most definitive evidence for obstruction and can be used in instances where conservative management has failed and surgical exploration is contemplated. The procedure can be performed safely only in experienced hands (91).

Differential Diagnosis: Conditions outside of the thoracic outlet rarely cause intermittent neurologic and vascular symptoms in the upper extremity. One should consider the possibility of tumors of the superior pulmonary sulcus (Pancoast's syndrome), impingement of a cervical nerve, cervical cord tumor, brachial plexus paralysis, carpal tunnel syndrome with retrograde symptomatology, peripheral neuropathies, syringomyelia, progressive muscle atrophy, reflex sympathetic dystrophy, and thrombosis or inflammation of the vascular tree (82).

The diagnostic workup for thoracic outlet syndrome is presented in Table 2.7, and a review of features that should warn of more serious disease is listed earlier in Table 2.2.

Complaints of a purely vascular obstruction, with objective swelling of the upper limb or Raynaud's phenomenon, are rare. Inflammatory diseases, such as giant cell arteritis, Takayasu's arteritis, and thrombosis of the subclavian vein (also called effort thrombosis or Paget-Schroetter syndrome) must be considered (82, 89).

Management: Aggravating factors can be remedied. For example, women with heavy pendulous breasts should obtain brassieres that provide proper support (Fig. 2.8). Sleep position should be reviewed with each patient. Patients should try to avoid sleeping with their arms hyperabducted or elevated. Some patients can be trained to avoid hyperabduction by tying each wrist with a stocking, which in turn

TABLE 2.7 DIAGNOSTIC WORKUP FOR THORACIC OUTLET SYNDROME

History
1. Intermittent pain, paresthesia, and swelling of part or all of an upper extremity
2. Aggravating factors, such as hyperabducting arms, at work or during sleep
3. Absence of specific features of carpal tunnel syndrome, cervical disc disease, or other systemic disease

Physical Examination
1. Observation for structural disorders (e.g., drooping shoulders, heavy pendulous breasts)
2. Check for masses in supraclavicular fossa
3. Perform special tests and maneuvers (e.g., Roos test, cervical rotation–lateral flexion test, Adson's test, hyperabduction, costoclavicular maneuvers
4. Absence of objective swelling or atrophy in most patients

Routine Tests
1. Cervical spine and chest roentgenograms
2. Tests for inflammation
3. Electrocardiogram if chest pain coexists
   A beneficial response to treatment may be the best test

Special Tests (rarely needed)
1. Electrodiagnostic studies
2. Vascular studies, including venography, venous flow rates, angiography, or magnetic resonance angiography
3. Neurography of brachial plexus

is safety-pinned to the bed sheet to allow some arm motion, but to restrict hyperabduction of the arms during sleep. (If the patient maintains his or her sanity, this can work. Most patients break the hyperabduction habit quickly!)

During sedentary activities, patients should learn to roll their shoulders up and backward to prevent drooping of the clavicle (Exercise 2.H). Hyperabduction required by employment may necessitate consultation with an occupational therapist. Other jobs that may require modification include those of letter carriers, painters, welders, and others who carry heavy loads on their shoulders or who work overhead. Repetitive abduction and adduction may result in hypertrophy of the subclavius and pectoral muscles, which may, in the susceptible person, compress the neurovascular bundle. Crane operators who push and pull levers can be at risk for thoracic outlet syndrome (99).

Trigger or pain points are frequently present along the trapezius ridge and, if palpable, can be relieved with injection of a nonaqueous steroid-anesthetic mixture (Fig. 2.6).

To perform an intralesional injection, prepare the area with soap and alcohol. Draw up to 40 mg of methylprednisolone acetate sterile aqueous suspension (or other equivalent corticosteroid agent suspension) with an equal amount of lidocaine hydrochloride 1%. The mixture will flocculate within the syringe. Using the shortest needle that can reach the required depth, use the needle as a probe. When the lesion is reached, pain is perceived. Inject 1 mL or less per lesion. Have the patient apply ice for 10 to 20 minutes after the injection. Up to a total of 60 mg of the methylprednisolone or equivalent can be injected but should not be repeated within 6 to 8 weeks.

Of paramount importance are exercises to strengthen and correct postural deficits (83, 99) (Table 2.6). The following exercises should be prescribed: shoulder elevation with resistance (Exercise 2.H); isometric neck strengthening (Exercises 2.C a–c; 2.D a, b; and 2.E a, b). If symptoms of chest wall pain are evident, chest wall stretching (Exercise 2.I) may be helpful. (Another technique for chest wall stretching is Exercise 7.C.) These exercises correct the forward inclination of the neck and stretch the pectoral musculature.

For patients with a positive test for subluxation of the first rib as described above, the following exercise to mobilize the first ribs is recommended (95). The patient pushes the head forward, to the side, and backward against the palm of the hand on the painful side. The patient pushes in each direction for 1 second and pauses between directions. Each direction is repeated ten times before pausing. The entire series is repeated up to ten times a day. The cervical rotation–lateral flexion test should return to normal and can be used to measure outcome. If sleep is disturbed, a muscle relaxant or sedative may be prescribed at bedtime for the first week or two (83).

Outcome and Additional Suggestions: Physical therapy and exercise, instructions in proper sitting, and proper work and sleep positions should provide relief in 50 to 90% of patients (83–85, 87, 88), usually within 6 weeks (5). Morning stiffness, hand congestion, and paresthesia are the first symptoms to improve.

Fewer than 5% of our patients require surgical treatment.

Before surgical exploration, consider the following:

1. Has carpal tunnel syndrome or cervical disc lesion been excluded?
2. Has a chest roentgenogram for tumor been reviewed recently?
3. Were aggravating factors eliminated (sleep position, sitting positions, improper work habits)?
4. Did the patient comply with the exercise program?

Whenever a carpal tunnel syndrome coexists, we would treat the carpal tunnel more aggressively before considering thoracic outlet surgery and then reassess the thoracic outlet symptoms after relief from median nerve entrapment has been effected.

Electrodiagnostic testing and electromyography should precede surgery in order to exclude other neurologic disorders that could result in dissatisfaction with the surgical outcome. If available, neurography may be the most definitive test for sites of obstruction in patients with disputable neurogenic features. Vascular studies and nerve conduction tests may be normal, yet surgical intervention is still undertaken because of persistent symptoms. At operation, compression has been found as low as the second rib (88), and the current surgical procedure of choice is resection of the first rib to provide more space for the neurovascular bundle.

Unfortunately, we have seen surgical failures. The symptoms have returned when the patient resumed work requiring hyperabduction. A change in jobs should have preceded operation. We have found that if cases are properly selected, first rib resection through the transaxillary approach gives good results in 85% of operated patients (100). Failure following first rib resection may result from surgical inexperience (101), coexisting reflux esophagitis, coronary artery disease, or carpal tunnel syndrome (84). It can also result from subluxation of the first rib stump with limitation of movement during the cervical rotation–lateral flexion test. Monotonous desk work has been thought to contribute to the subluxation (102). Finally, reflex sympathetic dystrophy can complicate surgery or be overlooked as a confounding coexisting problem.

REFERENCES

1. Bland JH, Boushey DR: Anatomy and physiology of the cervical spine. Semin Arthritis Rheum 20:1–20, 1990.
2. Teresi LM, Lufkin RB, Reicher MA, et al.: Asymptomatic degenerative disc disease and spondylosis of the cervical spine: MR imaging. Radiology 164:83–88, 1987.
3. Boden SD, Davis DO, Dina TS, et al.: Abnormal magnetic-resonance scans of the lumbar spine in asymptomatic subjects. J Bone Joint Surg 72A(3): 403–408, 1990.
3a. Ohlsson K, Attewell RG, Palsson B, et al.: Repetitive industrial work and neck and upper limb disorders in females. Am J Ind Med 27(5): 731–747, 1995.
4. Travell JG, Simons DG: Myofascial pain and dysfunction: the trigger point manual. Baltimore: Williams and Wilkins, 1983.
5. The American Academy of Craniomandibular Disorders: Craniomandibular disorders: guidelines for evaluation, diagnosis, and management. Charles McNeill, ed. Chicago: Quintessence Publishing Co., 1990.
6. Shiffman E, Fricton JR, Haley D, Shapiro BL: The prevalence and treatment needs of subjects with temporomandibular disorders. J Am Dent Assn 120:295–303, 1990.
7. Motegi E, Miyazaki H, Ogura I, et al.: An orthopedic study of temporomandibular joint disorders. Part 1: Epidemiological research in Japanese 6–18 year olds. Angle Orthod 62:249–256, 1992.
8. Jagger RG, Wood C: Signs and symptoms of temporomandibular joint dysfunction in a Saudi Arabian population. J Oral Rehabil 19: 353–359, 1992.
9. Harinstein D, Buckingham RB, Braun T, et al.: Systemic joint laxity (the hypermobility joint syndrome) is associated with temporomandibular joint dysfunction. Arthritis Rheum 31: 1259–1264, 1988.
10. Greene CS, Laskin DM: Long-term status of TMJ clicking in patients with myofascial pain and dysfunction. JADA 117:461–465, 1988.
11. Fricton JR: Clinical care for myofascial pain. Dental Clin North Am 35:1–28, 1991.
12. Forssell H, Kirveskari P, Kangasniemi P: Effect of occlusal adjustment on mandibular dysfunction. Acta Odontol Scand 44:62–69, 1986.

12a. Moss RA, Lombardo TW, Villarosa GA, et al.: Oral habits and TMJ dysfunction in facial pain and non-pain subjects. J Oral Rehabil 22(1): 79–81, 1995.

13. Guralnick W, Kaban LB, Merrill RG: Temporomandibular-joint afflictions. N Engl J Med 299: 123–129, 1978.

14. Freese AS: Costen's syndrome: a reinterpretation. AMA Arch Otol 70:309–314, 1959.

15. Trenouth MJ: The relationship between bruxism and temporomandibular joint dysfunction as shown by computer analysis of nocturnal tooth contact patterns. J Oral Rehabil 6:81–87, 1979.

16. Small EW: An investigation into the psychogenic bases of the temporomandibular joint myofascial pain dysfunction syndrome. In: Bonica JJ, Albe-Fessard DG, eds. Advances in pain research and therapy. New York: Raven Press, 1976:889–894.

17. Stein S, Loft G, Davis H, Hart DL: Symptoms of TMJ dysfunction as related to stress measured by the social readjustment rating scale. J Prosthet Dent 47:545–548, 1982.

18. Heloe B, Heiberg AN: A follow-up study of a group of female patients with myofascial pain–dysfunction syndrome. Acta Odontol, Scand 38:129–134, 1980.

19. Toller PA: Use and misuse of intra-articular corticosteroids in treatment of temporomandibular joint pain. Proc Roy Soc Med 70:461–463, 1977.

20. Greene CS, Laskin DM: Splint therapy for the myofascial pain–dysfunction (MPD) syndrome: a comparative study. JADA 107:235–238, 1983.

21. Goharian RK, Neff PA: Effect of occlusal retainers on temporomandibular joint and facial pain. J Prosthet Dent 44:206–208, 1980.

22. Kotani H, Abekura H, Hamada T: Objective evaluation for bite plate therapy in patients with myofascial pain dysfunction syndrome. J Oral Rehabil 21:241–245, 1994.

23. Zarb GA, Speck JE: The treatment of temporomandibular joint dysfunction: a retrospective study. J Prosthet Dent 38:420–432, 1977.

24. Hall LJ: Physical therapy treatment results for 178 patients with temporomandibular joint syndrome. Am J Otol 5:183–196, 1984.

25. Scott DS, Gregg JM: Behavioral-relaxation therapy. Pain 9:231–241, 1980.

26. Lovshin LL: Carotidynia. Headache 17: 192–195, 1977.

27. Lovshin LL: Vascular neck pain—a common syndrome seldom recognized: analysis of 100 consecutive cases. Cleveland Clin Q 27:5–13, 1960.

28. Fay T: Atypical facial neuralgia, a syndrome of vascular pain. Ann Otol 41:1030–1062, 1962.

29. Raskin NH, Prusiner S: Carotidynia. Neurology 27:43–46, 1977.

30. Couch JR, Ziegler DK, Hassanein R: Amitriptyline in the prophylaxis of migraine. Neurology 26:121–127, 1976.

31. Karlan MS, Beroza L, Cassisi NJ: Anterior cervical pain syndromes. Otol Head Neck Surg 87: 284–291, 1979.

32. Meyers-Stirling J: Calcium channel blockers in the prophylactic treatment of vascular headache. Ann Intern Med 120:395–397, 1985.

33. Eagle WW: Elongated styloid process. Arch Otol 25:584–587, 1937.

34. Blatchford SJ, Coulthard SW: Eagle's syndrome: an atypical cause of dysphonia. Ear Nose Throat J 68:48–51, 1989.

35. Krespi YP, Shugar JMA, Som PM: Stylohyoid syndromes: an uncommon cause of pharyngeal and neck pain. Am J Otolaryngol 2:358–360, 1981.

36. Travell J: Identification of myofascial trigger point syndromes: a case of atypical facial neuralgia. Arch Phys Med Rehabil 62:100–106, 1981.

37. Rask MR: The omohyoideus myofascial pain syndrome: report of four patients. J Cranioman Prac 2:256–262, 1985.

38. Salins PC, Bloxham GP: Bursitis: a factor in the differential diagnosis of orofacial neuralgias and myofascial pain dysfunction syndrome. Oral Surg Oral Med Oral Path 68:154–157, 1989.

39. Asher SW: Headache and facial pain. Hosp Med 16:33–40, 1980.

40. Stock SR: Workplace ergonomic factors and the development of musculoskeletal disorders of the neck and upper limbs: a meta-analysis. Am J Ind Med 19:87–107, 1991.

41. Rossignol AM, Morse EP, Summers VM, Pagnotto LD: Video display terminal use and reported health symptoms among Massachusetts clerical workers. J Occup Med 29(2):112–118, 1987.

42. Laban MM, Braker AM, Meerschaert JR: Airport induced "cervical traction" radiculopathy: the OJ syndrome. Arch Phys Med Rehabil 70:845–847, 1989.

43. McKinney LA: Early mobilisation and outcome in acute sprains of the neck. Br Med J 299: 1006–1008, 1989.

44. Gargan MF, Bannister GC: Long-term prognosis of soft-tissue injuries of the neck. J Bone Joint Surg 72B:901–903, 1990.

45. Schuyler-Hacker H, Green R, Wingate L, Sklar J: Acute torticollis secondary to rupture of the sternocleidomastoid. Arch Phys Med Rehabil 70:851–853, 1989.

46. Goldman S, Ahlskog JE: Posttraumatic cervical dystonia. Mayo Clin Proc 68:443–448, 1993.

47. Truong DD, Dubinsky R, Hermanowicz N, Olson WL, et al.: Posttraumatic torticollis. Arch Neurol 48:221–223, 1991.

47a. Van den Bergh P, Francart J, Mourin S, et al.: Five-year experience in the treatment of focal movement disorders with low-dose Dysport botulinum toxin. Muscle Nerve 18(7):720–729, 1995.

48. Barnsley L, Lord SM, Wallis BJ, et al.: Lack of effect of intraarticular corticosteroids for chronic pain in the cervical zygapophyseal joints. N Engl J Med 330:1047–1050, 1994.

49. Cohen A: Trends in human factors research. Occupational Health and Safety (June):30–36, 1982.

50. Deal CL, Schnitzer TJ, Lipstein E, et al.: Treatment of arthritis with topical capsaicin: a double-blind trial. Clin Therap 13(3):383–395, 1991.

51. Pronsati MP: Using microcurrents. Adv Phys Therap 2(17):8–9, 1991.

52. Peck CL, Kraft GH: Electromyographic biofeedback for pain related to muscle tension: a study of tension headache, back, and jaw pain. Arch Surg 112:889–895, 1977.

53. Jacobs A, Felton GS: Visual feedback of myoelectric output to facilitate muscle relaxation in normal persons and patients with neck injuries. Arch Phys Med Rehabil 50:34–39, 1969.

54. Hubbell SL, Thomas M: Postpartum cervical myofascial pain syndrome: review of four patients. Obstet Gynecol 65(3)(Suppl):56s–57s, 1985.

55. Kaganov JA, Bakal DA, Dunn BE: The differential contribution of muscle contraction and migraine symptoms to problem headache in the general population. Headache 21:157–163, 1981.

56. DeGowen EL, DeGowen RL: Bedside diagnostic examination. 5th ed. New York: Macmillan, 1987.

57. Lacroix JM, Clarke MA, Bock JC, Doxey NCS: Muscle-contraction headaches in multiple-pain patients: treatment under worsening baseline conditions. Arch Phys Med Rehabil 67: 14–18, 1986.

58. Cronen MC, Waldman SD: Cervical steroid epidural nerve blocks in the palliation of pain secondary to intractable tension-type headaches. J Pain Symptom Manage 5:379–381, 1990.

59. Waldman SD: Complications of cervical epidural nerve blocks with steroids: a prospective study of 790 consecutive blocks. Reg Anesth 14: 149–151, 1989.

60. Bywaters EGL: Lesions of bursae, tendons, and tendon sheaths. Clin Rheum Dis 5:883–918, 1979.

61. Bywaters EGL: Rheumatoid and other diseases of the cervical interspinous bursae, and changes in the spinous processes. Ann Rheum Dis 41: 360–370, 1982.

62. Katz AL, Pate D: Floppy head syndrome. Arthritis Rheum 23:131–132, 1980.

63. Resnik D: Hyperostosis and ossification in the cervical spine. Arthritis Rheum 27:564–569, 1984.

64. Williamson PK, Reginato AJ: Diffuse idiopathic skeletal hyperostosis of the cervical spine in a patient with ankylosing spondylitis. Arthritis Rheum 27:570–573, 1984.

65. Trojan DA, Pouchot J, Pokrupa R, et al.: Diagnosis and treatment of ossification of the posterior longitudinal ligament of the spine: report of eight cases and literature review. Am J Med 92: 296–306, 1992.

66. Sarkozi J, Fam AG: Acute calcific retropharyngeal tendinitis: an unusual cause of neck pain. Arthritis Rheum 27:708–710, 1984.

67. Karasick D, Karasick S: Calcific retropharyngeal tendinitis. Skel Radiol 7:203–205, 1981.

68. Newmark H, Zee CS, Frankel P, et al.: Chronic calcific tendinitis of the neck. Skel Radiol 7: 207–208, 1981.

69. Bouvet J, Le Parc J, Michalski B, et al.: Acute neck pain due to calcifications surrounding the odontoid process: the crowned dens syndrome. Arthritis Rheum 28:1417–1420, 1985.

70. Banergee A: The hanging head method for the treatment of acute wry neck [Letter]. Arch Emerg Med 8:71, 1991.

71. Bredenkamp JK, Maceri DR: Inflammatory torticollis in children. Arch Otolaryngol Head Neck Surg 116: 310–313, 1990.

72. Pagni CA, Naddeo M, Faccani G: Spasmodic torticollis due to neurovascular compression of the 11th nerve. J Neurosurg 63:789–791, 1985.

73. Freidman A, Fahn S: Spontaneous remissions in spasmodic torticollis. Neurology 36:398–400, 1986.

74. Borodic GE, Mills L, Joseph M: Botulinum A toxin for the treatment of adult-onset spasmodic torticollis. Plast Reconstr Surg 87:285–289, 1991.

75. D'Costa DF, Abbott RJ: Low dose botulinum toxin in spasmodic torticollis. J Roy Soc Med 84:650–651, 1991.

76. Lu CS, Chen RS, Tsai CH: Double-blind, placebo-controlled study of botulinum toxin injections in the treatment of cervical dystonia. J Formos Med Assoc 94(4):189–192, 1995.

77. Davis DH, Ahlskog JE, Litchy WJ, et al.: Selective peripheral denervation for torticollis: preliminary results. Mayo Clin Proc 66:365–371, 1991.

78. Viikari-Juntura E, Porras M, Laasonen E: Validity of clinical tests in the diagnosis of root compression in cervical disc disease. Spine 14: 253–257, 1989.

79. British Association of Physical Medicine: Pain in the neck and arm: a multicentre trial of the effects of physiotherapy. Br Med J 1:253–258, 1966.

80. Honet JC, Puri K: Cervical radiculitis: treatment and results in 82 patients. Arch Phys Med Rehabil 57:12–16, 1976.

81. Urschel HC, Razzuk MA, Hyland JW, et al.: Thoracic outlet syndrome masquerading as coronary artery disease (pseudoangina). Ann Thorac Surg 16:239–248, 1973.

82. Urschel HC, Razzuk MA: Management of the thoracic-outlet syndrome. N Engl J Med 286: 1140–1143, 1972.

83. Dale WA, Lewis MR: Management of thoracic outlet syndrome. Ann Surg 181:575–585, 1975.

84. McGough EC, Pearce MB, Byrne JP: Management of thoracic outlet syndrome. J Thorac Cardiovasc Surg 77:169–174, 1979.

85. Conn J Jr: Thoracic outlet syndromes. Surg Clin North Am 54:155–164, 1974.
86. Swift TR, Nichols FT: The droopy shoulder syndrome. Neurology 34:212–215, 1984.
87. Tyson RR, Kaplan GF: Modern concepts of diagnosis and treatment of the thoracic outlet syndrome. Orthop Clin North Am 6:507–519, 1975.
88. Roos DB: Experience with first rib resection for thoracic outlet syndrome. Ann Surg 173: 429–442, 1971.
89. Bertelsen S: Neurovascular compression syndromes of the neck and shoulder. Acta Chir Scand 135:137–148, 1969.
90. Makhoul RG, Machleder HI: Developmental anomalies at the thoracic outlet: an analysis of 200 consecutive cases. J Vasc Surg 16: 534–542, 1992.
91. Takeshita M, Minamikawa H, Iwamoto H, et al.: Neurography of the brachial plexus in the thoracic outlet syndrome. International Orthop 15:1–5, 1991.
92. Crawford FA: Thoracic outlet syndrome. Surg Clin North Am 604:947–957, 1980.
93. Roos D: Congenital anomalies associated with thoracic outlet syndrome. Am J Surg 132: 771–778, 1976.
94. Toomingas A, Hagberg M, Jorulf L, et al.: Outcome of the abduction external rotation test among manual and office workers. Am J Ind Med 19: 215–227, 1991.
95. Lindgren K, Leino E, Manninen H: Cervical rotation lateral flexion test in brachialgia. Arch Phys Med Rehabil 73:735–737, 1992.
96. Wilbourn AJ, Lederman AJ: Evidence for conduction delay in thoracic-outlet syndrome is challenged. N Engl J Med 310:1052–1053, 1984.
97. Urschel HC Jr: Letter to the editor. N Engl J Med 310:1053, 1984. [Reply to Wilbourn and Lederman, reference No. 96.]
98. Chengelis DL, Glover JL, Bendick P, et al.: The use of intravascular ultrasound in the management of thoracic outlet syndrome. Am Surg 60(8): 592–596, 1994.
99. Feldman RG, Goldman R, Keyserling WM: Peripheral nerve entrapment syndromes and ergonomic factors. Am J Ind Med 4:661–668, 1983.
100. Derkash RS, Goldberg VM: The results of first rib resection in thoracic outlet syndrome. Orthopedics 4:1025–1029, 1981.
101. Roos DB: Recurrent thoracic outlet syndrome after first rib resection. Acta Chir Belg 79: 363–380, 1980.
102. Lindgren K, Leino E, Lepantalo M, et al.: Recurrent thoracic outlet syndrome after first rib resection. Arch Phys Med Rehabil 72:208–210, 1991.

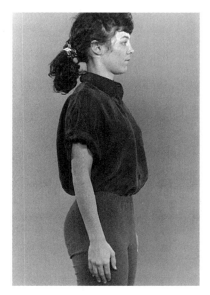

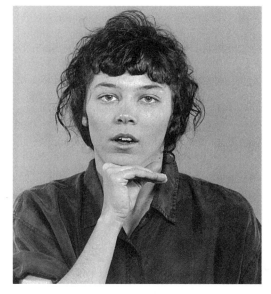

Exercise 2.A. Axial Extension

Also known as ''military press,'' ''posterior head/neck retraction,'' or ''posterior head/neck translation.''

This is the basic position for good head/neck alignment and should be the beginning position for all the exercises in this group. It can be performed in standing, sitting, and supine postures. Once mastered, the Exercise should be performed throughout the day and done regularly as a posture check.

Instructions: Tuck chin. Slowly move head backward, straightening and lengthening the neck. Movement should be slow and gentle. Hold the position 10–30 seconds and repeat, or perform the movement and proceed with another exercise.

Exercise 2.B. Jaw Balancing (Isometric)

Apply the resistance for these exercises with the open or loosely fisted hand. Begin with mouth open about an inch. Hold the resistance and muscle contraction 5–10 seconds, relax, and repeat five times per session. Exercises can be repeated with moderate resistance applied several sessions per day, or with maximum resistance one session per day.

2.B (a). Opening. Open the lower jaw against resistance, hold, and relax. Repeat five times per session.

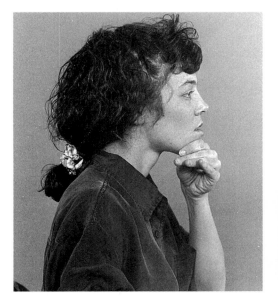

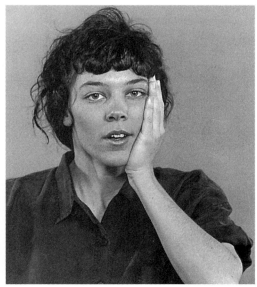

2.B (b). Forward Thrust. Push the jaw forward against the hand, hold, and relax. Repeat five times per session.

2.B (c). Lateral Thrust. Push the jaw sideward to the right against resistance, hold, and relax. Then push the jaw to the other side (left), hold, and relax. Repeat five times per side, five times per session.

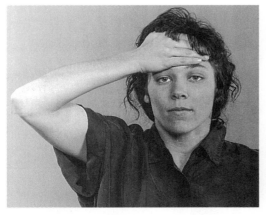

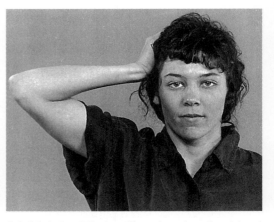

Exercise 2.C. Head/Neck Isometric Strengthening

In these exercises, apply resistance with the open or loosely fisted hand. Hold resistance 5–10 seconds. No movement of the head actually occurs during this exercise.

2.C (a). Flexion. Place hand on the forehead or under the chin. Tuck the chin, and push the head down and in the forward direction against resistance. Hold 5–10 seconds. Repeat five times per session.

2.C (b). Lateral Flexion. Place hand on the side of the head. Push the head as if the ear were to move toward the shoulder on the same side. Hold 5–10 seconds. Repeat five times per session.

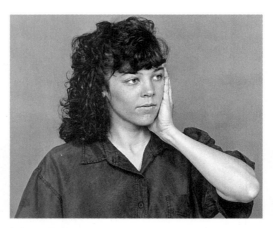

2.C (c). Rotation. Place hand in front of the ear or on the side of the head. Push the head in the rotary direction as if turning to one side. Hold 5–10 seconds. Repeat five times per session. Repeat on the other side.

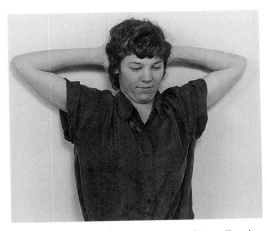

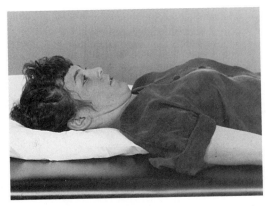

Exercise 2.D. Standing. Neck Erector Strengthening
2.D (a). Stand with the back to the wall, feet 6 inches from the wall. Place hands behind the head and push the head and shoulders against the wall. Hold 5–10 seconds. Repeat five times per session.

2.D (b). Lying supine. Lie supine with a pillow under the head and neck, knees bent. Tuck chin, straightening and lengthening the neck. Then push the head slowly against the pillow using the posterior neck muscles. Hold 5–10 seconds. Repeat five times per session.

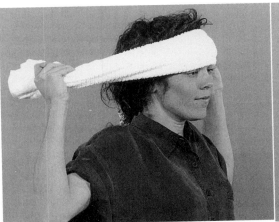

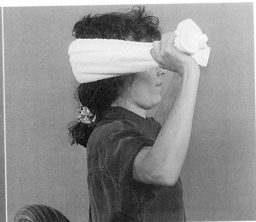

Exercise 2.E. Resisted Strengthening
   In these exercises, use a folded towel held between the hands for resistance.
2.E (a). Flexion. Place the towel across the forehead as illustrated. Push the head forward against the towel. Hold 5–10 seconds. Repeat five times per session.

2.E (b). Extension. Place the towel behind the head as illustrated. Push the head back into the towel. Hold 5–10 seconds. Repeat five times per session.

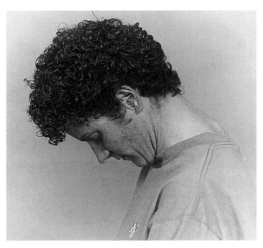

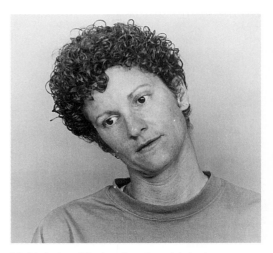

Exercise 2.F. Active Range of Motion (Flexibility)
   Perform the Axial Extension exercise (Exercise 2.A) to achieve the start position for this exercise. Repeat each movement at least five times per session.
2.F (a). Flexion. Tuck chin and bend neck, bringing head down and forward.

2.F (b). Lateral Flexion. Bend neck bringing one ear toward the shoulder on the same side.

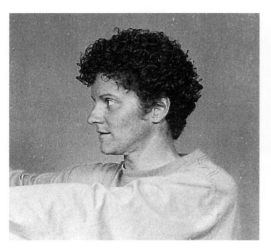

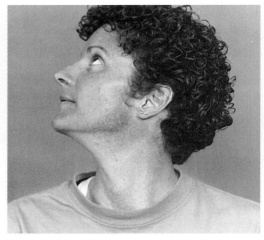

2.F (c). Rotation (straight plane). Rotate the head, turning toward one side and then toward the other.

2.F (d). Diagonal Rotation. Rotate the head looking up and toward one shoulder, then down and toward the opposite hip.

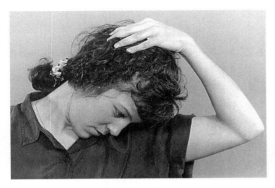

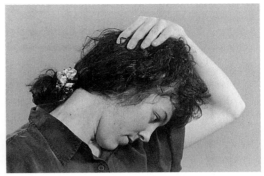

Exercise 2.G. Assisted Stretches
2.G (a). Sternocleidomastoid Stretch. Place one hand (left) over the opposite (right) ear, arm across the back of the head as illustrated. Next turn the face to the left and bend the neck bringing the head forward. Then, with the left hand, push the head farther forward and the toward the left armpit. Hold the position 5–10 seconds. The stretch should be felt along the right side of the neck. Repeat five times on each side.

2.G (b). Lateral Flexion. Place one hand (left) over the opposite (right) ear, arm over the top of the head as illustrated. With the left hand, pull the head to the left but not forward or downward. Hold the position 5–10 seconds. Repeat five times on each side.

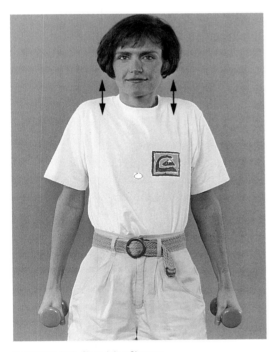

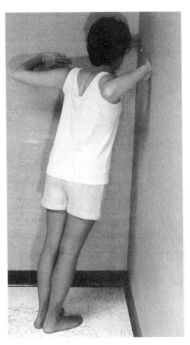

Exercise 2.H. Shoulder Shrugs
This exercise is performed standing or sitting, arms at the side, elbows straight. Hold a 2–5-pound weight in each hand as illustrated. Pull the shoulders slowly toward the ears and backward. Hold 5–10 seconds, and then relax completely between each shrug. Repeat five times per session. Exercise can be done with both shoulders at once or one at a time.

Exercise 2.I. Corner Stretch (Pectoral/Chest Wall Stretch)
Stand facing a corner with feet 12–36 inches from the corner, hands on the wall at shoulder level, elbows elevated. Lean into the corner until a stretching sensation is felt across the chest and shoulders. Hold 10–30 seconds with three to six repetitions. Perform two or three times daily.

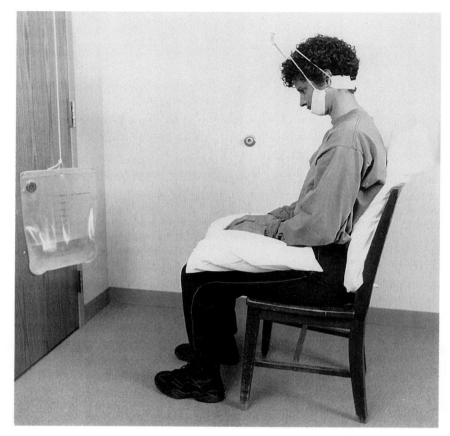

Exercise 2.J. Cervical Traction

Cervical traction is applied with the patient's head flexed 15–25 degrees. Traction should be performed at least twice daily for 5–10 minutes, gradually increasing the weight from 5 to 20 pounds. Discontinue if pain or other symptoms increase.

3: Upper Limb Disorders

Upper limb pain and disability may be intrinsic, referred from other structures, or part of systemic disease. Many disorders result from excessive force or movement or from improper work habits. New terms introduced in the past decade include cumulative movement disorders, cumulative trauma disorders, cumulative injury disorders, repetitive trauma disorders, or repetitive strain injury, all used interchangeably. Because specific diagnostic findings and pathology are often lacking, and because trauma or injury are pejorative terms to employers, the term cumulative movement disorders will be used here.

CUMULATIVE MOVEMENT DISORDERS (CMD) OF THE UPPER LIMB

Included in this grouping are ligament and tendon disorders, bursitis, myofascial pain, and nerve entrapment disorders. The incidence of these disorders has increased greatly in the past decade and in some countries has reached epidemic proportions. In one study of upper extremity work-related disability for 1989, Webster and Snook estimate the costs to have been $563 million (1). Societal attitudes toward work disability differ across the world. Work disability is far more likely in the technologically advanced countries of the Northern Hemisphere, primarily North America and Australia, than in less developed countries. Compensation is a major factor in symptom severity. Furthermore, psychologic factors, workplace politics, and perceived job stress are significant contributors to symptom onset and persistence (2). Behavior problems outside the workplace are also often major contributors to symptoms.

Naturally occurring diseases such as osteoarthritis, rheumatoid arthritis, or ganglia may be aggravated by repetitive tasks, but the tasks are not the primary reason that the disorder exists (3–6). The pathogenesis and a method for grading severity of cumulative movement disorders were presented in Chapter 1.

Cost-effective care must begin with a comprehensive appropriate history and physical examination (below). Only then can efficient further diagnosis and care be rendered.

Imaging, electromyography, and arthroscopy must be used judiciously. Magnetic resonance imaging (MRI), computed tomography (CT), arthrography, ultrasonography, and arthroscopy have become commonplace diagnostic tools in the past decade; but these procedures, like electromyography, have results that depend on the operator's skill and technique. The choice and timing of the diagnostic procedure will depend upon the clinical impression, response to past treatment, the potential duration of disability, and cost, as well as the availability of a skilled operator of the procedure (7).

Despite these limitations, office arthroscopy, made possible by the development of a small-caliber disposable arthroscope that is user-friendly, may provide much better definition of the cause for pain and disability. The preferred scope for shoulder evaluation is a 2.7 mm rigid arthroscope coupled with a high-resolution camera. Shoulder assessment with arthroscopy is currently an important methodology for identifying shoulder cuff lesions, instability, impingement, and early development of arthritis (7, 8). However, arthroscopy is invasive, expensive, and highly dependent on operator experience. Because of recent improvements in MRI technology, the choice between MRI and an invasive procedure like arthroscopy is not yet clear. In the United States, the cost of MRI is perhaps four times greater than that of arthrography, another invasive but less costly procedure; and because of additional costs for operating room time, anesthesia, and instrumentation, the cost for arthroscopy of the shoulder is perhaps as much as 10 times the cost of arthrography. MRI is not very sensitive to early articular cartilage lesions; significant cartilage lesions observed by arthroscopy were often missed on MRI. Studies of the sensitivity of these various diagnostic procedures are ongoing.

Shoulder impingement syndrome that fails conservative care may be further evaluated by either MRI or arthroscopy, but both procedures have limitations which become evident when findings are compared with observations at surgery.

HISTORY AND PHYSICAL EXAMINATION OF THE UPPER LIMB

A proper history of upper limb pain and disability should include:

- A general health history to determine if the problem might be referred from other locations or is part of a systemic rheumatic disease.
- A determination of what specific movements aggravate pain or disability and thus define which muscles or tissues might be affected.
- A personal history including hobbies, habits, sports, work tasks, previous injuries and disorders, use of alcohol or smoking (which might prolong recovery time).
- Other potential aggravating habits including neck, arm, and hand position when sleeping, using the upper limb to push off from the seated position, and hand or fist clenching.
- Functional assessment of those daily activities that are affected by the problem, activities that have been discontinued, and those activities that have been modified in order to be completed. A standardized functional assessment is useful.

Refer to Appendix A for a review of the elements of the history and physical examination for the rheumatic diseases. Of most importance is consideration of the whole person and not just a regional medical disorder. Table 3.1 lists the possibly critical signs that indicate more immediate attention; Table 3.2 provides helpful clues for aggravating factors that can prolong or cause recurrent pain and disability; and Table

TABLE 3.1 CRITICAL FEATURES FOR THE UPPER LIMB

1. Fever and chills
2. Lymphadenopathy
3. Constant and progressive pain
4. Pain in the axilla
5. Any visible swelling
6. Numbness and tingling above elbow
7. Inability to maintain active arm elevation
8. Shoulder pain unrelated to arm movement
9. Bruit over subclavian vessels
10. Other features of vascular impairment
11. Olecranon peribursal erythema and edema
12. Lateral instability during passive examination
13. Muscle atrophy
14. Nailfold infarcts (at the nail edges)
15. Diffuse swelling of a hand, with warmth
16. Clubbing

3.3 presents a differential diagnosis. Use these to construct a relevant history and physical examination.

Pain location should be ascertained: pain over the deltoid region can arise from the subacromial bursa or from a myofascial pain (trigger) point in the infraspinatus muscle. Pain in the triceps region may arise locally or from a pain (trigger) point in the serratus posterior superior muscle (9). You can also use a pain drawing to serve as a guide for diagnosis and to follow the patient's progress.

Pain pattern that is intermittent and disabling is likely the result of tendon injury or cumulative movement disorder. The list of aggravating factors (Table 3.2) should be reviewed with the patient. A new job, hobby, or aggravating resting positions may be contributing to cumulative movement disorder.

Abrupt onset of pain accompanied by limitation of active shoulder movement suggests a rotator cuff tear or shoulder joint dislocation.

Pain with specific movements may indicate the source. For example, pain during the first 30 degrees of arm abduction may originate in the deltoid muscle or subacromial bursa; pain during arm abduction between 60 and 120 degrees suggests supraspinatus involvement; pain with abduction and internal or external rotation suggests biceps and supraspinatus impingement under the acromion. Shoulder pain with arm pronation-to-supination movement indicates biceps involvement; pain during forward elevation can indicate subcoracoid bursitis, acromioclavicular osteoarthritis, glenohumeral arthritis, or biceps tendinitis.

TABLE 3.2 JOINT PROTECTION FOR THE UPPER EXTREMITY

Prevent cumulative movement disorders by frequently interrupting repetitive tasks such as washing windows, vacuuming, and working on an assembly line. Keep the elbow close to the body. Change the angle of shoulder motion when possible.

Sleep with the arms below the level of the chest.

If using crutches, adjust them properly to 2 inches (about 5 cm) below axillae; carry weight on ribs and hands, not under the arms. A forearm cane may be preferred.

Rise from a chair by pushing off with thigh muscles, not the hands.

Take frequent breaks when working with the arms overhead.

To grasp an object at your side or that is behind you, turn your body and face the object.

To reach a car seat belt, use the far arm and hand across the front of the body.

A swivel or wheeled chair may be useful when tasks done from a seated position are in various locations.

When driving, keep the hands below the 3 o'clock and 9 o'clock positions on the wheel. If possible, use a steering wheel that tilts.

Sports

Swimming: Strengthen and maintain shoulder muscles with proper exercises.

Tennis: Learn proper overhead and stroke technique.

　　Avoid tendinitis and impingement. Respect pain; avoid overuse; use frequent rest breaks. Relax your grip between strokes.

　　Maintain shoulder strength through exercise; be aware of proper posture and positioning of joints.

Cycling: Avoid falling onto an outstretched arm; learn to fall by pulling your arm in and rolling onto your shoulder.

Golf: To avoid golf shoulder injuries, perform conditioning exercises year-round. Learn proper swing and impact.

Elbow/Forearm

Avoid pressure and impact to the elbow

When sitting, do not contact any firm surface with the elbow.

In moving out of bed, use the abdominal muscles to help roll over.

　　When changing body position, do not push off with the elbow against a hard surface.

　　Use elbow pads for protection.

　　Use relaxation techniques focused on the hands and arms to protect the forearm muscles.

　　Recognize and avoid repetitive hand clenching or excessively hard gripping. For nocturnal hand clenching, wear stretch gloves with the seams to the outside.

　　Avoid forced gripping or twisting.

　　Use kitchen aids such as jar openers, enlarged grips on utensils, or power tools.

Take periodic breaks and alternate tasks during manual activities.

Use a light and two-handed grip when shaking hands repeatedly.

Avoid prolonged use of tools requiring twist/force motions.

Hold tools with a relaxed grip. Use foam/plastic pipe insulation (sold at hardware stores) on tool handles.

Take frequent short breaks.

Do not lean directly on elbows; stabilize with the forearms.

Change to a better work position or use elbow pads.

Sports

Use proper grip and play techniques with golf clubs, racquets, bats, or other pieces of sports equipment. For grip problems, consult a pro.

Use elbow protective equipment (hockey, roller-blading, skating).

Use stretch, strengthening, and relaxation exercises to condition the tissues that surround the elbow.

Hand/Wrist

Avoid cumulative movement patterns.

Interrupt repetitive tasks (e.g., typing, peeling vegetables, knitting, playing cards) by short breaks.

Rest the hands flat and open rather than tight-fisted.

Pad the handles on utensils, tools, and the steering wheel with pipe insulation.

Use the stronger, larger joints, especially the shoulders.

Use the palms and forearms to carry heavy objects.

Push, slide, or roll objects instead of lifting them.

Use pencil grips and pad the stapler.

Keep the hands off chairs when arising.

Be aware of hand clenching and wear stretch gloves to bed when nocturnal hand clenching is recognized.

Interrupt lengthy writing sessions by stopping for 1 to 2 minutes every 10 minutes.

Use relaxed grip on tools.

Enlarge the handles of work tools—2¼-inch diameter is optimum for most people.

(continued)

TABLE 3.2 JOINT PROTECTION FOR THE UPPER EXTREMITY (continued)

Texturize handle surfaces to provide an easy hold with less grip.
Bend and straighten (wiggle) your fingers and wrist often.
Wear stretch gloves while driving and at night if hand clenching is a habit.
Grasp objects with the hand and all fingers. Use both hands as much as possible when lifting heavy objects.
Use real tools, not the thumbs, to pinch and push in your daily job activities. Use pliers for hard-to-remove velcro fasteners.
Power tools (screwdriver, drill) are often preferable and easier to use than manual tools.
Avoid uncomfortable hand positions.
Keep hand and wrist extended for work activities. Adapt tools with handles designed so that the wrist is straight.
Use a wrist rest while working on a keyboard.
Use an appropriate tool to hit or move objects.
Fit the handles of vibrating tools with shock absorbers or rubber, or wear gloves with gel inserts.
If joints are painful, wear an appropriate splint for rest and activity.
Consult an occupational therapist about work-induced problems, splintering, and modifying or adapting tools and equipment.

Sports
For racquet sports or golf, use proper grip size. Relax the grip until just before ball impact.
For grip problems, consult a pro.
Use proper grip and play techniques with golf clubs, racquets, and other sports equipment.
Use a bowling ball with five finger holes. Bevel edges of the finger holes.
Golfers with arthritis should try using cushion grips and the baseball grip style (no interlocking fingers).

TABLE 3.3 DIFFERENTIAL DIAGNOSIS OF SHOULDER PAIN

Neurologic disorders	*Rheumatic disorders*
Brachial plexus neuritis	Aseptic necrosis of humeral head
Cervical nerve root compression	Crystal deposition diseases
Herpes zoster	Polymyalgia rheumatica
Nerve entrapment syndromes	Polymyositis
Shoulder-hand syndrome (reflex sympathetic dystrophy)	Rheumatoid arthritis
Spinal cord lesions	
Musculoskeletal disorders	*Referred pain*
Adhesive capsulitis	Heart
Bursitis, tendinitis	Lung
Myofascial pain disorders	Stomach
Fractures and dislocations	Aortic aneurysm
Infection	Gallbladder
Metabolic disorders	Diaphragm
Neoplasia	
Osteoarthritis	
Rotator cuff tear	
Thoracic outlet syndrome	

From Goodman CE, Serebro LH: Sorting out the shoulder syndromes. J Musculoskel Med 1 (June):37–45, 1984.

Pain quality should be considered. Burning pain that exceeds physical findings suggests reflex sympathetic dystrophy (shoulder-hand syndrome).

Personal factors such as attitude are important. Persons with the attitude, "I'm going to finish this task if it kills me!" are prone to tendinitis and recurrence.

Pain and disability attributed to the workplace may actually arise from a variety of factors: underlying congenital malformations, joint laxity, diseases which can predispose to symptoms, joint stresses outside the workplace, or excessive joint movement and loading dur-

ing work (10, 11). Shoulder pain may even result from playing one-armed bandits while on vacation, or from prolonged video game use! (12)

A patient's past history may suggest inflammation of the shoulder resulting from an inflammatory arthritis. Systemic rheumatic diseases, endocrine diseases, neurologic diseases, and cardiovascular disorders may contribute to shoulder pain, and the importance of a thorough knowledge of the patient's medical history is essential.

The shoulder is often the site for referred pain. Paresthesias accompanied by shoulder pain suggests pain referred from the neck or the carpal tunnel. Irritation of the anterior portion of the diaphragm may refer pain to the clavicle or to the front of the shoulder; pain from the posterior diaphragm may refer to the supraspinatus region of the shoulder; pain from the dome of the diaphragm may refer to the acromioclavicular joint area; and irritation of the central portion of the diaphragm may refer pain into both shoulder regions.

The elbow may be involved in systemic rheumatic diseases. It may also be the site of referred pain from the neck, shoulder, or wrist, and elbow pain may occur as a consequence of cumulative movement hand or wrist disorders. The history should include whether neck, shoulder, wrist, or hand position or movement aggravates the elbow problem. Paresthesia and pain suggest a local nerve entrapment arising anywhere in the neck, arm, elbow, or wrist. Refer to Table 3.1 for critical features of the upper limb.

Aggravating factors must be considered whether pain occurs during work, sport, hobby, or at rest (Table 3.2). Work habits, sleep positions, hand clenching while driving, using the elbow to push up from bed or as a prop when reading may contribute to perplexing pain or recurring complaints. Possible factors causing neuropathy (e.g., diabetes, alcoholism) should be elicited.

More than one condition may affect the elbow with comorbidity: Nirschl reported upon a series of 1213 patients with tennis elbow. Of these, 13 patients also had shoulder impingement (tendinitis), eight had a carpal tunnel syndrome, four had cervical or lumbar disc disease, and two had fibromyalgia (13).

Sometimes a soft tissue disorder of the elbow is superimposed upon other arthritis disorders, and relief of the local problem may relieve much of the disability that was attributed to the arthritis.

Soft tissue injury of the hand and wrist may arise from forgotten trauma, from unmentioned cumulative movement disorder outside the workplace, and from repeated exposure to a microwave oven while manipulating food being cooked (14).

Soft tissue inflammation and swelling, with inability to make a fist, can result from systemic inflammatory tenosynovitis of the flexor finger tendons (e.g., rheumatoid arthritis, psoriatic arthritis) before the joints become swollen. Morning stiffness that lasts longer than 30 minutes is an important clue.

Diabetes can lead to contracture of the metacarpophalangeal joints similar to Dupuytren's contracture but without the nodular thickening. A past history of frozen shoulder, carpal tunnel syndrome, or trigger finger should raise suspicion for diabetes.

Unconscious hand clenching may cause recurrent hand pain, weakness, and symptoms suggesting carpal tunnel syndrome. The clenching may occur during sleep or when driving or reading. Caffeine or theophylline intoxication may contribute to hand, jaw, and rectal clenching.

Writer's cramp, dystonia, and psychiatric problems may require a detailed history as described under the appropriate soft tissue heading.

Compression of the median nerve may give rise to variable signs and symptoms. A hand symptom diagram has been reported as a reliable inexpensive technique for diagnosis of carpal tunnel syndrome (Fig. 3.27, below). Pain and paresthesia usually occurs in the distribution of the median nerve but not always. Paresthesias and sensory deficits may involve the entire palmar aspect of the hand because of variable innervation. Onset of pain after several hours of sleep is usual; relief is often attempted by shaking the arm and hand, or elevating the arm. Symptoms may consist of sensory nerve complaints only, motor incoordination, or both. Burning pain suggests reflex sympathetic dystrophy (RSD). Sometimes RSD can occur concomitantly with a carpal tunnel syndrome and other nerve entrapments (15, 16).

Physical examination of the upper limb begins with observing how the patient uses the arm during the history. Specific functions to be observed include taking the coat or shirt off, pushing up from a chair with the arm, arm swing during gait, opening a door, unbuttoning/buttoning, and reaching overhead and behind the head as in combing the hair. Does the patient appear comfortable at rest? Is a tremor present? Are hair and skin color of the shoulder and arm normal? Is muscle mass symmetrical?

The *shoulder examination* is a complex but achievable art. Shoulder function depends on a scapulohumeral rhythm—an unhampered gliding and coordinated motion of humerus and scapula. This in turn depends on an intact shoulder cuff and its components. The sternoclavicular joint is the pivot on which the shoulder girdle moves on the trunk. Observe the patient from the rear during arm abduction and elevation. Observe the smoothness and symmetry of scapular motion. From the frontal view, note the symmetry of the acromioclavicular joints. Are they enlarged or swollen? Shoulder joint effusion is detected by ballottement with two hands, from posterolateral to anterior. Often the biceps tendon sheath will be swollen as well.

Range of motion is carried out with active movement (with the patient moving the arm), and then passive movement is noted (with the examiner moving the arm). Figure 3.1 indicates the normal range of abduction and elevation (0 to 180 degrees), internal and external rotation (45 degrees each). Internal and external rotation refer to the direction of rotation of the humeral head into or away from the glenoid fossa.

The examiner should keep one hand on the suprascapular ridge during passive examination in order to isolate true glenohumeral movement from scapulothoracic movement. Active movement may be restricted by pain; if the patient can be relaxed, sometimes by having the patient press the arm downward during abduction, then passive abduction and elevation can be determined without interference by muscle guarding.

Bursitis and tendinitis may interfere with active but not passive movement. Sometimes tendinitis will result in passive restriction as well, but only in one plane of movement. Adhesive capsulitis restricts both active and passive movement and usually in all planes of movement, except forward elevation.

The *painful arc syndrome* refers to shoulder pain and loss of active movement; when pain occurs between 60 and 100 degrees of active abduction, the problem is usually impingement beneath the acromion; but if it occurs at full elevation, a disorder of the acromioclavicular joint should be suspected.

Careful palpation should be carried out for synovitis, bicipital tenosynovitis, sternoclavicular joint disease, and shoulder joint crepitus. Using just enough force to cause blanching of the nail bed, the examiner searches for pain (trigger) points in the serratus, rhomboid, trapezius, teres minor, and supraspinatus muscles. To examine the medial border of the scapula, the patient should draw the scapula laterally by adducting the arm across the chest. This will expose the subscapularis muscle along the medial border of the scapula, where a pain (trigger) point can be exposed. Assessment for fibromyalgia tender points should also be pursued.

Whenever pain down the arm is present during normal active and passive movement, suspect referred pain. Most common is a trigger point in the infraspinatus muscle that refers pain into the arm (Traveling Salesman's Shoulder) (Figs. 3.2 and 3.3). Palpation of this point causes pain into the "target zone" over the deltoid region and even to the hand. The offending action is repetitive posterior arm motion, such as reaching back into the backseat of a car for a sample case or diaper bag.

Referred pain may be suspected when the physical findings of the shoulder region are normal. When paresthesia is present, the Spurling maneuver (see Chapter 2) should be performed to elicit features of cervical nerve root impingement. The Phalen maneuver for carpal tunnel syndrome may be useful as well (the technique is described below in the section "Carpal Tunnel Syndrome").

Maneuvers for Specific Disorders: The clinician often bases diagnosis on reproduction of pain during the examination or on the presence of tissue swelling. The examination may require some degree of experience. Refer to Plates III–VIII for anatomic detail.

Shoulder subluxation or dislocation usually follows trauma, and the patient feels the humeral head out of place. The dislocation is usually in the direction of the position of the arm at the time of trauma: extension–abduction–external rotation for anterior instability; adduction–forward flexion–internal rotation for posterior instability. Stress testing in these directions is positive in the direction of the instability. Radiographic confirmation is usual but may also demonstrate fracture, erosion, or ectopic calcification (17).

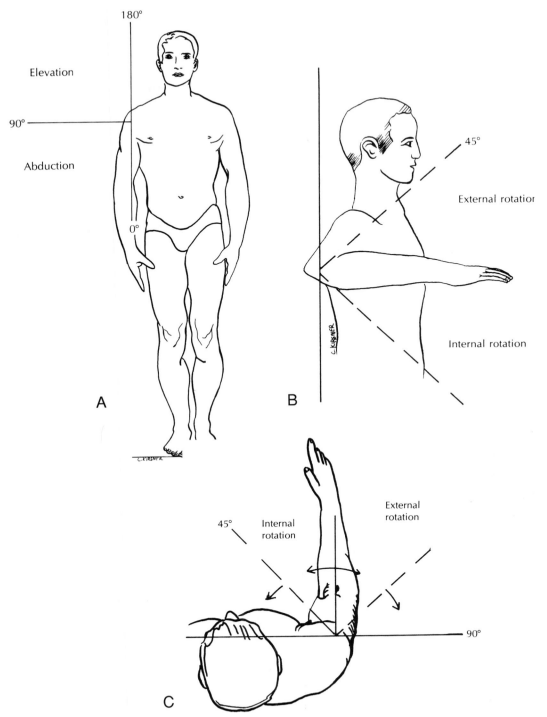

Figure 3.1. A. Active shoulder motion abduction from 0 to 90 degrees. Further raising of the arm (elevation) proceeds from 90 to 180 degrees. **B.** Rotation of the humerus, internally and externally. **C.** Internal and external rotation refer to the direction of movement of the humerus.

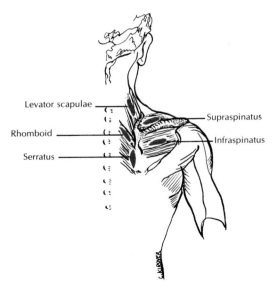

Levator scapulae

Rhomboid

Serratus

Supraspinatus

Infraspinatus

Figure 3.2. While the scapula is drawn laterally by having the patient bring the arm across the chest, palpation in the region of the supraspinatus, infraspinatus, serratus, rhomboideus, and levator scapulae muscles may establish the presence of myofascial pain (trigger) points with reproduction of pain in the "target zone."

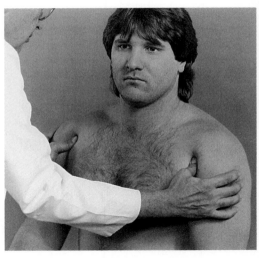

Figure 3.4. Detection of bicipital tendinitis by rolling across the long head of the biceps and comparing one side to the other.

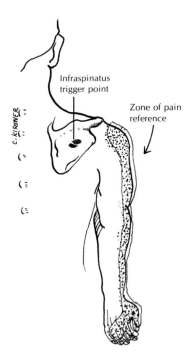

Infraspinatus
trigger point

Zone of pain
reference

Figure 3.3. Infraspinatus pain (trigger) point with target zone radiating from the deltoid region down as far as the hand.

In the throwing or overhead athlete, signs of occult anterior glenohumeral subluxation can be detected by the *apprehension test* and the *relocation test* (18):

Apprehension Test: With the patient supine and the arm in abduction and external rotation, the examiner pushes anteriorly on the posterior aspect of the humeral head. The test is positive if the patient becomes apprehensive, sometimes experiencing pain when previous recurrent dislocations have occurred. When anterior subluxation is present, the patient will experience pain.

The Relocation Test is then performed by administering a posteriorly directed force on the humeral head. The pain will be relieved when the subluxation has been reduced and the patient will then tolerate maximal external rotation of the shoulder (18).

Stress fracture of the acromion is indicated by tenderness over the tip of the acromion, in association with severe pain during active arm abduction.

Tests for the Impingement Syndrome: Begin with palpation of the biceps tendons; palpate both tendons for pain and tenderness (Fig. 3.4). Ask the patient to abduct with the palm down; abduction is usually painful. Impingement occurs between the acromion and the head of

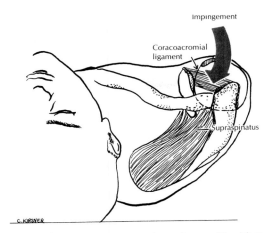

Impingement

Coracoacromial
ligament

Supraspinatus

C. KIRSNER

Figure 3.5. The impingement syndrome. Pinching
the supraspinatus or bicipital tendons between the
head of the humerus and the acromion.

the humerus (Fig. 3.5). The *impingement sign*
is determined as follows: Grasp the patient's
shoulder and stabilize the scapula with one
hand; then, with the other hand, passively
rotate the patient's arm internally and abduct
it slightly forward. Then have patient flex the
arms forward from the shoulder while keeping
the elbow extended and hands supinated (the
palmar aspect turned upward) (19, 20). If pain
is produced, subacromial impingement is
likely (21, 22) (Fig. 3.6).

The test for *Yergason's sign* for *bicipital
tendinitis* is performed by flexing the elbow
and having the patient forcefully supinate the
forearm against resistance (Fig. 3.7).

The *Moseley test* for *shoulder cuff tear* is
performed with active resistive motion in
which the patient abducts and elevates the arm
from 80 to 100 degrees against the examiner's
resistance. Simply have the patient initiate
abduction, then when 80 degrees is
approached, place your hand over the lower
arm and gently bear down as the patient attempts
to further elevate the arm. Often the arm will
drop (21).

Winging of the scapula (neurogenic paralysis of the serratus anterior muscle) may not be
obvious but is readily observed by having the
undraped patient face a wall and press the
outstretched arms to the wall; the involved
scapula projects away from the thorax. Paralysis may result from injury to the long thoracic
nerve or the brachial plexus.

The Elbow Examination: Inspection of the
elbow, active and passive movement, and
palpation will aid in differentiating systemic
disease, arthritis, or soft tissue disturbances.
Palpation may demonstrate swelling of the
tendon of the biceps anteriorly, swelling of the
olecranon bursa, tophi, or rheumatoid nodules
within the bursa. Points of tenderness at the
epicondyles should be compared with the uninvolved elbow.

Physical examination should include all
areas of the elbow for sites of tenderness,
which will be helpful in guiding treatment. The
epicondyles, the forearm flexors and extensors, the radial head during wrist pronation and
supination, and the triceps region during elbow
flexion and extension should be included in the
examination. Test for medial and lateral stability; elbow joint laxity suggests injury to the
anterior oblique portion of the ulnar collateral
ligament (23). The ability to move the elbow
through a full range of motion without difficulty helps to differentiate intraarticular disease
from other nonarticular entities such as olecranon bursitis.

The forearm muscles, approximately 1 to 2
inches distal to the elbow, should be palpated
for cord-like induration. This may provide the
examiner with evidence of a tear or adhesion
within one or more of the forearm tendons.

The presence of bilateral elbow tenderness
or swelling should alert the examiner to systemic diseases including fibromyalgia and rheumatoid arthritis.

Limitation of elbow extension is an important sign of underlying osteoarthritis. Pain on
wrist rotation may result from inflammation of
the annular ligament encircling the head of the
radius. Palpation of the area of the head of the
radius during wrist pronation-supination may
reveal crepitation and tenderness.

The Hand and Wrist Examination: Inspection of the hand and wrist should include hair
growth, skin and palm color, nail changes, and
finger deformity. Palmar or digital contracture
and other signs may signal systemic disease.
Skin tightness, looseness, and presence of telangiectasia are also important features suggesting systemic disorders. (See Anatomic
Plates VI–VIII.)

The normal wrist can flex and extend
approximately 80 degrees respectively from

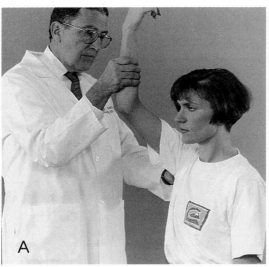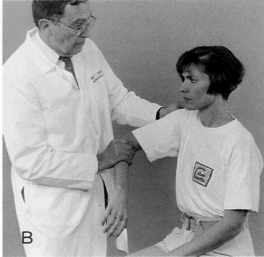

Figure 3.6. A. Test for impingement syndrome. Note arm is internally rotated at maximum elevation. **B.** Similar maneuver using compression of the greater tuberosity against the acromion.

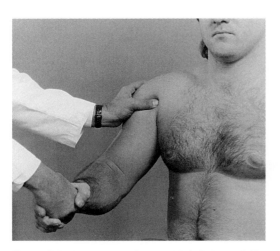

Figure 3.7. Yergason's sign for bicipital tendinitis. Patient forcefully turns the palmar aspect of the hand upward (supination) while the elbow is held in a flexed position. Supination is performed against the examiner's resistance. Pain is produced if bicipital tendinitis is present.

the horizontal. Ulnar wrist deviation is approximately twice the capability of radial wrist deviation (40 degrees versus 20 degrees, respectively). Finger flexion should be tested by having the patient bend the distal phalanx to approximate the proximal phalanx. Flexor tendon sheath swelling or true joint arthritis may cause limitation of flexion of proximal interphalangeal (PIP) or distal interphalangeal (DIP)

finger joints. Thumb abduction should approximate 80 to 90 degrees from a line drawn proximally along the index finger. Thumb adduction should reach to the base of the little finger. Flattening or atrophy of the thenar eminence should be noted (suggesting carpal tunnel syndrome with median nerve compression). Wasting of the interossei with "valleys" between the extensor tendons on the back of the hand may suggest ulnar nerve dysfunction. The metacarpophalangeal (MCP) collateral ligaments are tested for stability with the finger flexed to 90 degrees at the MCP joint. This tightens the collateral ligaments and allows little passive lateral finger motion (Fig. 3.8). Dorsal-volar motion of the wrist should be tested. The examiner attempts to move the patient's hand up and down within the horizontal plane of the patient's wrist. Wrist and PIP laxity may suggest the *hypermobility syndrome*. Joint laxity can be further determined by having the patient's thumb drawn into apposition to the forearm (Fig. 3.9).

MUSCULOTENDINOUS SHOULDER ROTATOR CUFF DISORDERS

Because of the tenuous vascular supply of the shoulder cuff and the restricted area within the coracoacromial arch, repetitive movement is a

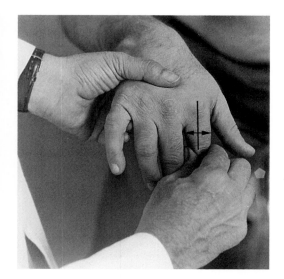

Figure 3.8. Metacarpophalangeal (MCP) collateral ligament stability test. The finger is flexed to 90 degrees at the MCP joint in order to tighten the collateral ligament. Normally, lateral finger motion is minimal in this position.

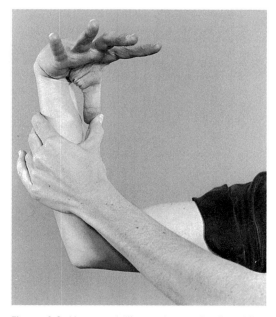

Figure 3.9. Hypermobility syndrome. Laxity of the wrist allows approximation of the thumb to the patient's ipsilateral forearm.

significant cause for upper limb shoulder disability. In addition, the use of exercise equipment, aging, longer work days (and more of them) in factories, upper limb disorders now rank second only to low back disorders in disability costs.

The musculotendinous rotator cuff portion of the shoulder capsule is the conjoint tendon of the supraspinatus, infraspinatus, and teres minor muscles, which insert onto the greater tuberosity, and the subscapularis, which inserts onto the lesser tuberosity (see Anatomic Plates IV and V). Injury generally occurs in young patients after a severe injury; in 40–60-year-olds after cumulative movements; and in seniors without any injury history. Seniors who use the upper limb to push off when arising from sitting are more prone to shoulder problems.

Calcific tendinitis, diabetes, and use of phenobarbital may affect the rotator cuff and lead to a frozen shoulder. More importantly, partial or complete tear of the rotator cuff may occur.

The Impingement Syndrome of the Shoulder

Impingement of the supraspinatus tendon and the biceps tendon and secondary involvement of the subdeltoid and subcoracoid bursae occur frequently. The site of injury often is against the coracoacromial arch, an unyielding structure consisting of the coracoid anteriorly, the strong coracoacromial ligament between the coracoid and the anterior leading edge of the acromion, and the acromion itself. Variation in size and shape of the acromion may contribute to impingement. The impingement may result from anatomic narrowing of the subacromial-subcoracoid interval or by an increase in the volume of the contents of this space (24). Using MRI measurement of the bony structures of the subacromial space, Sperner (24a) noted a significant difference in the space, with smallness noted in 25 patients with impingement syndrome when compared to age- and sex-matched controls. Neurovascular entrapment can also occur at this site (25).

During overhead arm elevation the tendon of the long head of the biceps and the supraspinatus muscle may become injured by the coracoacromial ligament and the anterior part of the acromion (Fig. 3.5). Shoulder instability allows an upward migration of the humeral head against the coracoacromial arch.

Most instances of bicipital tendinitis and supraspinatus tendinitis result from an associated impingement disorder. The biceps tendon aids in shoulder stabilization. Similarly, the supraspinatus muscle augments glenohumeral joint stability (26, 27). During action consisting of elbow flexion and supination, the biceps tendon does not slide in the intertubercular groove; rather, the humerus slides along the fixed biceps tendon, decreasing the intraarticular length of the tendon as the arm elevates. The loose-jointed athlete is more predisposed to an impingement disorder.

Presentation: The patient complains of painful motion of the shoulder in an arc from 60 to 75 degrees of abduction. Forward motion is generally unimpaired. Night pain is common. Pain is distributed generally throughout the shoulder region, often more anterior, and may vary from day to day or become constant. When the dominant involvement is biceps tendinitis or supraspinatus tendinitis, pain may be more anterior in the former, and more lateral in the latter.

Neurovascular entrapment has the added features of paresthesia and a sensation of swelling in the lower anterior arm and sometimes into the medial epicondyle area.

The *impingement sign* and other tests for impingement were described earlier (Fig. 3.6). Passive shoulder motion can usually demonstrate full normal range of motion. If restriction occurs in more than one plane, capsulitis or frozen shoulder is likely. Acute pain may restrict active but not passive motion.

Inability to elevate the abducted arm beyond 90 degrees despite normal passive arm elevation suggests a shoulder cuff tear, which can result from chronic impingement. Pain relief after injection of a local anesthetic beneath the acromion is a helpful diagnostic sign also (28) (Fig. 3.10).

Relationship of Tendinitis and Impingement Syndrome: Most instances of bicipital tendinitis are secondary to impingement. On the other hand, supraspinatus tendinitis may result from calcium apatite deposition disease, in which radiographic evidence of calcific tendinitis appears (29) (Fig. 3.11). Non-insulin dependent diabetes may predispose to calcific tendinitis (30). Acute bursitis may result from either

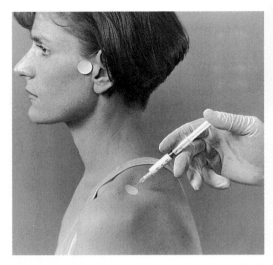

Figure 3.10. Having located the site of tendinitis beneath the acromioclavicular joint, a short No. 23 needle is threaded into the supraspinatus tendon and a corticosteroid–anesthetic mixture administered.

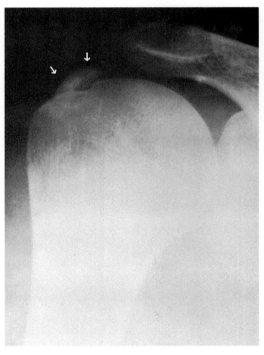

Figure 3.11. Calcification in the region of the subacromioclavicular bursa as noted by the arrows. (From the ACR Clinical Slide Collection, 1972. Used by permission of the Arthritis Foundation.)

impingement or from adjacent supraspinatus tendinitis.

Etiology: Biochemical, structural, and traumatic disturbances contribute to soft tissue shoulder disorders. Calcific tendinitis is not usually found in persons with an impingement syndrome. By age 40 to 50, degeneration of the shoulder cuff is usually present. Ischemic degenerative disruption of the shoulder cuff is common in the elderly, and small cuff tears are usual in the very old (31).

Pathologically, the impingement syndrome has been classified as follows:

Stage I: Edema and hemorrhage
Stage II: Fibrosis and tendinitis
Stage III: Tendon degeneration, bony changes, and tendon rupture (28)

Tendinopathies

Isolated *bicipital tendinitis* can occur. Pain is noted in the anterior shoulder and over the coracoacromial ligament. Either or both the long and short heads of the biceps may be affected. Impingement of the biceps in sports is common—for example, during the serve and overhead strokes of tennis, and in the follow-through stages of a golf swing. A painful catching sensation may occur and may be relieved by internal rotation of the shoulder, which clears the biceps tendon from under the coracoacromial arch (32). Biceps tendon instability can occur in youth during participation in throwing sports, or in the elderly as a result of a cuff tear. Palpation may reveal swelling of the biceps tendon sheath. Figure 3.4 illustrates a thumb-rolling method for examining the biceps tendon. Tenderness is often exquisite and the swollen sheath is palpable. Yergason's sign for bicipital tendinitis was described earlier (Fig. 3.7).

Biceps tendon rupture may result from a fall on the shoulder, following repeated corticosteroid injections of the biceps tenosynovium, abrupt pulling as when a lawn mower is recalcitrant and will not start. Visible swelling of the rolled up biceps' muscle belly is usually evident in the distal third of the arm. Usually, in the older person, the tear is partial, not complete, and treatment is not indicated.

Supraspinatus tendinitis may occur from carrying a heavy load, from impingement, or

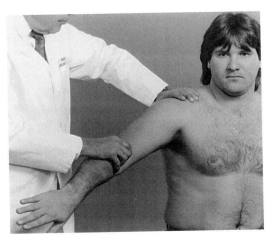

Figure 3.12. Examination of the supraspinatus muscle. With the arm held in 90 degrees of abduction and horizontally, rotate the arm into full internal rotation so that the back of the hand is rotated upward, then forward. Increased pain perception indicates impingement.

from metabolic derangement with calcification. The calcification may not be symptomatic and does not correlate with treatment outcome. Calcific tendinitis is usually acute in onset with pain lasting a few days until the calcium ruptures into the subacromial bursa. Pain is severe, constant, and immobilizing. *Dawbarn's sign* is present when tenderness is felt over the greater tuberosity while the arm is hanging down but not when the arm is abducted. Another technique for testing the supraspinatus tendon is performed with the arm held in 90 degrees of abduction and horizontally, then rotated into full internal rotation so that the back of the hand is rotated upward, then forward (33) (Fig. 3.12). The scapular rhythm may be altered due to muscle splinting. This results in a shrugging type motion of the shoulder.

Bursitis of the Shoulder

Subacromial bursitis may be acute or chronic and usually results from a preceding supraspinatus tendinitis. It can follow injury to other portions of the rotator cuff as well as cuff tear. The tear may involve the floor of the bursa with a buildup of pressure by synovial fluid (22). Pain is frequently referred to the insertion of the deltoid muscle at the junction of the upper third and middle third of the arm. Pain is present day and night and is aggravated by active abduction of the arm. Often the trauma is cumulative such as from carrying a heavy briefcase or performing a repetitive movement as when washing windows.

Subcoracoid bursitis produces pain over the coracoid process and medial shoulder. Swelling is rarely palpable; exquisite tenderness of the coracoid is usual. The bursa lies between the coracoid process and the joint capsule; it becomes irritated by pressure from the coracoid process against the head of the humerus during excessive arm movement.

Physical findings during an attack of bursitis depend on getting the patient to relax and allow the examiner to test passive shoulder movement. Subacromial bursitis restricts passive shoulder movement in abduction only. The tip of the shoulder is often tender, and tenderness just medial to the acromioclavicular joint suggests the presence of supraspinatus tendinitis. Subcoracoid bursitis may cause restricted forward arm elevation and arm adduction. Tenderness on the coracoid process is usually present. Treatment is described under ''Management.''

Shoulder Cuff Tear

Onset and etiology vary with age. Young persons rarely suffer a cuff tear unless the shoulder has had significant trauma. In the athlete, the cumulative movement of the arm in overhead sports, swimming, or in performing push-ups may further compromise the already tenuous vascularity of the supraspinatus muscle and tendons, leading to rupture (26). In addition, joint laxity may allow further impingement, also leading to rupture. In the elderly, the deficient vascularity may contribute to spontaneous rupture. In all patients with cuff tear, the shoulder performs elevation poorly. Pain is variable and probably depends on the degree of bursitis or tendinitis present at the time of rupture. The Moseley test (described earlier) is helpful when positive.

Laboratory and Imaging Procedures

In most patients who have no evidence of cuff tear and who are not engaged in sport activity, treatment should precede invasive or expensive tests. Only when treatment has failed can expensive intervention be justified. Furthermore, imaging probably should be considered *only if the diagnosis is in doubt, or if the patient has features indicating need for surgery, and the patient is likely to go forward with invasive treatment* (Table 3.4).

If limitation of shoulder movement in passive examination is evident, and polymyalgia or other inflammatory disease is suspected, a Westergren sedimentation rate and radiologic examination are appropriate.

If night pain persists after 7 to 10 days of treatment, a chest radiograph and blood chemistry tests are warranted.

Imaging of the Upper Limb in Cumulative Movement Disorders (Including Arthroscopy)

Although magnetic resonance imaging (MRI), computed tomography (CT), arthrography, ultrasonography, and arthroscopy have become commonplace in the past decade, these procedures, like electromyography, yield results that depend on the operator's skill and experience. The choice and timing of a procedure will depend upon the clinical impression, response to past treatment, potential duration of disability, cost, and availability of an experienced operator of the procedure; the skill of those in the community performing the procedure will be a major determinant (7). The finding of cuff tear does not imply causality of symptoms. Shoulder cuff tear occurs in asymptomatic persons of all ages, but increasingly in the elderly (34). In one study 54% of asymptomatic persons over the age of 60 (25 of 46 subjects) had rotator cuff tears on MRI; 13 of them had full-thickness tears (35).

If repeated episodes of shoulder dysfunction have occurred, radiologic examination should be performed with calcific tendinitis in mind (Fig. 3.11). If a calcium deposit is greater than 1.5 cm in diameter, irrigation of the bursa using a No. 15 needle is often helpful.

If axillary pain is present, chest radiographs with lateral views for the mediastinum are indicated, as tumor and other mediastinal lesions may refer pain to the axilla.

In patients in whom stage II impingement lesions are suspected and who must perform repetitive shoulder movement, anteroposterior

TABLE 3.4 DECISION CHART: UPPER LIMB

Problem	Action	Other Actions
A. Shoulder—Not acute, unilateral Use-related Tenderness + + B. Frozen Shoulder Diffuse, dull, episodic pain Aggravates sleep Motion limited actively and passively in all planes C. Tennis Elbow No visible swelling Pain with use/grip No numbness/tingling	Physical examination Conservative care Assess how activities at work and home/play are done Advise regarding correction of aggravating factors Exercise Medications—NSAIDs, ASA, acetaminophen Elbow—splint/rest initially, then exercise Local injection of crystalline steroid and local anesthetic mixture Vapocollant spray, use of ice Instructions to avoid reinjury	If conservative care not effective, reexamine patient, order roetgenograms, arthroscopy, test for inflammation For shoulder—consider arthrogram, MRI Examine for cervical disease Consult physical therapist Surgical consultation after at least 6 months no resolution, or consider arthrogram and pressure injection
D. Tendinitis 1. Shoulder—Unilateral Motion impaired in one plane only 2. Shoulder—Symmetrical or capsulitis Morning stiffness Little rest pain Palpable tendinitis or limited motion bilaterally	→ Oral or intralesional antiinflammatory Rx first Also begin workup for inflammatory rheumatic disease	CONSULTATION Rheumatologist Orthopaedist Physiatrist
3. Elbow No visible swelling Local tenderness Pain with finger motion against resistance	→ Splint/rest Oral or intralesional antiinflammatory Rx first	} Orthopaedic consultation
E. Bursitis 1. Shoulder—acute Constant severe pain Marked guarding to passive motion	→ Oral or intralesional antiinflammatory Rx first	
2. Elbow—visible swelling No joint limitation With or without warmth/ redness No skin penetration by injury	→ Immediate aspiration Examine fluid for Gram stain/ culture, sugar content, WBC, and diff/crystals	
F. Nerve Entrapment—Elbow Pain on finger extension or wrist supination Numbness/tingling Weakness of grip	→ Inject site of entrapment with crystalline steroid and local anesthetic mixture Rest	→ Surgical consultation
G. Disorders: Wrist and Hand 1. Pain and dysfunction: Thumb Trigger thumb de Quervain's disease Writer's cramp 2. Pain and dysfunction: Finger Collateral ligament callus Trigger finger 3. Pain, paresthesia, dysfunction Thoracic outlet syndrome Carpal tunnel syndrome Reflex dystrophy 4. Hypermobility syndrome; Dupuytren's contracture	Physical examination Conservative Care Assess how activities at work and home/play are done Advise regarding correction of aggravating factors Advise regarding splinting and joint protection Exercise, including stretching Tendon sheath or local injection of steroid and local anesthetic mixture Exercise Electrodiagnostic studies in selected cases Medications—NSAIDs Consider workup for inflammatory rheumatic disease if bilateral	Occupational therapist consultation Radiologic examination Tests for systemic rheumatic disease Orthopaedic or hand surgery consultation Rheumatology consultation Other appropriate consultation ↓

(continued)

TABLE 3.4 DECISION CHART: UPPER LIMB *(continued)*

Problem	Action	Other Actions

H. Danger List
    Swelling, warmth, fever, chills
    Numbness or tingling
    Aggravated neck movement
    Referred from elsewhere
    Axillary pain
    Erythema, cyanosis
    Nailfold infarcts
	→ Take immediate appropriate action to investigate serious local or systemic disease processes	→ CONSULTATION
		Rheumatologist
		Orthopaedist
		Physiatrist

roentgenographic views in neutral and internal rotation, axillary view, transscapular and supraspinatus outlet view of the shoulder should be obtained (36). Findings may include osteopenia or patchy cysts of the head of the humerus in the presence of supraspinatus tendinitis. *Cuff tear arthropathy* occurs when a massive capsule tear results in superior displacement of the humeral head, disuse atrophy and osteoporosis of the shoulder, and collapse of the proximal aspect of the humeral articular surface (37).

In older patients roentgenographic findings may demonstrate osteoarthritis of the glenohumeral joint or malignancy with loss of the distal end of the clavicle.

The acromioclavicular joint should be examined with oblique and tangential views, and tangential views of the bicipital sulcus should be obtained, when indicated, for persistent symptoms and signs of impingement of the biceps tendon (38). The presence of a spur either beneath the acromion or projecting from the acromioclavicular joint is not a contraindication to conservative treatment, and the presence of a spur is not predictive of outcome. On the other hand, severe osteoarthritis of the acromioclavicular joint is likely to require debridement.

Further imaging and/or arthroscopy is often indicated, in which case cost, invasiveness, and availability of a skilled operator must be considered. Diagnostic ultrasound is safe, noninvasive, less expensive, but highly dependent upon operator skill.

Findings on ultrasonographic evaluation of impingement disorders compared with findings at surgery in 102 patients revealed an overall sensitivity of 81% and specificity of 95%, but were less reliable in stage I and II lesions than in full-thickness tears (39).

Magnetic resonance imaging findings were reported in 80 patients who had subsequent shoulder surgery, in 13 asymptomatic subjects, and in six cadavers; the study revealed accurate diagnosis on the basis of marked contour abnormality and associated secondary findings on T2-weighted images. In some cases with intraoperative arthrograms, retracted tendons were concealed by intact synovial or bursal layers giving rise to a false-negative arthrogram. Overall, MRI with T2-weighted images are highly specific for full-thickness rotator cuff tears, and often demonstrate associated tendinitis and bursitis. MRI is indicated after conservative treatment has failed and can provide indications for appropriate surgery (40). In tendinitis (stage II impingement) MRI, using oblique coronal and axial views, allows complete evaluation of the tendon and the rotator cuff. For stage I and II impingement, Iannotti reported MRI sensitivity of 82% and specificity of 85% (41). When compared with arthrography (also invasive) MRI revealed abnormality in all full-thickness cuff tears discovered by arthrography, but arthrography missed a cuff tear in six patients in whom MRI was positive (42).

Ultrasound and arthrography were compared against surgical findings in 32 patients reported by Misamore and Woodward (43). Arthrography was correct in 87% but ultrasound in only 37% of patients. Incomplete tears are not readily apparent with ultrasound examination.

Arthroscopy allows gradation of the tendinitis, and with the use of a probe, the intertubercular portion of the tendon can be visualized. In 95% of cases, biceps tendinitis is seen as secondary to a primary impingement syndrome (44).

Management of Shoulder Disorders

- Performing a good history and examination is cost-effective and should exclude referred sources of pain.
- Provide the patient with an explanation of the problem, recognize aggravating factors for shoulder dysfunction, and discuss methods to avoid the aggravating habits. If necessary, refer the patient to a physical or occupational therapist, sports medicine specialist, or athletic trainer. (Review Tables 3.1 and 3.2.)
- Those patients without significant disability should receive conservative (noninvasive) treatment. All patients should be instructed in simple range-of-motion (ROM) exercises, particularly the Pendulum Exercise (Exercise 3.A). Many older patients with features suggestive of cuff tear will improve and recover, although slowly. Stretch tight tissues before initiating strengthening exercises; stretching and strengthening activities should be selected and sequenced so that muscles are not overstretched before strengthening can occur.
- To avoid reinjury: provide joint protection principles as detailed in Table 3.2. Some of the more commonsensical suggestions are to: restrict overhead use; avoid carrying heavy objects; avoid using the arm to assist arising from chairs (keep hands forward on thighs; sit on a higher stool if necessary); avoid repetitive chores, pacing such activities by rotating several chores, each for brief intervals.
- Provide pain relief as needed. Use local treatment with ice applications for 10 minutes several times a day and after workouts. Soft freeze packs are inexpensive and widely available. A package of frozen vegetables wrapped in a moist cloth provides a convenient cold pack. Ice massage should be used 4–5 minutes or for 1 minute after a burning sensation is achieved.

Nonsteroidal antiinflammatory drugs (NSAIDs) should be tried when stiffness and pain are present; these agents are used for at least several weeks. NSAIDs are moderately contraindicated in the elderly, in diabetics, in the presence of renal or hepatic diseases, and concomitantly with diuretics or anticoagulants.

Intralesional injection of a short-acting local anesthetic and a crystalline depository corticosteroid can provide rapid relief of pain and disability. When these are administered, heavy or repetitive arm use is contraindicated for at least 2 weeks. In patients with normal movement, the corticosteroid-anesthetic mixture provides pain relief in up to 90% of patients (30, 45–48). When compared to NSAIDs, injection has been found to be more helpful. Adebajo, Nash, and Hazleman (49) reported on 60 patients given placebo, diclofenac, or injection. In this double-blind study both interventions were better than placebo, but the triamcinolone and lidocaine hydrochloride subacromial bursa injections provided 50% more benefit. Similar findings were reported in a comparison of intralesional triamcinolone with naproxen (50). Intralesional injection may be better and cheaper than physiotherapy alone or in combination (51).

The importance of accurate diagnostic assessment before injection is stressed in a prospective study by Hollingworth et al. (52). In this randomized and double-blind study in 77 patients with local shoulder pain that could be reproduced on examination, the authors localized the individual tendon involvement by selective tissue tension using resisted active arm movements. Patients were randomly allocated into two groups, both of which received 80 mg methylprednisolone acetate mixed with a local anesthetic. One group received the injection into a specific anatomic area (tendon sheath, bursa, or joint space). The other group had a pain (trigger) point injection, in which the most tender point which reproduced pain was identified by deep palpation and then injected. After 1 week, 20% of the tender point injection group improved, whereas 60% of the anatomic injection site patients improved. A crossover was carried out for those still in pain. Overall, 12 of 63 tender point injections were successful, whereas 41 of 69 injections into more specific sites were successful (48).

Shoulder cuff injection requires selection of a crystalline steroid, either triamcinolone hexacetonide or methylprednisolone acetate, to be injected into the involved tissues. These include the supraspinatus tendon region, the

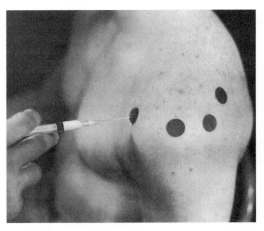

Figure 3.13. The four points for injection of the frozen shoulder. Using a suspension of a corticosteroid and local anesthetic, equal aliquots are injected into the supraspinatus tendon region, the subacromial bursa, the bicipital tendon sheath, and the joint capsule posteriorly. The latter site may be utilized also to inject the shoulder articulation.

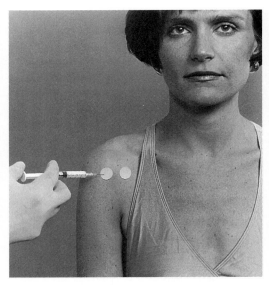

Figure 3.14. In performing injection for biceps tendinitis, the needle should be directed parallel to the tendon after puncturing the skin. If both the long and the short head of the biceps muscle are tender, both may be injected.

subacromial bursa, the biceps tendon sheath, and the shoulder capsule (Fig. 3.13).

Technique: Strict attention to injection principles is essential (see Appendix C). After preparation with surgical soap or povidone-iodine and alcohol, use gloves, and in a 3 mL syringe draw up a maximum of 20 to 40 mg methylprednisolone or equivalent steroid mixed with 1% lidocaine hydrochloride. A macroscopic flocculate occurs, thus further impeding absorption from the injection site. For the shoulder, a 1.5 or 2-inch No. 23 or No. 22 needle can be used. The sites for injection are:

- *Subacromial bursa:* Approached from the side. Find the distal end of the acromion and insert the needle just beneath this site. The usual depth is ½ to 1 inch. The bursa may also be approached posteriorly just proximal to the tip of the shoulder.
- *Subcoracoid bursa and coracoacromial arch:* Locate the coracoid process below the acromioclavicular joint. Insert the needle slowly, first above the coracoid process and then below it; take care not to inject the neurovascular bundle (Fig. 3.10).
- *Bicipital tenosynovium:* Can be located by careful palpation. The needle should be inserted parallel to the tendon. Both the long and short heads should be injected. Once the skin is penetrated about 2 inches

below the tendon insertion, the needle is directed upward and inward; inject as the needle is withdrawn, but keep the needle deep enough to reinsert it medially along the short head of the muscle to complete the injection (Fig. 3.14).

- *Intraarticular injection:* Best approached from a posterior site about 2 inches medial to the lateral shoulder, and below the outer end of the scapular spine. The needle should be advanced slowly and should slip into the valley between the head of the humerus and the glenoid fossa.

The shoulder should not be reinjected for 3 to 6 weeks, and only rarely are more than two injections required. Following the injection the patient should move the arm slowly in a small circle while bending forward and with the arm extended downward and forward (Exercise 3.A[b]). After a minute or so, the patient may try abduction and elevation; often pain is dramatically improved. Delay the exercise for a day after injection, however, in order to avoid injury and cause dispersal of the corticosteroid.

If the injection is successful and pain relief is achieved, the patient should initiate progressive range-of-motion and strengthening exer-

TABLE 3.5 UPPER LIMB EXERCISES

Condition	Exercise	Exercise Number
Impingement syndrome	Pendulum	3.A(a,b)
	Wand	3.B(a–d)
	Theraband Strengthening	3.D
	Self-Mobilization	3.I(a–d)
	Isometric Shoulder Strengthening	3.E
Biceps tendinitis	Biceps Stretch	3.L
	Triceps Strengthening	3.M
Bursitis/tendinitis	Pendulum	3.A(a,b)
	Wand	3.B(a–d)
	Wall Climb	3.C
	Theraband Strengthening	3.D
Cuff tear	Pendulum	3.A(a,b)
	Scapular Stretch	3.G
Scapulocostal/scapulothoracic syndrome	Pendulum	3.A(a,b)
	Scapular Stretch	3.G
	Subscapularis Strengthening	3.H
de Quervain's syndrome	Thumb Stretch	3.T
Trigger thumb	Thumb Stretch	3.T
Trigger finger	Finger Flexor Stretch	3.S
Myofascial pain	According to region	
Scapular pain	Scapular Stretch	3.G
	Infraspinatus Strengthening	3.F
	Subscapularis Strengthening	3.H
Upper arm	Triceps Strengthening	3.M
Epicondylitis (medial/lateral)	Forearm Extensor Stretch	3.J
(tennis elbow)	Forearm Flexor Stretch	3.K
	Wrist Extensor Strengthening	3.N
	Wrist Flexor Strengthening	3.O
	Manual Friction Massage	3.Q
Long thoracic nerve entrapment	Infraspinatus Strengthening	3.F
	Subscapularis Strengthening	3.H
Adhesive capsulitis	Pendulum	3.A(a,b)
	Wand	3.B(a–d)
	Wall Climb	3.C
	Theraband Strengthening	3.D
	Isometric Shoulder Strengthening	3.E
	Scapular Stretch	3.G
	Infraspinatus Strengthening	3.F
	Subscapularis Strengthening	3.H
	Self-Mobilization	3.I(a–d)
Carpal tunnel syndrome	Wrist Extensor Strengthening	3.N
	Wrist Flexor Strengthening	3.O
	Volar Carpal Ligament Stretch	3.P(a,b)
Fist clenching	Finger Extensor Strengthening	3.R
	Finger Flexor Stretch	3.S

cises such as the Pendulum, Wand, Theraband Strengthening, Self-Mobilization, and Isometric Strengthening exercises (Table 3.5, Exercises 3.A, 3.B, 3.D, 3.E, and 3.I). These exercises can be taught in the office with demonstration on the unaffected arm and provision of printed instructions with pictures provided in this chapter. Demonstration and brief guided practice are essential in teaching the exercises.

Other Rehabilitation Techniques

For patients with severe functional limitation who fail to respond to office management, additional measures often require an experienced physical therapist. Referral should be made if pain and limited range of motion persist after injection or when function does not return in spite of compliance with treatment recommendations. (*Frozen shoulder* is considered later in this chapter, but these measures should be considered for that disorder also, if office management has failed.)

The following guidelines can aid the physical therapist:

Assessment Procedures: Assessment for the plan of rehabilitation techniques should include measurement of shoulder range of motion and of scapular mobility, strength, and functional performance. Posture, alignment, and quality of movement should be observed in standing and sitting activities, with particular attention to the presence of protective patterns or guarding of the head, neck, or thorax. Excessive or improper trunk movement will often be substituted for a decrease in shoulder reach or strength. Observe scapulohumeral rhythm carefully to detect scapular dysfunction. Neck muscles may be hyperactive in the protective pattern. Breathing patterns should be observed and brought to the patient's attention.

Physical Modalities: Heat and cold modalities can be used for relief of pain and preparation for exercise and can be used in the home. Superficial heat or cold in the form of moist towels is effective. Simple thermal techniques that can be done in the home should be emphasized, but it is important that the patient limit the use to 20 minutes for heat or cool and 4–5 minutes for ice massage.

Physical therapy, under the direction of a licensed therapist, may entail the use of electrotherapeutic modalities such as interferential current, high voltage pulsed current, or microampere stimulation; these can be used for pain relief or as adjuncts to tissue repair for 2–4 weeks, but should be discontinued if benefit is not apparent. These electrotherapeutic modalities should be used in more acute cases and the cost-benefit ratio carefully considered. Ultrasound is often used in bursitis and tendinitis with some documented evidence of efficacy. Iontophoresis, the use of electric current to introduce chemical molecules into the body, and phonophoresis, the use of sound waves to introduce chemical ions to the body, are a means of treatment with medications. These techniques are used sparingly, as proof of efficacy is lacking. Emphasis should be placed on simple heat/cold modalities that the patient can use in the home in conjunction with an exercise program.

Manual Techniques: Manual techniques for treating shoulder dysfunction include massage of varying strokes and techniques, mobilization techniques to improve joint motion, and treatment of pain (trigger) or tender points with pressure and stretching. Shoulder pathology frequently produces associated pain (trigger) or tender points in the scapular or upper arm areas, causing increased discomfort and dysfunction. Impairments of scapular mobility can be addressed with a variety of manual techniques. Vertebral and costal alignment can be addressed with manual traction or muscle contraction techniques. Friction or deep tissue massage is recommended for tendinitis to mobilize tissue layers and improve circulation. Patients can be instructed in many self-treatment techniques for the shoulder area.

Breathing and Movement Reeducation: Shoulder pain and dysfunction often cause improper breathing patterns that should be addressed during the therapeutic process. Breathing techniques can be taught in the physician's or therapist's office or by means of video or audio tape programs. Relaxation and mobility of the thoracic structures are important components of proper breathing and are frequently impaired by shoulder pain. Techniques of movement awareness and education should be used to correct dysfunction in movement patterns. The Feldenkrais method, in which movements are initiated in small and gentle patterns, has many applications to shoulder dysfunction. Proprioceptive neuromuscular function (PNF) strategies, the use of diagonal patterns, is also very helpful in achieving proper and maximal shoulder function.

Exercise: All patients with shoulder dysfunction should be instructed in a program of progressive active and assisted exercise techniques as early as possible. Simple instructions for the Pendulum and Isometric Shoulder Strengthening exercises (Exercises 3.A and 3.E) should be provided in the physician's office. The importance of exercise for shoulder function should be iterated and reiterated by the physician and therapist. Simple exercise aids such as Theraband (Exercise 3.D) can also be provided in office settings. Instructions for the home program should be provided on the first visit, and the patient instructed to begin exercising gradually, several times per day. Range-of-motion and flexibility exercise are best performed several times per day rather than in one long session. In addition, careful attention to patterns of daily activity and function can uncover dysfunctional patterns. The unaffected shoulder can be used as a model to educate the patient about expected ranges, arcs, and functions. During the acute period of any shoulder function, the patient should perform gentle gravity-assisted (Pendulum) exercises and shoulder girdle movements (Scapular Stretch) to preserve humeral and scapular mobility and tissue health (Exercises 3.A, 3.F, 3.G, and 3.H). As acute pain resolves, the patient can progress to Wall Climbs (Exercise 3.C), Wand exercises (Exercise 3.B), mobilization activities (Exercise 3.I), and isometric and gentle resistive movements through partial range in all planes of movement (Exercise 3.E). Resistive activities through full range for strengthening are added only as pain and stability permit (Exercise 3.D). Full range-of-motion and flexibility movements can be done in side-lying positions or with gravity assistance to prevent impingement, or if scapular stabilization is weakened. Shoulder exercises should be done in single planes, combined movements, diagonal planes, and functional patterns. Because so many shoulder functions are done in diagonal planes, proprioceptive neuromuscular function (PNF) strategies are particularly useful (see Chapter 8).

Many aids to exercise can be used in shoulder programs. Devices such as the exercise wand, the pulley setup, therapeutic or Swiss balls, Theraband, and weights can be incorporated in exercise programs to improve performance and interest. Aquatic exercise programs can be designed to use the buoyancy and resistance of the water. The use of floats and paddles provides assistance and resistance in a supported environment (see Chapter 8).

Exercise programs should address specific functional needs of the patient in home and occupational settings. Ergonomic assessment can be helpful in planning for return to work or daily activity.

Outcome and Additional Suggestions

Of patients with these disorders, 90% will obtain satisfactory recovery within 3 to 6 weeks

(22, 28, 32, 53). Richardson reported that the prognosis of musculotendinous rotator cuff disorders correlated with passive range of movement. In nearly all patients in whom there was good passive range of motion of the shoulder at the start of treatment, a good result was seen following injection and exercise (54).

Prolonged immobilization for a tear of the rotator cuff may promote adhesive capsulitis (frozen shoulder). Early use of assisted passive range-of-movement exercise (Pendulum exercise) is the best preventive program. A trial of passive exercises followed by active exercises should be undertaken.

When an acromial spur or acromioclavicular joint arthritis is present, and if conservative measures fail after 6 months or so, then surgical debridement is indicated. Recognition of the source of the impingement by competent imaging or arthroscopy is essential to a good surgical result. Arthroscopy may be used for removal of loose bodies, debridement, and repair of partial-thickness rotator cuff tears. Full-thickness small shoulder cuff tears may also be treated with arthroscopic subacromial decompression and repair (8).

With proper patient selection and technical competence, arthroscopy can be carried out with a complication rate under 1%. Infection, traction neurapraxias, and bleeding are possible complications. Open techniques are still the ''gold standard'' and usually can be accomplished with a low incidence of complications and with a successful outcome.

One technique of reconstructing an irreparable massive rotator cuff tear is a latissimus dorsi transfer as described by Gerber (56, 57). Surgery consists of an acromioplasty including resection of the coracoacromial ligament, excision of the lateral clavicle or beveling of the undersurface of the lateral clavicle when necessary, and latissimus dorsi transfer.

Analysis of anterior acromioplasty failure in 67 cases reported by Ogilvie-Harris et al. (58) revealed diagnostic errors in 27 patients, operative errors in 28 patients, and no determined reason in 12 patients.

When a cuff tear is massive or has occurred in association with severe glenohumeral rheumatoid or osteoarthritis, pain can be managed (in the very elderly as well as in others) with a suprascapular nerve block (59, 60). Others report good results in massive cuff tear with decompression and debridement followed by strengthening exercises (61).

Scapulocostal (Scapulothoracic) Syndrome

The term "Traveling Salesman's Shoulder" links parascapular pain to overuse syndromes of the shoulder. The repetitive use of the stabilizers (serratus anterior, levator scapulae, pectoralis minor, and rhomboid muscles) when repeatedly reaching backward for a sample case in the backseat of the car is a common cause for the syndrome.

Pain and paresthesia over the medial border of the scapula, usually unilateral, occurs insidiously. Sometimes the pain radiates to the neck, upper triceps, deltoid insertion, the chest wall, and paresthesia may extend to the hand.

Physical examination may reveal diminished scapular motion on the involved side. Palpation reveals pain (trigger) points in the rhomboideus, infraspinatus, and subscapularis muscles. (To demonstrate this, the patient must draw the scapula laterally by reaching across the chest, placing the hand on the uninvolved shoulder, and rotating the involved shoulder forward). The pain (trigger) point along the medial scapular border is tender to palpation and reproduces much of the pain (62).

Injection of these points is carried out as follows (Fig. 3.15). Strict attention to injection principles is essential (see Appendix C). Prepare the area with surgical soap or povidone-iodine and alcohol, and apply gloves; then a 3 mL syringe containing a maximum of 20 to 40 mg of steroid is mixed with 1–2 mL 1% lidocaine hydrochloride. A 1 or 1.5-inch No. 23 or No. 25 needle can be used. The needle tip is used as a probe, and each site is injected with about 0.5 mL of the mixture. Often, the tenderness is quite diffuse, and the whole area can be needled. Infrared laser therapy may provide noninvasive relief (63).

In order to prevent recurrences, aggravating habits must be curtailed. Reaching for items stored behind (such as in the backseat), prolonged use of the telephone cradled between the neck and shoulder, or reaching behind for a seat belt are additional aggravating move-

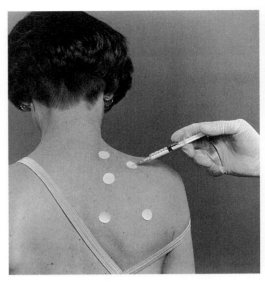

Figure 3.15. The scapular myofascial pain (trigger) points are injected with a nonaqueous steroid-anesthetic mixture.

ments. Refer to Table 3.2 for joint protection principles.

Exercises that mobilize these muscles are helpful (Exercises 3.A, 3.B, 3.D, 3.E, 3.F, 3.G, 3.H). Refer to the previous section on rehabilitation activities for additional treatment options.

Ice massage while stretching may be utilized but requires the assistance of others. A balloon filled with water and then frozen may be utilized for gentle stroking while the patient performs the stretching exercises. NSAIDs are helpful initially, in our experience, but should generally not be used for longer than a few weeks. Intralesional injection of a steroid mixed with a local anesthetic is less costly and more helpful in patients with gastrointestinal sensitivity to NSAIDs. Ultrasound has been advocated in persistent trigger points but is more expensive and requires several visits.

Other Scapular Region Myofascial Pain: Cumulative movement disorders may affect other muscles in this region. The supraspinatus muscle and the long head of the triceps muscle at the site of its attachment to the infraglenoid tubercle of the scapula may be injured by throwing motions. The infraspinatus and teres minor muscles may be injured during racquet sports. The serratus posterior superior muscle at the superior pole of the scapula and the levator scapulae may develop trigger points from recurrent forward trunk flexion during prolonged sitting. Ice massage, physical therapy, and good posture habits should provide improvement (62, 64, 65).

Tennis Elbow

The presentation of epicondylitis or "tennis elbow" can be acute, intermittent, subacute, or chronic; pain occurs at the lateral epicondyle of the elbow during grasping or supination of the wrist. The condition is usually unilateral and more common at the lateral epicondyle; when the medial epicondyle is the site of involvement it is often called "golfer's elbow."

Although usually due to a single factor, a painful elbow can result from gout or rheumatoid arthritis that prolongs tendinitis or bursitis at the elbow, and fibromyalgia may predispose to recurrent elbow pain.

Physical findings include local tenderness at the lateral epicondyle, tenderness along the conjoint extensor tendon about 1 or 2 inches distal to the epicondyle, weak grip, and increased pain when the patient extends the wrist, hand, or individual fingers against resistance. Often the clinician can detect a cord-like, firm band within one of the extensor tendons about two inches distal to the epicondyle. Passive stretching of the forearm extensor muscles (examiner grasps the ipsilateral hand and passively flexes the wrist with the elbow extended) will often produce a sensation of tautness or pulling on the involved side when compared to the uninvolved side. Elbow motion is usually normal.

When the medial epicondyle is involved, the findings include tenderness along the conjoint tendon of the flexor muscles of the forearm and extreme tenderness of the medial epicondyle. Passive stretching of the forearm flexor muscles (examiner grasps the ipsilateral hand and passively extends the wrist with the elbow also extended) will often produce a sensation of tautness or pulling on the involved side when compared to the uninvolved side.

Nirshl includes tendinitis at the insertion of the triceps muscle posteriorly under the term "tennis elbow" because the etiology and pathology are similar. In this location the pain is accentuated by posterior elbow extension against resistance and tenderness is noted along the distal triceps muscle (66).

Etiology includes repetitive movements or high torque strain in work or sport activities. Repetitive wrist turning or hand gripping, tool use, shaking hands, or twisting movements that may exceed tissue capacity. It is an occupational hazard in carpenters, gardeners, dentists, and politicians. Tennis players, particularly novices, suffer tennis elbow often as a result of pressure-grip strain or of backhand shots performed with a "leading elbow" in which the elbow is pointed to the net during racquet impact with the ball. The elbow and shoulder should be parallel to the net. Also, tennis elbow is more common in loose-jointed tennis players (67). Squash players with a "wristy backhand" or who play a lob from the front of the court are at risk for tennis elbow, as are badminton players. Many world class tennis players have suffered from tennis elbow, though most continued to play (68). Another possible cause is unconscious hand clenching, which may occur during sleep, while driving, or when reading.

Repetitive eccentric muscle overload, implicated in these movements, are those in which an applied force causes the muscle to lengthen as it is activated. The resulting higher muscle tension is more likely to produce muscle injury than concentric contractions (69).

Histopathology of tennis elbow includes edema and fibroblast proliferation of the subtendinous space, tendinopathy with hypervascularity, particularly involving the extensor carpi radialis brevis tendon, and spur formation with a sharp longitudinal ridge on the lateral epicondyle. Strain or tear of various portions of the extensor digitorum and extensor carpi radialis brevis muscles is thought to result in these findings (13, 66, 70–76). The inflammatory and vascular pathogenesis is supported by isotopic bone scanning and computerized infrared thermography findings (77).

Differential diagnosis should include cervical nerve root (C6–C7) impingement, posterior interosseous nerve entrapment (below in "Nerve Entrapment" section), degeneration or rupture of the superior segment of the medial collateral ligament (particularly in throwing

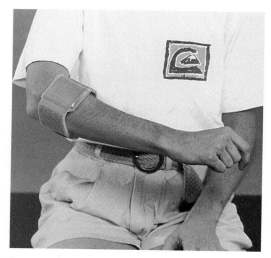

Figure 3.16. The tennis elbow band. The protective influence of a tennis elbow band during arm use is helpful in most patients with tennis elbow. This is one of many available styles.

sports), and ulnar nerve neurapraxia, all of which are uncommon (66). Thoracic outlet syndrome should be considered when the presentation includes bilateral medial epicondylar involvement. Retrograde pain from carpal tunnel syndrome could present as tennis elbow.

Laboratory and radiologic examination are not necessary unless the patient has features of systemic disease or fails to respond to conservative care. Radiologic examination is more important for excluding other factors when medial or posterior elbow symptoms occur or after trauma, if symptoms are severe and chronic, or when surgical treatment is contemplated. Local exostoses over the lateral epicondyle and soft tissue calcifications indicate chronicity; other lesions may be contributing to symptoms including radial-capitellar arthritis or loose bodies (78).

Management must begin with altering abusive elbow use (Table 3.2).

- Various tennis elbow bands and braces are helpful; if nothing more, they can remind the patient of proper elbow joint protection. These supports should provide gentle compression at the lateral epicondyle. The support should be used during any task requiring repetitive gripping and turning movements of the forearm (Fig. 3.16).
- Inflammation may be treated with NSAIDs, including aspirin. When persis-

tent local tenderness is present, local intralesional corticosteroid injections are helpful and with proper use can allow more rapid resolution of tennis elbow. Once the acute tenderness subsides, exercise can restore strength and movement.

- Basic exercise programs for epicondylitis can be selected from the forearm flexor/extensor stretch and wrist extensor/flexor strengthening exercises (Table 3.5, Exercises 3.J, 3.K, 3.N, and 3.O). Refer also to the previous section on rehabilitation activities. Patients whose disorders are function-related should rehabilitate the specific motions involved. For instance, tennis players should practice individual stroke movements, gradually increasing the speed and arc of movement. The motions can be done in an aquatic environment and/or with Theraband providing resistance in the direction opposite the stroke. Return to the actual function should be gradual, carefully monitored, and within the limits imposed by fatigue.
- Injections, when indicated, must be directed to all sites of tenderness, including the area of the tendon and ligament insertion (75). Methylprednisolone may be superior to triamcinolone (79, 80), and both have been found to be far superior to injection with local anesthetic alone in controlled studies (79, 80). The sites for injection can be identified with palpation and marked with the end of a ballpoint pen compressed against each site. The skin is prepared with soap and alcohol. A No. 25 needle is used as a probe, locating each tender site, into which small aliquots of the mixture are injected. We would not use more than 20 mg of methylprednisolone per site. A total of 40 mg of methylprednisolone and 1 mL 1% lidocaine hydrochloride should suffice (Fig. 3.17). After the steroid injection, heavy or repetitive arm use is contraindicated for at least 2 weeks. A postinjection crystal reaction may be seen, which is easily treated with ice packs; relief should be noted within 72 hours. Although longer-term series show no advantage with local injection, factors of overall cost and length of treatment are not reported or consid-

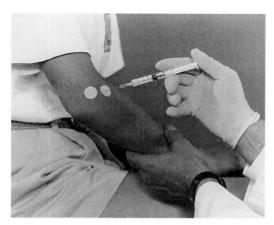

Figure 3.17. Injection of the lateral epicondyle and the band-like soft tissue pain (trigger) point in the extensor tendon for the patient with tennis elbow.

ered. Overall, 90% of patients are relieved with conservative care (13, 67, 70, 75, 81, 82). As soon as possible, an exercise program should begin (Table 3.5, Exercises 3.J, 3.K, 3.N, and 3.O).

Outcome and Additional Suggestions: Reinjection may be necessary in some patients but should not be performed in less than 3 weeks and no more than four injections should be made (82). When conservative office measures fail, referral to a physical therapist for ultrasound and physical therapy (Exercise 3.Q) will often provide relief. Splinting is used only during acute pain; normal use has been shown to be more helpful than further splinting (83).

Over 90% of patients obtain relief from these measures (13, 67, 69). Plaster immobilization is an additional therapeutic modality. Rarely, patients with persistent discomfort will prove to have a cervical nerve root impingement; electrodiagnostic studies should be considered. Fewer than 5% of patients require surgery for chronic recurrent tennis elbow. A "lateral release" of the common origin of the radial extensors is one of the surgical procedures recommended (84).

CUMULATIVE MOVEMENT DISORDERS OF THE WRIST AND HAND

During the past two decades gross physical labor has been replaced by robotics and computers, or at least by less physically challenging tasks. But the trade-off has been at the cost of wrist and hand use in and outside of the workplace. Home computers, the renewed interest in hand crafts, playing of musical instruments, use of video games, gaming devices, and sport activities must all be considered when evaluating a claim for work-related disability. Work elements to consider include posture, motion and repetition, material handling, work organization, and external factors (85).

Host factors of joint laxity, cross-sectional area within the carpal canal, congenital differences in innervation, muscularity, and head, neck, and shoulder positions may also contribute to hand problems. Psychosocial and work organization often are contributory factors but probably are not as important as physical effort (86).

de Quervain's Tenosynovitis

The tendons of the abductor pollicis longus and extensor pollicis brevis traverse a thick fibrous sheath at the radial styloid process. The abductor pollicis brevis often consists of two to four slips at its origin and may be subcompartmentalized, with perhaps greater tendency to suffer from cumulative movement disorder (87, 88). Thickening of the tendon sheath results in stenosis and inflammation.

The patient notes pain during pinch grasping or thumb and wrist movement. Palpation of the tendons in the anatomic "snuff box" area may reveal swelling when compared to the uninvolved side. Tenderness over the radial styloid is common. A positive Finkelstein test (Fig. 3.18), local tenderness and swelling in the vicinity of the radial styloid, is diagnostic (89); pain exacerbated with the Finkelstein test indicates tendinitis rather than osteoarthritis or other disorders.

Etiology: Although repetitive twisting movements are the usual cause, bilateral or unilateral tenosynovitis may accompany pregnancy (90), direct trauma, and systemic diseases such as rheumatoid arthritis and calcium apatite deposition disease.

Differential diagnosis includes osteoarthritis of the first carpometacarpal joint (which could be an innocent bystander, or the true cause for

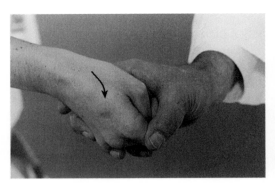

Figure 3.18. The Finkelstein test. The examiner gently rotates the patient's wrist ulnarly (*arrow*) while the patient's fingers are folded over the thumb. de Quervain's tenosynovitis can usually be distinguished from pain arising in the first carpometacarpal joint.

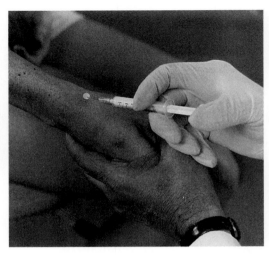

Figure 3.19. Injection of the tendon sheath in a patient with de Quervain's tenosynovitis. Use a No. 23 or No. 25 needle, 0.5 mL (10 mg) crystalline corticosteroid with 1 mL local anesthetic without epinephrine. Inject parallel to tendon.

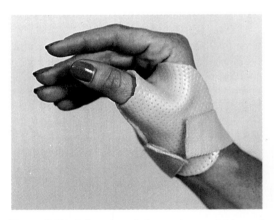

Figure 3.20. A thumb splint may be useful to rest the region of the first carpometacarpal joint for repetitive movement disorders including trigger thumb, de Quervain's tenosynovitis, and osteoarthritis.

symptoms); tendinitis of the wrist extensors (often detected by the presence of crepitation during palpation); and ganglia. Burning pain should suggest radial sensory nerve entrapment in the forearm. Other features of radial sensory nerve entrapment include paresthesia over the dorsum of the hand and a positive Tinel sign over the nerve in the mid-forearm just distal to the brachioradialis muscle belly. Also, forearm hyperpronation will often reproduce the symptoms (91).

Treatment includes wrist protection with a splint and one or two injections of a steroid–local anesthetic mixture into the tendon sheath. Often an adhesion will prevent the flow of the injected material proximally. Forced injection using a 3 mL syringe will often open the sheath and improve the prospects of recovery without operative intervention (Fig. 3.19).

To perform an intralesional injection, prepare the area with soap and alcohol. Draw up to 40 mg of methylprednisolone acetate sterile aqueous suspension (or other equivalent corticosteroid suspension) with 0.5 mL lidocaine hydrochloride 1%. The mixture will flocculate within the syringe. Use a ¾-inch No. 25 needle and direct it parallel to the tendon. The clinician should observe or palpate the proximal tendon sheath as the injection proceeds and note that the sheath distends during the injection. This assures proper placement of the needle. Have the patient apply ice for 10 to 20 minutes after the injection. Up to 90% of patients have improvement with this treatment

and can resume normal activities within 3 weeks, often within the first week. With care, complications are rare (92–97). Recurrence can be prevented with joint protection techniques (Table 3.2). When tendinitis of the thumb region is persistent, splinting and further care can be obtained with referral to an occupational therapist (Fig. 3.20). Also consider having the patient use a quilter's glove in the workplace (Fig. 3.21). If recurrence occurs after two injections, we would recommend surgery.

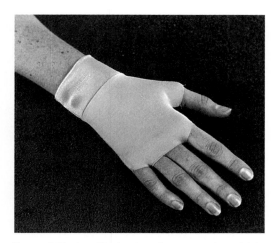

Figure 3.21. A quilter's glove has proved useful for persons who perform repetitive work and suffer from carpal tunnel syndrome, trigger finger, and other soft tissue disorders of the arm, wrist, and hand. They are sold at fabric stores (see Appendix E).

Ultrasound treatment and friction massage (Exercise 3.Q) may be beneficial. A simple thumb tendon stretching exercise (Exercise 3.T) is also helpful. Assessment of shoulder/trunk movement dysfunction may reveal more widespread effects of thumb pain. Correction of pain (trigger) or tender points and movement patterns is appropriate.

Intersection Syndrome

In intersection syndrome, pain and swelling occur at the crossing point of the first dorsal compartment muscles (abductor pollicis longus and extensor pollicis brevis) and the radial wrist extensors (extensor carpi radialis longus and brevis) (98). Peritendinitis crepitans may occur with crepitation palpable about 4 to 6 cm proximal to the radial carpal joint on the dorsal surface of the forearm. The condition is seen in those participating in rowing sports or weight training. Treatment includes splinting, NSAIDs, and local corticosteroid injection. Thumb immobilization may be required in severe cases (99).

Tendinitis about the Wrist and Hand

In addition to the above well-recognized forms of tendinitis, other tendons may be involved in cumulative movement disorders or systemic disease. The features include pain on active movement, local tenderness, and often crepitation during palpation. When the flexor wrist tendons are involved, the presentation may be symptoms of median nerve compression and carpal tunnel syndrome. But the forearm flexor tendinitis may be visible as a swelling proximal to the transverse carpal ligament.

Tenosynovitis may affect the extensor pollicis longus ("drummer boy's palsy"), common digital extensors in the fourth compartment accompanied by dorsal wrist pain, or the extensor digiti minimi. Treatment is similar to that described below under "Trigger Finger" (99).

Trigger Thumb

Snapping or triggering of the thumb can occur in children or adults. The flexor pollicis longus tendon may be compressed against a prominence of the head of the first metacarpal bone or a sesamoid bone. Thickening of the tendon sheath or tenosynovitis may follow repetitive movement or pressure. Tenderness is noted at the base of the thumb in the palmar aspect. Often, a nodule on the tendon can be palpated as it moves during thumb flexion and extension.

Detection and differentiation of a nodule from the normal sesamoid bones at the base of the thumb can be accomplished by having the patient flex and extend the PIP joint of the thumb while the examiner palpates and holds the metacarpophalangeal (MCP) joint straight. With the examiner's index finger palpating the flexor aspect of the MCP joint, the nodule can be felt to move with the tendon.

Trigger thumb and trigger finger are frequently seen in the industrial setting. Treatment and prevention are described under "Trigger Finger."

Bowler's Thumb

Presentation of bowler's thumb includes development of a soft tissue mass at the base of the thumb web and pain and stiffness of the digits that are used during bowling. Treatment lies in removing the cause: the bowling ball holes should be beveled in order to reduce friction (100).

Trigger Finger

Fusiform swelling of the flexor digitorum superficialis tendon over a metacarpal head accompanied by constriction of the tendon sheath results in the locking of a finger in flexion. Often, the patient first notices locking upon arising from sleep. When the bent PIP joint is passively returned to extension a popping sensation is sometimes perceived as the finger is straightened.

The etiology of trigger finger is repetitive movement. The number of movements the tendon performs per unit of time and the degree of clenching during use is important (13, 101–111). In some patients hand clenching can result from stress, from overuse by a compulsive person, or from performing tasks with the attitude, "I'm going to finish this if it kills me!" The "clencher syndrome" includes jaw clenching, hand clenching, and rectal clenching, often at different times but in the same individual. A worker who is a clencher, who drives a long distance to work, and who has a disagreeable supervisor is a likely candidate. Imagine clenching all three areas during the drive to work—by the time you get there, you are worn out! In this condition, it may be easy to blame a repetitive task for sore arms, sore coccyx (referred from the rectal muscles [M Sinaki, personal communication 1989]), and sore neck (referred from the temporomandibular joints).

Other potential causes to consider for recurrent trigger finger or trigger thumb are card playing, hand work, sports, recreational activity, prolonged reading with rapid turning of pages, prolonged horseback riding with a tight grip on the reins, and use of a musical instrument with prolonged practice and perhaps improper technique. Prolonged use of video games played with rapid repetition of action can lead to "arcade arthritis" with features of trigger finger, digital callosities, and arthralgia (12). Direct trauma is a rare cause (112). For additional potential causes (and behaviors to be modified or avoided), refer to Table 3.2 on joint protection.

Other associated disorders may include rheumatoid arthritis with presentation of symmetrical tenosynovitis, degenerative arthritis, Dupuytren's contracture, the "prayer hands" of diabetes, and ochronosis (113–115).

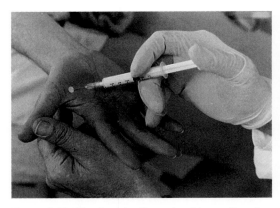

Figure 3.22. Site for injection of a trigger thumb. Use a No. 25 or No. 27 needle, 0.25 mL (10 mg) crystalline corticosteroid with 0.25 mL local anesthetic without epinephrine. Inject parallel to tendon.

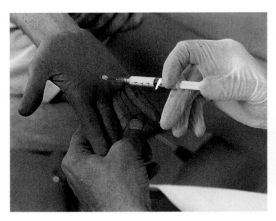

Figure 3.23. Site for injection of a trigger finger. Use a No. 25 or No. 27 needle, 0.25 mL (10 mg) crystalline corticosteroid with 0.25 mL local anesthetic without epinephrine. Inject parallel to tendon.

Differential diagnosis includes slipping of an extensor tendon, particularly in rheumatoid arthritis; a collateral ligament catching on a bony prominence on the side of a metacarpal head; traumatic splitting of the capsule or partial tendon rupture; tendon fibroma; and an abnormal sesamoid catching on a metacarpal head (116, 117).

Treatment for Trigger Finger and Trigger Thumb

- *Intralesional injection* with a local anesthetic and corticosteroid agent can provide prompt relief and the ability to return to work for trigger thumb (Fig. 3.22) or trigger finger (Fig. 3.23). To perform an intralesional injection, prepare area with soap or povidone-iodine and alcohol. Draw up 0.25 mL methylprednisolone acetate sterile aqueous suspension (40 or 80 mg/mL, or other equivalent corticosteroid suspension) with 0.25 mL lidocaine hydrochloride 1%. The mixture will flocculate within the syringe. Use a ¾-inch No. 25 needle and direct it parallel to the tendon. The clinician should observe or palpate the proximal tendon sheath as the injection proceeds and note that the sheath distends during the injection. This assures proper placement of the needle. Have the patient apply ice for 10 to 20 minutes after the injection. With careful administration of treatment, complications, including infection, tendon disruption, and sensitivity reactions, are rare. We have performed thousands of these injections safely.

- *Behavior modification* is foremost in preventive measures and treatment. Refer to Table 3.2 on joint protection.
- Use of an inexpensive *finger splint,* available at many pharmacies, or wrapping the PIP joint with ''Kling'' gauze, may help to remind the patient to protect the hand (118).
- Referral to an occupational therapist for further advice and splinting should be considered for patients with multiple tendon involvement or recurrences, or before referral for surgical intervention. Consider use of a quilter's glove (sold in fabric stores), which provides compression during repetitive movement (Fig. 3.21). Note also the section below on physical training.

Outcome and Other Suggestions

Patel and Bassini (119) compared 6 weeks of splinting trigger fingers (50 patients) with injection of betamethasone and lidocaine hydrochloride (50 patients). Thirty-three (66%) of patients treated with splints and 42 (84%) of those treated by injection were cured with follow-up longer than 1 year. Of the 17 who failed treatment with splinting, 15 were cured by injection. Patients with marked triggering, duration longer than 6 months before treatment, or with multiple involved digits were more likely to need surgery (119).

Whereas splinting, NSAIDs, and other conservative modalities are associated with return to work within 3 to 6 weeks (120), the addition of treatment by intralesional injection will provide pain relief within 4–7 days, and locking will usually cease within 14 days, saving several weeks of medical leave. Up to 90% of patients have a successful outcome with one to three injections (112, 121–126).

The cost and time savings of intralesional injection were compared with surgical results in one nonrandomized study, with results favoring injection. Younger patients and patients who refused injection and underwent surgery were compared to those willing to undergo injection. An average of 4 weeks of medical leave was saved by injection, and morbidity and success rates were comparable (125). In another comparative study, injection of the mixture of corticosteroid and local anesthetic agent had a fourfold greater success rate than that of a local anesthetic alone (127).

Percutaneous use of a No. 19 or No. 21 hypodermic needle to sever the horizontal fibers of the A1 pulley has been described (128); we have no experience in the technique.

Workplace layout and design and ergonomic hand tool design provide improved worker performance and well-being. An experienced occupational therapist, perhaps associated with a hand clinic, could be consulted for advice (129). Keyboard operators who are disabled often have myofascial shortening of muscles with impairment of wrist flexion and dorsiflexion to less than 70 degrees. They may also demonstrate ligamentous hypermobility of finger joints, as well as inefficient keyboard styles. Both the individual's physical characteristics and the workplace ergonomics must be addressed with physical exercise, technique retraining, and education (130).

Physical Training

Physical training for strength and endurance has been suggested for workers exposed to manual handling tasks. One such program, recommended by Peterson (131), is as follows: A weight ranging from 7 to 10 pounds is grasped, with the arm resting upon a table with the wrist hanging over the edge, palm down; the weight is raised as high as possible without lifting the arm from the table (Exercise 3.N). This is performed for 7 to 15 repetitions with increases in the weight and the number of repetitions each week. A second exercise is performed similarly but with palm up; the hand is raised as high as possible with the forearm maintained on a table (Exercise 3.O) (131). However, there are no longitudinal studies of the effect of physical training on physical work capacity. Studies have shown that training reduces absenteeism and employee turnover (132).

NERVE ENTRAPMENT DISORDERS

Features suggestive of nerve entrapment include a triad of pain, paresthesia, and weakness distal to the site of entrapment. Repetitive motion, overstretching, or direct force can result in formation of dense fibrous bands or tenosynovitis that compress a peripheral nerve.

The neurovascular bundle to the upper arm below the clavicle may be impinged within the coracoacromial space; peripheral nerves may become impinged at the elbow, wrist, or along one or more digits.

Impingement within the coracoacromial space was discussed earlier in association with shoulder impingement syndrome. In this condition, in addition to the triad of pain, paresthesia, and weakness, the patient may have the additional complaint of a sensation of swelling of the arm, or fullness within the medial epicondylar region of the elbow. Thoracic outlet syndrome often presents with similar features and should be considered if physical findings in the arm or hand are absent.

A diagnosis of nerve entrapment rests on demonstration and localization of a neuropathy. The techniques necessary for diagnosis are entirely operator dependent. The value and cost-benefit assessment of electrodiagnostic testing, imaging, or surgical exploration must be based on the impairment, not on results of tests. If pain and paresthesia are present without significant functional impairment, we would initiate symptomatic treatment and defer testing for later.

Long Thoracic Nerve Entrapment (Winging of the Scapula)

Arising from the fifth, six, and seventh cervical nerve roots, the long thoracic nerve runs beneath the subscapularis muscle and terminates in the serratus anterior muscle. Paralysis of the muscle is often painless, but the last 30 degrees of overhead arm extension is lost. The scapular rhythm is disrupted, and the scapula may be seen to draw away from the thoracic cage. To demonstrate this, the patient presses the outstretched arms against a wall, the physician observing the scapula from behind the patient. The involved scapula projects from the thorax. Injury to the brachial plexus or long thoracic nerve typically occurs from a direct blow or from compression. The condition is common in army recruits carrying heavy packs, or it may result from injury during a first rib resection for thoracic outlet syndrome (133). Stretching injury to the long thoracic nerve may follow heavy labor. Most such cases resolve spontaneously within 6 to 12 months. Strengthening exercises are recommended (Table 3.5, Exercises 3.F and 3.H).

Suprascapular Nerve Impingement

The suprascapular nerve carries pain fibers from the glenohumeral and acromioclavicular joints, and provides motor supply to the supraspinatus and infraspinatus muscles. Injury occurs from repetitive stretching as the nerve passes through the coracoid scapular notch. Injury may be bilateral, such as when it results from weight lifting exercise (134), or on the dominant side, such as in volleyball players (135). Diffuse shoulder pain is common. Painless paralysis may occur in volleyball players; the injury may not affect the sensory branch of the nerve (135). Atrophy of the supraspinatus and infraspinatus muscles is evident.

Suprascapular nerve compression by masses including ganglion or tumor can be identified by MRI imaging. Fritz et al. reported findings in 26 cases seen within a 12-month period. Five were malignant. MRI had been obtained because of ill-defined shoulder pain (136).

Treatment includes resting the affected arm and corticosteroid injection of the region of the suprascapular notch (137). If pain persists, surgical decompression may be helpful. In one study, 19% recurred postoperatively and reoperation revealed the nerve encased in scar tissue (138).

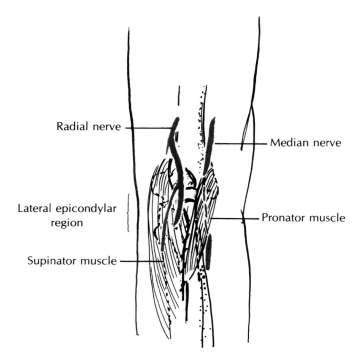

Figure 3.24. Nerve entrapment of the elbow region. The radial tunnel syndrome may result from radial nerve compression in the region of the lateral epicondyle. The pronator syndrome results from median nerve entrapment by the pronator muscle.

High Radial Nerve Palsy

Radial nerve compression in the arm above the elbow can cause weakness of wrist extension, stiffness in the dorsal arm and forearm, and inability to extend the fifth digit. Transient compression has been described in tennis players (139), and may occur from entrapment by the lateral head of the triceps. Electrodiagnostic study reveals denervation of the triceps (140).

Radial Tunnel Syndrome

The radial nerve pierces the lateral muscular septum (Fig. 3.24), where compression may cause pain and tenderness in the area of the lateral epicondyle. Chronic tennis elbow pain is not likely to be the result of radial nerve compression. Other symptoms include sensations of popping, paresthesia, and paresis. Particularly helpful to diagnosis in radial tunnel syndrome are the following:

- Pain reproduced by passive stretching or resisted extension of the middle finger (141)
- Pain reproduced by extreme forearm pronation with wrist flexion (142, 143)
- Pain reproduced by resisted forearm supination with an extended elbow (142, 143)
- Tourniquet test: when a tourniquet is applied above the pain area, pain and paresthesia may result (144)
- Palpation may generate intense tenderness over the posterior interosseous nerve under the proximal edge of the superficial head of the supinator muscle approximately 5 cm distal to the lateral epicondyle (145)
- A Hoffman-Tinel test performed over the radial head may produce tingling along the course of the nerve
- Involvement of the posterior interosseous nerve, a deep branch of the radial nerve, is suggested by the inability to extend the little finger (146)
- Temporary or permanent relief is seen following anesthetic injection

Electrodiagnostic tests are often normal when the compression is intermittent. High radial nerve compression may reveal denervation of the triceps. If the posterior interosseous nerve, a deep branch of the radial nerve, is involved, motor weakness of the extensors of the wrist and fingers may be evident.

Causes for entrapment include congenital anomalous structures, trauma, compression within a fibrous arcade of Frohse (147), compression by the supinator muscle, or against a bony prominence. The posterior interosseus nerve compression may result from forceful supination-pronation tasks or from carrying objects with the elbow fully extended, or from use of a heavy purse.

Most patients recover with rest and gentle exercise. If pain is persistent, and if the site of entrapment is established, surgical exploration is often helpful.

The Pronator Syndrome

Median nerve entrapment by the pronator teres muscle (Fig. 3.24) may result in diffuse arm pain, weakness of wrist pronation, and paresthesias along the median nerve distribution. Pain is reproduced by resistance to pronation of the forearm and flexion of the wrist (144), by a tourniquet test as described above, or by compression of the nerve under the pronator teres muscles for 30 seconds. Rest, injection with a corticosteroid and local anesthetic agent (10–20 mg methylprednisolone acetate and 1 mL 1% lidocaine hydrochloride) often provides relief (148). Surgical decompression is helpful if the disability persists despite these measures and if the site of entrapment is established.

Retrograde paresthesia into the forearm and arm, and even to the shoulder, may be caused by carpal tunnel syndrome (149). Symptoms may be reproduced by tapping over the median nerve at the wrist. Measurement of evoked mixed nerve action potentials may be helpful in diagnosis (150). Refer to the section ''Carpal Tunnel Syndrome'' below.

Lateral Antebrachial Cutaneous Nerve (LACN) Entrapment

Pain and paresthesia from the elbow crease to the thenar eminence, along the radial side of the forearm is the usual presenting complaint.

The etiology is trauma and entrapment occurs within the biceps tendon and the brachialis muscle. Diagnosis is aided by symptom relief after lidocaine hydrochloride injection into the region of the bicipital tendon and the elbow crease. Sensory nerve conduction often confirms the neuropathy. Surgical decompression is recommended (151).

Ulnar Nerve Entrapment at the Forearm (Cubital Tunnel Syndrome; External Compression Syndrome)

Ulnar nerve palsy, pain and paresthesia along the lateral forearm and wrist and 4th and 5th digits, and weakness, can progress to intrinsic muscle atrophy and flexion contracture of these digits. The etiology can be entrapment of the ulnar nerve in the cubital tunnel behind the medial epicondyle. The causes include repeated compression and minor trauma. Using the elbow to arise from bed or chair is a common cause. Compression may occur also from congenital bone abnormality, or from repeated subluxation of the nerve. Also common is retroepicondylar compression or compression by the humeroulnar arcade (144, 152–154). Direct trauma to the nerve is also common.

A positive Hoffman-Tinel test aids location of the site of entrapment. Sensory loss at the ulnar side of the 5th finger is often found. Other tests and maneuvers have limited value. If weakness or other motor signs are absent, local corticosteroid injection along the ulnar groove may be effective. Using a No. 25 ¾-inch needle, inject a mixture of 1 mL lidocaine hydrochloride and steroid (methylprednisolone 20–40 mg) cautiously into the groove, parallel with the nerve. When the needle is inserted ask the patient if there are any sensations of nerve penetration so that the injection is not into the nerve trunk.

If the patient needs to change the manner of getting up in bed, suggest a rope tied to the foot of the bed, carried up over the covers, with a loop on the end so the patient can use this to pull up and avoid pushing with the elbow.

Electrodiagnostic study is valuable if conservative measures fail. If surgery is indicated by disability or signs of weakness, operation should not be delayed. Results are less satisfactory when the condition has persisted for a year or longer (155).

Carpal Tunnel Syndrome (CTS)

The carpal tunnel is a narrow canal rigidly bounded by the carpal bones and roofed by the transverse carpal ligament. It contains nine flexor tendons with tendon sheaths, and the median nerve and adjacent vessels.

Features are variable but usually include pain and paresthesia in the distribution of the median nerve of the hand. Often these complaints awaken the patient several hours after retiring. The patient tries to obtain relief by elevating the arm, shaking the hand, or use of ice or NSAIDs. Motor incoordination is less common but can predominate, in which case the patient has difficulty performing pinch grasping, writing, or holding small utensils. Prolonged use as in writing or working at a handcraft may be followed by unbearable pain. Poor alignment of neck and upper body structures or poor head/neck/upper body posture with forward head and shoulders may accentuate symptoms (see Chapter 2). Because of variable innervation, paresthesia and sensory deficits may involve the entire palmar aspect of the hand. Raynaud's phenomenon may be seen. In severe or prolonged nerve entrapment, thenar flattening usually occurs.

Etiology of CTS includes host factors of tunnel size, local and systemic disease, nutrition, pregnancy, and habits. The pathophysiology includes increased carpal tunnel tissue pressure during exercise when compared with controls (156–158), sometimes as much as 10 times greater than the tissue pressure elsewhere in the upper limb. However, the increased pressure theory is not supported in all studies. Using contrast-injection studies, Cobb et al. demonstrated that the carpal tunnel communicates from the forearm flexor compartment to the palmar compartment and the whole space is an enclosed compartment. Shrinkage of the space in the elderly may occur, allowing nerve compression at lower pressure (159).

Synovial tissue study from 625 operated wrists rarely demonstrated inflammation, indicating that the contribution of tenosynovitis is uncommon (160).

Hand size does not correlate with development of carpal tunnel syndrome (161). Computed tomography has been used to demonstrate a smaller cross-sectional carpal tunnel area in patients than controls (162, 163), although Merhar et al. could not reproduce the difference (164). Magnetic resonance imaging can be used for this determination as well (165).

A Mayo Clinic study of 1016 patients found the following associated conditions: Colles' wrist fracture or other trauma, 13.4%; rheumatoid arthritis and other inflammatory rheumatic disease, 6.5%; menopause, 6.4%; diabetes, 6.1%; osteoarthritis wrist, 5.3%; pregnancy, 4.6%; myxedema, 1.4%; and other medical disorders, 7.3% (166).

Other associated medical conditions include acromegaly, amyloid, hepatic disease, fibromyalgia, or benign local tumors. Peripheral neuropathy can coexist in susceptible patients (diabetics, those who use alcohol excessively, or those who have malabsorption syndromes).

External factors include cumulative movement disorders and acute wrist flexion during resting positions when sleeping, reading, or driving; these occurred in 6% of patients in the Mayo series. Refer to Table 3.2 on joint protection.

Attribution is difficult. Older poultry workers with significant repetitive hand usage had median nerve sensory and motor latencies determined and compared to younger persons seeking employment at the company. No significant differences were detected (167). In other studies, obesity of the workers, age, or oophorectomy (surgical menopause) were personal factors confounding the data, and when these were eliminated from study, the corrected data showed no correlation of work type to nerve compression (168, 169).

Patients who are habitual clenchers (jaw, hand, rectum) and who drive long distances to work are more prone to work-related symptoms, particularly if the workplace is stressful.

Tests for Nerve Compression at the Wrist

Tests for nerve compression at the wrist include the Hoffman-Tinel test (Fig. 3.25) and the Phalen maneuver (Fig. 3.26) (170). Other assessment measures include a hand symptom diagram (Fig. 3.27) (171), compression of the

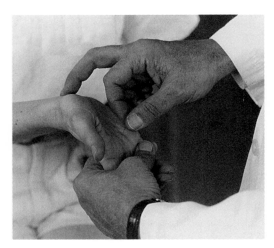

Figure 3.25. The Hoffman-Tinel test. Tapping over a compressed nerve at the wrist reproduces pain and paresthesia, proximal or distal to the site of compression.

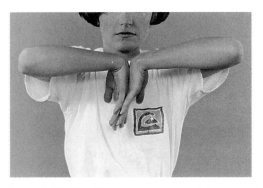

Figure 3.26. The Phalen maneuver. Acute wrist flexion maintained for 30 to 60 seconds reproduces symptoms in patients with nerve compression in the carpal canal (the carpal tunnel syndrome).

carpal tunnel, vibration testing, two-point discrimination, thermography, and nerve conduction measurement.

Because of a quantum leap in the incidence of carpal tunnel syndrome in the workplace in recent years, the methods for diagnosis are being continuously appraised. Each test is useful under specific conditions and is dependent upon operator ability and experience. The following is a review of the value of each technique for diagnosis.

In a study by Katz et al., a hand symptom diagram (Fig. 3.27) proved better than the Phalen and Tinel signs. While the sensitivity was 0.64 and specificity was 0.73, the negative predictive value of an "unlikely" diagram was 0.91 (171, 172).

The Hoffman-Tinel test was found in the Katz study to have a sensitivity of 0.60 and specificity of 0.67 when compared with median nerve conduction latency (172). Kuschner et al. found a positive Hoffman-Tinel test in 45% of normal control subjects (173).

The Phalen maneuver was found in the Katz study to have a sensitivity of 0.75 and a specificity of 0.47 when compared with median nerve latency. Kuschner et al. found a positive Phalen maneuver in 20% of normal control subjects (173).

Sensory testing abnormality is often a late finding (174). In experienced hands, the Semmes-Weinstein monofilaments test and the Weber two-point discrimination test are helpful earlier in the course of CTS (175). An automated tactile tester (ATT, Topical Testing, Inc., Salt Lake City, Utah) was compared with manual testing and with electrodiagnostic study in 61 patients with complaints suggesting carpal tunnel syndrome. When nerve conduction velocity was normal the ATT test was abnormal in 53%, whereas manual testing was abnormal in 28%. When nerve conduction velocity was abnormal the ATT test was abnormal in 82% and the manual testing was abnormal in 51%. In the same study, in a comparison of the ATT test with manual testing in fingers with definite nerve conduction abnormality, the ATT test was also abnormal in 82% and the manual test was abnormal in 51% of cases. Conversely, in the fingers with normal nerve conduction, the ATT test was normal in 53% and the manual study was normal in 28% of cases. The authors also noted that detection of localized warming was a good indicator of sensory abnormality (176).

Electrodiagnosis of carpal tunnel syndrome can be used for diagnosis and for localization of the entrapment. However, a false-negative result can occur in 10% of patients (177–179).

Other screening devices include a vibration threshold measurement device (Vibraton II, Physitemp Instruments Inc., Clifton, New Jersey) (180), and distal motor latency measurement (NervePace electroneurometer, Neurotron Medical, Lawrenceville, New Jersey) (180), but these have a high yield of false-negative values (180). The electroneurometer results were bet-

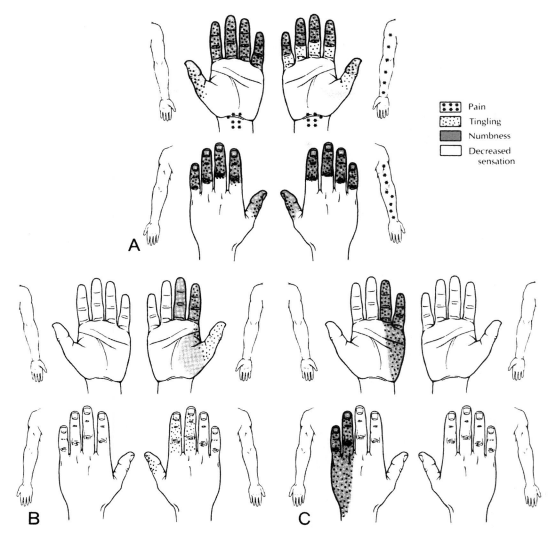

Figure 3.27. Hand symptom diagram for carpal tunnel syndrome (CTS). **A.** Diagram rated classic CTS for both hands; nerve conduction tests confirmed bilateral CTS. **B.** Diagram rated probable because of palmar symptoms; nerve conduction tests revealed right CTS. **C.** Diagram rated unlikely; nerve conduction tests indicated left ulnar nerve entrapment. (From Katz JN, Stirrat CR, Larson MG, et al. A self-administered hand symptom diagram for the diagnosis and epidemiologic study of carpal tunnel syndrome. J Rheumatol 1990;17:1495–1498.)

ter than vibration threshold determination but still had a 9% false-negative rate; the handheld device yielded results comparable with those of standard electrodiagnostic methodology (181). The use of the Bruel and Kjaer Vibrometer Type 1800/WH1763 over a range of frequencies appears to be more helpful, with one preliminary report demonstrating a clear separation of patients from controls using nerve conduction testing and surgical findings for definitive diag-

nosis (182). A carpal tunnel compression test method had a false-negative rate of 14% (183).

Current recommendations of the National Institute of Occupational Safety and Health (NIOSH) for work-related carpal tunnel syndrome include the following criteria:

One or more symptoms: paresthesias, hypesthesia, pain, or numbness affecting at least part of the median nerve distribution of the hand

Objective findings: either physical findings of a positive Tinel sign or a positive Phalen test, or diminished or absent sensation to pin prick in the median nerve distribution; or electrodiagnostic findings indicative of median nerve dysfunction across the carpal tunnel (184).

Use of screening methods during preemployment physical examinations using many of the screening tools is not useful as they are not predictive of future carpal tunnel syndrome (185).

A comparison of CT, MRI, and ultrasonography suggests that MRI will reveal mild degrees of nerve compression missed with ultrasonography as well as detecting tendon sheath thickening and ganglionic cysts (186). Imaging studies are highly dependent upon operator skill and experience and are costly and time-consuming. Three-dimensional imaging using MRI is under investigation (186a). These modalities and electrodiagnostic testing should be reserved for patients who have failed treatment after use of all conservative modalities. When synovitis is suspected within the carpal canal, ultrasonography is a recommended noninvasive diagnostic technique (187).

The use of laboratory testing for patients with carpal tunnel syndrome depends on the age of the patient and the mode of presentation. Most systemic diseases are associated with bilateral onset of carpal tunnel syndrome. When other features are present and onset is bilateral, we would order tests for rheumatoid arthritis; if Raynaud's phenomenon or other features of lupus are noted, then we would order antinuclear antibody test determinations. In all patients with persistent or recurrent carpal tunnel syndrome, a chemistry panel, complete blood count, Westergren sedimentation rate, and thyroid stimulating hormone determination should be considered.

Unilateral onset is often due to cumulative movement disorder but in rare instances can result from tuberculosis and other infectious agents, or from pseudogout, gout, osteoarthritis, or rheumatoid arthritis.

If infection is suspected, surgical intervention is essential; an underlying compartment syndrome can dissect into the carpal canal from the hand or forearm.

Management of Carpal Tunnel Syndrome

- Treatment for patients without motor nerve impairment should consist of splinting, instruction in joint protection principles and work modification (Table 3.2), antiinflammatory agents and posture alignment correction with appropriate stretching and strengthening exercises (Table 3.5).
- Initial *splinting* can be done with the use of an inexpensive splint containing a palmar ''spoon'' style metal support that maintains slight wrist extension. If osteoarthritis of the 1st carpometacarpal joint is prominent, consider referral to an occupational therapist for splinting for both this joint and the wrist. In one study, two-thirds of patients benefitted from splinting, and neither nerve conduction values nor job stress predicted the value of splinting (188). Consider use of a *quilter's glove,* which provides compression during repetitive movement (Fig. 3.21).
- *Exercise* to stretch the volar carpal ligament has been helpful in our experience. The exercise utilizes the bowstringing of the flexor retinaculum; benefit may occur in 6 weeks (189) (Exercise 3.P[a]). With fingers straight and wrist partially flexed, the patient presses the fingers against the opposite forearm or thigh. Although theoretically this position might increase the venous pressure in the carpal canal, we have not seen the exercise exacerbate the condition. Another technique to stretch the ligament requires a helper (Exercise 3.P[b]). Manual stretching of the carpal canal is carried out twice daily.
- *Occupational therapy* should be considered for work-related disability. Behavior on and off the job must be assessed. Resting positions during driving to and from work and while sleeping, reading, and using hands for crafts and hobbies may need modification. Ergonomic risk factors may be important but should be investigated by on-site inspection when possible. Tool modification, usage, and job rotation are possible modifications (185, 190–194). Attempts at prevention may include. the use of wrist motion (flexion/extension)

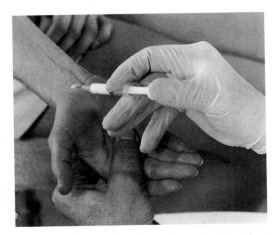

Figure 3.28. Carpal tunnel injection. Many clinicians consider carpal tunnel injection to be diagnostic and therapeutic. The site for injection should be to the radial side of the palmaris longus tendon. The needle may be directed proximally and then distally, with aliquots of the corticosteroid–anesthetic mixture injected in each direction. A ¾-inch, No. 25 needle to inject 20 mg methylprednisolone and 0.5 mL procaine hydrochloride may be used.

acceleration data to define high-risk tasks (195).

- *Local Injection:* If splinting and work simplification have not helped, the next step is a local injection of the volar carpal canal with corticosteroid and lidocaine hydrochloride. Patients likely to benefit include those over 50 years of age and those with constant paresthesias, intermittent paresthesias of longer than 10 months' duration associated with stenosing flexor tenosynovitis, and a Phalen test that is positive in less than 30 seconds (196). Using a No. 23 ¾-inch needle, inject a mixture of 1 mL 1% lidocaine hydrochloride and 20–40 mg methylprednisolone acetate cautiously into the radial side of the palmaris longus tendon or medial to the flexor carpi radialis tendon. To find this have the patient flex the wrist palm up with hand fisted; the tendon should bowstring. Prepare the site with soap and alcohol; wear gloves; make the injection parallel with the nerve (Fig. 3.28). When the needle is inserted ask the patient if there are any sensations of nerve penetration so that the injection is not made into the nerve trunk. Ice applied after the injection may prevent a crystal reaction

that is common at this site. After studies using cadaver injection of methylene blue, Minamikawa et al. recommend that 2 mL corticosteroid and local anesthetic agent be injected 3 cm proximal to the distal flexor wrist crease (197).

Injection can be repeated after 3 weeks but a third occurrence of symptoms indicates need for surgical treatment. Reports of long-term benefit after injection range from 20 to 92% (198). Inasmuch as over 90% have initial excellent night pain relief, Green suggests that the injection is at least as good as any other test for the presence of carpal tunnel syndrome (198), which Phalen said 20 years earlier (170). For the patient with constant symptoms, we would provide injection on the first visit. When performed with care, the injection is less hazardous and less expensive than the use of NSAIDs, in our experience. The injection is likely to provide relief and reduce the need for electrodiagnostic testing (198).

Injection of the carpal tunnel has variable results but, when used in conjunction with behavior modification and splinting, may provide prolonged relief.

- *Surgery:* If motor dysfunction with loss of grip or pinch grasping is present, or if the thenar eminence is flattened, proceed with electrodiagnostic testing or surgery. Many physicians reserve electrodiagnostic testing for patients with complex symptoms and those in whom compression at more than one site is suspected. Surgeons often want electrodiagnostic proof of nerve compression, sometimes for medicolegal reasons. However, as discussed earlier, significant rates of false-negative and false-positive test results occur depending upon electromyographer experience. Grundberg and others report good surgical results despite normal electrodiagnostic studies in patients with other features of carpal tunnel syndrome; surgery need not be withheld because of negative test findings (199, 200).
- *Techniques for surgery* include direct surgical exploration including the palm and forearm extensions of the canal. Surgery undertaken in patients with occupation-related carpal tunnel syndrome often fails regardless of surgical experience (201). Microsurgery may result in increased fail-

ure rate because of inability to inspect the area fully (202).

Brown has popularized an endoscopic carpal tunnel release procedure (203). Using a two-portal technique in 1236 procedures, only 2% were considered failures (longest follow-up was 30 months), and patients could return to work after 2 weeks (204). Complications included injury to the superficial palmar arch, wound hematoma, and severe paresthesias lasting up to 3 months (205). The technique has also been suggested to be safe and reliable (55). A multicenter randomized study of endoscopic surgery reported comparable results, and patients returned to work 3 weeks earlier than with the standard operation (206). Many report similar good results in carefully selected patients. Complications include tendon laceration, infection, bleeding, neurapraxias, median nerve laceration, and wound dehiscence. Choice of surgical technique is highly dependent upon surgical experience and cost. In most cases in which patients had conventional surgery on one hand and endoscopic release on the other, the latter was preferred (206).

After surgery, repetitive hand use at work may still not be tolerated. Surgery does not greatly improve motor function loss, but it usually aids in relieving nocturnal discomfort and preventing further motor dysfunction.

Digital Nerve Compression

Dobyns' experience at the Mayo Clinic establishes iatrogenic compression during treatment for another disorder as a very common cause for neuropathies of the hand (207). Tight splints and casts are common causes for digital neuropathies. Similarly, bowler's thumb, Frisbee finger, and the manacle wrist result from external compression.

Anterior Interosseous Nerve Syndrome (Drop Finger Deformity)

The usual presentation is the sudden loss of distal interphalangeal flexion of the thumb and distal interphalangeal flexion of the index finger. Etiology includes a lifting injury with strain and compression of the nerve by the flexor pollicis longus and flexor carpi radialis at the neck of the radius. A fibrous band may be found on the underside of the flexor digitorum superficialis.

Treatment measures include galvanic stimulation, splinting, and, if the problem persists after 3 months of onset, operative treatment. Neurolysis, interfascicular graft, internal neurolysis, and tendon transfer may be considered (208).

Ulnar Nerve Entrapment at the Wrist

The presentation is clumsiness and weakness of the hand. Nerve compression or entrapment may result either from a space-occupying lesion, often a ganglion, or from external compression. Five types of ulnar neuropathy are recognized on the basis of the level of the lesion. Lesions proximal to Guyon's canal before bifurcation (Guyon's canal lies beneath the volar carpal ligament and the pisohamate ligament; its radial distal wall is the hook of the hamate; its proximal ulnar wall is the pisiform) present with a mixed motor and sensory deficit. External compression is common among cyclists, workers who use pneumatic or vibrating tools, and avid video game players. A compression of the palmar cutaneous branch of the ulnar nerve with resulting pure sensory neuropathy may result from prolonged use of a mouse-directed computer (209). Diagnosis is established with nerve conduction study. Treatment usually requires surgical exploration and release of the nerve.

REFLEX SYMPATHETIC DYSTROPHY

The essential features of reflex sympathetic dystrophy (RSD), which may occur in either the upper or lower extremity, include *burning and sometimes throbbing pain,* diffuse uncomfortable aching, sensitivity to touch or cold, altered color or temperature of the involved extremity, localized edema, and erythema. Three stages in the course of RSD may occur. In the earliest stage, the presentation consists of hyperesthesia, hyperalgesia, localized edema, erythema, and altered skin temperature. In the second stage, 3 to 6 months from the time of onset, progression of the soft tissue edema, thickening of the skin and articular soft

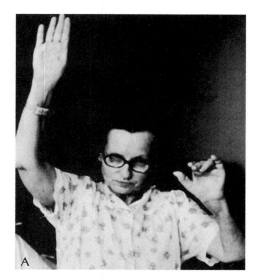

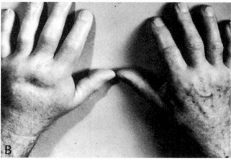

Figure 3.29. A. Shoulder-hand syndrome with presentation of frozen shoulder and cool, edematous swelling of the lower arm and hand. **B.** Note the flexion contractures and pitting edema of the hand. (From McCarty DJ, Koopman WJ, eds. Arthritis and allied conditions. 12th ed. Philadelphia: Lea & Febiger, 1993.)

tissues, muscle wasting, and brawny skin develop. In the third and most severe stage, the shoulder-hand syndrome manifestations of limitation of movement, contractures of the digits, waxy trophic skin changes, and brittle, ridged nails appear (210–214).

Other autonomic features include cyanosis, mottling, increased sweating, abnormal growth of hair, diffuse swelling in nonarticular tissue, and coldness (Fig. 3.29).

Terminology has included algodystrophy, causalgia, shoulder-hand syndrome, shoulder-hand syndrome variant, Sudeck's atrophy, and acute atrophy of bone. Often the syndrome follows injury, surgical intervention, or vascular accidents, such as heart attack or stroke. In a study of 140 patients, Pak reported that 40% of cases of RSD occurred following soft

tissue injury, 25% followed fractures, 20% occurred postoperatively, 12% followed myocardial infarction, and 3% followed cerebral vascular accidents (215). Of patients with RSD, 37% had significant emotional disturbances at the time of onset (215). Geertzen et al. report that 80% of dystrophy patients (26 patients) had a recent life-event (216). Myofascial trigger points are common in the area of trauma or about the shoulder girdle and trapezius (217, 218). Although only one extremity may appear involved, careful inspection may reveal symmetric synovitis (213, 218). The elbow is usually spared.

Etiology: The probability that central nervous system (CNS) disturbance plays a role in RSD causation is supported by the finding that unilateral sympathetic nerve blocks result in improvement in bilateral skin potential variations (pain thresholds) (217). This improvement lasts 48 hours, long after the pharmacologic effect of the anesthetic has worn off. Furthermore, myofascial trigger points also disappear (even in the limb contralateral to the sympathetic nerve block).

A feedback loop with involvement of skin, afferent input to the CNS, then feeding back via a sympathetic output to the skin is proposed as the method for CNS involvement (217). Nine patients with RSD were studied with a xenon-133 washout technique to measure blood flow, using the normal side as control. Changes in flow were compared with the arm first elevated and then dangling. The patients were found to have increased flow at rest but normal vasoconstriction responses. The authors concluded that patients with RSD have normal function of peripheral vascular mechanisms, increased resting blood flow, and therefore a decreased sympathetic activity (219).

Changes in the "gate controls" of Melzack and Wall are probable (211, 212, 220, 221) (see Chapter 14). A self-perpetuating "short circuiting" between pain fibers and sympathetic nerves is then established. This theory has been challenged in favor of a neuroendocrine dysfunction (222).

Quantitative electroencephalogram abnormalities have been described that are similar to those seen in minor head injury. In addition 7 of 10 patients demonstrated abnormal somatosensory evoked potentials. Thus cortical pathways appear to be involved in RSD (223). Serum norepinephrine level was found to be significantly lower in affected than in unaffected limbs (224).

Marrow edema has not been detected in RSD, whereas this finding is seen in regional migratory osteoporosis, which has been considered related to RSD (225).

Histologic findings in one study of three children with reflex sympathetic dystrophy revealed skin capillary endothelial swelling and basement membrane thickening and reduplication. Muscle findings suggest ischemic changes (226). Synovial changes include synovial edema, proliferation and disarray of synovial lining cells, proliferation of capillaries, fibrosis of the subsynovium, and slight perivascular infiltration with lymphocytes. The synovitis was more marked in the small finger joints of the affected side (227–229).

The occurrence of RSD following vascular or surgical insults has been mentioned. Reflex sympathetic dystrophy of a lower extremity in adolescents and following knee surgery may occur. The presentations were typical, often posttraumatic; pain was disproportionate to physical findings and typical skin changes occurred. Management consists of sympathetic nerve blocks or sympathectomy.

Excessive production or response of some prostaglandins is hypothesized. Interaction of products of inflammation that bind prostaglandin E_2, interleukin, histamine, bradykinin, and others, all linked to substance P, has been proposed by Kimbal (230).

Genetic predisposition is suggested by poor treatment outcome among affected Caucasian women. Of 15 women with RSD, a twofold increase of HLA A3, B7, and DR2(15) occurred compared to controls; those who had DR2(15) positive findings were more likely to have disease resistant to treatment (5/6 of patients). The authors suggest a possible genetic diathesis in RSD patients with poor treatment response (231).

Laboratory and Radiologic Examination: In the early stage, reflex sympathetic dystrophy may reveal no abnormal findings on laboratory testing. After 6 weeks' duration, scintigraphy, using technetium-99m pertechnetate ($^{99m}TcO_4$), may reveal increased uptake in the peripheral joints of the involved extremity (228, 232). In patients studied soon after onset of symptoms, scintigrams taken immediately postinjection usually show decreased perfusion of the affected areas (226). Three-phase scintigraphy was found to be of limited value when performed more than 6 months following onset of symptoms (232a). Laser Doppler measurement of skin capillary blood flow can aid diagnosis and was helpful in follow-up assessment (233).

Computed tomography may show focal areas of osteoporosis, a swiss cheese–like appearance that is quite striking (234). MRI, however, was nonspecific or normal in one study (235). However, skin thickening or edema is measurable by MRI study (225). RSD can also be studied with thermography or a quantitative sudomotor axon reflex test to measure sweat activity.

RSD in children may be on the increase and is perhaps due to the stress of sports participation. In one study (236) color change and edema was present in three-fourths of the 70 children reported. Three phase bone scans in 14 children reported by Goldsmith et al. (237) revealed diffusely decreased bone uptake at the symptomatic site.

Sedimentation rate and other tests of inflammation may increase in the later stages. In the third stage, roentgenographs of the involved extremities may reveal patchy osteoporosis, presumably due to increased blood flow to the involved extremity (228). A valuable test is the use of regional sympathetic nerve blocks (Bier block), for both therapy and diagnosis. Abrupt relief from pain and dysesthesia, although transient, is suggestive of a diagnosis of reflex sympathetic dystrophy. Tests to rule out insidious onset of a connective tissue disease should include rheumatoid and antinuclear antibody factor determinations. A chest roentgenogram for an occult neoplasm at the apex of the lung, on the involved side, should be performed. Electromyelography with a determination of nerve conduction velocity may be helpful if thoracic outlet syndrome or carpal tunnel syndrome is a consideration.

Differential Diagnosis: In the earliest stages, reflex sympathetic dystrophy is a difficult diagnosis. However, the qualities of *throbbing, burning pain, paresthesia,* and *altered skin temperature* are suggestive. Cervical nerve root impingement, Pancoast's syndrome, vasculitis, rheumatoid arthritis, peripheral neuropathy, migratory osteolysis, venous thrombosis, arteriovenous fistulae, progressive systemic sclerosis, and angioedema might be confused with early features of various presentations of RSD.

Management: Four modes of therapy are available, depending on the stage of the dystrophy at the time of the first visit:

1. For recent onset and with mild skin changes: myofascial trigger point injection and physical therapy; adrenergic blocking agents (guanethidine 10 mg three times daily) or α-receptor blocking agents (phenoxybenzamine 10–30 mg three times daily) (217, 238, 239), prazosin 1–6 mg/day, propranolol 10–90 mg four times daily, or nifedipine 10–30 mg three times daily; topical capsaicin or transcutaneous electrical nerve stimulation (TENS unit) may also be used. In addition, the tricyclic antidepressants may be helpful by providing improved sleep and less pain.
2. Sympathetic nerve blocks or regional Bier block.
3. Oral corticosteroids.
4. Sympathectomy when these more conservative measures are not effective or significant skin disease and contractures are occurring (212).

The best treatment is prevention. Early mobilization of the shoulder and arm after injury and following myocardial infarction or stroke should be encouraged. Prolonged use of intravenous therapy should be accompanied by intermittent passive shoulder motion. In the first stage, trigger-point injections with a corticosteroid–local anesthetic mixture, followed by physical therapy, including heat and exercise, may abort progression of the dystrophy. Guanethidine or phenoxybenzamine should be considered in first and second stage dystrophy. Smoking cessation is important in RSD as it is in many other soft tissue disorders (240).

The value of physical therapy is anecdotal but all agree that it appears beneficial. However, it must be individualized and supervised. A multicomponent program that includes desensitization, progressive graded loading (weightbearing), muscle strengthening and lengthening, aerobic exercise, and functional retraining is suggested. Hand splinting while at rest is useful to prevent contractures. Active stretching with the use of wand exercises, range-of-motion exercises, and in the acute stage, gentle passive motion, should be started.

In our experience, local steroid injections into tender soft tissues, particularly about the shoulder girdle and forearm, have been helpful in alleviating the throbbing, burning pain that interferes with any active exercise plan. Use of a TENS unit can be initiated after the initial visit; it is a noninvasive treatment and is worth trying before more complex treatment measures are utilized. Use of sedation or antidepressant medication may be helpful. Consideration for any possible missed diagnosis (e.g., a fracture) is important.

The key to success is to use whatever works quickly! Patients should respond within days; if they do not, move on to the next treatment level.

In second stage dystrophy, with incipient induration of the skin of the hand, resting hand and wrist splints may be helpful. At this point, stellate ganglion blocks performed at intervals of 1 to 4 days and repeated 6 to 12 times have been useful. If an immediate response (improved temperature, lessened pain) does not occur following the first or second nerve block, this treatment is abandoned (212, 227). An alternative therapy is to use oral corticosteroids in divided doses, ranging from 30 mg/day (227) to 80 mg/day (21). Steroid treatment has been found to be of most benefit in patients in whom positive technetium-99m bone scans suggested an active inflammatory lesion (227). The dose of corticosteroids is tapered quickly as the patient responds; continued low-dose corticosteroid treatment may be necessary for a prolonged period in severe cases. In all patients, at all stages of the disease, physical therapy should be performed twice daily at home, and the use of resting splints should be maintained.

Bier blocks (regional intravenous perfusion) can be tried before sympathetic blocks for upper limb involvement. Blocks can use bretylium (241), guanethidine, or reserpine combined with lidocaine hydrochloride; ketorolac and methylprednisolone can be added (241–243). However, at this time in the United States, neither guanethidine or reserpine are available for intravenous use. Guanethidine has been associated with severe side effects and should be used rarely (242a). Where available, the doses are: lidocaine hydrochloride 0.5% 35–45 mL; ketorolac 30–60 mg; methylprednisolone 80–120 mg; bretylium 1.5 mg/kg; reserpine 1.5–2 mg; or guanethidine 5–10 mg. Bier blocks may be performed at 48–72-hour intervals. One report states that intramuscular ketorolac was as helpful as Bier blocks (243).

When using Bier blocks or sympathetic blocks, oral medications and intensive mobilizing physical therapy should continue; each block should result in a longer duration of pain relief. At completion of the block, ice packs should be applied, followed by passive manipulation of any stiff joints. Intravenous sedation is often needed for additional analgesia when undertaking manipulation.

Epidural blocks with or without infusion pumps are used in some tertiary care centers. In general, the results have been disappointing and can be dangerous in the cervical region.

Daily ultrasound therapy has been used successfully for patients with lower limb dystrophy who refused sympathetic blocks or sympathectomy (244).

Sympathectomy may be considered if progression is apparent and a positive response to sympathetic nerve blocks occurs. A noninvasive technique using equipment that emits high frequency radio waves to perform upper thoracic sympathectomy may be applicable to the treatment of RSD (245). Others have used a transthoracic endoscopic electrocautery safely and beneficially (246). Patients with advanced dystrophic hands should have consultations with physical and occupational therapists. Occasionally, patients have both reflex sympathetic dystrophy and thoracic outlet syndrome, and may require surgical treatment for both conditions (resection of the first rib and cervical sympathectomy) (247).

Outcome and Additional Suggestions: Our experience with treatment of reflex sympathetic dystrophy prior to contracture has been excellent with either stellate ganglion blocks or corticosteroid therapy. As mentioned, if seen early after onset, pain (trigger) point injections may break the cycle. We have seen patients have an exacerbation several months after treatment, either upon exposure to cold or following emotional trauma. Small doses of tricyclic antidepressants (amitriptyline) and oral guanethidine have been helpful in treating recurrences.

RSD may occur in association with peripheral nerve entrapment. Jupiter et al. described nine patients with combined disorders diagnosed by electrodiagnostic study. Surgery to reduce scarring in the area, neurolysis, or repair and reconstruction with continuous sympathetic block resulted in improvement within 72 hours of surgery and during an average of 48 months of follow-up (248).

In late-stage dystrophy, with a practically immobilized hand, aggressive physical therapy is essential, and sympathectomy must be considered. We have seen late-stage dystrophy significantly improve without resorting to sympathectomy. Oral corticosteroids have not proven as helpful at this stage. A longitudinal study of a series of patients who are members of the Reflex Sympathetic Dystrophy Syndrome Association suggested incomplete recovery in the majority of those affected. The membership obviously is comprised of patients with an outcome that was less than satisfactory (249). The support group address is: Reflex Sympathetic Dystrophy Syndrome Association, P.O. Box 921, Haddonfield, NJ 08033.

OTHER SHOULDER REGION DISORDERS

Bursitis and other lesions that arise in soft tissues of the upper limb will be discussed here. Although the etiology may include cumulative movement disorder, these conditions frequently occur for other reasons.

Milwaukee Shoulder

The "Milwaukee shoulder," described by McCarty et al., is a syndrome in elderly women with calcium apatite deposition in the shoulder followed by cuff tear. The articular joint is usually severely eroded also. Soft tissue calcification is variable (250). Suprascapular nerve block for management should be considered before arthroplasty.

Frozen Shoulder (Adhesive Capsulitis)

The term "frozen shoulder" aptly describes the common disturbance of the shoulder with a limitation of shoulder motion in all directions with passive or active examination. Other terms used are periarthritis, adhesive capsulitis, adhesive bursitis, check rein disorder, and Duplay's disease (251). One or both shoulders may be involved as a result of diverse conditions.

Onset usually begins on one side and is insidious. Symptoms include pain at night in a shoulder that has lost range of motion particularly when reaching backward. Later, shoulder elevation is lost. Aching discomfort commonly involves the anterolateral aspect of the shoulder and arm, with radiation sometimes toward the neck and anterior chest area. Neuritic complaints are unusual. Patients are usually in their 50s or older. Untreated, the frozen shoulder goes through three stages: "freezing," "frozen," and "thawing." Spontaneous recovery is rarely complete (252, 253); pain improves but motion remains somewhat limited.

This painful arc is distinguishable from impingement syndrome by finding limitation in all planes during passive range-of-movement examination. However, at first, only elevation and internal rotation are lost; later, all ranges of movement are lost, with the exception of forward extension. The humeral head may be palpably felt higher in the shoulder joint. The tendons comprising the shoulder cuff are all tender.

Etiology: Frozen shoulder has been considered the result of an extension of inflammation of adjacent tendon structures. Reports suggesting a relation of frozen shoulder to trauma, stroke, myocardial infarction, pulmonary tuberculosis, thyroid disease, cervical disc disease, tumor, and scleroderma are viewed with skepticism by many. The relation of frozen shoulder to barbiturate use (254) is anecdotal but probable. The relation to diabetes (255) is both real and common, and in our experience outcome in diabetics is decidedly less satisfactory.

Etiology and Pathology: Diminished capsular volume and loss of capsular recesses as detected by arthrography are variable findings and arthroscopy may not reveal intraarticular adhesions in all cases (256–260). Arthroscopic findings include hypervascularity and inflammation, sometimes obliterating the opening between the subscapular bursa and the joint (260, 261). Also, often seen is a contracture of

the coracohumeral ligament and the rotator cuff interval, which is probably what produces the decreased rotation of the shoulder joint (262). In general, neither a synovitis nor a tendinopathy is regularly present; rather the capsule and capsular ligaments appear contracted (263). Synovial fluid is scant. Lundberg reported more fibroblasts and fibroplasia resembling that seen in Dupuytren's contracture (264).

Laboratory and imaging examination in frozen shoulder is nonspecific. The erythrocyte sedimentation rate may be elevated, sometimes suggesting polymyalgia rheumatica.

Radiologic examination is useful to exclude fractures, subluxation, osteoarthritis, calcific tendinitis, chondrocalcinosis, malignancy, avascular necrosis, and dislocation. In severe cases, the head of the humerus may be elevated in relation to the usual glenohumeral position. Arthrography is of value only to exclude a rotator cuff tear, but since cuff tear in the elderly is so common, the invasive procedure is rarely indicated. Similarly, scintigraphy will frequently demonstrate increased uptake in the involved shoulder, but the finding is not helpful. Experience with MRI is limited and not likely to be helpful.

Diabetes is a comorbid disorder and occurs in about 20% of patients. Diminished range of motion in upper limb joints by passive examination has been found to be significant when compared to matched nondiabetic controls (265). Other associated disorders include rheumatoid arthritis, polymyalgia rheumatica, and thyroid and parathyroid disorders.

Differential diagnosis of frozen shoulder depends upon mode of onset. When insidious and unilateral, and in the absence of constitutional features, the condition is unlikely to be related to an underlying disease. Rheumatoid arthritis, polymyalgia rheumatica, and endocrinopathies including diabetes, hypothyroidism, and hyperparathyroidism usually affect the shoulders symmetrically. Other uncommon problems that might simulate unilateral frozen shoulder include fracture, osteoarthritis, calcific tendinitis, chondrocalcinosis, Paget's disease, "Milwaukee Shoulder," malignancy, avascular necrosis, and dislocation. Polymyalgia rheumatica and giant cell arteritis would usually have additional features and involve the pelvic girdle as well.

Management: Goals of management are immediate relief of night pain, and pain-free motion with return to function over time.

Useful treatments plans include thermal modalities for short-term pain relief, graduated exercise, full-cuff injection with corticosteroid and local anesthetic, intraarticular distension, and manual techniques such as mobilization or manipulation.

- *Graded graduated exercise:* The importance of a graded graduated passive, then active, exercise plan is essential (266, 267). Treatment without a graded graduated exercise program is doomed to fail. Only 13 to 26% of patients recover without exercise (52, 268). Refer to Table 3.5 and appropriate exercises. Review the section "Other Rehabilitation Techniques," earlier in this chapter.

- *Pain management:* Although NSAIDs are about as effective as periarticular corticosteroid injections in terms of duration until normal range of motion is achieved, they are relatively contraindicated in the older age group, and if used for many months, they are more expensive (51). Oral prednisolone has been found to improve pain at night but did not relieve pain on movement or during rest and did not contribute to restored range of movement (269).

- *Shoulder cuff injection:* If the entire shoulder cuff can be injected with a corticosteroid and local anesthetic mixture, relief from night pain will occur within a few days, in our experience. Furthermore, therapeutic exercise can be performed more comfortably. Although much controversy exists on the sites for injection, the value of intraarticular and periarticular steroid injections for frozen shoulder in ultimately restoring normal function is noted by most practitioners and physical therapists. Anecdotal reports from our physical therapists treating referred patients with frozen shoulder report much better outcome in patients who have had intralesional corticosteroid injections just prior to initiation of therapy. Much of the literature still favors injection with a steroid and local anesthetic (46–52, 268, 270, 271). Use this treatment as soon as possible; the benefit is often lost if treatment is delayed more than 3 months (272). For 30 years, we have used three or four sites for injection; it takes no more time or quantity of steroid to inject these sites (Fig. 3.13).

- *Technique for shoulder cuff injection:* Shoulder cuff injection requires selection of a crystalline steroid, either triamcinolone hexacetonide or methyl prednisolone acetate, injected into the involved tissues. These include the biceps tendon sheath anteriorly, the subacromial bursa and supraspinatus tendon insertion anterolaterally, the teres minor area, and the shoulder capsule (Fig. 3.13). Strict attention to injection principles is essential (Appendix C). Prepare the area with surgical soap or povidone-iodine and alcohol and apply gloves. A 3 mL syringe containing a maximum of 20 to 40 mg steroid is mixed with 1–2 mL 1% lidocaine hydrochloride. A macroscopic flocculate occurs, thus further impeding absorption from the injection site. For the shoulder, a 1.5 or 2-inch No. 23 or No. 22 needle can be used. The shoulder should not be reinjected for 3 to 6 weeks, and no more than three injections should be required. Following the injection, the patient should move the arm slowly in a small circle while bending forward with the arm extended downward and forward for a minute or so.

- Gentle gravity assisted (Exercise 3.A[a,b]) and self-stretching exercise (Exercise 3.B[a–d]) and self-mobilization techniques (Exercise 3.I[a–d]) should begin at home within a few days. Patient instruction can be provided by photocopy from this chapter. If 90 degrees of passive range of motion on examination is not achieved with self-management techniques after the first 3 weeks, reinjection and referral to a physical therapist should be provided. If the patient is a diabetic and motion has shown no significant improvement, consider intraarticular distension treatment next. Comprehensive strengthening and posture/alignment training should be included in the final phases of treatment.

- *Intraarticular distension* performed by the radiologist following arthrography is a useful but invasive treatment. When motion is restricted in all planes and physical therapy has failed, this technique should be considered. The arthrogram is performed first and should demonstrate adhesive capsulitis. Then 40–80 mg methyl prednisolone acetate, 5–10 mL bupivacaine, and following this, up to 30 mL saline are injected until a loss of resistance is noticed (273–275). General anesthesia is used by some, but we have not found anesthesia to be necessary. However, the patient is prepared to expect transient pain. Jacobs reported that the inclusion of the steroid is more important than distension alone in restoring movement to the shoulder (274). In our experience, in patients for whom treatment with two injections and physical therapy has failed, only one treatment of intraarticular pressure injection is successful in 75% of cases.

- *Manipulation* may be performed by a physical therapist, chiropractor, or by an orthopaedist under a general anesthetic. The latter treatment should be reserved for those patients in whom all other less severe measures have failed, because of the cost and risk of tissue disruption. The addition of intraarticular corticosteroid at the time of manipulation has been shown to enhance the outcome of manipulation under anesthesia, in our experience and that of others (268). No prospective studies of manipulation are available, but in retrospective review, Hill and Bogumill reported 70% satisfactory results with orthopaedic manual manipulation under anesthesia in 17 patients in whom all previous measures had failed (276). Quick force techniques are more dangerous.

Outcome and Additional Suggestions: Normal or near normal range of movement is reported in 60–95% of patients treated with these multidisciplinary methods (253, 267, 277, 278). Once the patient can achieve 90 degrees of passive abduction (with the examiner assisting abduction), the shoulder motion usually will return to normal with home exercises. Some residual loss of motion can be seen in the elderly, but this may be "normal" for age. Fewer than 1% of patients with frozen shoul-

der will require manipulation under anesthesia. Diabetes and rheumatoid arthritis, as mentioned, are conditions associated with a poorer prognosis.

If adhesive capsulitis is severe and found in association with severe glenohumeral arthritis, a suprascapular nerve block may afford pain relief and allow physiotherapy to proceed (59, 60).

Abduction Contracture of the Shoulder

After repeated injections of any medication in large volume into the deltoid muscle, a band of dense scar tissue may form within the muscle and contracture may result. The patient presents with the inability to return the raised arm back down to the side of the body. Surgical excision may be required for relief (279).

Soft Tissue Enlargement of the Shoulder

Soft tissue thickening about the point of the shoulder may occur in amyloidosis (shoulder pad sign) or in acromegaly. Massive synovitis and effusion due to rheumatoid arthritis is ballottable, whereas the other conditions are not fluctuant. Amyloid infiltration has a rubbery feel upon examination.

Shoulder Girdle Lipomatosis

Two patterns may occur. Solitary fatty masses may occur between the bands of the muscles connecting the upper limb to the thoracic wall and deform the posterior shoulder region; a neuropathy or neuromyopathy of the affected arm may result from the nerve compression (280). A second type of lipomatosis consists of symmetrical fatty tumors about the upper arms with only cosmetic disturbance.

OTHER ELBOW REGION DISORDERS

Olecranon Bursitis

The olecranon bursa, at the posterior point of the elbow, has a synovial membrane that

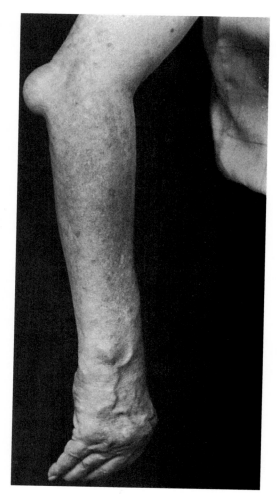

Figure 3.30. Olecranon bursitis.

may be affected by gout, rheumatoid arthritis, sepsis, hemorrhage, or trauma (Fig. 3.30). Traumatic bursitis occurs from pressure. Leaning on the elbow or using the elbow to arise from bed or as part of an occupation such as laying carpet, are common causes for olecranon bursitis. When of traumatic origin, onset is seldom acute, and the surrounding tissues are usually normal.

Acute septic bursitis, in contrast, presents with peribursal erythema and warmth. Similar findings may occur in rheumatoid arthritis, gout, pseudogout, and hemorrhage into the bursa. Peribursal edema and pain on movement favor a diagnosis of sepsis. Septic bursitis occasionally begins less acutely, and studies of the bursal fluid are essential for diagnosis. A surface temperature difference of 2.2°C

between the involved and uninvolved elbows has been found to be more reliable than bursal fluid leukocyte count in the recognition of septic bursitis (281). The temperature probe was obtained from IVAC Temp-Plus, San Diego, California (282). When septic bursitis has occurred, check for underlying disease including diabetes, alcoholism, use of corticosteroids, and other reasons for immunosuppression.

Laboratory and Radiologic Examination: When olecranon bursitis is of traumatic origin, the possibility of foreign body penetration should be considered, which may be revealed by radiologic soft tissue techniques. Aspiration of the bursal fluid with a No. 16 needle should be performed, and evaluation of the fluid should include white blood cell count and differential, Gram stain, sugar content (with comparison to a simultaneously drawn serum sample when possible), and culture. Predisposing causes for sepsis should be screened, including diabetes, rheumatoid arthritis, or hematologic disorders. Crystal identification with polarizing microscopy should be regularly performed and is especially important if the patient has had a history of gout or pseudogout, or recurrent olecranon bursitis.

Differential Diagnosis: Rheumatoid arthritis should be suspected when bilateral or nodular bursitis presents. Septic bursitis should be considered even if the bursal fluid white blood count is as low as 1400 cells/mm³. When the bursal synovium is very thick and sepsis is under consideration, surgical biopsy and debridement should be considered.

Management: Traumatic bursitis is managed with joint protection instruction (Table 3.2), aspiration of the bursal fluid with culture and synovianalysis, and antiinflammatory agents. Resolution is usual within a few weeks. However, if pain is not resolved, or fluid recurs, then a corticosteroid and local anesthetic agent can be used. Methylprednisolone acetate (20–40 mg) mixed with 0.5 mL 1% lidocaine hydrochloride will often prevent recurrence (282). Chronic persistent olecranon bursitis, often with a thick rubbery synovium should be considered for surgical removal. Recently, arthroscopic resection has been suggested; cost may determine surgical method (283).

Septic bursitis treatment requires identification of the organism and choice of appropriate antibiotic. Olecranon bursitis is more susceptible to oral antibiotics than is prepatellar bursitis. Antibiotic treatment for 5 days after fluid sterilization (10–14 days) plus repeated needle aspiration is usually successful.

Other Bursal and Cystic Swellings at the Elbow

Bursitis may also occur between the biceps insertion and the head of the radius. Pain presents at the elbow during wrist rotation. Tenderness is detected over the head of the radius and accentuated during wrist rotation. Response to local anesthetic injection at the site of tenderness aids in diagnosis. Methylprednisolone acetate 20 mg can then be injected.

Cubital Bursitis and Antecubital Cysts

Cubital bursitis and antecubital cysts may cause swelling and pain at the anteromedial border of the elbow or in the antecubital area. The median nerve may be stretched by the swelling, causing pain radiation into the forearm and hand. Repetitive movement and a roughened surface of the bicipital tuberosity are thought to contribute to the formation of cubital bursitis and antecubital cysts (284). Rheumatoid arthritis should also be considered (285). Aspiration and injection with methylprednisolone acetate 20 mg and 1 mL lidocaine hydrochloride 1% is often helpful. Excision may be required.

OTHER HAND AND WRIST DISORDERS

Ganglia of the Wrist and Hand

A ganglion is a cystic swelling overlying a joint or tendon sheath. Ganglia may be unilocular or multilocular, and are thought to result from herniation of synovial tissue from a joint capsule or tendon sheath. A jelly-like fluid can be aspirated from the lesion. Ganglia may spontaneously regress or recur. Common locations include the wrist (Fig. 3.31) and adjacent to finger joints. Ganglia transilluminate whereas solid tumors do not. Treatment includes any

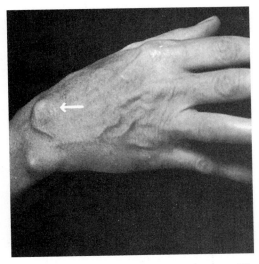

Figure 3.31. Ganglion (*arrow*) on the dorsum of the wrist. Aspiration reveals a clear gelatinous fluid.

of the following: leave it alone; aspirate and inject a crystalline steroid; or remove the ganglion surgically after tracing its connection to the tendon sheath or capsule, and repair the defect. In one study, intralesional hyaluronidase injection (up to 150 units in 1 mL) followed by fine needle aspiration resulted in cure at 6 months in 95% of 349 treated hand and wrist ganglia (286).

Other nodular conditions of the hand and wrist include epidermoid cysts or pearls, which are small, hard, pearl-like cysts several millimeters in diameter. They tend to disappear spontaneously over time. Lipomas, fibromas, neuromas, rheumatoid nodules (Fig. 3.32), dorsal exostoses, periarticular calcareous deposits, giant cell tumors, and synovial cysts are additional benign lesions that may occur as solitary or multiple lesions. Sarcomas are rare, but metastatic lesions to the digits can occur (287). Rheumatoid nodules sometimes are more distressing than the arthritis and can often be treated with intralesional injection of a corticosteroid. A mixture containing 0.1–0.3 mL of a corticosteroid and local anesthetic agent may be injected (the injection requires a fair amount of pressure) (288).

Soft Tissue Trauma of the Wrist and Hand

Whether from sport injury or from falling on the outstretched wrist, injury may involve

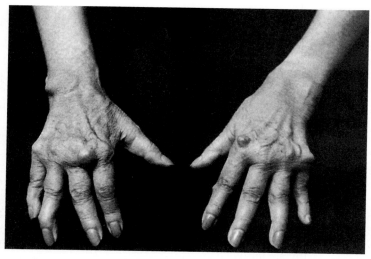

Figure 3.32. Rheumatoid nodulosis. In patients with rheumatoid arthritis, firm nodules may erupt and persist adjacent to joints or in the finger pulp. Similar lesions (pseudorheumatoid nodules) may occur on the extremities in the absence of rheumatoid arthritis.

the tendons, ligaments, or the articular disc at the wrist. Tendinitis crepitans, swelling, tenderness, and pain with specific movement may aid in diagnosis. Clicking may occur. Carpal instability as demonstrated by passive wrist dorsovolar movement or by lateral deviation, if significant, requires orthopaedic consultation.

A compartment syndrome, particularly after a crush injury, may occur and involve any of the fascial compartments of the hand and wrist. As elsewhere, a compartment syndrome may cause neurovascular compression, particularly involving the more radially situated muscles. Paresis, pain on passive motion of the metacarpophalangeal joint, and an elevated tissue pressure measurement are usual findings.

Prominence of the distal ulna with hypermobility ("piano key" motion) may occur spontaneously or as a result of injury or rheumatoid arthritis (Fig. 3.33).

The pisiform-triquetral joint may be sprained, resulting in the pisiform's being displaced distally. This results in pain with wrist flexion or ulnar deviation motions. The pisiform is tender to palpation in the hypothenar aspect of the palm. Reconstructive surgery may be indicated.

If trapezium–first metacarpal joint sprain results in subluxation with limitation of pinch grasping, it may suffice to inject the site of tenderness with a steroid–local anesthetic mix-

ture and to prescribe a thumb splint that allows pinch grasping, yet stabilizes the carpometacarpal joint (Fig. 3.20). For persistent symptoms, consider arthroplasty.

Patients who have suffered wrist sprain and have persistent symptoms should have repeat roentgenograms, including oblique views and special scaphoid roentgenograms in order to detect a fracture of the scaphoid. Imaging for suspected injury to the triangular fibrocartilage complex should be considered if pain is localized to the dorsoulnar side of the wrist (289, 290).

Infectious Tenosynovitis

Tuberculous tenosynovitis should be an immediate consideration if massive swelling of a single flexor tendon from the palm all the way out to the distal finger is noted. The absence of warmth or pain are additional features. Tuberculous tenosynovitis may also present as a "compound palmar ganglion" in which gradually enlarging rubbery masses are noted. These are slightly tender but without warmth or redness. Destruction of the enclosed tendons may occur. Acute septic tenosynovitis from gonococcal, staphylococcal, fungal, and syphilitic infections are considerations when warmth and erythema occur.

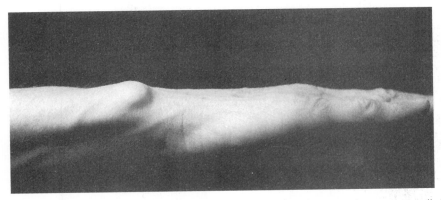

Figure 3.33. Posttraumatic laxity of the distal ulna. Examination with downward pressure results in ``piano key'' movement of the distal ulna.

Calcific Tendinitis

In the wrist, calcific tendinitis may involve the lateral wrist region with an attack of redness and swelling. Similarly, the palm and dorsum of the hand may swell. Fever, intense pain, redness and swelling may occur without regional adenopathy. Fluffy calcification may be evident on roentgenography (291). Calcium apatite deposition disease, the usual underlying disorder, may also involve the shoulder, hip, and Achilles tendon regions. Treatment consists of local ice packs and NSAIDs. Colchicine (0.6 mg twice daily) may prevent recurrences.

Calcific tendinitis can affect the digits as well as the wrist. The presentation may be mistaken for cellulitis. Radiologic evidence of calcification will clarify the situation (292).

Calcium pyrophosphate dihydrate crystal deposits in tendon sheaths of the digits has also been described. Chondrocalcinosis of an adjacent joint and synovial fluid microscopy with crystal identification (a red compensator lens is helpful) aid in diagnosis (293).

Psychophysiologic Disorders of the Hand

The habit of *hand clenching* (also called *fist clenching*) can lead to carpal tunnel syndrome, entrapment neuropathy, or a tennis elbow. This habit leads to hand fatigue, paresthesia, pain, and tendinitis. Often, the symptoms occur upon arising from sleep. The hand is clenched into a fist during sleep, often with both hands beneath the chin. Such symptoms should alert the clinician to ask about clenching during sleep and excessive hand grasping when driving, reading, or using tools. The patients may describe themselves as ``heavy-handed'' persons. Also, ask about jaw clenching, as the clencher syndrome is common with simultaneous hand clenching, jaw clenching, and rectal clenching. Sometimes these persons are driven by caffeine sensitivity or use of theophyllines. When in doubt, if the patient is relieved by sleeping with nylon stretch gloves (worn with the seams to the outside) as a therapeutic trial, the diagnosis is likely hand clenching (E Hess, personal communication, 1981). Exercises may be considered as well (Exercises 3.R and 3.S).

The clenched fist syndrome, considered a conversion syndrome (294), often follows a minor inciting incident. The patient has swelling, pain, and paradoxical stiffness in which the patient maintains the same degree of finger flexion despite changing the position of the wrist. Hand clenching is usually not noted on the first visit. Attempts to passively extend the fingers results in pain. The examiner can detect active contraction of the finger flexors. Secondary infection and maceration from the prolonged flexed position may be noted. The fingers can be extended under general anesthesia. No organic disease can be detected. Psychiatrically, the patient manifests severe anger and has poor defenses to stress. The prognosis is poor. Other similar disorders include violinist's cramp, trumpeter's lip, factitious lymphedema of the hand (294), and the syndrome of delicate self-cutting (295). The condition is often mistaken for a reflex sympathetic dystrophy, but prolonged observation will reveal normal use while dressing (295).

Writer's cramp may be of psychological origin, and can be divided into two types: simple and dystonic (296, 297). In both types muscular spasm and incoordination occur on attempts to write, play a musical instrument, or type at a keyboard or typewriter. Dystonic features include difficulty in picking up a pen, gripping it with a closed fist, and dystonic postures with a jerky motion. In walking, there may be loss of arm swing on the affected side. Features of dystonia may vary from time to time. Psychologic examination often fails to demonstrate abnormality (297). Some patients with dystonic writer's cramp respond to operant conditioning (6). Electrophysiologic studies demonstrate abnormalities of muscle control, with concurrent contraction of agonist and antagonist muscles. Documented cerebral lesions are notably absent in patients with occupationally determined focal dystonias. It may be an overuse syndrome. No treatment has been found to be helpful (298–300).

Dupuytren's Contracture

Usually painless, Dupuytren's contracture is a nodular fibrosing lesion within the palmar fascia that progresses to fibrous bands and usually radiates distally to the 4th and 5th fingers (Fig. 3.34). Ultimately the fingers are contracted by the taut bands. The flexor tendons are not intrinsically involved. Soft tissue pads over the PIP joints on the extensor surface (knuckle pads) may be associated findings. Nodular lesions within the plantar fascia of the feet may also develop concurrently. Males are more likely to develop the condition, and genetics is important; by late age, 68% of male relatives are reportedly affected. No definite relation to occupation has been accepted by investigators (301–303). Knuckle pads are benign thickened skin over the PIP joints. Although they may occur in unaffected normal individuals, they are four times more common in patients with Dupuytren's contracture. Diabetes and use of barbiturates are associated with development of the condition (21, 255). To be distinguished from Dupuytren's contracture are

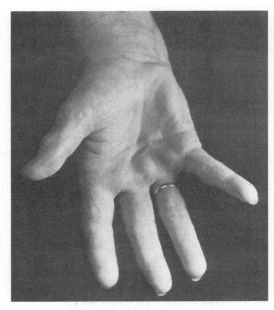

Figure 3.34. Nodular fibrosing lesion with bands radiating distally are features of Dupuytren's contracture.

diabetic cheiroarthropathy, camptodactyly, traumatic scars, Volkmann's ischemic contracture, and intrinsic joint disease. Shoulder-hand syndrome may present with a palmar fasciitis, and palmar fasciitis can be associated with a malignancy (304).

Treatment of patients with minimal Dupuytren's contracture includes instructing the patient to passively stretch the involved digits (hyperextending the digits), avoid a tight grip on tools and the like (by means of built-up handles, using pipe insulation or cushion tape) (C Goodwin, personal communication, 1980), and where possible, using a glove with padding across the palm during heavy grasping tasks. Intralesional injection with triamcinolone acetonide and lidocaine hydrochloride is helpful if local tenderness is bothersome. Allopurinol has been proposed as possibly helpful because of its potential to depress local xanthine oxidase activity (305). Because recurrence rates are high, surgery should be considered only when functional impairment is considerable.

Diabetic Cheiroarthropathy

Also known as the diabetic stiff hand syndrome, syndrome of limited joint mobility, and "prayer hands" of diabetes, the findings include

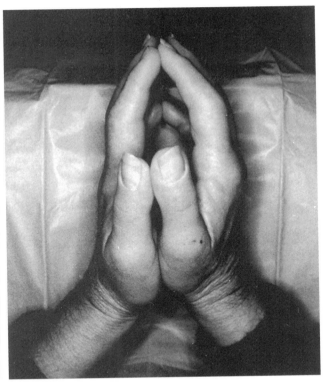

Figure 3.35. Syndrome of limited joint mobility or diabetic cheiroarthropathy. Contractures of digital joints result in a prominent "prayer sign." Skin changes may include sclerodactyly. (From McCarty DJ, Koopman WJ, eds. Arthritis and allied conditions. 12th ed. Philadelphia: Lea & Febiger, 1993.)

camptodactyly, palmar scarring, and associated tendon and nerve entrapments. Carpal tunnel syndrome, trigger finger, and tenosynovitis may also occur (306–309). The skin may have a waxy appearance over the dorsal surface of the fingers. The diabetes may be either type I or type II. These patients are at greater risk for diabetic microvascular disease. The skin and tendon changes may precede overt vascular complications. Nailfold capillary changes of scleroderma are not present, and inspection of the nailfold capillary morphology is helpful in the differential diagnosis. Diabetic cheiroarthropathy involves all four fingers, whereas Dupuytren's contracture more commonly involves just the 4th and 5th digits. Also, in cheiroarthropathy taut bands are not common (Fig. 3.35).

Treatment consists of passive palmar stretching, injection of flexor tendon sheaths with a corticosteroid–local anesthetic mixture, and good diabetic control, often including use of insulin. Insulin pump therapy may be important for control in severe cases (309). When steroid injection is to be made in a diabetic patient, he or she should be taught to check urine or blood sugar and utilize a sliding schedule of extra insulin dosage the following morning, consisting of two to six extra units of insulin, depending upon the level of test abnormality.

Sometimes tenolysis may be performed to provide full range of motion (310). Treatment with aldose reductase inhibiting agents is under investigation (311, 312).

Dorsal Edema of Secrétan (Secrétan's Syndrome)

Rarely, following injury to the dorsum of the hand, a peritendinous fibrosis may occur. This brawny, edematous swelling may gradually harden, and it often becomes painlessly persistent. Early, consistent elevation of the affected hand may be beneficial in preventing edema (C Goodwin, personal communication, 1992). Repeated injections of a corticosteroid may be helpful. Surgical excision has been shown not to shorten the period of disability and is rarely recommended (123, 313).

REFERENCES

1. Webster BS, Snook SH: The cost of compensable upper extremity cumulative trauma disorders. J Occup Med 36:713–717, 1994.
2. Feuerstein M, Callan-Harris S, Hickey P., et al.: Multidisciplinary rehabilitation of chronic work-related upper extremity disorders: long-term effects. J Occup Med 35:396–403, 1993.
3. Hadler NM: Coping with arm pain in the workplace. In: Occupational musculoskeletal disorders. New York: Raven Press, 1993:187–225.
4. Bird H, Hill J: Repetitive strain disorder: towards diagnostic criteria. Ann Rheum Dis 51:974–977, 1992.
5. Rempel DM, Harrison RJ, Barnhart S: Work-related cumulative trauma disorders of the upper extremity. JAMA 267:838–842, 1992.
6. Helliwell PS, Mumford DB, Smeathers JE, et al.: Work related upper limb disorder: the relationship between pain, cumulative load, disability, and psychological factors. Ann Rheum Dis 51: 1325–1329, 1992.
7. Halbrecht JL, Wolf EM: Office arthroscopy of the shoulder: a diagnostic alternative. Orthop Clin North Am 24:193–200, 1993.
8. Levy HJ, Gardner RD, Lemak LJ: Arthroscopic subacromial decompression in the treatment of full-thickness rotator cuff tears. Arthroscopy 7:8–13, 1991.
9. Travell JT, Simons DG: Triceps brachii muscle. In: Myofascial pain and dysfunction: the trigger point manual. Baltimore: Williams & Wilkins, 1983:462–476.
10. Bjelle A, Hagberg M, Michaelson G: Occupational and individual factors in acute shoulder-neck disorders among industrial workers. Br J Ind Med 38:356–363, 1981.
11. Luopajarvi T, Kuorinka I, Virolainen M, et al.: Prevalence of tenosynovitis and other injuries of the upper extremities in repetitive work. Scand J Work Environ Health 5 [Suppl 3]:48–55, 1979.
12. Myerson GE, Goldman J, Miller SB: Arcade arthritis: videogame violence. (Abstract #E83) Arthritis Rheum 25(4) [Suppl], 1982.
13. Nirschl RP, Pettrone FA: Tennis elbow: the surgical treatment of lateral epicondylitis. J Bone Joint Surg 61A:832–839, 1979.
14. Zambrano J, Boswick JA: Microwave injury to the upper extremity: a case report. Contemp Orthop 9:91–93, 1984.
15. Grundberg AB, Reagan DS: Compression syndromes in reflex sympathetic dystrophy. J Hand Surg 16A:731–736, 1991.
16. Jupiter JB, Seiler JG, Zienowicz R: Sympathetic maintained pain (causalgia) associated with a demonstrable peripheral-nerve lesion. J Bone Joint Surg 76A:1376–1384, 1994.
17. Goss TP: Shoulder and upper arm. In: Steinberg GG, ed. Ramamurti's orthopaedics in primary care. 2nd ed. Baltimore: Williams & Wilkins, 1992:36–39.
18. Jobe FW, Kvitne RS, Giangarra CE: Shoulder pain in the overhand or throwing athlete. Orthop Rev 18:963–975, 1989.
19. Misamore GW, Hawkins RJ: Shoulder impingement syndrome: when to suspect, what to do. J Musculoskel Med (July):55–63, 1984.
20. Hawkins RJ, Kennedy JC: Impingement syndrome in athletes. Am J Sports Med 8:151–158, 1980.
21. Matsen FA, Kirby RM: Office evaluation and management of shoulder pain. Orthop Clin North Am 13:453–475, 1982.
22. Bland JH, Merrit JA, Boushey DR: The painful shoulder. Semin Arthritis Rheum 7:21–46, 1977.
23. Whiteside JA, Andrews JR: Common elbow problems in the recreational athlete. J Musculoskel Med 6 (Feb):17–34, 1989.
24. Uhthoff HK, Sarkar K: Classification and definition of tendinopathies. Clin Sports Med 10: 707–720, 1991.
24a. Sperner G: Role of the subacromial space on development of the impingement syndrome. Unfallchirurg 98(6):309–319, 1995.
25. McIntyre DI: Subcoracoid neurovascular entrapment. Clin Orthop 108:27–30, 1975.
26. Scheib JS: Diagnosis and rehabilitation of the shoulder impingement syndrome in the overhand and throwing athlete. Rheum Dis Clin North Am 16:971–988, 1990.
27. Weiner DS, McNab I: Superior migration of the humeral head. J Bone Joint Surg 52B:524, 1970.
28. Neer CS, Welch RP: The shoulder in sports. Orthop Clin North Am 8:583–597, 1977.
29. Thompson GR, Ting M, Riggs GA, et al.: Calcific tendinitis and soft tissue calcification resembling gout. JAMA 203:464–472, 1968.
30. Mavrikakis ME, Drimis S, Kontoyannis DA, et al.: Calcific shoulder periarthritis (tendinitis) in adult onset diabetes mellitus: a controlled study. Ann Rheum Dis 48:211–214, 1989.
31. Rathbun JB, Macnab I: The microvascular pattern of the rotator cuff. J Bone Joint Surg 52B: 540–553, 1970.
32. Penny JN, Welsh RP: Shoulder impingement syndromes in athletes and their surgical management. Am J Sports Med 9:11–15, 1981.
33. Jobe FW, Radovich-Moynes D: Delineation of diagnostic criteria and a rehabilitation program for rotator cuff injuries. Am J Sports Med 10: 336–339, 1982.
34. Jerosch J, Muller T, Castro WH: The incidence of rotator cuff rupture: an anatomic study. Acta Orthop Belg 57:124–129, 1991.
35. Sher JS, Uribe JW, Posada A; et al.: Abnormal findings on magnetic resonance images of

asymptomatic shoulders. J Bone Joint Surg 77A: 10–15, 1995.

36. Frieman BG, Albert TJ, Fenlin JM: Rotator cuff disease: a review of diagnosis, pathophysiology, and current trends in treatment. Arch Phys Med Rehabil 75: 604–609, 1994.

37. Neer CS, Craig EV, Fukuda H: Cuff-tear arthropathy. J Bone Joint Surg 65A:1232–1244, 1983.

38. Kessel L, Watson M: The painful arc syndrome: clinical classification as a guide to management. J Bone Joint Surg 59B:166–172, 1977.

39. Farin PU, Jaroma H, Harju A, et al.: Shoulder impingement syndrome: sonographic findings. Radiology 176:845–849, 1990.

40. Rafii M, Firooznia H, Sherman O, et al.: Rotator cuff lesions: signal patterns at MR imaging. Radiology 177:817–823, 1990.

41. Iannotti JP, Zlatkin MB, Esterhai KP, et al.: Magnetic resonance imaging of the shoulder. J Bone Joint Surg 73A:17–29, 1991.

42. Morrison DS, Ofstein R: The use of magnetic resonance imaging in the diagnosis of rotator cuff tears. Orthopedics 13:633–637, 1990.

43. Misamore GW, Woodward C: Evaluation of degenerative lesions of the rotator cuff: a comparison of arthrography and ultrasonography. J Bone Joint Surg (Am) 73A:704–706, 1991.

44. Curtis AS, Snyder SJ: Evaluation and treatment of biceps tendon pathology. Orthop Clin North Am 24:33–43,1993.

45. Roy S, Oldham R: Management of painful shoulder. Lancet 1:1322–1324, 1979.

46. Weiss JJ: Intra-articular steroids in the treatment of rotator cuff tear: reappraisal by arthrography. Arch Phys Med Rehabil 62:555–557, 1981.

47. Berry H, Fernandes L, Bloom B, et al.: Clinical study comparing acupuncture, physiotherapy, injection and oral anti-inflammatory therapy in shoulder-cuff lesions. Curr Med Res Opin 7: 121–126, 1980.

48. White RH, Paull DM, Fleming KW: Rotator cuff tendinitis: comparison of local corticosteroid injections versus nonsteroidal therapy. (Abstract #63) Arthritis Rheum 28(4) [Suppl], 1985.

49. Adebajo AO, Nash P, Hazleman BL: A prospective double-blind dummy placebo controlled study comparing triamcinolone hexacetonide injection with oral diclofenac 50 mg TDS in patients with rotator cuff tendinitis. J Rheumatol 17: 1207–1210, 1990.

50. Petri M, Dobrow R, Neiman R, et al.: Randomized, double-blind, placebo-controlled study of the treatment of the painful shoulder. Arthritis Rheum 30:1040–1045, 1987.

51. Dacre JE, Beeney N, Scott DL: Injections and physiotherapy for the painful stiff shoulder. Ann Rheum Dis 48:322–325, 1989.

52. Hollingworth GR, Ellis RM, Hattersley TM: Comparison of injection techniques for shoulder pain: results of a double blind, randomised study. Br Med J 287:1339–1341, 1983.

53. Chard MD, Sattelle LM, Hazleman BL: The long-term outcome of rotator cuff tendinitis: a review study. Br J Rheumatol 27: 385–389, 1988.

54. Richardson AT: The painful shoulder. Proc Roy Soc Med 68:731–736, 1975.

55. Levy HJ, Soifer TB, Kleinbart FA, et al.: Endoscopic carpal tunnel release: an anatomic study. Arthroscopy 9:1–4, 1993.

56. Gerber C, Vinh TS, Hertel R, et al.: Latissimus dorsi transfer for the treatment of massive tears of the rotator cuff: a preliminary report. Clin Orthop 232: 51, 1988.

57. Gerber C: Latissimus dorsi transfer for the treatment of irreparable tears of the rotator cuff. Clin Orthop 275: 152–160, 1992.

58. Ogilvie-Harris DJ, Wiley AM, Sattarian J: Failed acromioplasty for impingement syndrome. J Bone Joint Surg (Br) 72:1070–1072, 1990.

59. Emery P, Bowman S, Wedderburn L, et al.: Suprascapular nerve block for chronic shoulder pain in rheumatoid arthritis. Br Med J 299: 1079–1080, 1989.

60. Milowsky J, Rovenstine EA: Suprascapular nerve block. Anesthesiology 2:541–545, 1941.

61. Rockwood CA Jr, Williams GR Jr, Burkhead WZ Jr: Debridement of degenerative, irreparable lesions of the rotator cuff. J Bone Joint Surg 77A:857–866, 1995.

62. Reynolds MD: Myofascial trigger points in persistent posttraumatic shoulder pain. Southern Med J 77:1277–1280, 1984.

63. Olavi A, Pekka R, Pertti K, et al.: Effects of the infrared laser therapy at treated and non-treated trigger points. Acupunct Electrother Res 14:9–14, 1989.

64. Travell J, Rinzler S, Herman M: Pain and disability of the shoulder and arm. JAMA 120: 417–422, 1942.

65. Simons DG, Travell JG: Myofascial origins of low back pain. 1. Principles of diagnosis and treatment. Post Grad Med 73:66–108, 1983.

66. Nirschl RP: Elbow tendinosis/tennis elbow. Clin Sports Med 11:851–870, 1992.

67. Bernhang AM, Dehner W, Fogarty C: A scientific approach to tennis elbow. Orthop Rev 4:35–41, 1975.

68. Priest JD, Jones HH, Tichenor CJC, Nagel DA: Arm and elbow changes in expert tennis players. Minn Med 60:399–404, 1977.

69. Galloway M, Demaio M, Mangine R: Rehabilitative techniques in the treatment of medial and lateral epicondylitis. Orthopedics 15:1089–1097, 1992.

70. Boyd HB, McLeod AC Jr: Tennis elbow. J Bone Joint Surg 55A:1183–1187, 1973.

71. Gunn CC, Milbrandt WE: Tennis elbow and the cervical spine. Can Med Assoc J 114: 803–806, 1976.

72. Nirschl RP: Tennis elbow. Primary Care 4: 367–382, 1977.

73. Goldie I: Epicondylitis lateralis humeri (epicondylalgia or tennis elbow): a pathologic study. Acta Chir Scand [Suppl] 339:110–112, 1964.

74. Sartar K, Uhthoff HK: Ultrastructure of the common extensor tendon in tennis elbow. Virchows Arch A Pathol Anat Histopathol 386:317–318, 1980.

75. Bernhang AM: The many causes of tennis elbow. NY State J Med (Aug):1363–1366, 1979.

76. Begg RE: Epicondylitis or tennis elbow: frequent finding of gunsight type spur in lateral epicondyle of distal humerus. Orthop Rev 9:33–42, 1980.

77. Thomas D, Siahamis G, Marion M, et al.: Computerised infrared thermography and isotopic bone scanning in tennis elbow. Ann Rheum Dis 51:103–107, 1992.

78. Warhold LG, Osterman AL, Skirven T: Lateral epicondylitis: how to treat it and prevent recurrence. J Musculoskel Med 10 (June):55–73, 1993.

79. Day BH, Govindasamy N, Patnaik R: Corticosteroid injections in the treatment of tennis elbow. Practitioner 220: 459–462, 1978.

80. Price R, Sinclair H, Heinrich I, et al.: Local injection treatment of tennis elbow: hydrocortisone, triamcinolone, and lidocaine compared. Br J Rheumatol 30: 39–44, 1991.

81. Nevelos AB: The treatment of tennis elbow with triamcinolone acetonide. Curr Med Res Opin 6:507–509, 1980.

82. O'Donoghue DH: Treatment of injuries to athletes. 4th Ed. Philadelphia: WB Saunders, 1984.

83. Little TS: Tennis elbow: to rest or not to rest. Practitioner 228:457, 1984.

84. Rosen MJ, Duffy FP, Miller EH, et al.: Tennis elbow syndrome: results of the "lateral release" procedure. Ohio State Med J 76:103–109, 1980.

85. Hagberg M: Exposure variables in ergonomic epidemiology. Am J Ind Med 21:91–100, 1992.

86. Bernard B, Sauter SL, Fine LJ, et al.: Psychosocial and work organization risk factors for cumulative trauma disorders in the hands and wrists of newspaper employees. Scand J Work Environ Health 18 [Suppl] 2:119–120, 1992.

87. de Quervain F: Uber eine Form von chronischer Tendovaginitis. Correspondenz-Blatt fur Schweizer Arzte 25:389–394, 1895.

88. Minamikawa Y, Peimer CA, Cox WL, et al.: de Quervain's syndrome: surgical and anatomical studies of the fibroosseous canal. Orthopedics 14:545–549, 1991.

89. Pick RY: de Quervain's disease: a clinical triad. Clin Orthop 143:165–166, 1979.

90. Schumacher HR Jr, Dorwart BB, Korzeniowski OM: Occurrence of de Quervain's tendinitis during pregnancy. Arch Intern Med: 145: 2083–2084, 1985.

91. Saplys R, Mackinnon SE, Dellon AL: The relationship between nerve entrapment versus neuroma complications and the misdiagnosis of de Quervain's disease. Contemp Orthop 15: 51–57, 1987.

92. Carlson CS, Curtis RM: Steroid injection for flexor tenosynovitis. J Hand Surg 9A:286–287, 1984.

93. Cooney WP III: Bursitis and tendinitis in the hand, wrist, and elbow. Minn Med 66:491–494, 1983.

94. Wilson DH: Tenosynovitis, tendovaginitis, and trigger finger. Physiotherapy 69:350–352, 1983.

95. Otto N, Wehbe MA: Steroid injections for tenosynovitis in the hand. Orthop Rev 15:290–293, 1986.

96. Anderson BC, Manthey R, Brouns MC: Treatment of de Quervain's tenosynovitis with corticosteroids. Arthritis Rheum 34:793–798, 1991.

97. Witt J, Pess G, Gelberman RH, et al.: Treatment of de Quervain's tenosynovitis. J Bone Joint Surg 73A:219–222, 1991.

98. Dobyns JH, Sim FH, Linscheid RL: Sports stress syndromes of the hand and wrist. Am J Sports Med 6:236–253, 1978.

99. Kiefhaber TR, Stern PJ: Upper extremity tendinitis and overuse syndromes in the athlete. Clin Sports Med 11:39–55, 1992.

100. Moidel RA: Bowler's thumb. Arthritis Rheum 24:972–973, 1981.

101. Hartwell SW Jr, Larsen RD, Posch JL: Tenosynovitis in women in industry. Cleve Clin Q 31:115–118, 1964.

102. Reed JV, Harcourt AK: Tenosynovitis: an industrial disability. Am J Surg 62:392–396, 1943.

103. Hadler NM: The influence of repetitive tasks on hand structure. Occup Health Safety 50:57–64 1981.

104. Hadler NM: Industrial Rheumatology: clinical investigations into the influence of pattern of usage on the pattern of regional musculoskeletal disease. Arthritis Rheum 20:1019–1025, 1977.

105. Greenberg L. Chaffin DB: Workers and their tools: a guide to the ergonomic design of hand tools and small presses. Midland, Mich.: Pendell Publishing Co., 1978.

106. Kuorinka I, Koskinen P: Occupational rheumatic diseases and upper limb strain in manual jobs in a light mechanical industry. Scand J Work Environ Health 5 [Suppl]: 3:39–47, 1979.

107. Maeda K, Hunting W, Grandjean E: Localized fatigue in accounting machine operators. J Occup Med 22:810–816, 1980.

108. Fahey JJ, Bollinger JA: Trigger-finger in adults and children. J Bone Joint Surg 36A: 1200–1218, 1954.

109. Chuinard RG: The upper extremity: elbow, forearm, wrist, and hand. In: D'Ambrosia, RD, ed. Musculoskeletal disorders. Philadelphia: JB Lippincott, 1977.

110. Burton RI: The jammed finger or thumb. Contemp Orthop 1:56–81, 1979.

111. McCue FC III, Baugher H, Burland WL, et al.: The "jammed finger:" how to prevent permanent disability. Consultant 19:29–38, 1979.

112. Quinnill RC: Conservative management of trigger finger. Practitioner 224:187–190, 1980.

113. Stewart GJ, Williams EA: Locking of the metacarpophalangeal joints in degenerative disease. Hand 13:147–151, 1981.

114. Parker HG: Dupuytren's contracture as a cause of stenosing tenosynovitis. J Maine Med Assoc 70:147–148, 1979.

115. Seradge H: Ochronotic stenosing flexor tenosynovitis: case report. J Hand Surg 6:359–360, 1981.

116. Rayan GM, Elias L: "Trigger finger" secondary to partial rupture of the superficial flexor tendon. Orthopedics 3:1090–1092, 1980.

117. Sammarco GJ, Sabogal J: Fibroma of the flexor tendon presenting as carpal tunnel syndrome and trigger finger. Orthopedics 4:299–300, 1981.

118. Swezey RL, Spiegel TM: Evaluation and treatment of local musculoskeletal disorders in elderly patients. Geriatrics 34:56–75, 1979.

119. Patel MR, Bassini L: Trigger fingers and thumb: when to splint, inject, or operate. J Hand Surg 17:110–113, 1992.

120. Johns AM: Time off work after hand injury. Br J Accident Surg 12:417–424, 1980–81.

121. Clark DD, Ricker JH, MacCollum MS: The efficacy of local steroid injection in the treatment of stenosing tenovaginitis. Plast Reconstr Surg 51:179–180, 1973.

122. Janecki CJ: Extra-articular steroid injection for hand and wrist disorders. Postgrad Med 68: 173–181, 1980.

123. Wolin I: The management of tenosynovitis. Surg Clin North Am 37:53–62, 1957.

124. Anderson B, Kaye S: Treatment of flexor tenosynovitis of the hand ("trigger finger") with corticosteroids. Arch Intern Med: 151:153–156, 1991.

125. Kraemer BA, Young L, Arfken C: Stenosing flexor tenosynovitis. Southern Med J 83: 806–811, 1990.

126. Panayotopoulos E, Fortis AP, Armoni A, et al.: Trigger digit: the needle or the knife. J Hand Surg 17:239–240, 1992.

127. Lambert MA, Morton RJ, Sloan JP: Controlled study of the use of local steroid injection in the treatment of trigger finger and thumb. J Hand Surg (Br) 17: 69–70, 1992.

128. Eastwood DM, Gupta KJ, Johnson DP: Percutaneous release of the trigger finger: an office procedure. J Hand Surg 17A:114–117, 1992.

129. Johnson SL: Ergonomic hand tool design. Hand Clin 9 299–311, 1993.

130. Pascarelli EF: Soft-tissue injuries related to use of the computer keyboard: a clinical study of 53 severely injured persons. J Occup Med 35: 522–532, 1993.

131. Peterson RR: Prevention! A new approach to tendinitis. Occup Health Nursing 27:19–23, 1979.

132. Genaidy AM, Karwowski W, Guo L, et al.: Physical training: a tool for increasing work tolerance limits of employees engaged in manual handling tasks. Ergonomics 35:1081–1102, 1992.

133. Wood VE, Frykman GK: Winging of the scapula as a complication of first rib resection: a report of six cases. Clin Orthop 149:160–163, 1980.

134. Saeed MA, Kraft GH: Bilateral suprascapular neuropathy. Orthop Rev 11:135–137, 1982.

135. Ferretti A, Cerullo G, Russo G: Suprascapular neuropathy in volleyball players. J Bone Joint Surg 69A:260–263, 1987.

136. Fritz RC, Helms CA, Steinbach LS, et al.: Suprascapular nerve entrapment: evaluation with MR imaging. Radiology 182:437–444, 1992.

137. Torres-Ramos FM, Biundo JJ: Suprascapular neuropathy during progressive resistance exercises in a cardiac rehabilitation program. Arch Phys Med Rehabil 73:1107–1111, 1992.

138. Post M, Grinblat E: Nerve entrapment about the shoulder girdle. Hand Clin 8:299–306, 1992.

139. Prochaska V, Crosby LA, Murphy RP: High radial nerve palsy in a tennis player. Orthop Rev 22:90–92, 1993.

140. Nakamichi K, Tachibana S: Radial nerve entrapment by the lateral head of the triceps. J Hand Surg 16A: 748–750, 1991.

141. Moss SH, Switzer HE: Radial tunnel syndrome: a spectrum of clinical presentation. J Hand Surg 8:414–420, 1983.

142. Weinstein SM, Herring SA: Nerve problems and compartment syndromes in the hand, wrist, and forearm. Clin Sports Med 11:161–186, 1992.

143. Lister GD, Belsole RB, Kleinert HE: The radial tunnel syndrome. J Hand Surg 4: 52–59, 1979.

144. Dan NG: Entrapment syndromes. Med J Aust 1:528–531, 1978.

145. Verhaar J, Spaans F: Radial tunnel syndrome. J Bone Joint Surg 73A:539–544, 1991.

146. Feldman RG, Goldman R, Keyserling WM: Peripheral nerve entrapment syndromes and ergonomic factors. Am J Ind Med 4:661–681, 1983.

147. Papadopoulos N, Paraschos A, Pelekis P: Anatomical observations on the arcade of Frohse and other structures related to the deep radial nerve: anatomical interpretation of deep radial nerve entrapment neuropathy. Folia Morphol 37: 319–327, 1989.

148. Seror P: Forearm pain secondary to compression of the medial antebrachial cutaneous nerve at the elbow. Arch Phys Med Rehabil 74:540–542, 1993.

149. Kummel BM, Zazanis GA: Shoulder pain as the presenting complaint in carpal tunnel syndrome. Clin Orthop 93:227–230, 1973.

150. Uchida Y, Sugioka Y: Electrodiagnosis of retrograde changes in carpal tunnel syndrome. Electromyogr Clin Neurophysiol 33: 55–58, 1993.

151. Patel MR, Bassini L, Magill: Compression neuropathy of the lateral antebrachial cutaneous nerve. Orthopedics 14:173–174, 1991.

152. Wadsworth TG, Williams JR: Cubital tunnel external compression syndrome. Br Med J 1: 662–666, 1973.

153. Clark CB: Cubital tunnel syndrome. JAMA 241:801–802, 1979.

154. Campbell WW, Pridgeon RM, Riaz G, et al.: Variations in anatomy of the ulnar nerve at the cubital tunnel: pitfalls in the diagnosis of ulnar

neuropathy at the elbow. Muscle Nerve 14: 733–738, 1991.

155. Barrios C, Ganoza C, de Pablos J, et al.: Post-traumatic ulnar neuropathy versus non-traumatic cubital tunnel syndrome: clinical features and response to surgery. Acta Neurochir (Wien) 110:44–48, 1991.

156. Sunderland S: The nerve lesion in the carpal tunnel syndrome. J Neurol Neurosurg Psychiatry 39:615–626, 1976.

157. Werner CO, Elmqvist D, Ohlin P: Pressure and nerve lesion in the carpal tunnel. Acta Orthop Scand 54:312–314, 1983.

158. Luchetti R, Schoenhuber R, DeCicco G, et al.: Carpal-tunnel pressure. Acta Orthop Scand 60: 397–399, 1989.

159. Cobb TK, Dalley BK, Posteraro RH, et al.: The carpal tunnel as a compartment. Orthop Rev 21:451–453, 1992.

160. Kerr CD, Sybert DR, Albarracin NS: An analysis of the flexor synovium in idiopathic carpal tunnel syndrome: report of 625 cases. J Hand Surg (Am) 17:1028–1030, 1992.

161. Armstrong TJ, Chaffin DB: Carpal tunnel syndrome and selected personal attributes. J Occup Med 21:481–486, 1979.

162. Dekel S, Papaioannou T, Rushworth G, Coates R: Idiopathic carpal tunnel syndrome caused by carpal stenosis. Br Med J 120:1297–1303, 1980.

163. Bleecker ML: Medical surveillance for carpal tunnel syndrome in workers. J Hand Surg 12A:845–848, 1987.

164. Merhar GL, Clark RA, Schneider HJ, et al.: High-resolution CT scans of the wrist in patients with carpal tunnel syndrome. Radiology 15: 549–552, 1986.

165. Cobb TK, Dalley BK, Posteraro RH, et al.: Establishment of carpal contents/canal ratio by means of magnetic resonance imaging. J Hand Surg 17A:843–849, 1992.

166. Stevens JC, Beard CM, O'Fallon WM, et al.: Conditions associated with carpal tunnel syndrome. Mayo Clin Proc 67:541–548, 1992.

167. Schottland JP, Kirschberg J, Fillingim R, et al.: Median nerve latencies in poultry processing workers: an approach to resolving the role of industrial "cumulative trauma" in the development of carpal tunnel syndrome. J Occup Med 33:627–631, 1991.

168. Nathan PA, Keniston RC, Myers LD, et al.: Obesity as a risk factor for slowing sensory conduction of the median nerve in industry: a cross-sectional and longitudinal study involving 429 workers. J Occup Med 34:379–383, 1992.

169. Nathan PA, Keniston RC, Myers LD, et al.: Longitudinal study of median nerve sensory conduction in industry: relationship to age, gender, hand dominance, occupational hand use, and clinical diagnosis. J Hand Surg 17A:850–857, 1992.

170. Phalen GS: The carpal tunnel syndrome. J Bone Joint Surg 48A:211–228, 1966.

171. Katz JN, Stirrat CR, Larson MG, et al.: A self-administered hand symptom diagram for the diagnosis and epidemiologic study of carpal tunnel syndrome. J Rheumatol 17:1495–1498, 1990.

172. Katz JN, Larson MG, Sabra, A: The carpal tunnel syndrome: diagnostic utility of the history and physical examination findings. Ann Intern Med 112:321–327, 1990.

173. Kuschner SH, Ebramzadeh E, Johnson D, et al.: Tinel's sign and Phalen's test in carpal tunnel syndrome. Orthopedics 15:1297–1302, 1992.

174. Spindler HA, Dellon AL: Nerve conduction studies and sensibility testing in carpal tunnel syndrome. J Hand Surg 7:260–263, 1982.

175. Szabo RM: Carpal tunnel syndrome. In: Szabo RM, ed. Nerve compression syndromes: diagnosis and treatment. Thorofare, NJ: Slack Inc., 1989: 101–120.

176. Hardy M, Jiminez S, Jabaley M: Evaluation of nerve compression with the Automated Tactile Tester. J Hand Surg 17A: 838–842, 1992.

177. Bendler, EM, Greenspun B, Yu J, Erdman WJ: The bilaterality of carpal tunnel syndrome. Arch Phys Med Rehabil 58:362–364, 1977.

178. Harris CM, Tanner E, Goldstein MN, Pettee DS: The surgical treatment of the carpal tunnel syndrome correlated with preoperative nerve conduction studies. J Bone Joint Surg 61A:93–98, 1979.

179. Kimura J: The carpal tunnel syndrome: localization of conduction abnormalities within the distal segment of the median nerve. Brain 102: 619–635, 1979.

180. Grant KA, Congleton JJ, Koppa RJ, et al.: Use of motor nerve conduction testing and vibration sensitivity testing as screening tools for carpal tunnel syndrome in industry. J Hand Surg 17A:71–76, 1992.

181. Steinberg DR, Gelberman RH, Rydevik B, et al.: The utility of portable nerve conduction testing for patients with carpal tunnel syndrome: a prospective clinical study. J Hand Surg 17A: 77–81, 1992.

182. Jetzer TC: Use of vibration testing in the early evaluation of workers with carpal tunnel syndrome. J Occup Med 33:117–120, 1991.

183. Durkan JA: A new diagnostic test for carpal tunnel syndrome. J Bone Joint Surg 73A: 535–538, 1991.

184. Occupational disease surveillance: carpal tunnel syndrome. MMWR 38:485–489, 1989.

185. Katz JN, Liang MH: Carpal tunnel syndrome and the workplace: epidemiologic and management issues. Internal Med Spec 9(5):64–73, 1988.

186. Buchberger W, Judmaier W, Birbamer G, et al.: Carpal tunnel syndrome: diagnosis with high-resolution sonography. Am J Roentgenol 159: 793–798, 1992.

186a. Howe FA, Saunders DE, Filler AG, et al.: Magnetic resonance neurography of the median nerve. Br J Radiol 67(804):1169–1172, 1994.

187. Nakamichi K, Tachibana S: The use of ultrasonography in detection of synovitis in carpal tunnel syndrome. J Hand Surg (Br) 18: 176–179, 1993.

188. Kruger VL, Kraft GH, Deitz JC, et al.: Carpal tunnel syndrome: objective measures and splint use. Arch Phys Med Rehabil 72:517–520, 1991.

189. Wiley BC: Exercise therapy for carpal tunnel syndrome. Aches Pains (Feb): 41–42, 1984.

190. Birkbeck MQ, Beer TC: Occupation in relation to the carpal tunnel syndrome. Rheumatol Rehabil 14:218–221, 1975.

191. Kaplan PE: Carpal tunnel syndrome in typists. JAMA 205:821–822, 1983.

192. Cannon LJ, Bernacki EJ, Walter SD: Personal and occupational factors associated with carpal tunnel syndrome. J Occup Med 23:255–258, 1981.

193. Emlen W, Dugowsen C: A new occupational association with carpal tunnel syndrome. (Abstract #107) Arthritis Rheum 26(4) [Suppl], 1983.

194. Wick WJ: Carpal tunnel syndrome: retailing. J Occup Med 23:524–525, 1981.

195. Marras WS: Toward an understanding of dynamic variables in ergonomics. Occup Med 7:655–677, 1992.

196. Omer GE, Jr: Median nerve compression at the wrist. Hand Clin 8:317–324, 1992.

197. Minamikawa Y, Peimer CA, Kambe K, et al.: Tenosynovial injection for carpal tunnel syndrome. J Hand Surg 17A:178–181, 1992.

198. Green DP: Diagnostic and therapeutic value of carpal tunnel injection. J Hand Surg 9A: 850–854, 1984.

199. Grundberg AB: Carpal tunnel decompression in spite of normal electromyography. J Hand Surg 8:348–349, 1983.

200. Louis DS, Hankin FM: Symptomatic relief following carpal tunnel decompression with normal electroneuromyographic studies. Orthopedics 10: 434–436, 1987.

201. Tountas CP, Macdonald CJ, Meyerhoff JD, Bihrle DM: Carpal tunnel syndrome a review of 507 patients. Minn Med 66:479–483, 1983.

202. Editorial: Surgical treatment of carpal tunnel syndrome. Lancet 1:1125, 1979.

203. Brown MG, Keyser B, Rothenberg ES: Endoscopic carpal tunnel release. J Hand Surg (Am) 17: 1009–1011, 1992.

204. Brown MG, Rothenberg ES, Keyser B, et al.: Results of 1236 endoscopic carpal tunnel release procedures using the Brown technique. Contemp Orthop 27: 251–258, 1993.

205. Brown RA, Gelberman RH, Seiler JG, et al.: Carpal tunnel release: a prospective randomized assessment of open and endoscopic methods. J Bone Joint Surg 75A:1265–1275, 1993.

206. Agee JM, McCarroll HR, Tortosa RD, et al.: Endoscopic release of the carpal tunnel: a randomized prospective multicenter study. J Hand Surg 17A:987–995, 1992.

207. Dobyns JH: Digital nerve compression. Hand Clin 8:359–367, 1992.

208. Young C, Hadson A, Richards, R: Operative treatment of palsy of the posterior interosseous nerve of the forearm. J Bone Joint Surg 72A: 1215–1219, 1990.

209. Deleu D: Mouse-directed computers and ulnar sensory neuropathy. J Neurol Neurosurg Psychiatry 55: 232–239, 1992.

210. Homans J: Minor causalgia: a hyperesthetic neurovascular syndrome. N Engl J Med 222: 870–874, 1940.

211. deJong RH, Cullen SC: Theoretical aspects of pain: bizarre pain phenomena during low spinal anesthesia. Anesthesiology 24:628–635, 1963.

212. Bonica JJ: Causalgia and other reflex sympathetic dystrophies. Postgrad Med 53:143–148, 1973.

213. Steinbrocker O, Argyros TG: The shoulder-hand syndrome: Present status as a diagnostic and therapeutic entity. Med Clin North Am 42: 1533–1553, 1958.

214. Mowat AG: Treatment of the shoulder-hand syndrome with corticosteroids. Ann Rheum Dis 33:120–123, 1974.

215. Pak TJ, Martin GM, Magness JL, Kavanaugh GJ: Reflex sympathetic dystrophy. Minn Med 53:507–512, 1970.

216. Geertzen JHB, deBruijn H, de Bruijn-Kofman AT, et al.: Reflex sympathetic dystrophy: early treatment and psychological aspects. Arch Phys Med Rehabil 75:442–446, 1994.

217. Procacci P, Francin F, Zoppi M, et al.: Role of sympathetic system in reflex dystrophies. In: Bonica JJ, Albe-Fessard DG, eds. Advances in pain research and therapy. Vol 1. New York: Raven Press, 1976.

218. Edeiken J, Wolferth CC: Persistent pain in the shoulder region following myocardial infarction. Am J Med Sci 191:201–210, 1936.

219. Christianssen K, Henriksen O: The reflex sympathetic dystrophy syndrome: an experimental study of blood flow and autoregulation in subcutaneous tissue. (Abstract #E42) Arthritis Rheum 25(4) [Suppl], 1982.

220. Bonica JJ: Neurophysiologic and pathologic aspects of acute and chronic pain. Arch Surg 112:750–761, 1977.

221. Melzach R, Wall PD: Pain mechanisms: a new theory. Science 150:971–979, 1965.

222. Schott GD: An unsympathetic view of pain. Lancet 1:634–636, 1995.

223. Ritchlin C, Chabot R, Kates S, et al.: Cortical abnormalities in patients with reflex sympathetic dystrophy. Abstract #690) Arthritis Rheum 37(9) [Suppl]:S275, 1994.

224. Harden RN, Duc TA, Williams TR, et al.: Norepinephrine and epinephrine levels in affected versus unaffected limbs in sympathetically maintained pain. Clin J Pain 10:324–330, 1994.

225. Schweitzer ME, Mandel S, Schwartzman RJ, et al.: Reflex sympathetic dystrophy revisited: MR

imaging findings before and after infusion of contrast material. Radiology 195:211–214, 1995.

226. Nickeson R, Brewer E, Person D: Early histologic and radionuclide scan changes in children with reflex sympathetic dystrophy syndrome. (Abstract #C38) Arthritis Rheum 28(4) [Suppl], 1985.

227. Kozin F, McCarty DJ, Sims, J, et al.: The reflex sympathetic dystrophy syndrome. I. Clinical and histologic studies: response to corticosteroids and articular involvement. Am J Med 60: 321–331, 1976.

228. Kozin F, Genant HK, Bekerman C, McCarty DJ: The reflex sympathetic dystrophy syndrome. II. Roentgenographic and scintigraphic evidence of bilaterality and of periarticular accentuation. Am J Med 60:332–338, 1976.

229. Kozin F, Ryan LM, Carerra GF, et al.: The reflex sympathetic dystrophy syndrome. III: Scintigraphic studies, further evidence for the therapeutic efficacy of systemic corticosteroids, and proposed diagnostic criteria. Am J Med: 70:23–30, 1981.

230. Kimball ES: Involvement of cytokines in neurogenic inflammation. In: Kimball ES, ed. Cytokines and inflammation. Boca Raton: CRC Press, 1991:169–189.

231. Mailis A, Wade J: Profile of caucasian women with possible genetic predisposition to reflex sympathetic dystrophy: a pilot study. Clin J Pain 10:210–217, 1994.

232. Carlson DH, Simon H, Wegner W: Bone scanning and diagnosis of reflex sympathetic dystrophy secondary to herniated lumbar disks. Neurology 27:791–793, 1977.

232a. Lee GW, Weeks PM: The role of bone scintigraphy in diagnosing reflex sympathetic dystrophy. J Hand Surg (Am) 20(3):458–463, 1995.

233. Irazuzta JE, Berde CB, Setha NF: Laser Doppler measurements of skin blood flow before, during, and after lumbar sympathetic blockade in children and young adults with reflex sympathetic dystrophy syndrome. J Clin Monit 8:16–19, 1992.

234. Sambrook P, Champion GD: Reflex sympathetic dystrophy: characteristic changes in bone on CT scan (letter). J Rheumatol 17:1425–1426, 1990.

235. Koch E, Hofer HO, Sialer G, et al.: Failure of MR Imaging to detect reflex sympathetic dystrophy of the extremities. Am J Roentgenol 156: 113–115, 1991.

236. Wilder RT, Berde CB, Wolohan M, et al.: Reflex sympathetic dystrophy in children. J Bone Joint Surg 74A:910–919, 1992.

237. Goldsmith DP, Vivino FB, Eichenfield AH, et al.: Nuclear imaging and clinical features of childhood reflex neurovascular dystrophy: comparison with adults. Arthritis Rheum 32:480–485, 1989.

238. Tabira R, Shibasake H, Kuroiwa Y: Reflex sympathetic dystrophy (causalgia) treatment with guanethidine. Arch Neurol 40:430–432, 1983.

239. Ghostine SY, Comair YG, Turner DM, Kassell NF, Azar CG: Phenoxybenzamine in the treatment of causalgia. J Neurosurg 60:1263–1268, 1984.

240. An HS, Hawthorne KB, Jackson WT: Reflex sympathetic dystrophy and cigarette smoking. J Hand Surg (Am) 13:458–460, 1988.

241. Hord AH, Rooks MD, Stephens BO, et al.: Intravenous regional bretylium and lidocaine for treatment of reflex sympathetic dystrophy: a randomized, double-blind study. Anesth Analg 74:818–821, 1992.

242. Duncan KH, Lewis RC, Jr, Racz G: Treatment of upper extremity reflex sympathetic dystrophy with joint stiffness using sympatholytic Bier blocks and manipulation. Orthopedics 11: 883–886, 1988.

242a. Jadad AR, Carroll D, Glynn CJ, McQuay HJ: Intravenous regional sympathetic blockade for pain relief in reflex sympathetic dystrophy: a systematic review and a randomized, double-blind crossover study. J Pain Symptom Manage 10(1):13–20, 1995.

243. Farah BA: Ketorolac in reflex sympathetic dystrophy. Clin Neuropharm 16:88–89, 1993.

244. Portwood MM, Lieberman JS, Taylor RG: Ultrasound treatment of reflex sympathetic dystrophy. Arch Phys Med Rehabil 68:116–118, 1987.

245. Wilkinson HA: Radiofrequency percutaneous upper-thoracic sympathectomy. N Engl J Med 311:34–48, 1984.

246. Samuelsson H, Claes G, Drot C: Endoscopic electrocautery of the upper thoracic sympathetic chain: a safe and simple technique for treatment of sympathetically maintained pain. Eur J Surg [Suppl] 572:55–57, 1994.

247. Dale WA, Lewis MR: Management of thoracic outlet syndrome. Ann Surg 181:575–585, 1975.

248. Jupiter JB, Seiler JG, Zienowicz R: Sympathetic maintained pain (causalgia) associated with a demonstrable peripheral-nerve lesion. J Bone Joint Surg 76A:1376–1384, 1994.

249. Greipp ME, Thomas AF: Reflex sympathetic dystrophy syndrome: a longitudinal study. Medsurg Nursing 3:378–381, 384, 1994.

250. Halverson PB, Cheung HS, McCarty DJ, et al.: ''Milwaukee shoulder:'' association of microspheroids containing hydroxyapatite crystals, active collagenase, and neutral protease with rotator cuff defects. I. Clinical aspects. Arthritis Rheum 24:464–473, 1981.

251. Duplay ES: De la périarthrite scapulohumérale et des raideurs de l'épaule qui en sont la conséquence. Arch Gen Med 20:513–542, 1872.

252. Clarke GR, Wilis LA, Fish WW, Nichols PJR: Preliminary studies in measuring range of motion in normal and painful stiff shoulders. Rheumatol Rehabil 14:39–46, 1975.

253. Reeves B: The natural history of the frozen shoulder syndrome. Scand J Rheumatol 4: 193–196, 1975.

254. Mattson RH, Cramer JA, McCutchen CB, et al.: Barbiturate-related connective tissue disorders. Arch Intern Med 149:911–914, 1989.

255. Bridgman JF: Periarthritis of the shoulder and diabetes mellitus. Ann Rheum Dis 31:69–71, 1972.

256. Loyd JA, Loyd HM: Adhesive capsulitis of the shoulder: arthrographic diagnosis and treatment. Southern Med J 76:879–883, 1983.

257. Wiley AM, Older MWJ: Shoulder arthroscopy. Am J Sports Med 8:31–38, 1980.

258. Ha'eri GB, Maitland A: Arthroscopic findings in the frozen shoulder. J Rheum 8:149–152, 1981.

259. Neviaser JS: Adhesive capsulitis of the shoulder: a study of the pathological findings in periarthritis of the shoulder. J Bone Joint Surg 27:211–222, 1945.

260. Wiley AM: Arthroscopic appearance of frozen shoulder. Arthroscopy 7:138–143, 1991.

261. Fareed DO, Gallivan WR Jr: Office management of frozen shoulder syndrome. Clin Orthop 242:177–183, 1989.

262. Ozaki J, Nakagawa Y, Sakurai G, et al.: Recalcitrant chronic adhesive capsulitis of the shoulder. J Bone Joint Surg (Am) 71A: 1511–1515, 1989.

263. Uhthoff HK, Sarkar K: Periarticular soft tissue conditions causing pain in the shoulder. Curr Opin Rheumatol 4:241–246, 1992.

264. Lundberg BJ: The frozen shoulder. Acta Orthop Scand [Suppl] 119, 1969.

265. Schulte L, Roberts MS, Zimmerman C, et al.: A quantitative assessment of limited joint mobility in patients with diabetes. Arthritis Rheum 36:1429–1443, 1993.

266. McCarty DJ, Halverson PB, Carrera GF, et al.: ''Milwaukee shoulder:'' association of microspheroids containing hydroxyapatite crystals, association with rotator cuff defects. II. Synovial fluid studies. Arthritis Rheum 24:474–483, 1981.

267. Weiser HI: Painful primary frozen shoulder mobilization under local anesthesia. Arch Phys Med Rehabil 58:406–408, 1977.

268. Thomas D, Williams RA, Smith DS: The frozen shoulder: a review of manipulative treatment. Rheum Rehabil 19:173–179, 1980.

269. Binder A, Hazleman BL, Parr G, et al.: A controlled study of oral prednisolone in frozen shoulder. Br J Rheumatol 25:288–292, 1986.

270. Binder AI, Bulgen DY, Hazleman BL, Roberts S: Frozen shoulder: a long-term prospective study. Ann Rheum Dis 43:361–364, 1984.

271. Bulgen DY, Binder AI, Hazleman BL, et al.: Frozen shoulder: prospective clinical study with an evaluation of three treatment regimens. Ann Rheum Dis 43:353-360, 1984.

272. Rizk TE, Pinals RS, Talaiver AS: Corticosteroid injections in adhesive capsulitis: investigation of their value and site. Arch Phys Med Rehabil 72:20–22, 1991.

273. Ekelund AL, Rydell N: Combination treatment for adhesive capsulitis of the shoulder. Clin Orthop 282:105–109, 1992.

274. Jacobs LGH, Barton MA, Wallace WA, et al.: Intra-articular distension and steroids in the management of capsulitis of the shoulder. Br Med J 302:1498–1501, 1991.

275. Morency G, Dussault RG, Robillard P, et al.: Distention arthrography in the treatment of adhesive capsulitis of the shoulder. Can Assoc Radiol J 40:84–86, 1989.

276. Hill JJ Jr, Bogumil H: Manipulation in the treatment of frozen shoulder. Orthopedics 11: 1255–1260, 1988.

277. Steinbrocker O, Argyros TG: Frozen shoulder: Treatment by local injections of depot corticosteroids. Arch Phys Med Rehabil 55:209–213, 1974.

278. Russek AS: Role of physical medicine in relief of certain pain mechanisms of shoulder. JAMA 156:1575–1577, 1954.

279. Groves RJ, Goldner JL: Contracture of the deltoid muscle in the adult after intramuscular injections. J Bone Joint Surg 56A: 817–820, 1974.

280. Enzi G, Carraro R, Alfieri P, et al.: Shoulder girdle lipomatosis. Ann Intern Med 117: 749–750, 1992.

281. Smith DL, McAfee JH, Lucas LM, et al.: Septic and nonseptic olecranon bursitis. Arch Intern Med 149:1581–1585, 1989.

282. Smith DL, McAfee JH, Lucas LM, et al.: Treatment of nonseptic olecranon bursitis. Arch Intern Med 149:2527–2530, 1989.

283. Kerr DR, Carpenter CW: Arthroscopic resection of olecranon and prepatellar bursae. Arthroscopy 6:86–88, 1990.

284. Karanjia ND, Stiles PJ: Cubital bursitis. J Bone Joint Surg 70B:832–833, 1988.

285. Ehrlich GE: Antecubital cysts in rheumatoid arthritis: a corollary to popliteal (Baker's) cysts. J Bone Joint Surg 54A:165–169, 1972.

286. Otu AA: Wrist and hand ganglion treatment with hyaluronidase injection and fine needle aspiration: a tropical African perspective. J Roy Coll Surg Edinb 37:405–407, 1992.

287. Fogel GR, Younge DA, Dobyns JH: Pitfalls in the diagnosis of the simple wrist ganglion. Orthopedics 6:990–992, 1983.

288. Ching DW, Petrie JP, Klemp P, et al.: Injection therapy of superficial rheumatoid nodules. Br J Rheumatol 31:775–777, 1992.

289. Cerofolini E, Luchetti R, Pederzini L, et al.: MR evaluation of triangular fibrocartilage complex tears in the wrist: comparison with arthrography and arthroscopy. J Comput Assist Tomogr 14:963–967, 1990.

290. Sullivan PP, Berquist TH: Magnetic resonance imaging of the hand, wrist, and forearm: utility in patients with pain and dysfunction as a result of trauma. Mayo Clin Proc 66:1217–1221, 1991.

291. Watson FM, Purvis JM: Acute calcareous deposits of the hand and wrist. Southern Med J 73:150–151, 1980.

292. Dilley DF, Tonkin MA: Acute calcific tendinitis in the hand and wrist. J Hand Surg 16B: 215–216, 1991.

293. Gerster JC, Lagier R: Upper limb pyrophosphate tenosynovitis outside the carpal tunnel. Ann Rheum Dis 48:689–691, 1989.

294. Simmons BP, Vasile RG: The clenched fist syndrome. J Hand Surg 5:420–427, 1980.

295. Swift DW, Walker SA: The clenched fist syndrome. Arthritis Rheum 38:57–60, 1995.

296. Sanavio E: An operant approach to the treatment of writer's cramp. J Behav Ther Exp Psychiatry 13:69–72, 1969.

297. Sheehy MP, Marsden CD: Writer's cramp: a focal dystonia. Brain 105:461–480, 1982.

298. Marsden CD, Rothwell JC: The physiology of idiopathic dystonia. Can J Neurol Sci 14 [Suppl 3]:521–527, 1987.

299. Newmark J, Hochberg FH: Isolated painless manual incoordination in 57 musicians. J Neurol Neurosurg Psychiatry 50:291–295, 1987.

300. Lockwood AH: Medical problems of musicians. N Engl J Med 320:221–227, 1989.

301. James JIP, Wynne-Davies R: Genetic factors in orthopaedics. In: Apley AG, ed. Recent advances in orthopaedics. London: J & A Churchill, 1969.

302. Vilijanto JA: Dupuytren's contracture: a review. Sem Arthritis Rheum 3:155–176, 1973.

303. Ling RSM: The genetic factor in Dupuytren's disease. J Bone Joint Surg 45B: 709–718, 1963.

304. Leslie BM: Palmar fasciitis and polyarthritis associated with a malignant neoplasm: a paraneoplastic syndrome. Orthopedics 15: 1436–1439, 1992.

305. Murrell GAC: Free radicals and Dupuytren's contracture. Br Med J 295(6610):1373–1375, 1987.

306. Rosenbloom AL, Silverstein JH, Lezotte DC, et al.: Limited joint mobility in childhood diabetes mellitus indicates increased risk for microvascular disease. N Engl J Med 305:191–194, 1981.

307. Knowles HB Jr: Joint contractures, waxy skin, and control of diabetes. N Engl J Med 305: 217–218, 1981.

308. Fitzcharles MA, Duby S, Waddell RW, et al.: Limitation of joint mobility (cheiroarthropathy) in adult noninsulin dependent diabetic patients. Ann Rheum Dis 43: 251–257, 1984.

309. Sibbitt WL, Jr: Diabetic stiff hand syndrome. Int Med Specialist 10(9):71–86,1989.

310. Robertson JR, Earnshaw PM, Campbell IW: Tenolysis in juvenile diabetic cheiroarthropathy. Br Med J 2:971–972, 1979.

311. Eaton RP, Sibbitt WL, Harsh A: The effect of an aldose reductase inhibiting agent on limited joint mobility in diabetic patients. JAMA 253:1437–1440, 1985.

312. Giugliano D, Marfella R, Quatraro A, et al.: Tolrestat for mild diabetic neuropathy. Ann Intern Med 118:7–11, 1993.

313. Redfern AB, Curtis RM, Wilgis EFS: Experience with peritendinous fibrosis of the dorsum of the hand. J Hand Surg 7:380–382, 1982.

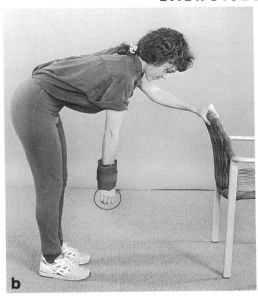

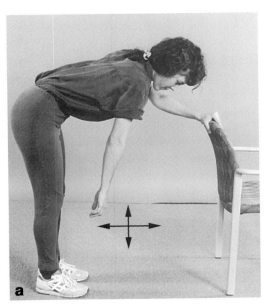

Exercise 3.A. Pendulum (Codman's) Exercise for Shoulder Mobility

Bending over with the affected arm hanging down, the patient swings the arm from the shoulder **(a)** forward and backward, side to side and **(b)** in 6–12-inch circles. A 3–5-pound weight on the wrist or in the hand provides additional traction and momentum to the swing.

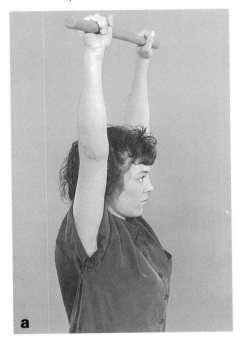

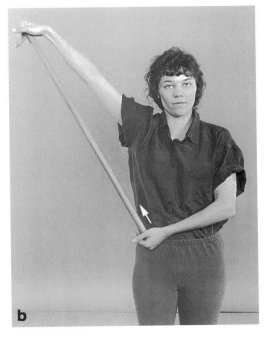

Exercise 3.B. Wand Exercises

Wand (or broomstick/yardstick) exercises help to mobilize the affected shoulder as the unaffected shoulder performs various movements, such as **(a)** wand flexion, **(b)** wand abduction, and **(c)** wand

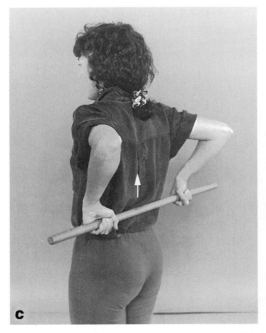

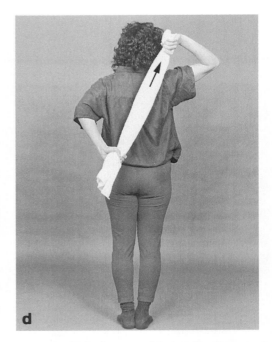

internal rotation. The patient performs the desired movement with both arms while holding the wand between both hands. **(d)** Towel internal rotation. The exercises above can be varied by using a towel stretched between the hands instead of a wand.

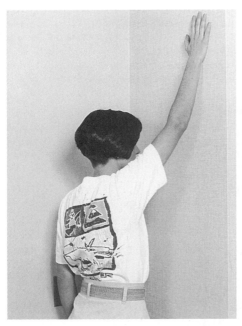

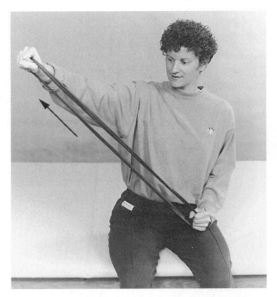

Exercise 3.C. Wall Climb Exercise for Shoulder Mobilization

The patient stands 1–2 feet away and facing the wall. The fingers "walk" up the wall, assisting shoulder flexion, abduction, and external rotation. Exercise effects can be varied by changing the patient's angle to the wall; external rotation will be increased as the patient turns away from the wall toward the 90-degree angle.

Exercise 3.D. Theraband (patented) Strengthening Exercise

As the Theraband is stretched by the exercising limb, it provides resistance in the direction of the pull. In this illustration, resistance is provided to right shoulder abduction, flexion, and the scapular stabilizers as the left arm secures the Theraband.

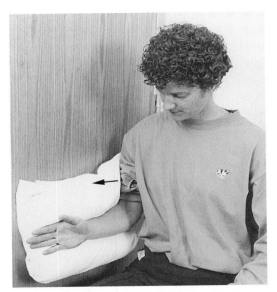

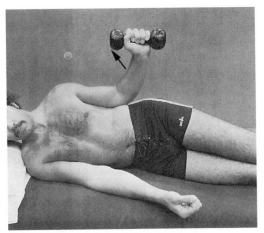

Exercise 3.E. Isometric Shoulder Strengthening

The patient pushes against a stable surface such as a wall so that the muscle is contracted, but no movement actually occurs. Shoulder abduction is illustrated. Shoulder flexion or extension can be strengthened by rotating the body toward or away from the wall and altering the direction of the contraction.

Exercise 3.F. Infraspinatus/Teres Minor Strengthening

Move the weight in the direction of the arrow to strengthen the infraspinatus and teres minor muscles. (From Jobe FW, Radovich-Moynes D: Delineation of diagnostic criteria and a rehabilitation program for rotator cuff injuries. Am J Sports Med 10:336–339, 1982.)

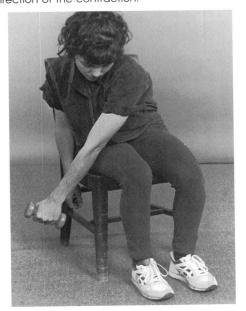

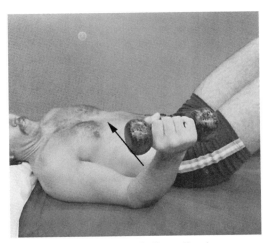

Exercise 3.G. Scapular Stretch

From a seated position, the patient grasps a 2–5-pound weight on the side of the pain and slowly moves (thrusts) the arm forward, then leans forward with the trunk straight and brings the arm across the chest so that a stretching sensation is felt in the painful parascapular region. The weight is allowed to approach but not to touch the floor. The stretch is held 10–30 seconds and repeated several times per day.

Exercise 3.H. Subscapularis Strengthening

The patient moves (lifts) the weight in the direction of the *arrow* to strengthen the subscapularis muscle. (From Jobe FW, Radovich-Moynes D: Delineation of diagnostic criteria and a rehabilitation program for rotator cuff injuries. Am J Sports Med 10:336–339, 1982.)

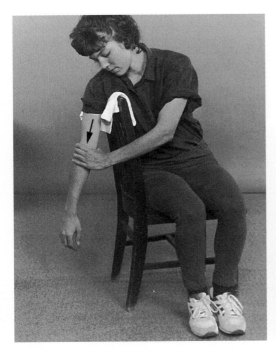

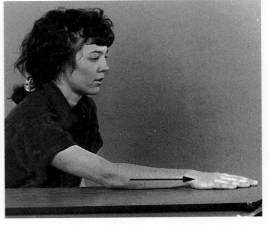

Exercise 3.1 (a). Distraction/Inferior Glide. The patient sits sideways at the edge of the seat with the right arm over the padded back of the chair as illustrated, axilla firmly placed on the top edge of the chair. Using the left hand, the patient grasps the *right* arm just above the humeral condyles or, alternatively, just above the *right* wrist. The patient pulls directly down toward the floor with the *left* arm with repeated rhythmic movements, exerting gentle distracting forces on the *right* shoulder. Alternate method: patient holds a 3–5-pound weight in the *right* arm, allowing the weight to stretch the shoulder capsule.

3.1 (b). Flexion. Patient sits with the arm supported, elbow straight, palm down. Patient bends forward, sliding the arm forward so that the arm is passively flexed.

Exercise 3.1. Self-Mobilization Techniques for the Shoulder Capsule

In these exercises the patient uses self-applied and carefully directed forces to gently mobilize and stretch the shoulder capsule. In the illustrations the right shoulder is to be mobilized.

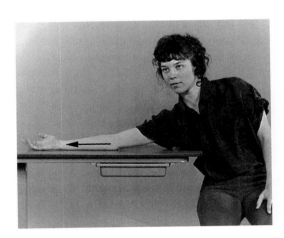

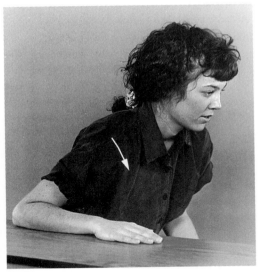

3.1 (c). Abduction biceps tendon stretch. Patient is seated with the forearm supported, palm up, elbow straight. Patient leans toward the *right* side, stretching the inferior and anterior capsule.

3.1 (d). Anterior capsule stretch. Patient is seated with the *right* forearm supported at the side as illustrated. Keeping the *right* arm fixed and stable, the patient leans the trunk forward, creating a gentle stretch at the anterior capsule (front of the shoulder). Trunk movements can be continued in a slow rhythmic series.

Exercise 3.1. Self-Mobilization Techniques for the Shoulder Capsule

In these exercises the patient uses self-applied and carefully directed forces to gently mobilize and stretch the shoulder capsule. In the illustrations the right shoulder is to be mobilized.

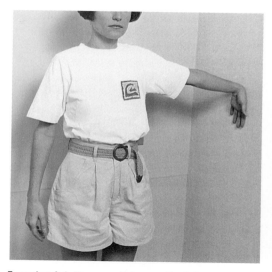

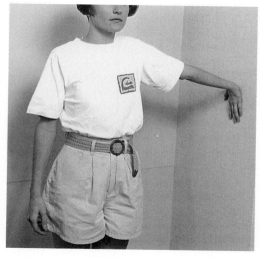

Exercise 3.J. Forearm Extensor Stretch
   The patient places the back of the hand (dorsal surface) against the wall and applies gentle pressure to achieve a stretch to the forearm extensor tissues. Hold 1 minute and do one repetition 3 times per day. This exercise is useful in the rehabilitation of lateral epicondylitis.

Exercise 3.K. Forearm Flexor Stretch
   The flexor tissue groups are stretched as in Exercise 3.J, but with gentle pressure on the palm of the hand. This exercise is useful in medial epicondylitis.

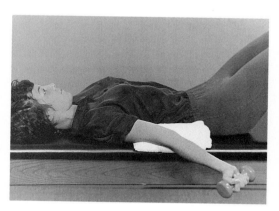

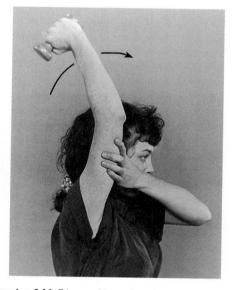

Exercise 3.L. Biceps Stretch
   This exercise provides a gentle stretch to the biceps and elbow capsule. The weight should not exceed 4 pounds, and the upper arm is stabilized on a firm surface. The position should be held 3–5 minutes and the exercise repeated 3 times per day.

Exercise 3.M. Triceps Strengthening
   Resistance exercise for strengthening the triceps muscle. Straighten arm as indicated with a 3–5-pound weight, 10 times per daily session.

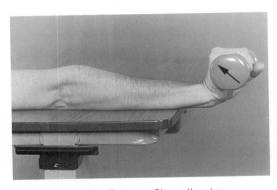

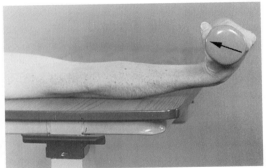

Exercise 3.N. Wrist Extensor Strengthening
   With the palm down, the patient extends the wrist against the resistance of a 1–5-pound weight held in the hand. Exercise is repeated 8–10 times per daily session. Decrease weight and/or repetitions if elbow or epicondylar pain increases.

Exercise 3.O. Wrist Flexor Strengthening
   With the palm up, the patient bends the wrist against resistance to strengthen flexor groups.

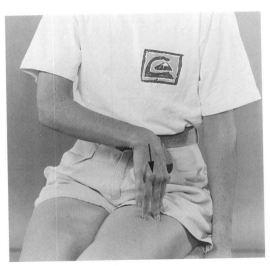

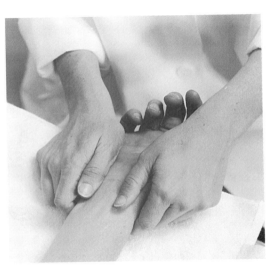

Exercise 3.P. Exercises to Stretch the Volar Carpal Ligament

3.P (a). Wiley's technique. Use forced wrist flexion to "bowstring" the flexor tendons, stretching the volar capsular tissues. The patient first holds the wrist, hand, and fingers of the involved side straight, then flexes the wrist, and then presses the straight fingers against the thigh, arm, or other stable surface with maximum force while slowly flexing the involved wrist to at least 45 degrees and holding the position 5 seconds. The exercise is to be repeated 3 times in succession, every few hours throughout the day.

3.P (b). Manual stretch of the volar carpal ligament. The operator's thumbs pull apart and the operator's fingers press upward on the patient's wrists. Continue for 10–20 seconds, six repetitions, several times a day.

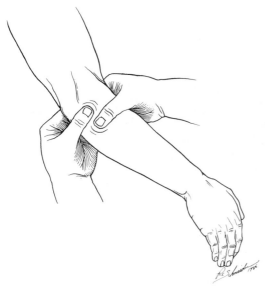

Exercise 3.Q. Friction Massage Technique for Tendinitis

The therapist uses deep massage across the musculotendinous fibrous tissues.

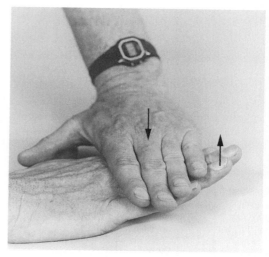

Exercise 3.R. Finger Extensor Strengthening

Finger extension exercises are performed against the other hand/arm. The fingers are extended (straightened) against the other hand/arm for resistance. Exercise is repeated 5–10 times per daily session, using maximum force. The movement can also be used as a strategy to relax the hand throughout the day, using less than maximum force. The patient is then instructed to extend the fingers 3–5 times several times per day.

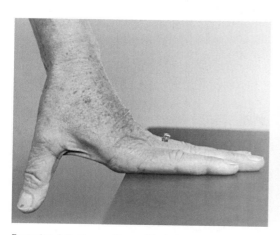

Exercise 3.S. Finger Flexor Stretch

Place hand palm down on table, fingers flat. Lift palm while keeping fingers flat. Stretch will be felt across palm and at finger/palm joint.

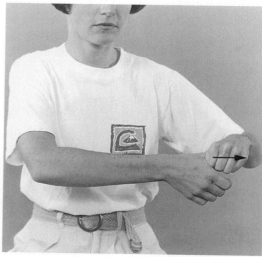

Exercise 3.T. Thumb Stretch (for de Quervain's Syndrome or Trigger Thumb)

The patient stretches the affected thumb by grasping it firmly with the other hand and applying gentle traction while moving it in straight and circular movements.

4: Thoracic and Chest Wall Pain Disorders

Chest wall pain disorders may occur as primary entities or may be secondary manifestations of other systemic disorders, or they may coexist with other serious underlying disorders. Myofascial chest wall pain syndrome is a symptom disorder with one or more tender points palpable on the chest wall that reproduce the chest discomfort.

The history and physical examination remain the most important and reliable diagnostic tools. Numerous questionnaires that would differentiate chest wall pain from intrathoracic causes for chest pain have been researched, yet none are as good as a probing finger (1, 2).

In the assessment of chest pain, examiners are very much influenced by the patient's body language and other nonverbal messages. The patient's style of presentation can have a profound effect on the examining physician. In one study, three groups of internists observed a videotaped interview of a "patient," an actress, who gave each group the same history, verbatim. One group witnessed the patient in a business-like presentation, the second group witnessed a histrionic characterization, and the third group simply read a verbatim transcript of the interview. Initial diagnostic impressions differed dramatically: a cardiac cause was suspected by 50% of physicians viewing the business-like portrayal, but only by 13% of those viewing the histrionic portrayal. A cardiac workup was undertaken by 93% of the physicians viewing the business-like portrayal presentation versus only 53% for the histrionic portrayal (3). Those who read only the transcript made a cardiac diagnosis 36% of the time and 73% undertook a cardiac workup.

Panic attacks often present with severe chest pain and fear of impending death. A history of previous episodes suggesting panic must be obtained.

Important critical signs and symptoms must be delineated (Table 4.1). Myocardial infarction is occurring more frequently in women, yet consideration for cardiac origin of chest pain is often delayed in women compared to men. Women who smoke or have hypertension or other risk factors for heart disease are prime candidates for cardiac origin of chest pain.

Chest pain may arise from structures superior to the chest, within the chest (intrathoracic), inferior to the chest, posterior to the chest, or from structures involving the chest wall. A hands-on examination must not end with the use of the stethoscope! Careful palpation for local areas of exaggerated tenderness (pain points) is potentially the most fruitful component of the physical examination. Myofascial chest wall pain is common, but is often the last condition to be considered, and then only after thousands of dollars have been needlessly expended. Table 4.2 presents a decision chart for chest pain.

TABLE 4.1 POTENTIALLY CRITICAL FEATURES FOR CHEST PAIN

1. Fever, chills, sweats
2. Lymphadenopathy
3. Weight loss
4. Bruits or significant murmurs
5. Pericardial rub
6. Pleural rub
7. Retrosternal chest pain during effort
8. Pain localized to a single site, and worsening
9. Limitation of chest expanse
10. Pain that radiates to the midthoracic spine
11. Pain that radiates to the neck, or to the left or both arms, or to the axilla
12. Hemoptysis
13. Any unexplained laboratory abnormality

TABLE 4.2 DECISION CHART: CHEST PAIN

Problem	Action	Other Actions

1. Chest pain, unilateral, nonacute
   Duration for hours
   Not only effort-induced
   Trigger points present
	General examination
	ECG and chest roentgenogram
	Assess how activities at work and
	   home/play are done
	Advise regarding correction of
	   aggravating habits
		Bone scan
		NSAIDs trial
		GI workup

2. Chest pain, bilateral, nonacute
   Tender costochondral joints,
   symmetric
   Chest expanse limited (<4 cm)
	Exercises, including stretching
	Medications: nitroglycerine,
	   antidepressants, relaxants,
	   serotonin reuptake inhibitors
		Trial NSAIDs

3. Chest pain, bilateral, nonacute
   Numbness of upper limbs
   present
	Local injection of steroid and local
	   anesthetic mixture
	Advise to stop smoking
	+ Bone scan, tests for
	     inflammation
	+ Examine for thoracic outlet
	     syndrome	

4. DANGER LIST
   Fever, chills
   Effort pain
   Pain radiation to midthorax,
     shoulder
   Numbness and weakness,
     upper limb
   Hemoptysis
   Pleural pain
   Axillary pain
	→ Chest roentgenogram
	Workshop as appropriate
	Cardiac stress testing
	Urgent consultation →
		GI workup
		Cardiac workup
		Roentgenograms
		   of chest and
		   neck

CHEST PAIN ARISING FROM STRUCTURES SUPERIOR TO THE CHEST

Panic and other psychophysiologic disorders deserve special emphasis. In patients who were urgently admitted for the first time with chest pain, Kisely et al. noted that patients with normal coronary angiograms, when compared to those with abnormality, were more likely to smoke and drink alcohol excessively; in addition, these patients had twice as many psychiatric disorders in the follow-up period (4).

In a study of 334 patients with acute chest pain presenting at an emergency room, one-third had evidence of panic disorder or depression, and this group of patients was more likely to have had multiple visits to an emergency room compared to those without psychiatric disorder (5). A five-year follow-up of younger patients with chest pain lacking organic cause demonstrated that those with tension and anxiety continued to suffer chest pain for several years with continued use of urgent care centers. Intervention had no significant impact on pain (6).

Cervical disc disease and thoracic outlet disturbance may give rise to referred pain that involves the chest region. Active neck motion aggravating neuropathic chest pain (pain and paresthesia) suggests a C6-C7 disc compression causing chest pain (7). Precordial chest pain and features of angina may be caused by cervical nerve root irritation (8). The Spurling maneuver may be useful when cervical origin for pain is suspected (9, 10) (see Chapter 2).

When chest wall pain results from thoracic outlet syndrome, additional symptoms of paresthesia in the upper extremities and a sensation of arm swelling occur. The Roos test or modified Adson test is helpful (see Chapter 2).

CHEST PAIN ARISING FROM INTRATHORACIC STRUCTURES

A brief list of intrathoracic causes for chest pain is presented in Table 4.3. A careful history of the quality, duration, radiation, and precipitating causes of the pain must be undertaken. Anginal pain classically occurs in the retrosternal region and may radiate into the neck, the left arm, and occasionally into the medial aspect of

TABLE 4.3 SOURCES OF CHEST PAIN OF INTRATHORACIC ORIGIN

1. Classic Heberden's angina (arteriosclerotic heart disease)
2. Angina of pulmonary hypertension or aortic stenosis
3. Prinzmetal's angina (arteriosclerotic heart disease)
4. Acute myocardial infarction
5. Dressler's syndrome (post–myocardial infarction syndrome)
6. Postpericardiotomy syndrome
7. Pericarditis
8. Mitral valve prolapse
9. Dissection of the aorta
10. Diseases of the pleura
11. Pulmonary embolism
12. Pneumothorax
13. Disease of the esophagus
14. Mediastinal or pulmonary neoplasms
15. Diaphragmatic irritation

both arms. Angina is usually distinguishable from pain of chest wall origin by its brief duration, its aggravation by cold and exertion, and its relief with rest. Chest wall pain, by contrast, lasts for hours or days, occurs at rest, and may improve with general activity. In one study, 11% of patients with a history of true angina had chest wall tenderness and normal angiograms (11).

Pericardial pain, which is retrosternal, is often worse in the recumbent position and improves when the patient sits up and forward, and may be accentuated by deep breathing. Complaints of chest discomfort, fatigue, dyspnea, palpitations, tachycardia, anxiety, and neurotic behavior have been described in the past under various labels, including "neurocirculatory asthenia," DaCosta's syndrome, or "effort syndrome" (12). These symptoms also occur in the hyperventilation syndrome, panic attack, and panic disorder.

Chest pain may be part of an autonomic nervous system dysfunction. Mitral valve prolapse is often asymptomatic. Some patients have a constellation of symptoms that includes sudden severe aching in the chest and extremities and vasomotor instability. The pain is not angina in most instances. Inasmuch as 25% of subjects have mitral valve prolapse, attribution of this disorder to the etiology of chest pain is difficult. Autonomic nervous system dysfunction is suggested by abnormal response to a tilt table, Valsalva maneuver, and cold pressor tests. The symptomatic patients may demon-

strate a wildly oscillating heart rate or prolonged bradycardia (13). Chest wall pain points are common (14). Treatment with beta blockers has been helpful. Others have suggested serotonin reuptake inhibitors. Mitral valve prolapse may be a manifestation of Ehlers-Danlos syndrome, Marfan's syndrome, or the marfanoid syndrome.

Pleural pain is generally located on one side of the chest, is accentuated by breathing, and is generally not aggravated by movement.

Hiatus hernia and reflux esophagitis are common causes for anterior chest pain. Chest wall tenderness may occur. The discomfort is often accentuated by recumbency. If the examiner exerts pressure to the epigastrium, just below the xiphoid process, this maneuver frequently reproduces the pain of esophageal origin. Patients with mild esophageal motor dysfunction also have a high prevalence of psychiatric disorder and often respond to psychopharmacologic treatment (15).

CHEST PAIN ARISING FROM STRUCTURES INFERIOR TO THE CHEST

Chest pain may result from gas entrapment syndromes, biliary tract disease, peptic or gastric ulcer, pancreatitis, and subphrenic abscess. Gastric ulcers and gastritis may occur with marked variability in history, severity, and chronicity. Nevertheless, a history of bowel dysfunction, weight loss, stool changes, or dietary indiscretion should provide clues to these conditions.

Myofascial pain points in the rectus abdominis, serratus posterior inferior, iliocostalis, and other torso muscles may give rise to pain in the anterolateral chest or posterior chest areas (16).

CHEST PAIN ARISING FROM DISORDERS POSTERIOR TO THE CHEST

Chest pain may arise from herpes zoster, lesions of the dorsal spine such as osteoporosis, costovertebral joint dysfunction, tumor, Scheuermann's disease, and, rarely, thoracic disc disease.

Osteoporosis often presents with pain that radiates from the back to the front around both sides of the chest, and is often aggravated by sitting. Tumor pain and disc pain are highly variable; neurologic findings of the lower limbs must be carefully appraised. Intermittent long tract signs are common.

Costovertebral joint dysfunction may follow medical or surgical procedures with trauma to the chest wall or repetitious twisting movements. The pain typically follows the involved intercostal nerve pathway and is aggravated by twisting movement. Tenderness is elicited by firm palpation over the involved costovertebral joint. Relief following injection with a local anesthetic confirms the diagnosis.

CHEST PAIN ARISING FROM THE CHEST WALL STRUCTURES

Rib trauma or fracture, metastatic tumors, and other lesions evident on radiologic examination may cause pain and local tenderness.

Costochondritis is rarely a pathologic finding. The term should be reserved for inflammatory disease of the costosternal joints. Whenever *bilateral* anterior chest pain and tenderness is noted in a younger patient, consider spondyloarthropathy (nonspinal involvement of the musculoskeletal system in association with HLA-B27 antigen). Tests of inflammation may be normal, yet scintigraphy will often demonstrate bilateral uptake at the costosternal joints. Tietze's syndrome presents with swelling of the upper costosternal region and will be discussed more fully below. Infections may involve the costosternal joints, particularly among intravenous drug abusers; *Aspergillus* was found to be the offending organism in three such reported patients. Scintigraphy may be more accurate than computed tomography for assessing septic costosternal joints (17). When inflammation is not present, the term *costosternal syndrome* is preferred.

The clinician should also consider diseases of the breasts and the regional lymph nodes.

LABORATORY TESTS AND IMAGING

As discussed, the history and physical examination remain the most significant diagnostic tools for evaluating chest pain. The clinician must consider the psychosocial milieu as well as what past treatment measures have been attempted and with what results. A therapeutic trial with medication for suspected acid reflux and other gastrointestinal diseases may be performed if clinically feasible before expensive or invasive diagnostic procedures are used. As mentioned, psychotropic agents may improve patients with manometric evidence for esophageal dysfunction.

The edrophonium test has been used, but it should be noted that results may be more abnormal when patients are told that the test is expected to reproduce symptoms than when the patients are told that the medication is given to observe changes in the tracing (18). Many other tests are used to induce esophageal symptoms or to measure motility, but the results may have little relation to outcome and may therefore be irrelevant (19).

When the patient has atypical angina, a recommended approach is to combine treadmill exercise with thallium-201 imaging, two-dimensional echocardiography, or positron emission tomography. The latter may in time become the procedure of choice; however, it is expensive and not widely available. Coronary angiography and Doppler flow studies provide functional assessment (20). Again, when psychiatric disease is present, even with objective coronary disease, psychopharmacology will be important to the outcome.

The decision chart presented in Table 4.2 may be helpful for the workup.

MYOFASCIAL CHEST WALL SYNDROMES

Included here are subacute and chronic painful conditions of the anterior chest wall associated with tenderness of the chest wall structures (Fig. 4.1; see also Anatomic Plate XIV). Swelling does not occur.

The commonly described myofascial chest wall syndromes include the *costosternal syndrome,* the *sternalis syndrome, xiphodynia,* and the *rib-tip syndrome.* Each of these descriptive syndromes is characterized by local chest wall tenderness with accompanying pain, of a severity ranging from a dull ache to a throbbing intense discomfort.

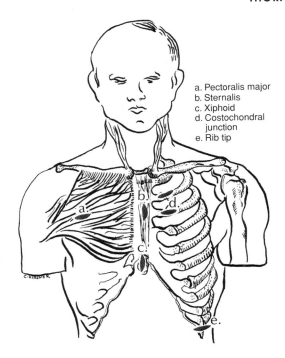

a. Pectoralis major
b. Sternalis
c. Xiphoid
d. Costochondral
   junction
e. Rib tip

Figure 4.1. Myofascial chest wall pain. Myofascial trigger points may be found (a) at the second or third left costochondral junction in the upper outer chest quadrant within the pectoralis major muscle; (b) at the manubriosternal junction; (c) at the tip of the xiphoid process; (d) at the center of the sternum in the sternalis muscle; or (e) on a lower rib tip.

In these myofascial chest wall syndromes, pain is present at rest and during chest movement; it lasts up to several hours or days, and it may be related to breathing. Anxiety and hyperventilation may occur. Occasionally myofascial chest wall pain syndrome is superimposed upon true angina and causes severe disability (21). Nitroglycerin may relieve myofascial chest wall pain unrelated to angina (22). The response to nitroglycerin is therefore not always helpful in differential diagnosis.

Although occasionally considered as one entity, *chest wall pain syndrome* (21), most physicians prefer individual terminology, depending on points of maximum tenderness in the chest wall. These syndromes require consideration for multifactorial diagnosis and treatment.

Costosternal Syndrome

This term applies to conditions involving and limited to pain in the anterior part of the chest wall. The pain sometimes radiates to the whole anterior chest region and may be accentuated by deep inspiration (23). The pains are usually intermittent, last a few days, and occur intermittently for months or years. *The specific feature of costosternal syndrome is the presence of tenderness and pain reproduction during palpation at one or more costosternal junctions.* Tenderness may also be noted along the nearby intercostal muscles. Relief from pain by a local anesthetic or anesthetic-corticosteroid injection of the involved costochondral joint area is an additional feature of the syndrome (23). Treatment should include posture correction and chest wall stretching (refer to exercises below).

The Sternalis Syndrome

The sternalis syndrome is the only myofascial disorder in which a pain point gives rise to bilateral anterior chest pain (24). The pain point is in the sternal synchondrosis, or in the sternalis muscle overlying the body of the sternum (Fig. 4.1). Pain is noted in the center of the chest wall, and usually the patient recognizes that the origin of the pain is in the chest wall region, rather than within the thorax. The symptoms tend to be less intermittent and the severity less frightening than in those disorders associated with the costosternal syndrome.

Xiphodynia

Xiphodynia is a syndrome characterized by spontaneous pain in the anterior chest associated with distinct discomfort and tenderness of the xiphoid process of the sternum (25). Pressure over the xiphoid reproduces the pain, which is intermittent and often aggravated by eating a heavy meal, lifting, stooping, bending, or twisting. Intralesional injection with a local anesthetic can provide prompt temporary or permanent relief, and will aid in diagnosis (26). "Tack hammer" deformity of the xiphoid is another cause for xiphoid pain and may require surgical excision (27).

Rib-Tip Syndrome

Rib-tip syndrome differs from others in that the patient presents with severe lancinating pain

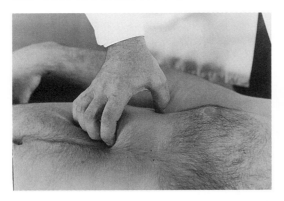

Figure 4.2. The hooking maneuver. The examiner's curved fingers are hooked under the lower ribs, then the rib cage is gently pulled anteriorly. This reproduces a snapping sensation and pain.

associated with hypermobility of the anterior end of a costal cartilage, most often the tenth rib but occasionally involving the eighth or ninth rib (28). The syndrome, variously called slipping rib, slipping rib cartilage syndrome, or clicking rib, is characterized by hypermobility of a rib-tip. Digital pressure over the involved rib may reproduce a painful clicking. The slipping rib syndrome results from recurrent subluxation of a costal cartilage, and is associated with a stabbing or lancinating pain (29). The pain is easily confused with abdominal visceral disease (30). Injury or indirect trauma due to lifting or twisting is often the cause (31, 32). Other features of the syndrome include pain aggravated by arm abduction, audible clicking sensation in the chest wall, and relief of pain by lying down (32).

Physical examination includes the ''hooking maneuver''—the examiner's curved fingers are hooked under the ribs at the costal margin and the examiner gently pulls the rib cage anteriorly (30) (Fig. 4.2); this reproduces the snap and pain. Excision of the involved rib has been recommended, but a steroid–local anesthetic injection into the intercostal muscles adjacent to a slipping rib may be of value. In other cases, only the rib-tip of the lower ribs is tender, and the pain is self-limited. Many patients can learn maneuvers to reposition the rib with muscle contraction and small movement patterns.

Physical examination for myofascial chest pain should include a measurement of chest expansion. Inflammatory rheumatic disease of the chest wall (e.g., ankylosing spondylitis) restricts chest expansion, and may indicate inflammation of the sternocostal joints (13).

Tests and Maneuvers for Myofascial Chest Wall Pain Syndromes

Thoracic spine motion, spinal curves, and symmetry of the chest wall and the breasts should be evaluated. Careful palpation of the supraclavicular fossae and axillae for lymphadenopathy should be performed. Palpation is best performed beginning with the acromioclavicular joints, continuing to the sternoclavicular joints, and then down each of the costosternal joints. The sternal synchondrosis, the overlying sternalis muscle, and the xiphoid process should be palpated. Xiphodynia must be distinguished from the deeper epigastric tenderness of gastrointestinal disease. A helpful way to distinguish these is to compare the tenderness to palpation in the epigastrium while the patient performs a partial sit-up, with the severity of discomfort during palpation while the patient is relaxed and recumbent. Xiphodynia and superficial lower chest wall pain are worse during the partial sit-up. Conversely, true intraabdominal lesion tenderness is diminished during contraction of the superficial abdominal muscles, and worsens when the abdominal muscles are relaxed.

The distinguishing characteristic of myofascial chest pain is the ability to reproduce the pain state by local pressure (21). Associated pain points may also be found over the pectoralis muscles, the lower sternocleidomastoid muscle area (25), the tip of the lower costal cartilages (28), and most commonly, the third left costochondral joint (33). Bilateral chest wall pain may result from a pain point in the sternalis muscle (24). ''If local pressure applied to the anterior part of the chest wall becomes a routine procedure in the physical examination of all patients with precordial pain, a surprisingly large number of cases of costosternal syndromes will be discovered'' (23). This statement was published in 1976, and remains true today. A finger poke on the chest wall is more valuable than questionnaires or imaging in most instances. When present, chest wall tenderness indicates treatment first, testing later.

Etiology. Inflammatory rheumatic disease can cause myofascial symptoms and must be excluded. Anxiety is common in patients with chest wall pain syndrome. However, psychologic investigations suggest that pure psychogenic chest pain is uncommon (34). On the other hand, acute anxiety and panic may result from episodes of myofascial chest wall pain. Injection of the pain point, performed as a therapeutic test, may alleviate both the pain and the anxiety.

Myofascial chest wall pain syndrome usually results from "misuse" activity or improper postures similar to those which cause myofascial pain in other body regions. An attack of chest wall pain may follow prolonged sitting in a slouched position or assuming a bent-over position (35). Chest pain has been a common complaint in users of video display terminals. Whether the pain arises from the chest wall or the gastrointestinal tract remains unknown (36). The pectoral muscles may be overworked in activities that require repeated adduction of the arm across the chest (e.g., stacking logs, polishing a car). Older persons may excessively use the trunk muscles when pushing off from chairs.

A pain-spasm-pain cycle may ensue, which is aggravated by anxiety (37). The clinician must consider household chores, job, and hobbies as possible aggravating factors. Smokers who cough are not only at risk for developing these syndromes, but often their response to treatment is less satisfactory unless smoking is curtailed. Table 4.4 presents some of the common aggravating factors.

Laboratory and Radiologic Examination. Myofascial chest wall pain has no specific laboratory abnormalities. An erythrocyte sedimentation rate determination is useful to exclude tumors or other inflammatory processes. A roentgenogram of the chest and an electrocardiogram are required for most patients. However, the highest yield for chest roentgenogram is found in patients with cough, dyspnea, or pleuritic chest pain (7). Calcification of costal cartilages is commonly present, and any association to the pain is speculative (L Lovshin, personal communication, 1960). Scintigraphy may be considered for patients with bilateral tender costochondral joints. When costochondritis is due to a spondyloarthropathy, the scan

TABLE 4.4 AGGRAVATING FACTORS FOR DISORDERS OF THE CHEST

Posture: practice good body alignment, especially during reading, writing, keyboarding, and sewing. The head, neck, and shoulders should be supported by the trunk and in line with it.

Use good breathing patterns to maintain chest wall flexibility.

Smoking-induced cough aggravates chest wall pain. *STOP SMOKING.*

Sleeping with the arms overhead can pinch nerves, thus causing chest wall pain. Sleep with the arms below chest level, not overhead.

When working with the arms overhead (e.g., painting a ceiling), place the body strategically so as to work upward and forward. Perform shoulder strengthening and spine extension exercises.

Sports

Improper weight lifting techniques can cause chest wall muscle strain. Use supervised conditioning and warm-up procedures.

Use appropriate protective equipment during sports activities.

may demonstrate involvement of symmetric costochondral joints as well as other axial skeletal joints.

If significant psychiatric disturbance is absent, and features suggest possible gastrointestinal disorder, an edrophonium test, an esophageal motility study using radionuclide esophageal transit testing, and acid perfusion testing may be indicated (38–40). Electrodiagnostic testing of the upper extremities occasionally helps to delineate chest wall pain that results from cervical nerve root impingement.

Differential Diagnosis. In most cases, chest wall pain syndromes can be differentiated from other, more serious disorders (41). In one community hospital emergency room, only 7 of 50 consecutive patients seen for chest pain had coronary artery disease (LA Mohan, personal communication, 1981). Myofascial chest wall pain was the cause for chest pain in the majority of the remaining patients, and in another study was responsible for approximately 2% of all office visits (33).

Chest wall pain in association with psychiatric disturbance is atypical and bears no relation to activity, time of day, or thoracic structures. The pain is usually centered over the cardiac apex. Often there are no discrete pain points that reproduce the pain, and sometimes all areas are exquisitely tender (the "touch-me-not'' syndrome). Such pain frequently accompanies anxiety and depression, has an emotional precipitant, and generally does not awaken the patient during sleep (34).

A chest wall pain syndrome may be the presenting feature of fibromyalgia. Such patients will demonstrate tenderness in tender point locations and not in control sites, and have post-sleep fatigue and widespread aching (Chapter 7).

Management. Most attacks of myofascial chest wall pain are self-limited, and the patient may require only reassurance. For patients with subacute and chronic recurring myofascial chest wall pain, these six steps for management should be followed:

1. Exclude other organic disease.
2. Provide the patient with an explanation of the pain. The presence of a local tenderness goes far to demonstrate to the patient that the pain does indeed originate outside of his or her head or heart. The physician should briefly describe the pain-spasm-pain cycle and its aggravation by fatigue or emotion.
3. Recognize and eliminate aggravating factors (Table 4.4). These include improper posture while sitting or working, misuse of pectoralis major muscles, and prolonged sedentary activities, such as typing (Exercise 4.A). Smokers should be encouraged to quit; group therapy is often available for this purpose.
4. Instruct the patient on self-help techniques and appropriate exercises to lengthen, strengthen, and retrain muscles. Chest wall stretching can be accomplished easily (Exercises 4.B and 4.C). Posture retraining and correction exercises may also be necessary (Exercises 4.D, 4.E, and 4.F).
5. Provide for relief from pain. Pain originating from myofascial chest wall pain points may be relieved either by applying local pressure, massage, or ice (25, 37), or by local injection with a steroid–local anesthetic mixture (Fig. 4.3). At least two-thirds of patients obtain good results with these methods (23). Intralesional injection is best carried out with a 1-inch No. 23 needle, 1 or 2 mL 1% lidocaine hydrochloride mixed with 10–40 mg

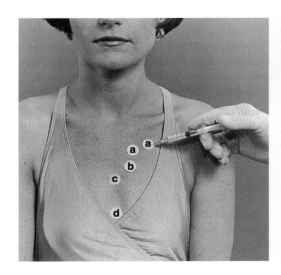

Figure 4.3. Sites for injection: (a) second and third costochondral junctions; (b) pectoralis major muscle; (c) sternalis muscle; and (d) xiphoid process.

methylprednisolone or similar nonaqueous crystalline steroid. After careful skin preparation, the needle is used as a guide to locate the point of maximum tenderness. When multiple lesions are present, 10–15 mg methylprednisolone can be used on each lesion, the total dose not to exceed 40 mg methylprednisolone. If fibromyalgia is contributing to the pain, the use of relaxation tapes, tricyclic antidepressants, cyclobenzaprine, or carisoprodol may be helpful. Self-help techniques should be used regularly.

6. Project an expected outcome. Most patients with myofascial chest wall pain who follow these management principles obtain good relief in 3 to 6 weeks. The exercises should be kept up for at least 6 weeks following relief. The patient must conscientiously avoid improper posture or repeated misuse of chest wall muscles.

When the chest wall pain syndrome and underlying arteriosclerotic heart disease coexist, careful attention to treatment of both disorders is essential. Smoking should be discontinued, since a chronic cough may cause chest wall muscle fatigue and subsequent spasm. Similarly, patients with chest wall pain superimposed upon chronic bronchitis and emphysema should stop smoking. Relaxation techniques and biofeedback training along with physical therapy are helpful. Patients with no other underlying cause for continued distress should be closely reevaluated for other causes. A trial of tricyclic antidepressant medication may be rewarding. Although muscle relaxants have not proved helpful, drugs to control anxiety may be useful in an overly anxious patient. Amitriptyline and other tricyclics may be beneficial for sleep disturbances or as anxiolytic agents for nocturnal panic that sometimes occurs in these patients. The value of analgesic compounds is limited, but prescribing a nonsteroidal antiinflammatory agent may be worthwhile, especially if tests of inflammation suggest the possibility of a spondylarthritis underlying the chest pain syndrome. In some patients a therapeutic trial using a nitroglycerine compound may provide relief but the relief should not be considered as proof of the presence of arteriosclerotic heart disease (21).

TIETZE'S SYNDROME

Costochondral region pain associated with enlargement of an upper costochondral cartilage characterizes Tietze's syndrome (42, 43) (Fig. 4.4). Tietze's syndrome may be acute, intermittent, or chronic. The swelling is firm to bony-hard, slightly elongated, or, less often, round. This feature of swelling, not seen in other myofascial chest wall pain syndromes, must be emphasized. It is for this reason that Tietze's syndrome is considered separate from other chest wall pain syndromes. In approximately 80% of cases the lesion is single. Most often it occurs in the second costochondral junction, and less often in the third costochondral junction on one side or the other (44). The swelling is nonsuppurative and tender, and histological examination reveals increased vascularity with proliferation of columns of cartilage. Cleft formation with mucoid debris is seen (45). The etiology is unknown. Some believe it is a rheumatoid variant (46). Radiologic examination usually reveals little, and tests for inflammation are generally normal.

Differential diagnosis includes mainly sepsis or tumors of the underlying rib, or pain from intrathoracic structures. Radiologic examination may be required periodically to exclude other diseases. Although spontaneous remission generally occurs, months or years may elapse before improvement is noted. Biopsy of the rib may be required for reassurance. We have found local injections with a corticosteroid-anesthetic mixture to be effective. Patients with persistent symptoms should have a bone scan to exclude sepsis and evidence of systemic inflammation. Persistent symptoms may be helped by local physical therapy, including hot or cold applications, and by nonsteroidal antiinflammatory drugs.

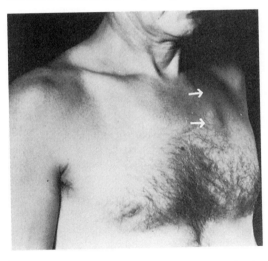

Figure 4.4. The Tietze's syndrome lesion. Costochondral swelling is observed. (Photograph courtesy Dr. John Calabro, Worcester, Mass.)

REFERENCES

1. Wise CM, Semble CM, Dalton CB: Musculoskeletal chest wall syndromes in patients with noncardiac chest pain: a study of 100 patients. Arch Phys Med Rehabil 73:147–149, 1992.
2. Buntinx F, Truyen J, Embrechts P, et al.: Evaluating patients with chest pain using classification and regression trees. Fam Pract 9: 149–153, 1992.
3. Birdwell BG, Herbers JE, Kroenke K: Evaluating chest pain. Arch Intern Med 153: 1991–1995, 1993.
4. Kisely SR, Creed FH, Cotter L: The course of psychiatric disorder associated with non-specific chest pain. J Psychosom Res 36: 329–335, 1992.
5. Yingling KW, Wulsin LR, Arnold LM, et al.: estimated prevalences of panic disorder and

depression among consecutive patients seen in an emergency department with acute chest pain. J Gen Intern Med 8:231–235, 1993.

6. Roll M, Kollind M, Theorell T: Five-year follow-up of young adults visiting an emergency unit because of atypical chest pain. J Intern Med 231: 59–65, 1992.

7. Butcher BL, Nichol KL, Parenti CM: High yield of chest radiography in walk-in clinic patients with chest symptoms. J Gen Intern Med 8:115–119, 1993.

8. Myers G, Freeman R, Scharf D, et al.: Cervico-precordial angina: diagnosis and management (Abstract). Am J Cardiol 39:287, 1977.

9. Nachlas W: Pseudo-angina pectoris originating in the cervical spine. JAMA 103:323–325, 1934.

10. Yeung MC, Hagen NA: Cervical disc herniation presenting with chest wall pain. Can J Neurol Sci 20:59–61, 1993.

11. Levine PR, Macette AM: Musculoskeletal chest pain in patients with "angina:" a prospective study. Southern Med J 82:580–585, 1989.

12. Wooley CF: Where are the diseases of yesteryear? Circulation 53:749–751, 1976.

13. Coghlan HC, Phares P, Cowley M, et al.: Dysautonomia in mitral valve prolapse. Am J Med 67: 236–244, 1979.

14. Maresca M, Galanti G, Castellani S, et al.: Pain in mitral valve prolapse. Pain 36:89–92, 1989.

15. Clouse RE: Psychopharmacologic approaches to therapy for chest pain of presumed esophageal origin. Am J Med 92(5A):106S–113S, 1992.

16. Simons DG, Travell JG: Myofascial origins of low back pain. 1. Principles of diagnosis and treatment. Postgrad Med 73;66–108, 1983.

17. Massie JD, Sebes JI, Cowles SJ: Bone scintigraphy and costochondritis. J Thorac Imaging 8:137–142, 1993.

18. Rose S, Achkar E, Falk GW, et al.: Interaction between patient and test administrator may influence the results of edrophonium provocative testing in patients with noncardiac chest pain. Am J Gastroenterol 88:20–24, 1993.

19. Richter JE: Overview of diagnostic testing for chest pain of unknown origin. Am J Med 92(5A):41S–45S, 1992.

20. Hackshaw BT: Excluding heart disease in the patient with chest pain. Am J Med 92(5A): 46S–51S, 1992.

21. Epstein SE, Gerber LH, Borer JS: Chest wall syndrome: a common cause of unexplained cardiac pain. JAMA 241:2793–2797, 1979.

22. Master AM: The spectrum of anginal and noncardiac chest pain. JAMA 187:894–899, 1964.

23. Wolf E, Stern S: Costosternal syndrome. Arch Intern Med 136:189–191, 1976.

24. Pace JB: Commonly overlooked pain syndromes responsive to simple therapy. Postgrad Med 58:107–113, 1975.

25. Whermacher W: The painful anterior chest wall syndromes. Med Clin North Am 42:111–118, 1958.

26. Sklaroff HJ: Xiphodynia—another cause of atypical chest pain: six case reports. Mt Sinai J Med 46:546–548, 1979.

27. Howell JM: Xiphodynia: a report of three cases. J Emerg Med 10:435–438, 1992.

28. McBeath AA, Keene JS: The rib-tip syndrome. J Bone Joint Surg 57A:795–797, 1975.

29. Davies-Colley R: Slipping rib. Br Med J 1:432, 1922.

30. Heinz GJ, Zavala DC: Slipping rib syndrome: diagnosis using the "hooking maneuver." JAMA 237:794–795, 1977.

31. Holmes JF: A study of the slipping rib cartilage syndrome. N Engl J Med 224:928–932, 1941.

32. Ballon HC, Spector L: Slipping rib. Can Med Assoc J 39:355–358, 1938.

33. Benson EH, Zavala DC: Importance of the costochondral syndrome in evaluation of chest pain. JAMA 156:1244–1246, 1954.

34. Billings RF: Chest pain related to emotional disorders. In: Levene DL, ed. Chest pain: an integrated diagnostic approach. Philadelphia: Lea & Febiger, 1977.

35. Swezey RL: Arthritis: rational therapy and rehabilitation. Philadelphia: WB Saunders, 1978.

36. Schnorr TM, Thun MJ, Halperin WE: Chest pain in users of video display terminals (Letter). JAMA 257:627, 1987.

37. Travell J, Rinzler SH: Pain syndromes of the chest muscles: resemblance to effort angina and myocardial infarction and relief by local block. Can Med Assoc J 59:333–338, 1948.

38. Rokkas T, Anggiansah A, McCullagh M, et al.: Acid perfusion and edrophonium provocation tests in patients with chest pain of undetermined etiology. Digestive Dis Sci 37:1212–1216, 1992.

39. Smout AJ, Lam HG, Breumelhof R: Ambulatory esophageal monitoring in noncardiac chest pain. Am J Med 92(5A):74S–80S, 1992.

40. Elloway RS, Jacobs MP, Nathan MF, et al.: The clinical utility of provocative radionuclide oesophageal transit in the evaluation of non-cardiac chest pain. Europ J Nucl Med 19:113–118, 1992.

41. Greenfield S, Nadler MA, Morgan MT, Shine KI: The clinical investigation and management of chest pain in an emergency department: quality assessment by criteria mapping. Med Care 15: 898–905, 1977.

42. Tietze A: Uebver eine eigenartige Haufung von Fallen mit Dystrophie der Rippenlenorpel. Klin Wehnschr 58:829–831, 1921.

43. Pinals RS: Traumatic arthritis and allied conditions. In: McCarty DJ, ed. Arthritis and allied conditions. 10th ed. Philadelphia: Lea & Febiger, 1985.

44. Levey GS, Calabro JJ: Tietze's syndrome: report of two cases and review of the literature. Arthritis Rheum 5:261–269, 1962.

45. Cameron HU, Fornasier VL: Tietze's disease. J Clin Pathol 27:960–962, 1974.

46. Kurguzov OP, Solomka IaA, Kuznetsov NA: Tietze's syndrome. Khirurgiia 9:161–167, 1991.

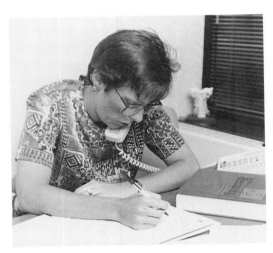

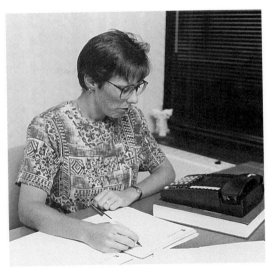

Exercise 4.A (a). The subject must be able to recognize aggravating factors contributing to chest wall pain. Notice the hunched position in this illustration. Consider the ramifications after an eight-hour work day.

4.A (b). The subject must learn to correct aggravating postural factors which may contribute to chest wall pain.

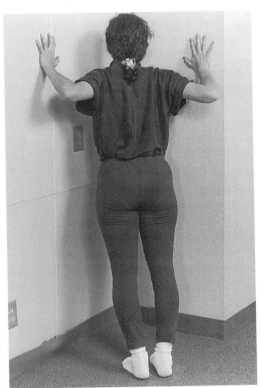

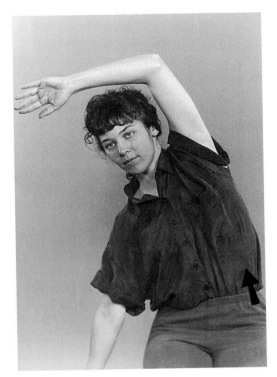

Exercise 4.B. Corner Stretch

Face corner with hands on adjoining walls as illustrated. Feet are 12 to 24 inches from the corner and elbows are at shoulder height. Keeping feet flat and cervical spine aligned with thoracic spine, gently ``fall'' into the corner. Hold 10 to 30 seconds. Repeat 1–3 times twice daily. Stretch is felt across upper chest as well as down calves into ankles.

Exercise 4.C. Lateral Chest Wall Stretch

Sit in an armless chair and raise one arm over the head, bending to opposite side. Do not lean forward or backward. Hold 5 to 30 seconds. Repeat 1–3 times twice daily. Stretch is felt along lateral rib cage as indicated by *arrow*.

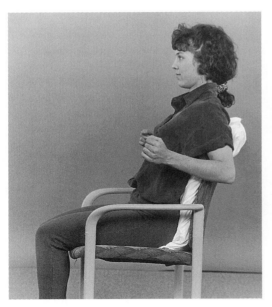

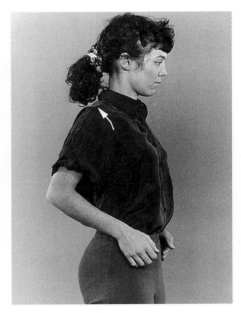

Exercise 4.D. Isometric Thoracic Extension

Sit in a straight chair with a pillow behind the back. Simultaneously push the upper back into the pillow and squeeze the shoulder blades together. Hold 5 to 30 seconds. Repeat 1–3 times twice daily.

Exercise 4.E. Shoulder Curls

Stand straight and curl the shoulders up and back as the *arrow* indicates. Do not push the head forward. Repeat slowly for 5 to 10 repetitions.

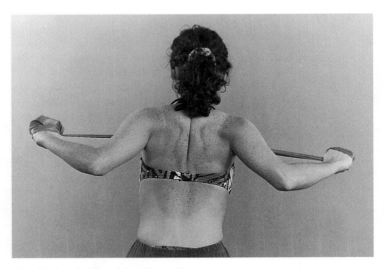

Exercise 4.F. Resistive Horizontal Shoulder Abduction

Hold Theraband and spread arms apart as indicated. A slow, rhythmic stretch to full range for ten repetitions is suggested. Resistance to stretch is felt along the anterior chest wall. This effectively strengthens the scapular adductor muscles, allowing for proper shoulder alignment.

5: Low Back Pain

The social and economic costs of back pain include not only the costs of medical diagnosis and management but also those of loss of job productivity and income. Since 1960, costs for disability have risen six times faster than the work force needed to pay for them (1). Partly because of high costs and partly because of stoicism, as few as 3% of people suffering back pain seek medical attention, and most continue to work despite pain (2). Therefore, for every patient seen with disabling back pain, there are many others with similar complaints who are coping without any treatment.

Only a small minority of patients have serious or life-threatening underlying disease; the work-up can cost thousands of dollars, yet it does little to increase the likelihood of finding a significant causally related underlying disease.

Most persons with an attack of low back pain recover within a week, and only 5% remain disabled longer than 3 months (3). In one study of patients with proved herniated nucleus pulposus (Fig. 5.1) with radiculopathy and moderate nerve encroachment on imaging,

more than 90% recovered following noninvasive active treatment measures including back schooling, lumbar stabilization training, and general upper and lower body strengthening and flexibility exercises (4).

Coping abilities, fear of being laid off, and the psychosocial milieu may be more important to chronicity of back pain than either medical or surgical management (5).

Chronic persistent back pain is often the result of psychosocial factors, including secondary gain (e.g., sick leave, disability benefits), repetitive or inappropriate personal habits leading to misuse injury at work or at home. The severity of back symptoms leads to a disproportionate use of medical care, unrelated to the severity of the medical condition (6).

Cost-effective care for low back pain requires rapid identification of any serious causative disease (which is rare) and, in patients without any underlying causative disease, early and comprehensive management intervention with prompt return to usual activities. Bed rest for longer than 2 days is wasteful in most instances (7).

Rarely are back pain diagnoses scientifically valid (8). The presence of *degenerative arthritis* of the apophyseal joints, *disc degeneration* with narrowed intervertebral disc space, and *fibrofatty nodules* in the sacral region (Fig. 5.2) are often unrelated to outcome from treatment of low back pain.

A ''classic sciatica'' history also does not necessarily mean intraspinal origin for pain; assumptions concerning any connection between sciatica features and the cause of pain in a particular patient must be made with caution. Sciatica is a symptom and not a disease. It may result from herniation of the nucleus pulposus (ruptured disc), from extrinsic disorders in the pelvis or thigh such as an entrapment neuropathy, or from a myofascial pain syndrome (9, 10). Often multiple etiologic factors are operating in an individual patient.

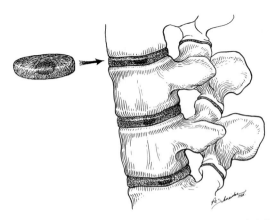

Figure 5.1. The spinal unit consists of a three-joint complex comprising two posterior apophyseal joint articulations and the vertebral body with interposed disc. Within the disc is the nucleus pulposus.

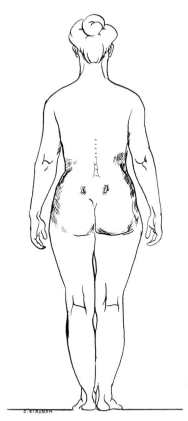

Figure 5.2. Episacroiliac lipomas. These fleshy fibro-fatty nodules commonly occur over the sacroiliac joints at the insertion of the erector spinae muscles.

PATHOPHYSIOLOGY OF LOW BACK PAIN

What is relevant in the source of back pain? Since 1934, when Mixter and Barr described the ruptured disc as a cause for sciatica (11), most etiologic considerations for back pain have revolved around a structural concept such as discogenic pain, degenerative disease of the spine, facet joint disturbance, nerve entrapment, spinal stenosis, or vertebral bony disorders. Today we believe that many cases of back pain have little direct correlation with any structural abnormality evident on roentgenographs. Nevertheless, it is important to consider the known and demonstrable abnormalities that can give rise to back pain.

The Spinal Articulations

The spinal unit consists of a three-joint complex comprising two posterior apophyseal joint

articulations and the vertebral body with interposed disc (12, 13) (Fig. 5.1; see also Anatomic Plates III, IX, and XV). Pathologic changes may be due to apophyseal joint synovitis or degeneration, injury or degenerative changes within the articular disc, apophyseal joint laxity, or traumatic subluxation. The result is entrapment of the nerve root as it exits through this complex. Also, stenosis of the spinal canal or additional new instability of articulating units above or below the level of involvement can be relevant. "Lumbosacral strain" is often misused as a catch-all term.

The sacroiliac joint can be a source for low back pain, and recent imaging findings support a role for functional sacroiliac instability as a cause of low back pain (14).

Fissures and tears of lumbar discs are common with advancing age (15). The occurrence of multiple fissures led Jayson (16) to speculate that a systemic disease process might be operative in cases of degenerative disc disease. A fibrinolytic defect attributable to mechanical derangement of the lumbar spine has been suggested by Klimiuk et al. (17), as determined by prolongation of the euglobulin clot lysis time; the results paralleled clinical outcome with persistent abnormality during chronic pain, and return to normal following recovery. They speculate that the abnormality might lead to a failure to clear fibrin, resulting in further inflammation and fibrosis.

Pressure studies have suggested that only discs that are already fissured will undergo rupture from external trauma. On the basis of these findings, it was postulated that a disc that prolapses after some heavy work would likely have prolapsed anyway, with the particular incident only precipitating its onset early (16).

In 1933 Ghormley (13) emphasized the importance of abnormalities of the posterior facet joint (zygapophyseal joint) as a cause for back pain. The posterior facet joints are innervated by the posterior rami of two spinal nerve levels. Instillation of hypertonic saline into a facet joint was found to produce low back pain, as well as pain radiating into the trochanteric area and down the posterolateral thigh. Furthermore, a local anesthetic injection of the facet joint restored normality. Ashton et al. (18) examined innervation of the ligamentum flavum and the lumbar facet joint capsule using antisera to a general neuronal marker protein gene product and to peptide markers of sensory nerves. The facet capsule but not the ligamentum flavum was found to be substantially innervated by sensory and autonomic nerves; the authors doubt the contribution of the ligamentum flavum to pain perception.

Pelvic lateral tilt, scoliosis, kyphosis, and lumbar lordosis often are not correlated with the presence of back pain (19). Shortness of a leg and body asymmetry may contribute to back pain. Disc degeneration, as evidenced by discography, is also poorly correlated with low pack pain. Rather, pain probably results only if the vertebral end plate is also fractured (20).

Spinal mobility includes ventroflexion, extension, lateral flexion, and rotation. Movement is restricted by various ligaments and other skeletal structures. The ''stiffness'' of aging is often the result of degenerative expansion of the apophyseal joints, spur formation, disc degeneration, and ligamentous changes.

Soft Tissue Factors

Although low back pain appears to originate in the spinal musculature, more likely the pain is referred from ligaments or articular structures (21). The posterior thoracolumbar fascia covers the posterior aspects of the back muscles; the fascia provides a series of accessory posterior ligaments that anchor the L2 to L5 spinous processes to the ilium and resist lumbar flexion (22). Presumably, injury of the fascia can become a source for myofascial pain disorder.

Biomechanical Factors

Introduction of pressure transducers into the nucleus pulposus of human subjects assuming various positions and performing various tasks reveals complex forces in the spine (23). Pressure measurements in the third lumbar disc, investigated while the subject was standing, were used as a standard, and then the intradisc load in other body positions was measured and compared. Sitting increased the load by 30%, walking by 15%, coughing by 50%, jumping by 50%, bending 20 degrees in forward flexion by 85%, lifting a 20-kg weight with the knees

bent by 300%, and lifting a 20-kg load with the knees straight by 500% (24). Sitting with a backrest inclined greater than 90 degrees reduced the load on the lumbar L3 disc by 10 to 20% (25). Lumbar disc pressure is also positively correlated with body weight (23).

Using a cannulated screw to measure interosseous pressure within a vertebral body, Esses and Moro (26) confirmed these findings of lumbar intradisc pressure related to body position, again finding pressures to be greatest in the sitting position, lowest in the prone position, and intermediate in the standing position. Improper lifting (back bent, legs straight) can result in the generation of 1000 to 2000 lb/in^2 of intradisc pressure (27). If the annulus of the lumbar disc has been previously injured, the disc can rupture at 700 lb/in^2 (23–28).

The role of abdominal and chest musculature in back support was investigated using an inflatable corset and measuring a balloon placed within the stomach. This demonstrated that lumbar disc and thoracic disc pressures could be reduced 30 to 50% by tightening abdominal and chest muscles while performing various activities and while assuming different positions (28, 29). The abdominal muscles minimize torquing, bending and shearing stresses in the lumbar spine, thus protecting it (30).

Muscle Strength

The thoracolumbar trunk may be considered a hollow, cylindrical chamber. If the pressure of this chamber is increased by compression of abdominal musculature, the cylinder can withstand greater stress.

Trunk muscle strength and fatigue have been the subject of more recent studies which affirm the importance of good muscle tone (31, 32). Using an encapsulated transmitter (a radio pill) and electromyographic data, measurements were made in healthy student volunteers of trunk stress and intradisc pressures during the performance of several occupational tasks that required spinal movement and trunk stress. Lumbar disc pressure and myoelectric back muscle activity during effort were found to be correlated with symptoms (33–35). These studies support the concept of the trunk as a cylinder and of the role of the trunk muscles in spinal stress and work. Flor et al. (36) noted that patients with chronic back and neck pain were less able to perceive muscle tension (contraction) levels than normal subjects, suggesting that some workers may overly contract muscles in the performance of a work effort.

Gracovetsky et al. (37) used an optimized model of the lumbar spine based on data from a weight lifter performing a "dead-lift" exercise. The study results suggested that in handling heavy loads the stress at each intervertebral joint is identical, and with maximal voluntary effort the weight lifter does not exceed 67% of the ultimate strength of his or her tissues.

Persons with back pain have weak trunk musculature compared to that of normal subjects. Using isokinetic measurements, which are sensitive and reliable quantification measurements of trunk muscle performance, many studies report muscular insufficiency in persons with chronic low back pain (38–46), though others disagree (47, 48). In addition, restoration of strength did not necessarily result in return to work (49, 50, 50a). Furthermore, strength deficits are not predictors of poor work performance (51, 52), and restoration of strength may not reduce pain (53). Strength training, therapy to restore flexibility (particularly hamstring lengthening), and work hardening will be discussed later.

Reactive muscle spasm occurs in stages. Spasm is no more common than strain or fatigue but is more persistent, with an average duration of 3 weeks. Spasm is involuntary and may be viewed as having a natural, protective role. This first stage of muscle spasm may proceed into *hypertonia.* Muscles in hypertonia come under voluntary control, but increased tone may persist for years if the provocative source is not removed. The final stage may be *physiologic adaptation* after prolonged disuse. Adaptive shortening may also result from posture, pain, or chronic fatigue of muscle groups. If the hamstring muscles shorten, the lumbar erectors will be affected as well, and often a tight, painful back will improve simply through the performance of exercises that stretch the hamstring muscles. (See Chapter 1, section "Myofascial Pain Disorder and Fibromyalgia.")

Predictors of Low Back Pain

Physical impairment cannot be predicted by any test other than a history of past low back pain (54). Assessment of current functional limitation is not correlated with anatomic or structural impairment, which suggests that disability is more likely rather to be the result of psychosocial factors (55).

In an effort to determine the predictive value of various physical findings for future back pain, not necessarily disabling pain, Biering-Sorensen (56) examined 920 patients and followed them prospectively for 12 months. The examination included abdominal and trunk strength measurements and tests of endurance. Of those with a past history of back pain, predictors of future back pain were (*a*) tightness in the hamstrings, and (*b*) lack of endurance of back muscles. First occurrence of back pain was correlated with spinal laxity, lack of trunk muscle strength, and lack of trunk muscle endurance. Patients who had a past history of back pain but without recurrence in the study period were noted to have leg length inequality, to be obese, or to be tall.

The patient's number of children born has been found in a number of studies to have a poor correlation with future low back pain. However, the number of children *raised* was found to be correlated with future back in *both men and women* in one retrospective study (56a). The trend was linear and the strength of association to child-raising was greater in men than in women!.

Workplace Ergonomics

Workplace injuries are often not the primary pathogenetic factor in low back pain, only the setting in which underlying disease becomes manifest (57). Driving long distances, improper seating, slipping accidents, frequent lifting, lifting more than 25 pounds combined with twisting, and lifting in an asymmetrical plane are stressors in such occupations as truck driving, nursing, and material handling (57–61).

Work posture and resting posture may impair disc nutrition and increase stress on the posterior articulations (62). Back pain is as common among clerical workers in jobs requiring prolonged sitting as in workers whose jobs require heavier workloads (63).

Psychosocial Factors

In comparing back pain to actual workloads on the lumbar spine, Magnusson et al. (64) noted that many complaints of back pain could not be attributed to high peak workloads, repetitiveness of lifts, or large loads. Rather, monotony, stress, and low job satisfaction were thought to be factors of greater importance. Similar findings were noted in a Swedish study (65). Back pain chronicity and disability have little relation to objective physical findings, mode of onset, severity of initial pain complaint, or imaging findings (6). Outright malingering is rare in clinical experience. Patients with hypochondriasis may be more likely than others to complain of back pain, and they do poorly with manipulation treatment (66), but most are not disabled.

A remarkable body of evidence has accumulated in the past decade demonstrating the importance of the following psychosocial factors to work disability.

Lack of job control and fear of layoff (67)
Monotony and job dissatisfaction (68, 69)
Unsatisfactory employee appraisal rating by supervisor (70)
Distress and dissatisfaction with coworkers or bosses (71)
Poor coping strategies (72)
Divorce, low income, less education (73–75)
Compensation benefits (76)

Early intervention for back pain management must include both assessment of psychosocial factors and development of interventions that are tailored to the individual.

Smoking

Smoking has long been recognized as a risk factor for back pain (77). Smokers have more pain complaints in limb areas also (78). In pigs exposed to tobacco smoke, measurement of radioactive isotopes and tissue oxygen revealed 30–40% reduction in diffusion of oxygen, sulphate, and methyl glucose in the intervertebral disc (79). Disc nutrition and tissue hypoxia may lead to impairment of fibrinolytic activity with impaired healing (80). In one study, if smoking is stopped and nonsmoking status persists, the risk of future back pain was found to return to normal after 10 years (81).

CLASSIFICATION OF LOW BACK PAIN

Back pain can be classified as:

Traumatic or Nontraumatic, with or without neurologic impairment.

Primary or Secondary, with or without neurologic impairment.

Acute or Chronic (longer than 3 months' duration), with or without neurologic impairment.

Specific or Nonspecific, with or without neurologic impairment.

Formerly, a long list of primary nontraumatic diagnoses were provided and based upon anatomic derangements. Then, when imaging demonstrated ''lesions'' within the spine, additional diagnoses were made. But with further experience, low back pain has been designated more often as a symptom disorder with outcome that has no relationship to any structural abnormality. In most instances the term ''nonspecific low back pain'' qualified by ''acute'' or ''chronic'' (longer than 3 months' duration), is appropriate.

Table 5.1 details those features that should be quickly apparent or searched for to identify low back pain secondary to another critical illness or a neurologic impairment that if not rapidly improved with conservative treatment would lead to urgent surgical evaluation.

TABLE 5.1 POTENTIALLY CRITICAL SIGNALS FOR LOW BACK DISEASE

Bladder or bowel dysfunction or impotence
Weakness of ankle dorsiflexion
Ankle clonus
Color change in the extremity
Considerable night pain
Constant and progressive symptomatology
Fever and chills
Weight loss
Lymphadenopathy
Distended abdominal veins
Buttock claudication

TABLE 5.2 NONDISC CAUSES OF SCIATICA

A. Entrapment Neuritis
   1. Obturator neuritis
     a. obturator hernia
     b. osteitis pubis
   2. Meralgia paresthetica
     a. arthritis
     b. psoas abscess
     c. traction injury
     d. obesity
     e. external pressure
   3. Lumbar spinal stenosis
   4. Spinal degenerative joint disease
     a. Apophyseal joint spur formation
     b. Facet syndrome
     c. Root sleeve fibrosis
   5. Ankylosing spondylitis
   6. Lumbosacral and sacral cysts and tumors
B. Trauma
   1. Iatrogenic injections
   2. Contusion
C. Sciatic Neuritis (rare)

Sciatica (pain and paresthesia in the buttock and/or leg in the distribution of the sciatic nerve) may be a clue to intraspinal disease, and when accompanied by evidence of weakness or reflex change, is strongly suggestive of nerve root compression. Table 5.2 lists intraspinal and extraspinal causes of sciatic pain. When sciatica is aggravated by coughing, sneezing, or defecating, an intraspinal cause is more likely.

Pseudosciatica refers to unilateral or bilateral sciatic pain and paresthesia not aggravated by coughing, sneezing, or defecating, and with normal neurologic findings. Causes include bursitis and other soft tissue conditions near the sciatic nerve (Table 5.2).

LOW BACK PAIN SYNDROMES

Certain features may be found during the examination that can result in more rational treatment and prevention. For example, when low back pain is below the sacroiliac joints, diffusely across the sacrum, and the glutei are tender to palpation, the cause is often repetitious improper bending with knees straight. Such tasks as making a bed, using the bottom file drawer, gardening, or improper calisthenic exercise may lead to such pain. Pseudosciatica and trochanteric bursitis also often result from the same improper bending. Table 5.3 lists other lifestyle factors as well as methods to correct them.

Myofascial Low Back Pain

Characteristic features of myofascial low back pain include: pain worse after rest, pain relieved by movement, pain after sitting, stiffness, a sensation of tightness in the back, and a flattened appearance of the lumbar spine during forward bending. The onset of aching discomfort is gradual, and the pain is felt diffusely throughout the low back, often worse after rest or sitting and improved by walking or moving about. Pain is aggravated by cold and relieved by warmth. Bilateral leg pain and paresthesia may occur. Limping and listing do not usually occur. Tenderness is present within the affected muscle and soft tissues, and often the sacroiliac joints are tender (Fig. 5.3). Range of movement is often restricted. Pain (trigger) points may be present but, to many clinicians, are too variable to be important (refer to the discussion of trigger points and tender points in Chapter 1). When the piriformis muscles are tender and involved, sciatica is usually a prominent complaint. Neurologic deficits are absent. The importance of recognizing myofascial pain disorder is the value of treatment and prevention. Lifestyle factors, such as lack of conditioning, smoking, or overuse, are always to be considered; behavior change is essential in order to prevent recurrences. Soft tissue injections or other local treatment techniques combined with counseling are cost-effective and safe (82–86a).

Facet Joint Syndrome

Osteoarthritis or other derangement within the facet joints (also called posterior joint complexes or apophyseal joints) are thought to give rise to a characteristic syndrome of acute back pain with sciatica, often with immobilizing pain. Hyperextension accentuates the pain. Tenderness to deep palpation is found in the vicinity of the posterior joint complex.

The acute "locked up" back may occur without provocation or warning. Listing of the spine is usually present. Often seen in younger

TABLE 5.3 JOINT PROTECTION FOR THE LOW BACK

Strengthen and use the abdominal muscles that support the back.
Attain and maintain ideal weight.
Avoid prolonged periods of sitting or standing.
Wear supportive cushion-soled shoes when standing or walking on concrete surfaces.
Use proper rest and sleep positions.
Perform trunk and hamstring flexibility exercises regularly.
To release a ``locked back,'' lie on the back and elevate the legs to the 90/90 position (Exercise 5.A). Rest the lower legs on a chair or piano stool.
Turn the body while moving the feet in alignment so that the toes point in the direction you are facing.
To move objects at your side, rotate the entire body by moving the feet.
To lift large or heavy objects, move the object to the chest, lift it with the arms, and use the thigh muscles for strength. Hold the object close and centered in front of you.
When lifting children or pets, be prepared for sudden shifts of weight. Do not carry a child on your side. Carry the child Indian or Oriental style on your back, or use a front or back harness pack.
For a sore ``tailbone,'' protect the point of tenderness at the tip of the coccyx. Sit on a foam cushion 3 inches thick and the size of the seat cushion. Cut a 3-inch circle out of the cushion center for pressure relief. Place the cushion under the tailbone whenever seated or doing exercises on the floor.
Sleep side-lying with the legs slightly bent and a pillow between the knees, or back-lying with the knees and feet elevated with a cushion or pillow.
Do not sleep on the stomach. Place a tennis ball in a pocket sewn onto the front of a tee shirt so that the pressure will awaken you if you roll onto the stomach.
A leg length discrepancy more than 0.5 inches may be the cause of back pain. Try a corrective insert to raise the shorter leg, and determine if pain is improved.
Avoid prolonged sitting. Use active sitting techniques such as ``wiggling the pelvis'' and rocking to activate and relax the pelvic muscles.
Break up seated tasks like desk work and card games by standing and moving around for 2 minutes every 15 minutes or so.
Use cruise control when driving long distances.
Do not carry a large wallet in a back pocket. Check for pressure placed on the pelvic bones by a wallet, tight belt, or constricting jeans that can squeeze nerves in the pelvis or groin.
Always bend at the knees, not at the waist.
When lifting an object, bend the knees, keeping the back straight. Use the palms of both hands or the forearm, rather than one hand, to pick up and carry an object.
Do a regular strengthening and lengthening program for abdominal and back muscles.
Use a step stool to reach overhead objects.
When standing for prolonged periods, place one foot on a higher surface (stool, brick, phone book) for a while and then alternate.

Sports
Do trunk stretching and leg stretching warm-up exercises before the sport activity.

patients with joint laxity, it is not rare in others. Usually 48 hours of rest, supine with legs elevated, followed by manipulation or physical therapy and exercises, will bring improvement. Interestingly, the attacks occur less frequently with time. During intercritical periods, the back examination is usually normal.

Sacroiliac Strain Disorder

Unilateral buttock pain following a traumatic event is the usual presentation of sacroiliac strain disorder (87). Local tenderness is present. A number of methods for stress testing have been described, but the best test appears to be the response to a local corticosteroid agent mixed with a local anesthetic. In one report of 72 patients, 81% were relieved at follow-up 9 months later (88).

Herniation of the Nucleus Pulposus

Because imaging evidence of disc herniation is common and often asymptomatic and occurs with increasing frequency with age, evidence for nerve impairment is essential for diagnosis. The classic features of a symptomatic herniated nucleus pulposus are aching pain in the buttock and paresthesias radiating into the posterior thigh and calf, or into the posterolateral thigh and lateral foreleg. Paresthesia may be noted all the way to the heel, or within a zone of the lateral foreleg. When the S1 nerve root is compressed, the pain often radiates into the poste-

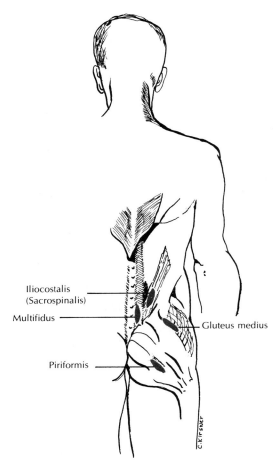

Iliocostalis
(Sacrospinalis)

Multifidus

Gluteus medius

Piriformis

Figure 5.3. Myofascial pain (trigger) points of the low back region. Points arising in the erector spinae muscles, the gluteal fascia, and the presacral fascia are common in patients with low back pain.

walking some distance; pain is relieved somewhat by bending forward. Severe involvement is suggested when the patient cannot walk farther than one block before claudication begins, but can walk farther when using a grocery cart (with forward spinal tilt). In addition, the patient may have learned to relieve pain by leaning over a table, or resting with the trunk prone upon the stairway. Reflexes are usually symmetrical and present but proximal leg weakness is common. Buttock muscle mass may be diminished. Flattening of the lumbar spine is evident. Bilateral spasm within the piriformis muscles may also be found (89).

Cauda Equina Syndrome

Compression of the lower spinal nerve roots, the cauda equina, leads to radicular symptoms in both legs and impaired sphincter and sexual function. Back pain may be absent.

Psychogenic Back Pain

Back pain of psychosomatic origin, as well as true malingering, are rare (19). In these instances the patient's history is vague, and the patient often places emphasis on blaming others for his or her plight. The term "compensation neurosis" is a rather ambiguous one, yet these patients often continue to be disabled after their claims for financial gain are settled.

Psychogenic back pain may present with complaints of pain of obscure origin, with hypochondriasis, and with pain out of proportion to the physical findings. Review of systems is often positive with complaints from head to toe. Often, around the time of onset, a significant stressful event has "charged up" the nervous system, or depression may have begun, often following a loss of a loved one. Hand or jaw clenching may be a clue to underlying stress. The misery guide (below) may be out of proportion to the presentation.

Somatoform disorder, the "touch-me-not" syndrome, may be observed during the physical examination. Such patients will overreact and withdraw from palpation everywhere they are touched. Consider the possibility of malingering or pain of psychogenic origin if somatoform complaints are observed during the physi-

rior gluteal fold and down the posterior thigh into the calf and heel. Indications of a large herniated disc include back pain at onset, then improvement in back pain but increased buttock and leg pain and paresthesia. Significant weakness and a limping gait occur. Pain is usually aggravated by coughing or defecating, a symptom usually absent in nondisc causes for sciatica. Tables 5.4 and 5.5 summarize the examination features of nerve entrapment at various levels.

Lumbar Spinal Stenosis

In addition to the features suggestive of herniation of the nucleus pulposus, significant lumbar stenosis results in buttock claudication after

TABLE 5.4 BACK EXAMINATION (105, 135)

Position	Test	Impairment
Standing	Alignment	Scoliosis; pelvic asymmetry
Standing	Trendelenberg	Hip muscle weakness
Bending	Schober test	Spasm, arthritis, DISH, disc degeneration
Extension	Pain aggravation	Facet joint disease
Twisting actively	Range of motion	Discogenic pain, muscle spasm
Twisting passively	Psychogenic response	Should be pain-free
Stand up on toes ten times	Plantar flexion	S1
Walking	Gait	Weakness, cerebellar dysfunction pes planus
Kneeling	Ankle reflex[a]	S1
Sitting with feet on floor	Toe/ankle dorsiflexion	L5
Sitting with feet on floor	Toe/ankle dorsiflexion	Malingering if cogwheel action is noted
Sitting with feet on floor	Abduct hip with resistance	Piriformis muscle irritation
Sitting with legs hanging free	Knee reflex[a]	L4
Arising from chair	Quads, hip extensors	Muscle weakness
Bending forward over table	Palpation	Spasm, episacroiliac nodules, trigger points, piriformis syndrome
Bending forward over table	Percussion	Intraspinal impingement (disc or tumor)
Lying supine	Hip, abdominal exam	Referred pain disorder
Lying supine	Straight-leg-raising	Sciatic nerve root irritation; tight hamstrings
Lying supine	Leg length	Structural disorder
Lying on side, hip extended and knee flexed	Ober test	Hip flexor contracture, psoas muscle, fascia lata contracture
Lying on side, upper leg extended	Hip abduction	L5
Lying on side, upper leg flexed	Trochanteric bursitis	Pseudosciatica
Lying prone (on abdomen)	Hip extension	L2, 3, 4 (Pain); S1 (Weakness)
Lying prone (on abdomen)	Hamstring reflex	L5
Lying prone (on abdomen)	Reversed SLR	L4, 5; S1

[a]Hyperreflexia: Test for Babinski reflex, other signs of segmental cord compression above lesion.

TABLE 5.5 NEUROLOGIC TABLE FOR LOW BACK DISORDERS

Nerve Root	Sensory Loss	Motor Weakness	Reflex Change
L2	Proximal lateral thigh	Iliopsoas	Normal
L3	Distal anteromedial thigh	Hip adduction	Normal
L4	Medial calf	Foot dorsiflexion, quadriceps	Normal Knee jerk
L5	Lateral calf, first toe web	Toe extension	Hamstring, posterior tibial
S1	Lateral dorsal and plantar foot	Foot eversion, stand on toes	Ankle jerk

cal examination (below). Alcoholism can present as back pain from the many falls that occur during times of intoxication.

Fibromyalgia should be considered in patients with myofascial back pain. Examination for tender points may be essential for establishing a more comprehensive management program (see Chapter 7).

Psychosocial indicators of disability include (90):

Low education, limited skills, low income

Smoking, drug dependence

Attitude problems, irrational beliefs, depression

History of many pain workups

Unlimited compensation

Deconditioning

Several disability determination questionnaires are available for identifying workers who could become disabled (75, 91–95). However, in a prospective study psychologic profiles were not found to predict future outcome or disability

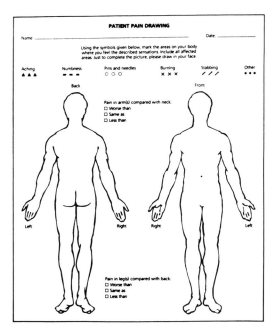

Figure 5.4. Pain drawing for documenting back pain history. (From Mooney V: Evaluating low back pain disorders in the primary care office. J Musculoskel Med 1:16–26, 1984.)

(96). Pain drawings are another simple and reliable tool that can be used to distinguish organic from nonorganic pain (97, 98).

The pain drawing (Fig. 5.4) provides a permanent record of the location, quality, type, depth, and intensity of pain (99) and can assist in decision making (Table 5.6). It can also suggest psychologic disturbance (100). In one study, the accuracy of the pain drawing was more useful in assessing psychogenic disorders (85%) and spinal stenosis (58%), than for other diagnoses (101). Using three scoring methods, Parker et al. found that the pain drawing of pain sites was of limited value as a predictor of psychological distress, and that the pain drawing body map did not differentiate between organic and nonorganic pain patterns (100a).

MacNab described two other syndromes of interest. The "racehorse syndrome": a tense, hard-working, hyperreactive person who tends to hyperextend the spine; and the "razor's edge syndrome," which signifies persons on the razor's edge of emotional stability who present outlandish appearances and complaints (102). Even when these syndromes are suspected, however, the clinician must neverthe-

less perform a careful examination, provide reassurance, and when necessary, suggest counseling.

HISTORY AND PHYSICAL EXAMINATION

The history is the most cost-effective diagnostic intervention. Most practice parameters and practice guidelines depend upon the history and physical findings for determining diagnostic and treatment interventions. In one study of patients seen for low back pain, 6% did not meet criteria for expensive interventions and accounted for 27% of the total charges. The initial examination should be based on a solid and objectively derived foundation in an effort to determine which patients should receive consultation, physical therapy, or imaging interventions (102a).

The history-taking will vary with the mode of presentation and age of the patient, but it should quickly recognize those critical features that are listed in Table 5.1.

Severity of symptoms often may not relate to severity of illness. For example, nonspecific low back pain of improper use may be more painful and disabling than the back pain resulting from a herniated disc or tumor. In a prospective study of 174 patients with low back pain, the elements of patient history were evaluated for their sensitivity and specificity in identifying patients requiring surgical intervention. The most important warning symptoms were found to be the combination of inability to sleep, awakening and inability to fall back to sleep, medication required to sleep, and pain worsened by walking (102b).

Acute injury should be distinguished from simple work stresses that are individually benign, but when performed repetitively, become cumulatively harmful (103).

Try to "suffer vicariously" with the patient with low back pain in order to entertain the various modalities of diagnosis and treatment (99, 104, 105, 106). Ask five basic questions:
1. Where is the pain? (A pain drawing (Fig. 5.4) can record the patient's pain experience.)
2. What loss of function has occurred? Is bowel or bladder function affected?

TABLE 5.6 DECISION CHART: THE LOW BACK

Problem	Action	Further Action

1. Acute recurrent
No neurologic loss
Spinal motion restricted
No major trauma
 	
2. Acute onset
With sciatica
With weakness
Reflexes normal
	General examination
	Assess how activities at work/
	   home/play are done
	Advise correction of
	   aggravating factors
	Exercise and rest
	Provide pain relief:
	   Cold, spray, stretch regimen
	   Traction, supports, relaxants
	   Medications including
	     acetaminophen,
	     cyclobenzaprine, NSAIDs,
	     antidepressants
	   Local injection of steroid and
	     anesthetic mixture
	Nerve block
	Electrodiagnostic study if >6
	   weeks
	Roentgenograms if age >50
		Rheumatology/Physiatry
		   consultation
		Bone Scan
		CT Scan, MRI
		Electrodiagnostic study

3. Chronic backache
Myofascial trigger points
   present
Rest aggravates,
   movement helps
	Add manipulation
	Rule out fibromyalgia
	Bone scan if persistent	

4. Chronic backache with
   stiffness
Morning stiffness
Onset under age 40
3 months' duration
Limited lumbar motion/
   chest expansion
	Rule out spondylarthropathy
	HLA-B27 determination	

5. Acute or subacute With weakness With reflex loss Positive spinal punch or root signs	Consultation with surgeon	

6. Danger signs present
Night pain, paralysis
Fever, weight loss
Bladder/bowel dysfunction
Color change in limb
Constant and progressive
   symptomatology
	Immediate action or
	   consultation
		→ Neurosurgical or
		   Orthopaedic
		   consultation
		Vascular study

3. When does it hurt—is pain continuous or intermittent? Does pain awaken the patient from sleep? (Fibromyalgia and myofascial pain are aggravated by rest, and often improve with walking or stretching.) Is pain worse upon arising, when walking, bending, reaching, or sitting? Is pain aggravated by coughing, sneezing, or defecating? Is this the first episode? How long has this episode been present?

4. How and why—is there a definite injury history or repetitive movement disorder? Has the patient recently engaged in a new sport, hobby, or task?

5. What is the patient's past history? Cancer, urinary tract disease, and past history of back pain are essential parts of the history. What was done therapeutically, and with what result?

Stiffness or gelling, duration, and location could indicate inflammatory disease and help to distinguish it from noninflammatory disease. However, fibromyalgia and Parkinson's disease can cause "all over" stiffness.

Constitutional features of fever, chills, sweats, or weight loss indicate need for urgent diagnosis and treatment.

Weakness is a common complaint but must be objectively quantified and distinguished from fatigue. Test the patient's ability to arise unassisted from a chair, arise from a crouched position, and stand on heels, toes, and one leg.

If the onset followed trauma, elicit information regarding the extent of trauma (e.g., was the car totalled?), presence of abrasions, lacerations, or fractures at the time of injury, and availability of radiographs. Is litigation pending?

What pain words are used? Are they appropriate? No easy, reliable, verified method exists for determining the significance of psychologic factors or for assessing disability (107–109).

The *misery index* (90) as described below can be used to assess quickly the appropriateness of the presentation of symptoms. Sometimes the patient perceives disability that does not fit your findings, or more serious disease may be suspected in a more stoic patient. The misery index is determined by assessing the patient as follows:

In front of the patient, place your hands in front of you, one about two feet above the other, with palms facing one another, and ask: "If you were so bad that you could not get out of bed, and if that is like being in the bottom of a pit" (indicate this by wiggling your lower hand) "and being restored to perfect is like being out of the pit" (indicate this by wiggling your upper hand); "now put your hand somewhere between mine to indicate how miserable you have been this week."

This version of a pain scale can discriminate irrational pain concern or alert you to search more closely for evidence of critical disease. It has not been validated or tested for reliability, but we offer it as a simple guide to the patient's sense of suffering.

The symptom of *stiffness* should be considered separately from pain. Stiffness that begins insidiously and occurs during the night or early morning hours may suggest inflammatory diseases of the spine (e.g., ankylosing spondylitis) (110). In addition to stiffness, characteristic clinical findings suggestive of ankylosing spondylitis include: insidious onset, symptoms more than 3 months' duration, age less than 40 years, and pain improvement with motion.

A history of aching, numbness, and tingling radiating posteriorly or posterolaterally into the lower extremity below the knee (sciatica),

or pain and burning that radiate anteriorly into the groin or anterior hip region, is often present in herniated disc disease. Aggravation by coughing, sneezing, or straining during defecation also suggests intraspinal disease.

Certain symptoms may suggest a diagnosis or location of disease origin:

- Night pain that awakens the patient could indicate an intraspinal tumor or disease within abdominal or retroperitoneal structures
- Chills or fever suggest infection, often from renal or retroperitoneal areas, or even intraspinal abscess
- Changes in bowel and sexual function or urination suggest lesions of the cauda equina
- Claudication followed by numbness and tingling suggests spinal stenosis

Spinal stenosis often causes the patient to stop walking because of aching in the buttock and calf regions; numbness and tingling may occur in one or both lower extremities. Relief in these patients may occur with bending forward, such as leaning over a table. In one study, greater age, severe lower-extremity pain, and the absence of pain when seated were also found most strongly associated with the diagnosis of lumbar spinal stenosis (110a).

Physical examination can demonstrate relevant structural disorders (Table 5.4). The value of the back examination lies in its use as a screening method for disease identification, not severity or prognosis (105, 106, 110, 111). In fact the reliability of the examination is directly related to keeping it simple and basic (112, 113).

1. *Observation:* The examination begins with observation of the appearance of the patient while sitting, rising, standing, walking, and bending. Observing the patient undressing can be helpful. Structural abnormalities can only be demonstrated with the patient completely disrobed. The examiner proceeds to search for such objective findings as back or pelvic asymmetry, unequal leg length, spasm, scoliosis, loss of range of motion, loss of muscle mass, weakness, or abnormal reflexes. Pes planus should be noted. Mobility can be observed as the patient bends over. Joint laxity may be deter-

mined by asking the patient to try to touch the palms to the floor with the legs straight. This is an important clue to the hypermobility syndrome (see Chapter 7).

Scoliosis, when present, should be described as occurring to the right or left, depending on the convexity direction of the curve. Leg length discrepancy greater than 2 cm should be noted. Pelvic tilt during forward bending may indicate leg length inequality (114).

2. *Movement:* Restriction of chest expanse may suggest ankylosing spondylitis or other inflammatory disease of the spine or rib cage. Using a tape measure, the examiner measures the chest circumference at the breast line, after expiration and again after inspiration. A difference of 2 inches or more is normal (115). The spinal curvatures are examined with forward flexion, extension, and lateral flexion (Fig. 5.5). The examiner notes rigidity, spasm, pain, or listing of the

body to one side. Symmetric loss of spinal motion may occur in degenerative disease of the posterior joints or ankylosing spondylitis, whereas asymmetric loss of movement suggests disc disease—though this is not a hard-and-fast rule (21).

Deyo et al. (116) point out the limited value of findings of lumbar movement for diagnosis, but the finding of limited movement does help to determine the methods to use for physical therapy. In a prospective study of flexibility of the spine and hamstring muscles in men with and without back pain, the indicators useful to identify those with back pain included limitation of sagittal motion and straight leg raising (117) (see below, item 6).

To record mobility of the lumbar spine, the modified Schober test may be recorded: with the patient standing erect, mark the skin in the midline of the patient's back at the level of the lumbosacral junction in line with the "dimples of Venus" (at the level of the posterior superior iliac spines); place another mark 10 cm above the first, and a third mark 5 cm below the first. Ask the patient to bend forward as if to touch his toes. Then measure the distance between the upper and lower marks. Normal is greater than 20 cm (118–120). In addition to ankylosing spondylitis, less common disorders associated with loss of motion include diffuse idiopathic skeletal hyperostosis (DISH), the rigid spine syndrome (121), and severe myofascial pain disorders.

Use of the modified Schober test for spine flexion is questioned by Miller et al. (122) and by Merritt et al. (120), who used a blind interrater "worst case" protocol; but the studies used only normal subjects without comparison to those with symptoms. Certainly, the Schober test would be more useful in cases in which the patient's measurement before onset of back pain is available for comparison. Others use a double inclinometer system; we have not used this technique.

Range of hip movement should always be determined in order to identify back pain resulting from intrinsic hip disease. The foot of the involved extremity is placed on the opposite knee. The examiner then presses the knee and thigh downward: pain results if intrinsic hip disease is present (see Chapter 6).

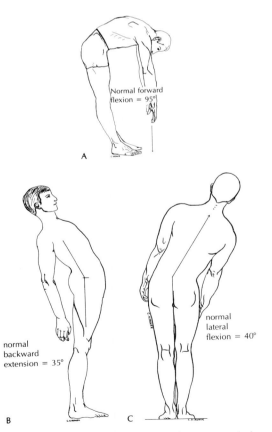

Figure 5.5. Normal ranges of spinal movement: **A.** Flexion. **B.** Extension. **C.** Lateral flexion.

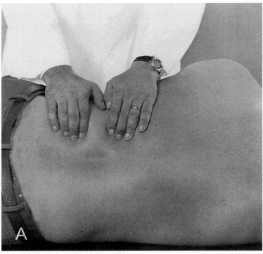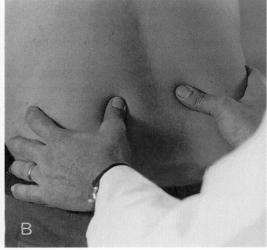

Figure 5.6. Physical examination for myofascial pain points is best performed with the patient side-lying or lying across an examining table with knees bent. This relaxes the hamstrings and allows careful palpation for the pain points that reproduce the pain. **A.** Erector muscles. **B.** Presacral fascia, gluteal fascia, and episacroiliac nodules.

In most patients with a diseased hip, the examination reveals limitation of internal rotation and abduction.

3. *Palpation:* Soft tissue examination can indicate whether to try local injection therapy with a corticosteroid and local anesthetic mixture to relieve tenderness and pain (trigger) points. With the patient bent over a table, or side-lying, soft tissue tenderness is determined and pain reproduction is sought (123) (Fig. 5.6). Also, when gentle skin pinching performed over the site of pain causes the patient to withdraw with exaggerated response, psychogenic back pain is suggested. Diffuse tenderness surrounding the sacroiliac joints and across the low sacrum indicates low back strain from repetitive bending at the waist. Palpation for areas of tenderness is carried out after testing with skin pinching. Using enough force to cause blanching of the fingernail, palpate the erector spinae muscles, glutei, sciatic notch region, sacroiliac joint region, and hip areas in order to identify areas of exaggerated tenderness. These can be marked with the blunt end of a ballpoint pen for injection (see below).

Pain (trigger) points (where pain is reproduced at a distance from the palpated "trigger point") are uncommon, and tender points could be part of the more widespread fibromyalgia disorder. In one study of physical therapists' examining for trigger points at a variety of locations, interobserver reliability of trigger point examination was poor regardless of the therapist's experience (124).

Bone tenderness may be more reliable and reproducible (125). Njoo and van der Does used modified criteria for a trigger point, then prospectively compared 61 patients with chronic nonspecific low back pain with 60 controls, utilizing five blinded examiners. Inclusion criteria were local tenderness in the quadratus lumborum and gluteus medius and back pain of at least 3 months' duration with no other cause. Trigger points with referred pain and twitch response were found in 10% of patients and 3% of controls. However, back pain patients were differentiated from controls by the occurrence of localized tenderness, "jump sign" (patient vocalizes or exhibits withdrawal during palpation), pain recognition, and a palpable band. Thus a trigger point symptom is significant, whereas the palpable trigger point is not (125a). Another finding, episacroiliac nodules, has little relation to the cause of pain. The nodules are common and they can change in size without any relation to symptoms (126–129) (Fig. 5.2).

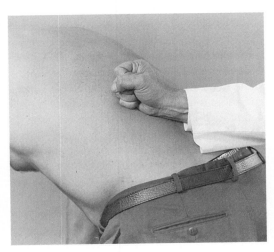

Figure 5.7. Firm spinal percussion should be performed over each vertebra in the midline and to the symptomatic side as well as the side opposite. A positive test, which occurs with pain reproduction in the symptomatic hip or limb, is highly suggestive of herniated nucleus pulposus (ruptured disc).

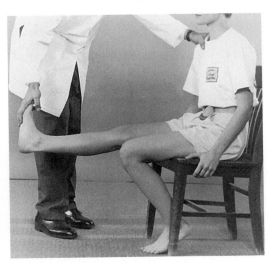

Figure 5.8. Straight leg test in seated position. Probably a better test for sciatic nerve impingement. Positive test occurs when pain is reproduced in the back and leg.

Tenderness in the sciatic notch in patients with sciatica is often due to herniated nucleus pulposus (ruptured disc), but may also occur in the piriformis or other myofascial syndromes.

4. *Percussion:* While the patient is standing on the floor and bending over the examining table with knees flexed, or side-lying, firm percussion in the center and to each side of the lumbar vertebrae may reproduce sciatica (Fig. 5.7). In our experience, a positive percussion test is as good an indicator of lumbar disc disease as is a positive straight-leg-raising maneuver in the seated position (Fig. 5.8) or a reflex change. When percussion above the site of a suspected nerve impingement reproduces sciatica, the sciatica is often caused by a lesion requiring surgery.

5. *Other Features:* While the patient is supine on the examining table, the examination continues with careful palpation of the abdomen. Auscultation for bruits over the abdominal, iliac, and femoral vessels is performed. Peripheral pulses are palpated. Rectal and pelvic examinations are also part of the back examination. Tender (trigger) points of the iliopsoas can be searched for in this position.

Gait abnormalities should be noted. A patient's inability to walk on his or her toes

or heels provides evidence of weakness in the gastrocnemius or tibialis anterior muscle groups, respectively. Active foot and toe dorsiflexion testing against the examiner's resistance may reveal more subtle weakness of involved muscle groups.

6. *Neurologic Examination:* Tests for nerve root compression should be carried out regardless of pain distribution. Maneuvers that stretch the nerve trunk include straight-leg-raising (Lasègue's sign), and the reversed straight-leg-raising test (130). The straight-leg-raising test is usually performed with the patient lying flat on his or her back with the uninvolved knee bent 45 degrees, and that foot resting on the table. The involved leg is raised straight up, while the ankle is kept at 90 degrees of flexion (Fig. 5.9). Generally, if hamstring muscles are not tight, straight-leg-raising can reach 90 degrees of upright vertical position. In a positive test, pain and tingling are reproduced. The test is nonspecific, and any type of irritation of the sciatic nerve may yield a positive result. Dorsiflexion of the foot increases the pain during the straight-leg-raising maneuver. If medial hip rotation is added during straight leg raising the reliability is also improved (131).

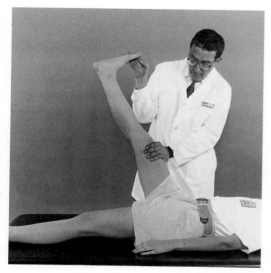

Figure 5.9. The straight-leg-raising maneuver (Lasègue's sign). After gradually raising the straight leg to the maximum tolerated position, the foot is then drawn to a 90-degree angle. Paresthesias are accentuated if the sciatic nerve has been irritated. Tightness of the hamstring muscles may result in a false positive straight-leg-raising maneuver.

Straight leg raising is often limited by tightness of the hamstring muscles rather than by sciatic nerve irritation and, as an isolated finding, is poorly correlated with the presence or absence of herniated disc disease. Shortening of the hamstring muscle itself is frequently found in patients with low back pain.

A positive straight-leg-raising (SLR) test in conjunction with other features may indicate the level of lumbar intervertebral disc herniation. Shiqing et al. (132) report that when the passive SLR test is performed with the patient lying supine, the degree of limitation of the SLR test was closely related to the size of the protrusion; also, when the angle of SLR was less than 40 degrees, the protrusion lay anterior or anterolateral to the spinal nerve in 87% of cases; and when limitation of SLR of the uninvolved limb occurred, the protrusion was in the axilla of the spinal nerve in 77% of cases.

Perhaps more reliable is the SLR test performed with the patient seated: the leg is passively raised as the patient bends forward while seated on a firm chair (Fig. 5.8).

Reversed straight leg raising is performed with the patient lying prone and the legs raised backward, one at a time. Pain over the involved

nerve root (caused perhaps by compression) may be reproduced regardless of which leg is posteriorly raised.

Interobserver error has demonstrated little value in the sensory nerve examination when compared to pain drawings; the sensory examination findings were poorly correlated with final diagnosis (112); neurologic deficits may have little relation to outcome (111).

Special maneuvers to increase intraspinal pressure, using jugular compression (Naffziger's test), may prove useful in some patients.

When the L5 nerve root is compressed, pain radiates into the posterolateral hip, and numbness and tingling may be noted in a lateral zone of the foreleg (133). Impingement of the L3-L4 nerve roots is associated with depression of the knee jerk; impingement of the first sacral nerve root is associated with depression of the ankle jerk; and impingement of the L5 nerve root may be associated with depression of the posterior tibial tendon reflex. Asymmetric hamstring reflex (for L5 nerve root) may be determined with the patient prone. The examiner percusses the conjoint tendon of the semitendinosus and biceps femoris muscles at the ischial tuberosity and notes muscle contraction at the popliteal region (134) (Table 5.5).

In the presence of a symptomatic herniated nucleus pulposus, the pain is often complicated by reflex spasm, which results in pain during rest and flattening of the lumbar spine. Trigger points may be present; atrophy is usually not evident.

Limb strength and circumference above and below the knee should be determined and compared. The dominant side is usually 1 to 2 cm larger than the other.

Table 5.4 provides a review of examination techniques in the various body positions. Table 5.5 reviews the usual findings of various nerve root disturbances.

7. *Tests for Malingering:* If malingering is suspected, two tests may be helpful. If the patient complains of weakness of a leg, have the patient lie supine, the examiner standing at the foot of the examination table. Grasp both of the patient's legs and hold them about 6 inches up from the table with the patient's heels supported on your palms. Now ask the patient to lift the uninvolved leg. When this is

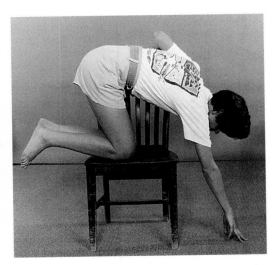

Figure 5.10. The test for malingering is done by asking the patient to kneel on a chair and lean forward, which relaxes the sciatic nerve. The patient is then told to hold onto the chair with the left hand and reach to the floor with the right hand. Because the sciatic nerve is relaxed and the patient's back is supported, no pain should result and the patient should be able to reach within 5 cm of the floor, even when sciatic nerve impingement is present. In malingering patients, however, pain will be described, and motion limited.

attempted, the opposite leg should depress the examiner's hand. Now reverse the procedure and ask the patient to lift the involved limb. If the patient is not making a true effort, the opposite limb will not reflexively depress that palm.

Another technique, described as the Burns test (135), is done by asking the patient to kneel on a chair and bring the buttocks as close to the heels as possible. This, of course, relaxes the sciatic nerve. The patient is then told to hold onto the chair with the left hand and reach to the floor with the right hand (Fig. 5.10). Because the sciatic nerve is relaxed and the patient's back is supported, no pain should result and the patient should be able to reach within 5 cm of the floor, even when sciatic nerve impingement is present. In malingering patients, however, pain will be described, and motion limited.

Disability Determination

Examinations for purposes of disability determination do not have to be difficult if the examination includes appropriate consideration from objective information. In the Code of Federal Regulations of the United States *disability* is defined as the "inability to engage in any substantial gainful activity by reason of any medically determinable physical or mental impairment or impairments which can be expected to result in death or which have lasted, or can be expected to last, for a continuous period of not less than 12 months." *Impairment* is defined as "an impairment that results from anatomic, physiologic, or psychologic abnormalities which are demonstrable by medically acceptable clinical and laboratory diagnostic techniques. Statements of the applicant, including his own description of his impairment (symptoms) are, alone, insufficient to establish the presence of a physical or mental impairment."

Primary consideration is given to the severity of the individual's impairment, age, education, and work experience. Medical considerations alone (including the physiologic and psychologic manifestations of aging) can justify a finding that the individual has a disability and his impairment is one that meets the duration requirement and is listed in the Code of Federal Regulations. Payment is made for the amount of "disease," whereas illness may be independent, according to Hadler. The same severity of disease may cause little illness or disability in one person, yet might be associated with severe illness behavior in another. He accepts low back pain as a disease (136), but the *illness impact* on behavior may result from such other factors as lifestyle and quest for medical attention (109).

Illness is the perception of disease. According to Hadler, the physician should not have a role in judging whether a particular injury arose out of or during work; neither can we determine causality with any degree of precision (137). Unfortunately, the physician is given the task of stating causality in industrial cases. As has been pointed out, more than an injury is often involved when disability occurs. Impairment can be considered to be an anatomic or functional loss, and disability to be the loss of capacity to work in gainful employment. The physician assists in determining:

1. compensability, a subjective assessment;

2. termination of the healing period (when no further medical recovery is feasible), also subjective; and

3. the degree of permanent impairment (138). The American Medical Association (AMA) guidelines for rating disability (permanent impairment) use only objective determinants. Most orthopaedists use this guide but also add other attributes that are subjective (138). Problems arise from the fact that injury may result from "normal" work in which the repetitive task or activity results in rapid degeneration of tissue, or when a structural disorder is additive to job stress, or when injury is not really definable and separate from other underlying or predisposing causes (137).

LABORATORY AND RADIOLOGIC EXAMINATION

Tests of inflammation, such as the Westergren erythrocyte sedimentation rate and C-reactive protein, are inexpensive and excellent screening tests for the presence of tumors, infection, and inflammatory diseases of the spine. Urinalysis, blood counts, serum acid and alkaline phosphatase, serum protein electrophoresis, HLA-B27 determination, and other tests should be performed as appropriate.

HLA-B27 determination should be considered for patients under age 40 with spinal distress that has had an insidious onset, has had a duration greater than 3 months, is accompanied by stiffness that follows resting, and is improved with exercise (110). In such individuals, particularly in the absence of imaging abnormalities, an HLA-B27 determination may support a working diagnosis of spondylarthritis (19). The sedimentation rate may be normal in 20% of symptomatic patients. A chemical battery of tests should be obtained in patients with persistent back pain and disability. Cushing's syndrome, Paget's disease, tumor, hematologic disorders, and osteomalacia are some of the systemic disorders that should be ruled out. A urinalysis should be part of the back examination. For older patients, in whom the sedimentation rate elevation may be non-specific, the C-reactive protein test may be more helpful.

Routine roentgenographic back examination should generally be reserved for patients with a history of major trauma, patients in whom physical examination has revealed an abnormality, older patients, or patients whose medication or treatment could result in skeletal disorders (e.g., steroids) (113, 139). Spurs and other evidence of degenerative changes of the articular structures are so prevalent (140, 141) that the clinician should analyze the relationship of radiologic findings to symptoms with caution (19).

In one study, findings of joint space narrowing, sclerosis, and spur formation were found to bear no relationship to type of work, absence from work, sex, race, or sport activity. The findings were correlated only with age (142). In another study of 292 men with back pain graded as none, mild, or severe, the findings of transitional vertebrae, Schmorl's nodule, disc sign, disc space narrowing at L3-L4, and L5-S1, and spurs were similar in all three symptom groups. Traction spurs (in which the spur points directly anteriorly or away from the disc space and is separated from the adjacent osseous end plate by 3 to 5 mm) in association with disc space narrowing at the L4-L5 interspace were significantly related to symptoms of severe low back pain (143).

When indicated, roentgenographic examination of the lumbar spine should include anteroposterior (AP) and lateral views of the lumbosacral spine, and a true AP view of the pelvis in order to detect silent hip disease that refers pain to the low back. Additional views that may be helpful in certain circumstances include sacroiliac joint films, and left and right oblique views of the spine.

Attempts to prove spinal instability with flexion-extension roentgenographs have not been found to be reliable (144). The addition of side-bending views may improve reliability but further study is needed (145).

Osteoarthritis with marginal vertebral and apophyseal joint spurs is likely to be significant if the neuroforamina are encroached upon. Osteoarthritis, if severe, does result in limitation of spinal motion. Most patients with proved herniation of the nucleus pulposus have normal roentgenograms. Congenital deformities of the low lumbar and lumbosacral spinal areas are seen in up to 30% of radiographic surveys.

Changes in the neural arch, abnormality of the transverse process of the fifth lumbar vertebra, with or without sacralization, or a spina bifida occulta often are unrelated to symptoms (25). Rarely, after trauma, symptoms may occur in relation to such structural changes in younger individuals.

Roentgenographic examination may also reveal squaring of the vertebral bodies, erosion, sclerosis characteristic of ankylosing spondylitis, and other spondylarthritides (21). Spinal roentgenographic examination reveals the occasional abscess, with soft tissue swelling adjacent to an involved disc and its adjacent vertebra. Specialized radiographic techniques include tomograms and computed tomography for determining the size of the spinal canal and for identifying tumors (146).

Scintigraphy is of value in diagnosis of adolescent sport injuries to the pars interarticularis in which a stress fracture might have occurred (147), or if inflammatory arthritis of the spine, osteoporosis with fracture, osteomalacia, osteomyelitis, disc space infections, tumor, or Paget's disease are suspected (148).

Computed tomography (CT) with or without contrast media has been helpful in diagnosing many diseases of the spine, including herniated disc, facet degeneration, and spinal stenosis (149). When compared to computed tomography in cases of herniated disc, myelography was accurate in 83% and computed tomography in 72% of 122 patients who had surgically confirmed herniated disc (150). Elective contrast myelography is reserved for patients with atypical pain, or for localization of the site of pathology preceding operative intervention. Discography is still a controversial diagnostic procedure.

Magnetic resonance imaging (MRI) can be particularly helpful in the diagnosis of disc degeneration, disc space infection, and soft tissue lesion (151). Disc bulges and protrusions are found commonly in studies of asymptomatic individuals; in one study it was found that only extrusions of disc material were indicative of pain (152). In comparing MRI with postmyelogram CT scan and with operative findings in 102 disc lesions, Janssen et al. report 96% accurate predictions for MRI compared to 57% with postmyelogram CT scan (153).

Arthrography of facet joints with instillation of steroids and local anesthetic agents using fluoroscopic control has been advocated for diagnostic study (154). However, its value is questioned, and the procedure is rarely indicated. Dory (155) noted that the articular capsule nearly always burst following the procedure! Others state that arthrography findings do not differentiate a pain-producing joint from a normal one; the subjective response to an anesthetic facet joint injection must serve as the diagnostic end point (156).

Less expensive techniques, if available, include routine and pulsed-echo ultrasound, and are useful if the technician is experienced (157).

Thermography has had technical enhancement in recent years but remains a tool of uncertain value. Certainly it cannot be used alone in the diagnosis of back pain etiology (158).

Electrodiagnostic Studies

An electromyogram (EMG) may be falsely normal if performed too soon after onset of symptoms. This test cannot detect nerve compression until demyelination has occurred. Later it may help to confirm nerve root compression. EMG and nerve conduction studies may be helpful in patients with atypical sciatica, nerve root entrapment syndromes, peripheral neuropathy, and herniated nucleus pulposus. Motor nerve conduction velocities, H reflexes, and F wave responses occur depending upon levels of electrical stimulation. Motor unit activity is zero electrically at rest; with contraction, electrical activity is seen. Fasciculations represent discharges of the entire motor units, and fibrillations and positive sharp waves may signify denervation. The reliability of electrodiagnostic testing is dependent upon the clinical expertise of the electromyographer (159). If critical findings for spinal cord compression are present, do not wait for an electrodiagnostic determination; obtain imaging or surgical consultation promptly.

Most patients have acute or subacute soft tissue injury as the predominant etiology of their back pain. In patients with no critical findings, the *best test* may be the injection of tender soft tissues with a local anesthetic–corticosteroid mixture, in association with a back exercise program, as a test as well as a treatment. Rapid relief of pain by this method may be more revealing than a roentgenogram of the back.

Physician variation in the use of imaging varies with specialty and locality. Thus, in a study of patients with back pain without neurologic findings, surgeons used imaging more often than nonsurgeons, and physiatrists used more electrodiagnostic tests. Rheumatologists ordered more laboratory studies than others (160).

DIFFERENTIAL DIAGNOSIS

Systemic infections cause few local findings on back examination, and local tenderness is rarely significant. Weight loss, fever, and elevation of the erythrocyte sedimentation rate should raise suspicion of an infectious origin of low back pain.

Fractures, congenital spinal deformities, spondylolysis, spondylolisthesis, spondylarthritides, Paget's disease, osteitis condensans ilii, osteoporosis, osteomalacia, and tumors are other disorders that are suggested by clinical and radiologic examination. Intraspinal neoplasms, including ependymoma, neurofibroma, or metastatic tumors, usually cause constant pain without relief when the patient is recumbent. Benign bone tumors, such as giant cell tumors, hemangioma, and osteoma, are rare. (Refer to Table 5.1 on critical signs for the low back, and to Table 5.6, a decision chart for low back pain.) Less common causes for stiffness of the spine include alkaptonuria, interspinous bursitis (Brastrup's syndrome), and Forestier's disease (161). Keep in mind, too, that herpes zoster may be a cause for unilateral back pain.

Back pain may be referred from the hip, and physical examination should detect the limitation of hip motion. Hip pain often limits the patient's ability to cross the leg while putting on a stocking (162).

Many other disorders can cause *referred pain* in the back. Peptic ulcer disease produces pain localized near the midline of the lower thoracic region; kidney disease causes flank pain with radiation into the groin; and neurofibromatosis (with café-au-lait spots) may cause sciatica-like pain that radiates into the legs. Pelvic disease and aortic aneurysms may be manifested initially as low back pain. Renal colic (stone) often refers pain into the testicle, in addition to producing back distress. Retroperitoneal fibrosis may raise the erythrocyte sedimentation rate, and prostatitis or pyelonephritis may cause a dull, persistent, ill-defined back pain.

MANAGEMENT OF LOW BACK PAIN

Acute low back pain differs from chronic low back pain (longer than 3 months' duration) in responsiveness to simple home measures. Chronic back pain is seldom due to a single structural disorder. More often social and psychologic factors equally contribute to "injury." Treatment requires that the patient have the desire to recover; the patient must have goals that he or she wishes to achieve (163).

Applying our six-point management program to low back pain should provide rational and cost-effective management.

1. Exclude serious disease (Table 5.1)
2. Recognize and eliminate simple aggravating factors (you can review Table 5.3 with the patient)
3. Provide an explanation for the patient
4. Provide pain relief (medication and physical measures)
5. Provide physical therapy and exercise advice with referral to other health professionals as appropriate
6. Provide an expected outcome for the patient

Two overriding principles of management are (a) the effect of behavior and attitude on chronicity, and (b) the fact that most patients recover if provided a spectrum of treatment modalities. Do not keep repeating the same treatment if prompt benefit has not occurred. Many of the treatment measures should be taught for home use; patients should not have to pay for things they can do at home, such as hot or cold packs, rest activities, or exercise repetitions done after the exercises have been learned (164).

Use imaging modalities to confirm a diagnosis only when critical features are present and when the patient is willing to undertake surgical treatment, if recommended.

Also be aware of the limitations of current outcome measurements. Gill and Feinstein suggest that quality of life can be measured only by determining the opinions of patients, which are not included in current instruments (165). As Lawrence et al. point out, the burden of illness is not accurately measured. Moreover, little is known about such factors as provider and patient compliance. They note, too, that the economics of therapy can guide us when no therapy is clearly superior; return-to-work and patient self-management programs should be considered as well as other therapeutic options (166).

MANAGEMENT OF AN ACUTE ATTACK OF BACK PAIN

Spontaneous improvement occurs in most acute back disorders within a few days. Therefore:

- Look for critical features (Table 5.1). If none are present, provide treatment, and then if improvement has not occurred in a timely fashion, consider further diagnostic study
- Provide instruction on changes in daily living habits, posture improvement, weight control, and other physical improvements
- Bed rest should be of limited duration, perhaps not longer than 2 days, until physical therapy or manipulation can be started (7)
- Provide pain relief
- Provide instruction on exercises or manipulation

Pain relief begins with reassuring the patient that you have found no structural damage that would cause lifelong pain. In addition, the comprehensive examination is reassuring and can convey to the patient the fact that he or she can improve. Pain relief is only an adjunct to the exercise and behavioral changes that must occur. For acute attacks of pain, teach the patient to lie down on the floor and elevate the legs on a chair in the 90/90 position whenever an attack occurs (Acute Rest Position, Exercise 5.A). Instruct the patient on proper sleep or resting positions also (Exercise 5.B). Then have

the patient begin progressive Posterior Pelvic Tilt, pelvic clock or "active sitting" (described later in this chapter), Abdominal Curls, Single and Double Knee-to-Chest exercises, and gentle Extension exercises (Exercises 5.C, 5.G, 5.D, 5.E, and 5.K, respectively; refer to Table 5.7, below). These exercises constitute a basic program that should be performed at least twice daily in the acute phase of back pain for diagnoses such as myofascial low back pain, facet joint syndrome, and the "tight back" syndrome. For persons with a "loose back," exercises should emphasize stabilizing or isometric activities, rather than stretching. Instruct the patient to progress the exercise slowly but on a consistent and regular basis. Exercise progression should remain within the patient's limits of pain and fatigue. Repetitions should be adjusted and new exercises added so that the exercise session lasts no more than 30 minutes, including warm-up and cool-down and relaxation. General warm-up can be done with slow gentle movements—a sort of "loosening up" process. Warm-up to each exercise can be done by performing the movement slowly and through only part of the range.

An alternative to floor rest and exercise would be a warm water pool program in which the patient begins with suspension in the water for 30 minutes and progresses with gentle pelvic mobility exercises in the suspended position. Relaxation and breathing exercises are important for pain management and restoration of sleep pattern, particularly in acute phases of back syndromes.

Help the patient develop a program of active self-care, even though the patient may be experiencing acute pain. In several studies the outcome for self-care was found to have better outcome, higher patient satisfaction, and lower costs than programs providing pain medication and bed rest (167, 168).

Muscle relaxants for acute pain are often helpful (169). Cyclobenzaprine is of value when muscle spasm is present. Gradual buildup of dosage from 10 mg twice daily to four times a day, or 10 mg in the morning and 20 to 30 mg in the evening, can be helpful. In a study in which cyclobenzaprine was combined with diflunisal for treatment of 7 to 10 days' duration, greater benefit and global rating improvement could be seen with the drug combination than

TABLE 5.7 EXERCISES FOR THE LOW BACK

Condition	Exercise	Exercise Number
Myofascial low back pain	Posterior Pelvic Tilt	5.C
	Single Knee-to-Chest	5.D
	Double Knee-to-Chest	5.E
	Sitting Chest-to-Knees	5.F
	Abdominal Curl	5.G
	Standing Lumbar Extension	5.K
	Straight Leg Stretch	5.L
	Wall Slide	5.M
	Back Flexibility—Arch Back	5.N(a)
	Back Flexibility—Sag Back	5.N(b)
	Tai Chi Squat	5.O
	Trunk Rotation	5.P
	Therapeutic Ball—Prone	5.R
	Aquatic Exercise	5.S
	Chinning Bar Exercise	5.T
	Piriformis Stretch	5.U
	(see also ``Nonspecific low back pain'' below)	
Facet joint syndrome	Acute Rest Position	5.A
	Supine Rest Position	5.B
	Posterior Pelvic Tilt	5.C
	Single Knee-to-Chest	5.D
	Double Knee-to-Chest	5.E
	Sitting Chest-to-Knees	5.F
	Abdominal Curl	5.G
	Straight Leg Stretch	5.L
	Wall Slide	5.M
	Back Flexibility—Arch Back	5.N(a)
	Supine Lumbar Stabilization	5.Q
	Aquatic Exercise	5.S
	Chinning Bar Exercise	5.T
Herniated nucleus pulposus (discogenic disease and sciatica)		
Acute	Acute Rest Position	5.A
	Posterior Pelvic Tilt[a]	5.C
	Elbow Prop[a]	5.H
Resolving	Acute Rest Position	5.A
	Supine Rest Position	5.B
	Single Knee-to-Chest	5.D
	Prone Push-up	5.I
	Standing Lumbar Extension	5.K
	Straight Leg Stretch	5.L
	Prone Lumbar Extension	5.J
Chronic	Any of the above in a graded progression. The following can be introduced as tolerated:	
	Supine Rest Position	5.B
	Posterior Pelvic Tilt	5.C
	Prone Push-up	5.I
	Prone Lumbar Extension	5.J
	Standing Lumbar Extension	5.K
	Straight Leg Stretch	5.L
	Wall Slide	5.M
	Back Flexibility—Arch Back	5.N(a)
	Back Flexibility—Sag Back	5.N(b)
	Tai Chi Squat	5.O
	Trunk Rotation	5.P
	Supine Lumbar Stabilization	5.Q
	Therapeutic Ball	5.R
	Chinning Bar Exercise	5.T
	Piriformis Stretch	5.U

(continued)

TABLE 5.7 EXERCISES FOR THE LOW BACK *(continued)*

Condition	Exercise	Exercise Number
Lumbar spinal stenosis	Acute Rest Position	5.A
	Supine Rest Position	5.B
	Posterior Pelvic Tilt	5.C
	Single Knee-to-Chest	5.D
	Double Knee-to-Chest	5.E
	Sitting Chest-to-Knees	5.F
	Abdominal Curl	5.G
	Straight Leg Stretch	5.L
	Wall Slide	5.M
	Aquatic Exercise	5.S
	Chinning Bar Exercise	5.T
Piriformis syndrome	Single Knee-to-Chest	5.D
	Double Knee-to-Chest	5.E
	Straight Leg Stretch	5.L
	Piriformis Stretch	5.U
Psychogenic back pain	See ''Nonspecific low back pain'' according to symptoms	
Nonspecific low back pain (LBP)		
1. ''Loose'' Back	Posterior Pelvic Tilt	5.C
	Prone Push-up	5.I
	Prone Lumbar Extension	5.J
	Standing Lumbar Extension	5.K
	Straight Leg Stretch	5.L
	Tai Chi Squat	5.O
	Supine Lumbar Stabilization	5.Q
	Therapeutic Ball—Prone	5.R
	Aquatic Exercise	5.S
2. ''Tight'' Back	Posterior Pelvic Tilt	5.C
	Single Knee-to-Chest	5.D
	Double Knee-to-Chest	5.E
	Sitting Chest-to-Knees	5.F
	Abdominal Curl	5.G
	Straight Leg Stretch	5.L
	Back Flexibility—Arch Back	5.N(a)
	Back Flexibility—Sag Back	5.N(b)
	Trunk Rotation	5.P
	Aquatic Exercise	5.S
	Chinning Bar Exercise	5.T
	Piriformis Stretch	5.U

[a]Pain tolerance is the determining factor.
Note: Aquatic and Therapeutic Ball programs can be designed for any stage.

with either drug alone, or with placebo. Peak benefit occurred at day 4 (170). Other nonsteroidal antiinflammatory agents (NSAIDs) may be similarly utilized. Analgesics may be necessary. If osteoarthritis is present, a nonaspirin NSAID can be useful, but many patients respond to acetaminophen or nonacetylated salicylate when used first.

As soon as acute pain begins to resolve and the patient tolerates more movement and activity, exercise time should increase as well as the number and variety of exercises performed.

Manipulation of the spine has been utilized for nearly a century, and a major segment of the patient population with chronic back pain utilizes this treatment.

Seven techniques of manipulation that include thrusting, hyperextension, rotation, torsion, and pelvic rock are commonly in use; in general, rotational and mobilizing types are also used (171, 172). Increasing interest in the various ''hands-on'' forms of therapy has led to numerous books and articles describing the techniques. Swezey (173) has provided a comprehensive review of this subject including massage, traction, mobilization, and manipulation.

Manipulation combined with behavior modification is a valid treatment (174, 175). Compared with all other forms of treatment, manipulation for acute and subacute onset of back pain is effective with earlier onset of pain relief, and at significantly lower cost (172, 176–185).

Meta-analysis of spinal manipulation reveals a positive correlation of this treatment with recovery at 3 weeks (186). Also, manipulation was found to be more effective than mobilization (187). Hadler et al. (188) report a prospective controlled trial of manipulation versus mobilization for nonindustrial back pain of a duration of 1 month or less. Manipulation was found to be modestly better, with earlier onset of pain relief. Multimodalities have been found to be more effective than manipulation or mobilization alone (189–191). Blomberg et al. studied the effect of local pain (trigger) point corticosteroid injections added to manual therapy. The combined therapy result was found to be superior to conventional treatment in Swedish primary health care in improving the everyday function of patients with low back pain. The combined treatment was also more cost-effective: both groups (manual therapy alone versus combined therapy) had an average of 3.8 and 3.5 physician visits, but the manual therapy alone group had an average of 8.6 physiotherapy visits versus only 2.0 visits for those having the combined therapy (86, 86a). Two studies of the cost-effectiveness of chiropractic manipulation, however, found that the number of visits required by the chiropractor, as well as the tendency to use more radiologic studies, resulted in higher cost than physical therapy (191a). In another prospective and randomized study of 1633 patients with low back pain, primary care practitioners provided less costly care than that provided by orthopaedists or chiropractors, with similar outcomes for all three groups (191b).

TREATMENT FOR HERNIATED NUCLEUS PULPOSUS

Selection for surgery should be based upon a definite diagnosis and indications for a specific surgical procedure (e.g., laminectomy, fusion, abscess drainage). Most patients with a herniated nucleus pulposus do not require surgical intervention.

Indications for surgery usually require imaging. Indications for imaging and myelography include presence of a cauda equina syndrome, sciatic pain, a corresponding neurologic deficit, or failure to respond to conservative management.

In the absence of neurologic weakness, back pain should be treated conservatively and imaging considered for those who fail a 6-week comprehensive treatment program that can be provided in the office setting. Examination for critical findings should be repeated if symptoms persist beyond 2 or 3 weeks.

The importance of using multiple modalities in treatment is emphasized. Saal and Saal reported that of 64 patients with sciatica, a positive EMG, and a positive CT scan demonstrating a herniated nucleus pulposus without significant stenosis, 90% had good or excellent results, with 92% returning to work. But to achieve this, the patients had a multiple modality treatment program including a back school, spinal stabilization with exercise training for postural control, trunk and general body strengthening, and flexibility exercises. Epidural and selective nerve root blocks were used when indicated for pain control (192). A meta-analysis of low back pain demonstrated the positive value of a multimodality program in returning patients to work without surgery (37 studies) (192a).

Specific exercises useful in the management of the herniated nucleus pulposus are listed in Table 5.7, including activities for the acute, resolving, and chronic stages. The patient's tolerance for pain and movement are the deciding factors in the progression of the exercises, as well as in choosing the exercises that relieve rather than exacerbate the pain. Exercises that promote mobility and flexibility of the spine and trunk (Pelvic Tilt, Exercise 5.C; Prone Push-up, Exercise 5.I; and Lumbar Extension, Exercises 5.J and 5.K) should be started as early as possible; they may be performed in partial ranges if that is all that the patient can tolerate. These exercises can also aid in relaxation of spasm and muscle tension. Strengthening exercises to maintain trunk (abdominal and extensor) stability (Wall slides, Exercise 5.M; Tai Chi Squat, Exercise 5.O; and Lumbar Stabilization, Exercise 5.Q) should be introduced as soon as the patient can tolerate the exertion. Exercises to maintain length and flexibility of the hamstring muscles and trunk muscles should be introduced as soon as the patient can tolerate movement and mild stretching (these include Sitting Straight Leg Stretch, Exercise 5.F; Back Flexibility, Exercise 5.N; Standing Trunk Rotation, Exercise 5.P; Therapeutic Ball Exercises, Exercise 5.R; Chinning Bar Exercise, Exercise 5.T; and Piriformis Stretch, Exercise 5.U).

Patients with chronic pain and poor muscle tone and those with spinal degenerative disorders often do well with an aquatic program that includes water walking and mild pool aerobics. If lower limb or foot disorders hamper the aquatic program, a flotation program may be helpful (Exercise 5.S).

Chemonucleolysis and disc surgery are reserved for patients with critical findings that are severe or have persisted beyond 6 weeks of therapy (193). Chemonucleolysis results are less satisfactory in cases with a free (sequestered) segment (194). Considering total costs, surgery is more cost-effective than chemonucleolysis (195). Chemonucleolysis with chymopapain has significant risk and toxicity and is used less commonly now. However, it has been approved for selected patients with established herniated nucleus pulposus. Criteria for treatment include the presence of at least four of the following five features:

1. Leg pain greater than back pain
2. Paresthesia localized to a dermatome
3. Straight leg raising reduced 50% or more, or positive tibial nerve sign
4. Two or more neurologic findings: atrophy, motor weakness, reflex loss, diminished sensory appreciation
5. Radiologic evidence of abnormality

Chymopapain was compared with placebo in a double-blind randomized study. Thirty-one of 53 placebo-treated patients failed to benefit, whereas 40 of 53 chymopapain-treated patients were improved. Of the placebo failures, all were then given chymopapain, and 91% improved (196). In another randomized prospective study without selection, less success with chymopapain was reported: those treated with chymopapain had a 52% failure rate, whereas those operated upon had an 11% failure rate (197). Chymopapain has adverse reactions including anaphylaxis. Only experienced surgeons who carefully screen patients for the procedure should be given referrals. In their

hands, up to 80% beneficial results have been reported (198).

Surgical results parallel the size of defect seen on myelograms (i.e., the larger the defect, the greater the chances of a good outcome). *The severity of a patient's pain is a poor indicator for surgical outcome.* Surprisingly, surgical outcome has not been found to be well correlated with psychopathology as evidenced by personality inventory determination (199). Resumption of normal activity postoperatively was 16 days when no secondary gain (i.e., reduced work stress, compensation) was present, compared to 36 days if secondary gain was evident. Also, surgical failures were twice as common in those having secondary gain (200). When sciatic pain or neurologic impairment is present and imaging provides evidence of significant stenosis, surgery is successful in up to 96% of cases (194).

TREATMENT FOR CHRONIC OR RECURRENT LOW BACK PAIN

Comprehensive care involves using multiple resources—and the earlier, the better. Even the most severely disabled can be returned to gainful employment or removed from a dependency position if all facets of the physical and psychosocial milieu are considered and addressed (191, 201–203). Restoration of physical and mental hardiness is essential for long-term benefit. Treatment may also be structured according to pain intensity, pain-related disability, and pain persistence (204). The patient who has some good or well days would seem more likely to benefit with fewer modalities, but data are not available. As mentioned, questionnaires that might indicate a more tailored approach for individual patients are undergoing refinement. Treatment programs might include:

- Behavior change
- Back schools
- Corsets and braces
- Physical therapy and exercises
- Medications such as mood altering drugs
- Work-hardening
- Soft tissue injections
- Lumbar epidural injections

Behavior Change: Psychosocial factors must be considered at the outset of management.

As Fordyce (205) has pointed out, we must not merely treat the experience of pain, we must also treat the disability of pain behavior. Dissatisfaction with job and coworkers, marriage or relationships, or problems that seem to have no solutions should be revealed (206). Drug dependency, including smoking, is also important. Work habits, home activities, and sports should be considered too. Cognitive-behavioral therapy for chronic low back pain should be reserved for patients with severe illness behavior and should be used in conjuction with other treatment programs. Only an experienced psychologist should be consulted. In one study comparing cognitive-behavioral therapy with EMG feedback, both were found to be moderately effective (206a). Both are costly.

Aggravating factors to be determined include lifting, stooping, bending, prolonged sitting, stair climbing, use of high-heeled shoes, and strains resulting from occupational sources or new hobbies. Nachemson has stressed consideration for the strain involved in lifting with the knees straight instead of flexed, and the back flexed instead of straight (25). (In nearly all cases of gluteal area pain, a history of lifting with straight knees can be obtained.)

Proper sitting positions should be provided. The trunk-thigh angle should be 105 degrees or greater (207). Thus, the upright portion of the chair should be tilted slightly backward from the vertical position, the seat should be convex, and support for the lumbar region should be present across the back of the chair. Sitting forward or backward from this position increases lumbar flexion and thereby increases lumbar disc compression. The height of the chair should allow frequent changes in position, and the distance of eye level to a work surface should be approximately 16 inches (eyeglasses are set for this distance). There should be an open space beneath the seat of the chair to allow knee flexion beyond 90 degrees (207). The patient's feet should be able to touch the floor or a footrest. The end of the seat should be approximately 5 inches from the posterior aspect of the knee. The seat fabric should be porous. The height of the table or work surface may have to be adjustable also, allowing the arms to be comfortable as the patient sits back. Inexpensive seating supports can be temporarily devised with folded towels, sheets, or papers. Trial and error is often the best procedure for developing seating adaptation.

Proper resting positions for patients with back pain should reduce lumbar lordosis. Such positions are detailed in Exercises 5.A and 5.B (25, 208). Use of a bed pan actually increases lumbar lordosis and disc pressure, and is more aggravating than allowing the patient to use a bedside commode (21). Proper bed rest as the only treatment of low back pain should be used for no longer than a 1 or 2 days (7). Patients should avoid sleeping on the stomach, or straight out, flat on the back; both positions cause hyperextension of the lumbar spine. Preferred sleep positions include side-lying or supine with legs elevated so that hips and knees are both flexed to 90 degrees.

Patients who work on concrete floors or walk with a heavy heel-strike may benefit from the use of viscoelastic shoe inserts (209) or running shoes.

Back schools have become increasingly popular. These programs teach groups of patients techniques for symptomatic management as well as prevention. Ergonomic analysis of job tasks can be provided. Patients have a fair degree of satisfaction with this approach (210, 211), but they must be able to comprehend the information (208, 212). In one study, employment status doubled after back school education (212). However, patients with acute back pain do not benefit (58). Back schools should provide follow-up reinforcement of the behavior modification. The physician should perform this task for patients who have attended a back school.

In a study of a back school program that was individualized to a production line or company, the reported incidence of low back pain was not reduced, but the company absenteeism was reduced by at least 5 days per year per employee (213).

Back schools should be combined with work-hardening, labor and management input, and preventive techniques (210a). A California controlled study of county government employees who had a high rate of absenteeism for back pain revealed that the intervention group showed a modest decline in back pain prevalence rates but a significant improvement in satisfaction and reduction in risky behaviors at 1 year postintervention. The return on investment at 1 year was calculated to be 179% (214).

Corsets and Braces: If a corset is used, it should provide abdominal compression and generally be utilized for a limited time. The patient should learn to depend on stronger abdominal muscle tone for back support (123, 215). In general, fewer than 5% of patients with back disease follow through on wearing the corset after purchase (174).

A back brace differs from a corset in having horizontal rigid elements, producing more restriction of spinal motion. A brace is utilized predominantly for patients with osteoporosis and vertebral compression fractures, or for posttraumatic vertebral fractures. The lumbosacral support corset with a heat-moldable plastic insert can be used in older patients with osteoporosis, those with lumbosacral junction anomalies, or in young patients with joint laxity until they develop good abdominal tone with exercise.

Physical Therapy and Exercises: Patients with chronic or repeated pain occurrences should be referred for a comprehensive back rehabilitation and protection program provided by physical and occupational therapists. Strong encouragement should be offered for the development of a lifelong exercise habit that includes daily exercises done at home and participation in community exercise programs. In addition to those exercises that are aimed at the back structures, activities that produce results such as cardiovascular conditioning, neuroendocrine effects, and general flexibility are important. Movement programs such as dance, Tai Chi, aquatics, walking or hiking, bicycling, and yoga can provide recreational as well as remedial benefits.

Physical modalities such as heat, cold, electrotherapy, and ultrasound should be recommended as adjuncts to physical exercise, and expensive modalities limited to those that produce obvious benefits within a short period of time.

A variety of manual techniques such as massage, trigger or pain point pressure techniques, and myofascial release can be beneficial for short-term relief. These techniques should be combined with restorative exercise programs.

Posture retraining and movement education can address problems of alignment and movement dysfunction. Back pain of any duration causes compensatory adjustments in movement and posture that can further complicate function. Movement education techniques such as those of Feldenkrais (''Movement Awareness'') incorporate relaxation, breathing, and progressive movement patterns to return integrated function. Posture retraining should address total patterns, including neck and thoracic spine, rather than simply pelvic position. The soft tissues that encompass the ''low back'' actually have attachments in the upper spine and neck so that compensatory patterns are complex and wide-reaching.

A wide variety of exercise programs and philosophies has been proposed to address low back pain, including those that emphasize flexion, extension, lumbar stabilization, or the use of special equipment such as a therapeutic ball. Programs using isokinetic equipment have been popularized in some centers. All programs have had some benefit when properly carried out—none is clearly superior to the others in controlled studies. The best program is clearly the one that the patient will carry out over a long period of time, without expensive equipment, producing the desired results under the guidance of a health or exercise professional who is available for ongoing consultation when necessary. Table 5.7 lists specific exercises that are recommended for some of the diagnoses discussed in this chapter.

For the patient with chronic or persistent back pain due to these conditions, the exercises should be arranged in a program that includes the easier, basic exercises as warm-up activities and then progresses to the more difficult activities. For instance, in myofascial back pain, Exercises 5.C to 5.G and 5.K can be done in the first few minutes of a session. Then Exercises 5.F, 5.L through 5.P, 5.T, and 5.U can be arranged so that the existing problems are addressed. As the patient progresses, exercises can be moved to the ''warm-up'' phase with only a few repetitions and more attention given to specific problems such as tight hamstrings, quadriceps weakness, and so on. Consultation with a physical or occupational therapist can be helpful in determining the composition of an exercise program, and it should be expected that the program will change over time. Similar program development should occur with the patient who has a diagnosis of facet joint syndrome or nonspecific low back pain.

Several types of aquatic therapy and exercise programs are available for patients with back pain, addressing acute as well as chronic conditions, with both preventive and rehabilitative goals. For the acute injury, suspension in warm water (traction effect) with gentle progressive exercise can provide early comfort and mobility. The properties of water (thermal, buoyancy, resistance, and drag) provide an excellent medium for comprehensive programs. Progression to calisthenic exercise done in water, water walking, or water aerobics can occur as the patient's abilities permit. Exercise activities can vary the arc of motion, the number of movements in a particular pattern, the speed of movement, surface exposed, equipment used, and length of time of exercise in order to produce the desired effects. Water exercise programs can vary from very gentle to extremely vigorous. Aquatic therapists with appropriate training are skilled professionals who utilize the properties of water with other techniques to address specific problems and goals in treatment. Pool programs have the advantage of providing recreational as well as therapeutic benefits.

''Active sitting'' is a technique in which the person alternately contracts the abdominal muscles, arches the low back and hikes one hip then the other while in a sitting position. It is done in any sitting position and provides excellent relief from muscle tension and fatigue. Teach this technique in the office setting and urge frequent performance.

The health care professional can provide a home exercise program on the first visit. The exercises can be selected on the basis of muscle tightness (with flattening of the lumbar spine), presence or absence of sciatica, posture, and degree of strength and tone. Table 5.7 and the exercise illustrations at the end of the chapter are provided for guidance. All illustrations may be photocopied for this purpose. The clinician should demonstrate the exercise, not just hand out the illustration. The number of repetitions and the number of times a day to perform them should be individualized. If the patient is given much more than 10 to 30 minutes of exercise per session, many patients, in our experience, will not cooperate.

Medications: Acetaminophen, salicylates, nonacetylated salicylates, other NSAIDs, and mild analgesics, with or without muscle relaxants, are useful to most patients. The use of tricyclic antidepressants for nocturnal sedation as well as for depression has been helpful for many patients with chronic back pain. There is a growing recognition of the value of mood altering drugs, such as amitriptyline, in providing improvement in back pain (133, 169, 174, 215). These agents should be started slowly, and are often prescribed as a single bedtime dose. Side effects of morning hangover or daytime dry mouth may be diminished with a regimen consisting of dosage given every 2 hours for two or three doses each evening (e.g., 6 PM, 8 PM, 10 PM). In a prospective study of chronic back pain in which amitriptyline was tested against atropine (used as a placebo), MMPI scales normalized and analgesic use dropped by 50% in the treatment group (216).

NSAIDs may be helpful in some patients with chronic myofascial back pain, especially those with associated degenerative arthritis of the posterior apophyseal joints. Benefit is related to analgesic or antiinflammatory effects or both. When significant lumbar stenosis with sciatica is also present, lumbar epidural steroid injections may be helpful (see below).

There is no place for long-term oral corticosteroids in any nonspecific disorder of the low back. Therapeutic exercise is the cornerstone of management.

Work-hardening: The injured worker can benefit from work-hardening. The technique identifies movements specific to each job task, and then an exercise program is developed for strengthening the muscles used in the task. This program is supervised by an occupational therapist. The patient is guided through highly structured simulated work tasks. Work-hardening may help the patient achieve a level of productivity that is acceptable in the competitive labor market (217).

Soft Tissue Injections: Indications include:
1. Patients with persistent pain of several weeks' duration or longer, with either very localized pain within soft tissues or diffuse pain across the sacrum and glutei

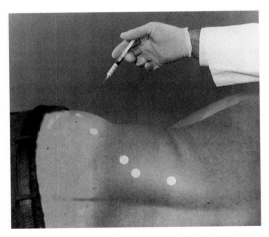

Figure 5.11. Myofascial pain point injection. Using the needle as a probe, the points of tenderness are located. Following skin penetration, aliquots of a corticosteroid–local anesthetic mixture are injected. Needle length varies with the size of the patient and ranges from a 1½-inch No. 22 needle to a 4-inch No. 20 spinal needle. Often both sides require injection at the same time, but we seldom exceed a volume of 5 mL or a total of 80 mg steroid.

2. Tenderness localized in the sacroiliac joint region
3. Pain at rest that is worse than pain during movement or walking
4. Stiffness and tightness of the low back that has not responded to oral medication and stretching

Steindler (218) advocated in 1938 the use of local anesthetic injections within the soft tissue of the low back, and claimed lasting relief in the vast majority of patients with low back pain. He emphasized the importance of using the needle as a probe; contact of the needle with the area of tenderness must reproduce the patient's pain before injection (Fig. 5.11, below).

In a controlled study comparing the effects of long-acting local anesthetics versus saline solution, patients were assessed as follows: by a subjective pain scale; the effect of pain on physical activity; on limitation of movement; and the effect of pain on mood and sleep at the following intervals: before, 15 minutes after, 24 hours after, and 7 days after injections. Benefit was noted in the control group only at 15 minutes; but the treatment group had significant pain relief and global improvement at each assessment. Bupivacaine 0.5%,

up to 36 mL per patient visit, was used; no adverse reactions were reported (219). Using bupivacaine alone may require up to 12 visits (220, 221). Also, cardiac and other sensitivity reactions to bupivacaine are not uncommon.

Collee et al. (222) noted little difference in a 2-week double-blind, randomized study comparing the efficacy of a single injection of 5 mL lignocaine 0.5% with that of 5 mL isotonic saline in 41 patients with tenderness over the medial part of the iliac crest. Pain score results favored lignocaine injection, though the difference was not appreciable.

The addition of a corticosteroid agent combined with a local anesthetic may reduce the frequency of visits and shorten the duration of disability. The corticosteroid agent should be a long-acting preparation (13, 123, 133, 174, 223, 224).

The efficacy of local soft tissue injections of an anesthetic and corticosteroid mixture has not been well studied but it is safe and should be considered as a cost-effective measure in the individual patient. Garvey (225) reported little added benefit in using the combined corticosteroid and local anesthetic agents for treatment of lumbosacral strain in patients who did have a localized point of maximum tenderness, and duration longer than 1 month. On the other hand, Bourne (226) reported results in patients with nonspecific chronic low back pain followed for longer than 10 years; injections consisted of triamcinolone acetonide 10 mg and 1 mL lidocaine hydrochloride 1% into the point of maximum tenderness in 22 patients. Pain relief for a minimum of 5 weeks per injection was the minimum criterion for ''success.'' Over the 10-year period the average patient received a total of 44 mg triamcinolone. When the sacroiliac joint region was the major pain site, the result was good in 51%, fair in 28%, and a failure in 21% of patients. For soft tissue pain in other areas of the back, the results were 52%, 24%, and 24%, respectively. Overall, these 22 patients had a total of 115 points of tenderness injected, in which 77% good or fair results were obtained. Similar results were reported by Sonne et al. (227).

In our experience, patients with pain of 3 months' duration or longer will often have relief of symptoms for 3 weeks or more when a maximum of 20 mg methylprednisolone or triamcinolone mixed with a local anesthetic is injected per lesion. Do not exceed a total of 80 mg steroid at one visit. We do not inject more than six times per year.

To perform a soft tissue injection, prepare area with soap and alcohol. We prefer to use up to 80 mg methylprednisolone acetate sterile aqueous suspension with an equal amount of lidocaine hydrochloride 1% because the mixture will flocculate within the syringe and may prolong the local effectiveness of the injection. Using the shortest needle that can reach the required depth, use the needle as a probe. Lumbar, sacroiliac, and gluteal areas usually require a 2-inch depth. When the lesion is reached, pain is perceived. Inject 20 mg steroid or less per lesion. Some patients will have a concomitant trochanteric bursitis; check the area of the trochanteric bursae; if tender, the area should be injected as well. Have the patient apply ice for 10 to 20 minutes after the injection. Up to a total of 80 mg of the corticosteroid can be injected but should not be repeated within 6 to 8 weeks (Fig. 5.11). The presacral fascia, trochanteric bursa region, and sacroiliac joint areas often contain tender areas and all may be injected if symptomatic; a No. 20 3.5-inch spinal needle may be required in obese persons.

The *piriformis syndrome* (see section on this topic, below) may similarly benefit from such injection therapy. Steroid injection may be tried in patients with *spinal stenosis*. We have seen many patients who failed lumbar epidural block treatment who have ongoing benefit with soft tissue injections; failure with epidural injections does not mean failure with soft tissue injections. Using the needle as a probe (2-inch No. 20 or 3.5-inch spinal needle), injecting deep into the erector spinae, at the region of the apophyseal joints L3-L4, L4-L5, and L5-S1, into the sacroiliac joints and, if tender, into the deep gluteal muscles on each side may provide several months of relief.

The patient with low back pain associated with episacroiliac lipoma may have substantial and lasting pain relief by an injection of the areas of tenderness, including the lipomas. The presacral fascia beneath the lipoma is the probable site for tenderness (127, 128).

Facet Joint Injections: Although facet joint injections with corticosteroids have been advocated (154), results are mixed, and their high cost is a deterrent to their use (171, 228–232). In one study, a 23% long-term placebo effect was noted (232). Lynch and Taylor noted that facet joint injection requires the routine use of arthrography, with added cost and risk (154). Murtagh reported success with a CT-guided injection technique (233). Since the publication in 1988 of a well-done study that questioned the reliability of the diagnosis of facet joint syndrome as a specific entity and the cost-effectiveness of facet joint treatment, the use of injections for facet joint syndrome has largely been abandoned (234).

Lumbar Epidural Injections: Caudal epidural injections of triamcinolone plus procaine hydrochloride is reserved for patients with intractable sciatic pain, spinal stenosis, and inoperative disc herniation. It is also effective in some patients with reflex sympathetic dystrophy. Controlled studies have demonstrated mixed results (235). Resolution of psychosocial factors has been found to be more important when epidural blocks were administered to persons with work-related injury (236). Complications following epidural steroid therapy are rare; they include bacterial meningitis, anesthetic toxicity, steroid toxicity, and improper needle placement (237). The nerve blocks are frequently administered in a series of three, 1 month apart. Cost is a significant factor as well, and epidural blocks should generally be used only after a comprehensive regimen of psychosocial interventions, physical therapy, and medications have been used. Intradisc steroid injection has not proved effective (238).

OUTCOME AND ADDITIONAL SUGGESTIONS

Return to the previous accepted level of function represents a "satisfactory outcome." This, of course, is modified by age and other health situations (174, 239). Outcome often depends on the motivation of the patient and good communication between all involved parties (employer, insurer, physician, attorney, patient, and the patient's family) (174).

The importance of a comprehensive program for low back pain was reported by Reed and Harvey in 1964 (239). In this study, medical, psychologic, sociologic, and vocational evaluations were performed on 185 persons, all of whom were on welfare although previously employed. Of these, after treatment, only 69 patients were felt likely to be employable full-time; 31 of these 69 welfare recipients did become fully employed; in addition, 16 became part-time employees. Interestingly, 33 other patients left the evaluation program prematurely because they had obtained full-time employment. Only four were believed to be malingering.

In a more recent study of a series of 100 patients with chronic low back pain, 80% were reportedly improved; however, of those previously working, only three actually returned to work (174). Yet, in most series, fewer than 2% of patients with back pain are found to be malingering. These reports offer conflicting return-to-work results, and the issue bears further scrutiny, perhaps both methodologically and sociopolitically.

Transcutaneous Electrical Nerve Stimulation (TENS): This modality provides short-term benefit in patients with postsurgical back pain, but benefit has been found not to last beyond 2 months (240). TENS did not add to the benefit of an exercise program when compared with sham TENS in a controlled study of chronic low back pain (241). Many insurance companies will not cover this treatment anymore.

Acupuncture: Acupuncture (recommended by Osler 50 years ago! [19]) has come and gone in the treatment of low back pain in this country. In one study, when the acupuncture therapist provided no suggestion of benefit to the patient, only 4% of the patients had lasting relief (242). This failure of acupuncture was confirmed by others (243).

Radiofrequency denervation, and *posterior rhizotomy* have been advocated but are investigational in the opinion of many authors and clinicians (244–248).

Pain Centers and Spas: Pain centers are utilizing multiple treatment modalities in an inpatient setting. The eight points of treatment listed by Gottlieb (249) are: biofeedback relaxation, self-control techniques to handle stress and anxiety, patient-regulated medication, case conferences, physical therapy education, vocational rehabilitation, patient education, and a

therapeutic milieu. Some critics of pain clinics view them as a graduate school for professional pain patients (250)! European spas provide a relaxing and graded exercise program, diet, and frequently include injections with phenylbutazone.

A comprehensive back therapy program requires active patient participation. Structural causes for pain, if present, are treated with anesthetic blocks or corticosteroid-anesthetic blocks and injections. Such programs include patient participation in daily activities under the direction of a psychologist, a physical therapist, an occupational therapist, a recreational therapist, and a physician. Should the patient fail on the initial program, he or she then may enter a cognitive behavior modification program led by a psychologist. The patient obtains positive reinforcement support for demonstrating improvement, which includes decreased dependency on drugs other than psychotropic agents. Discharge goals are set by the patient in group therapy sessions (251). Patients learn to recognize manipulative factors of chronic pain complaints and their effects on interpersonal relationships. A 10-month follow-up in one program revealed that 70% of the patients had increased their activity or were working. In an 80-month follow-up of 36 patients in a similar pain clinic program, despite verbal reports of continued pain, most patients reported that they were coping much better with back pain, and they displayed a marked reduction in their utilization of medical resources (252). However, most of these patients still regard themselves as failures, and require praise and further encouragement for the smallest improvements (251). No controls were used.

It should be obvious to the physician that a pain center must provide a multifaceted program. "Center" programs that provide only one or two modalities, such as biofeedback training or acupuncture, do not suffice and can only delay comprehensive care.

Most patients with low back pain require supportive and preventive therapy. They usually do not have a complex esoteric disease. A treatment regimen, readily provided in an outpatient setting, includes (*a*) recognition and modification of aggravating factors, sometimes involving vocational guidance personnel or an occupational therapist; (b) physical therapy and exercise to restore proper soft tissue support for the spine; (c) relief from pain with mild analgesics, NSAIDs, ice massage, vapocoolant spray, and stretch, or with local soft tissue injections using an anesthetic-corticosteroid mixture; (d) proper instructions in rest, with or without a corset or traction; and (e) possible use of mood altering drugs for nocturnal sedation and for altering pain perception. Even the patient with chronic long-standing back pain can be helped in most instances by the personal physician.

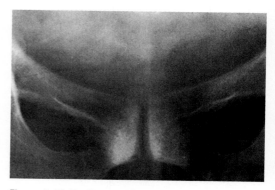

Figure 5.12. Radiographic features of osteitis pubis include erosion, sclerosis, and widening of the symphysis pubis.

PAIN SYNDROMES OF THE PELVIS

Postpartum and Nongynecologic Pelvic Pain Disorders

Nongynecologic somatic pelvic pain is a common problem; in one study of 183 women, 47% were thought to have a musculoskeletal origin for the pain. These women had a better outcome than those with other etiologies (253).

Chronic back pain following epidural anesthesia has also been a common concern. A small retrospective study comparing outcome following extradural or general anesthesia found a greater incidence of chronic back pain occurring after extradural anesthesia (254). Similar findings were noted in a much larger retrospective study of 11,701 women: 19% had chronic back pain following epidural anesthesia versus 10% without epidural anesthesia. Of these, 26 women had persistent buttock and leg paresthesias, and 23 of those 26 had an epidural anesthetic (255).

Osteitis Condensans Ilii

Sclerosing densities occur on the iliac side of the pelvis. These are usually readily distinguishable from the radiographic features of ankylosing spondylitis in which the lesion involves both the sacrum and ilium. Blaschke, however, reviewed 109 patients with the finding of osteitis condensans ilii and discovered that one-third suffered from sciatica, two-thirds had a diffuse fibromyalgia syndrome, and nearly half of the patients had an elevation of

the erythrocyte sedimentation rate (256). The symptoms often are self-limited and may respond to NSAIDs. HLA-B27 typing is reported to be positive in 25% of these patients (257). Findings of osteitis condensans ilii may be seen in patients with familial chondrocalcinosis and calcium apatite deposition disease. Two involved families, reported by Arturi et al. (258), with a total of nine affected persons, demonstrated osteitis condensans ilii (3/9), costal cartilage calcification (7/9), intervertebral disc calcification (4/9), and articular calcifications (3/9).

Osteitis Pubis

Inflammation on each side of the periosteal bone of the symphysis pubis is detectable clinically by local direct point tenderness, and radiographically by erosion, sclerosis, and widening of the symphysis pubis (Fig. 5.12). This disorder may result from regional spread of sepsis following surgery of the prostate gland or bladder, or inguinal herniorrhaphy. However, it often occurs insidiously without any known provoking cause. The vast majority of patients are females aged in the 20s through the 40s. The presentation consists of pain in the low anterior pelvis with radiation into the adductor muscles of both thighs. The patient may assume a duck-waddling gait. Local tenderness with reproduction or accentuation of pain by pressure over the symphysis pubis is diagnostic. Tenderness may occur before radiographic changes are evident. Later, the radiographic features of bone rarefaction and erosion, with

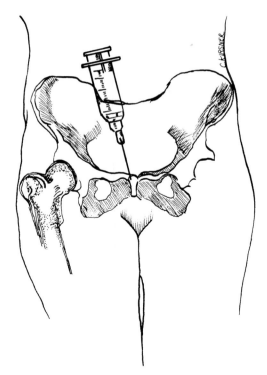

Figure 5.13. Injection for osteitis pubis. After proper preparation, a 1½-inch No. 22 or No. 23 needle is used as a probe. The corticosteroid–local anesthetic mixture is injected at the proximal symphysis pubis region along the bony surface. Strict aseptic technique is essential.

separation of the symphysis pubis and subsequent new bone repair, are revealed (259).

Osteitis pubis may be secondary to ankylosing spondylitis, chondrocalcinosis (259, 260), or polymyalgia rheumatica (261). When the condition is associated with arthritis, pain frequently has no relation to radiographic change. In female patients, subluxation and irregularity of the medial surfaces were found to be correlated with number of children born and not to arthritis (260). Often the condition is self-limited, and symptomatic benefit may be obtained from use of NSAIDs (262), or from local corticosteroid injections into the tender regions of the symphysis pubis (Fig. 5.13) if sepsis has been excluded.

To perform an injection, prepare area with soap and alcohol. Shaving is not necessary. Draw up to 40 mg methylprednisolone acetate sterile aqueous suspension (or other equivalent corticosteroid suspension) with an equal amount of lidocaine hydrochloride 1%; the mix-ture will flocculate within the syringe. Identify the point of maximum tenderness on the pubic bone at the symphysis pubis. Using the shortest needle that can reach the required depth, use the needle as a probe. When the lesion is reached, pain is perceived. Inject 1 mL or less per lesion. Have the patient apply ice for 10 to 20 minutes after the injection. Up to a total of 40 mg of the corticosteroid can be injected but should not be repeated within 6 to 8 weeks. Usually only one injection is necessary.

Use of a sacral belt to stabilize the pelvis has also provided symptomatic benefit. Obviously, when radiographic progression suggests osteomyelitis, surgical consultation should be obtained (259). Some surgeons advocate wedge resection of the symphysis pubis for persistent symptoms, but pelvis instability can result in up to one-third of operated patients (263).

Traumatic osteitis pubis, the *gracilis syndrome,* is a fatigue fracture of the bony origin of the gracilis muscle at the pubic symphysis. Surgery, in one case, suggested that the lesion resulted from an avulsion fracture (264). Similarly, osteitis pubis may result from injuries of the adductor longus muscle origin. Pain usually radiates to the perineal region or to the adductor region of the thigh. Athletic activities associated with traumatic osteitis pubis include fencing, basketball, track, hockey, soccer, and bowling. A bony lesion on the lower margin of the pubis at the symphysis is often the only roentgenographic finding. Spontaneous relief has been reported; others recommend local corticosteroid injection; surgical procedure is recommended only if symptoms persist beyond 6 months and a definite lesion is evident (264).

Chronic groin pain, usually unilateral, at the pubic insertion of the inguinal ligament, may be an enthesopathy from overuse. Treatment with a corticosteroid and local anesthetic mixture was found in one study to be beneficial in patients who agreed to the injection, as compared to those who deferred treatment. When it is effective, the injection may spare the patient elaborate investigation or surgery (264a).

Coccygodynia

This disorder may occur secondary to low back disorders with referred pain to the coccyx region; from visceral, rectal, or genitourinary disturbances with regional muscle spasm; from local myofascial injury with point tenderness at the sacrococcygeal joint; from rectal clenching (M Sinaki, personal communication, 1986), or from local inflammatory or posttraumatic lesions involving the coccyx and its ligamentous attachments (265, 266). Rectal clenching, like jaw clenching, may be a chronic subconscious act.

A lumbar disc herniation of the nucleus pulposus may result in pain in the coccyx region but is rare. Percussion over the L4 region often reproduces such pain. Falling or sitting down abruptly onto a hard surface may precipitate the problem.

Physical examination requires a careful rectal examination. Grasp the coccyx and note excessive anterior displacement suggesting traumatic displacement. Then move the coccyx forward and backward, noting any unusual motion and pain on motion. Normal movement is up to 30 degrees anteriorly, and 1 cm laterally. Pain during movement is more important diagnostically (267). Next, palpate the sacrococcygeal joint and determine if the pain is arising from the joint. Lastly, palpate the muscles and ligament of the pelvic floor. Unusual tenderness here suggests unconscious rectal clenching.

The most common aggravating factor is improper sitting posture (268). A 5-year prospective study of 120 patients rarely identified a definitive cause; 20% of patients ultimately had coccygectomy.

Local treatment measures include injection with a local anesthetic–corticosteroid mixture into soft tissue at several levels. If the spinal percussion test is positive or other features of L4 nerve root impairment are noted, injection at the L4 region is included. When point tenderness occurs at the sacrococcygeal joint, pain may be alleviated by a local anesthetic–corticosteroid injection directly into the tender area. Finally, if the tip of the coccyx is tender, that area is included. The area should be prepared well. A 2-inch No. 22 needle may be used for the L4 region, then after a partial aliquot is injected at that site, the needle may be changed to a ¾-inch No. 23 needle for the remaining sites. A total of 40–60 mg methylprednisolone or equivalent steroid mixed with lidocaine

hydrochloride 1% can be used. In one prospective study of 120 patients, physical therapy with diathermy and ultrasound was found not to be helpful. However, injection of the soft tissues adjacent to the coccyx and the top of the coccyx with 40 mg methylprednisolone and bupivacaine (10 mL 0.25%) resulted in pain relief in 60%; the addition of manual manipulation of the coccyx for 1 minute in a flexion/extension motion provided relief in 85%. Coccygectomy was performed in 20%, resulting in success in over 90% (268a).

The use of a 3- or 4-inch thick, soft, foam rubber cushion with a 3-inch hole cut out of the center provides additional comfort. The cushion may prevent a pain-spasm-pain cycle. A Silastic or water-filled cushion has also proved to be helpful. Surgical resection of a radiographically normal coccyx is rarely necessary. Persistent pain raises suspicion for a lumbar disc herniation.

The *levator syndrome,* in which coccygodynia and a sensation of a high, vague pain in the rectum occurs in association with tenderness of the left levator ani muscle, may respond to high-voltage electrogalvanic stimulation. This can be administered by rectal probe that is reported to be commercially available (269, 270). Alternatively, with conscious effort, the patient can often willfully relax these muscles.

Ischial (Ischiogluteal) Bursitis

''Weaver's bottom'' or ''tailor's bottom'' refers to pain in a bursa overlying the ischial tuberosity, and irritation of the sciatic nerve may coexist (271). The patient often has exquisite pain when sitting or lying. Such patients often are given floor exercises to do, but find them painful. Point tenderness with pain reproduction is suggestive. Occasionally we have seen similar pain accompany silent prostatitis, ankylosing spondylitis, or Reiter's syndrome. Rectal examination for prostate irritation should be considered in patients with atypical symptoms. Ankylosing spondylitis or other spondylarthritides should be excluded. Tenosynovitis of the hamstring muscle at this site must be distinguished; the ischium is not the site of tenderness. Rather, the upper muscular tissue is tender and straight leg raising is painful, and the end point is usually less than 60 degrees of elevation. Local anesthetic–corticosteroid injection into the site of maximum tenderness, followed by use of a 3-inch foam rubber cut-out cushion, is helpful. The cushion should have two holes cut for the ischial tuberosities. Each hole should be about 3 inches in diameter and they should be about 3 inches apart (i.e., their centers should be about 6 inches apart). This condition is intractable, and may last many months. Exercises should be done while lying on the cushion. These consist of stretching (Exercise 5.L) and knee-to-chest exercises (Exercises 5.D or 5.E).

When injecting the bursa, warn the patient to call out if neuritic pain occurs, since the sciatic nerve is nearby and should not be injected (271). A 2 or 3-inch No. 20 needle with 20 mg methylprednisolone and procaine hydrochloride is used.

The Piriformis Syndrome

The piriformis muscle fills the greater sciatic foramen. Six features of the piriformis syndrome are described (272):

1. A history of traumatic injury to the sacroiliac and gluteal region.
2. Pain in the region of the sacroiliac joint, greater sciatic notch, and piriformis muscle extending down the lower limb and causing difficulty walking.
3. Acute exacerbation by lifting or stooping.
4. A palpable, sausage-like swelling of the muscle.
5. A positive straight-leg-raising test.
6. Gluteal atrophy if the condition is long-standing.

When associated with spinal stenosis the symptoms are bilateral. Neurologic examination is normal (89). The sign of Pace and Nagle—pain and weakness on resisted abduction–external rotation of the thigh—is helpful (273). Enlargement of the piriformis has been reported with imaging, either by CT scan or MRI (274). EMG may be helpful (275).

Treatment includes rectal muscle massage (274) and local injection with a corticosteroid-anesthetic mixture.

To perform the piriformis muscle injection, have the patient bent across the examination table or side-lying on the table, and palpate the area of tenderness. Often the muscle belly is indurated. Mark the area and prepare it with soap and alcohol. We prefer to use 40–60 mg methylprednisolone acetate sterile aqueous suspension with an equal amount of lidocaine hydrochloride 1% because the mixture will flocculate within the syringe and may prolong the local effectiveness of the injection. Using the shortest needle that can reach the required depth, use the needle as a probe. When the lesion is reached, pain is perceived. Have the patient apply ice for 10 to 20 minutes after the injection. A single injection often suffices, and injection should not be repeated within 6 to 8 weeks. Initiate intensive piriformis stretching exercise when the acute phase has resolved (Exercise 5.U). Additional exercises that should be used in the rehabilitation program include single and double knee-to-chest exercises (Exercises 5.D and 5.E), and straight leg stretches (Exercise 5.L). Occasionally, after all conservative measures have been utilized without success, exploratory surgery with section of a fibrous band or other nerve entrapment release may be necessary (276).

ENTRAPMENT NEUROPATHIES

In addition to nerve entrapments already described, others are also common. Meralgia paresthetica is described in Chapter 6.

Abdominal Cutaneous Nerve Entrapment

The patient is often a teenage girl who notes a dull, burning pain with sharp exacerbations. The pain radiates transversely across the lower abdomen to the midline, and often the patient can localize the origin of pain with one finger (277, 278). The abdominal cutaneous nerves arise from the thoracoabdominal nerve trunks and divide into anterior, lateral, and posterior branches. The nerves pass through a tough fibrous ring in the abdominal wall. Traction of the nerve against this ring may result in a burst of pain. In some patients the nerve is overstretched and angulated as a result of spinal, rib, or other skeletal structures. Symptoms may also result from abdominal distension, but often no apparent cause is found (277, 278). The nerve is easily put under tension and angulated within the abdominal wall's fibrous ring. Most cases involve the anterior cutaneous branch at the rectus margin. Examination with careful palpation of the rectus abdominis usually localizes and reproduces the pain at the fibrous ring. Local anesthetic injection of the region is both diagnostic and therapeutic (277).

Similarly, trigger points with resulting neuritic pain can arise in the vulva, vagina, and sacrum. Injection with a local anesthetic is both diagnostic and therapeutic (279).

Obturator Nerve Entrapment

Often following a pelvic fracture, osteitis pubis, or development of an obturator hernia, the patient notes pain and paresthesia in the groin that travels down the inner aspect of the thigh; these symptoms are aggravated during passive (examiner moves the limb) or active hip motion (patient moves limb himself or herself). Local nerve block is necessary to establish the diagnosis. MRI of the spine, abdomen, and pelvis may be important and necessary to exclude surgically amenable causes (280).

Ilioinguinal Pain Syndrome

Chronic pain across the low anterior pelvis, perineum, groin, thigh, or testicle may result from cicatricial adhesions which entrap the ilioinguinal nerve following herniorrhaphy, appendectomy, urologic, or gynecologic surgery. Treatment with local injection, nerve block, TENS, tricyclic antidepressants, or biofeedback are often not helpful. The condition can arise from faulty posture associated with hip or spine disease in which gait must rely heavily on abdominal muscle support (281).

REFERENCES

1. Institute of Medicine: Pain and disability. Washington, DC: National Academy Press, 1987:38.
2. Wood PHN: Back pain in the community. Clin Rheum Dis 6:3–16, 1980.
3. Papageorgiou AC, Rigby AS: Review of UK data on the rheumatic diseases. Br J Rheumatol 30:208–210, 1991.
4. Saal JA, Saal, JS: Nonoperative treatment of herniated lumbar intervertebral disc with radiculopathy. Spine 14(4):431–437, 1989.
5. Clemmer DI, Mohr DL: Low-back injuries in a heavy industry. II: Labor market forces. Spine 16:831–834, 1991.
6. Yelin EH, Henke CJ, Epstein WV: Work disability among persons with musculoskeletal conditions. Arthritis Rheum 29(11):1322–1333, 1986.
7. Deyo RA, Diehl AK, Rosenthal M: How many days of bed rest for acute low back pain? N Engl J Med 315(17):1064–1070, 1986.
8. Nachemson, AL: Newest knowledge of low back pain: a critical look. Clin Orthop 279:8–20, 1992.
9. King JS, Lagger R: Sciatica viewed as a referred pain syndrome. Surg Neurol 5:46–50, 1976.
10. Swezey RL: Pseudo-radiculopathy in subacute trochanteric bursitis of the subgluteus maximus bursa. Arch Phys Med Rehabil 57:387–390, 1976.
11. Mixter JW, Barr JS: Rupture of the intervertebral disc with involvement of the spinal canal. N Engl J Med 211:210–215, 1934.
12. Kirkaldy-Willis WH: Five common back disorders: how to diagnose and treat them. Geriatrics 33:32–41, 1978.
13. Mooney V, Robertson J: The facet syndrome. Clin Orthop 115:149–156, 1976.
14. Aprill C, Bogduk N: Diagnostic conservative management. Br J Radiol 65(773):361–369, 1992.
15. Hilton RC, Ball J, Benn RT: Annular tears in the dorsolumbar spine. Ann Rheum Dis 39:533–538, 1980.
16. Jayson MIV: Back pain: some new approaches. Med J Aust 1:513–516, 1979.
17. Klimiuk PS, Pountain GD, Keegan AL, Jayson MI: Serial measurements of fibrinolytic activity in acute low back pain and sciatica. Spine 12:925–928, 1987.
18. Ashton IK, Ashton BA, Gibson SJ, et al.: Morphological basis for back pain: the demonstration of nerve fibers and neuropeptides in the lumbar facet joint capsule but not in ligamentum flavum. J Orthop Res 10:72–78, 1992.
19. Quinet RJ, Hadler NM: Diagnosis and treatment of backache. Sem Arthritis Rheum 8:261–287, 1979.
20. Hirsch C: The mechanical response in normal and degenerated lumbar discs. J Bone Joint Surg 38A:242–243, 1956.
21. Matthews JA: Backache. Br Med J 1:432–434, 1977.

22. Bogduk N, Macintosh JE: The applied anatomy of the thoracolumbar fascia. Spine 9:165–170, 1984.

23. Nachemson A, Morris JM: Lumbar discometry: lumbar intradiscal pressure measurements in vivo. Lancet 1:1140–1142, 1963.

24. Nachemson A, Morris JM: In vivo measurements of intradiscal pressure: discometry, a method for the determination of pressure in the lower lumbar discs. J Bone Joint Surg 46A: 1077–1092, 1964.

25. Nachemson A: Towards a better understanding of low-back pain: a review of the mechanics of the lumbar disc. Rheumatol Rehabil 14: 129–143, 1975.

26. Esses SI, Moro JK: Intraosseous vertebral body pressures. Spine 17:S155–S159, 1992.

27. Fahrni WH: Conservative treatment of lumbar disc degeneration: our primary responsibility. Orthop Clin North Am 6:93–103, 1975.

28. Bartelink DL: The role of abdominal pressure in relieving the pressure on the lumbar intervertebral disc. J Bone Joint Surg 39B:718–725, 1967.

29. Morris JM, Lucas DB, Bressler B: Role of the trunk in stability of the spine. J Bone Joint Surg 43A:327–351, 1961.

30. Farfan HF: Muscular mechanism of the lumbar spine and the position of power and efficiency. Orthop Clin North Am 6:135–144, 1975.

31. Addison R, Schultz A: Trunk strengths in patients seeking hospitalization for chronic low-back disorders. Spine 5:539–544, 1980.

32. Suzuki N, Endo S: A quantitative study of trunk muscle strength and fatigability in the low-back-pain syndrome. Spine 8:69–74, 1983.

33. Andersson GBJ: Epidemiologic aspects on low-back pain in industry. Spine 6:53–60, 1981.

34. Davis PR: The use of intra-abdominal pressure in evaluating stresses on the lumbar spine. Spine 6:90–92, 1981.

35. Ortengren R, Andersson GBJ, Nachemson AL: Studies of relationships between lumbar disc pressure, myoelectric back muscle activity, and intraabdominal (intragastric) pressure. Spine 6:98–103, 1981.

36. Flor H, Schugens MM, Birbaumer N: Discrimination of muscle tension in chronic pain patients and healthy controls. Biofeedback Self Regul 17(3):165–177, 1992.

37. Gracovetsky S, Farfan HF, Lamy C: The mechanism of the lumbar spine. Spine 6:249–262, 1981.

38. Spengler DM, Szpalski M: Newer assessment approaches for the patient with low back pain. Contemporary Orthopaedics 21:371–378, 1990.

39. Delitto A, Rose SJ, Crandell CE, Strube MJ: Reliability of isokinetic measurements of trunk muscle performance. Spine 16:800–803, 1991.

40. Limburg PJ, Sinaki M, Rogers JW, et al.: A useful technique for measurement of back strength in osteoporotic and elderly patients. Mayo Clin Proc 66:39–44, 1991.

41. Allen ME: Clinical kinesiology: measurement techniques for spinal disorders. Orthop Rev 17:1097–1104, 1988.

42. Kishino ND, Mayer TG, Gatchel RJ, et al.: Quantification of lumbar function. Part 4: Isometric and isokinetic lifting simulation in normal subjects and low-back dysfunction patients. Spine 10:921–927, 1985.

43. Smith SS, Mayer TG, Gatchel RJ, Becker TJ: Quantification of lumbar function. Part 1: Isometric and multispeed isokinetic trunk strength measures in sagittal and axial planes in normal subjects. Spine 10:757–764, 1985.

44. Smidt G, Herring T, Amundsen L, et al.: Assessment of abdominal and back extensor function. Spine 8:211–219, 1983.

45. Robinson ME, Cassisi JE, O'Connor PD, MacMillan M: Lumbar iEMG during isotonic exercise: chronic low back pain patients versus controls. J Spinal Disord 5:8–15, 1992.

46. Szpalski M, Federspiel CF, Poty S, et al.: Reproducibility of trunk isoinertial dynamic performance in patients with low back pain. J Spinal Disord 5:78–85, 1992.

47. Shiado O, Kaneda K, Ito T: Trunk-muscle strength during concentric and eccentric contraction: a comparison between healthy subjects and patients with chronic low-back pain. J Spinal Disord 5:175–182, 1992.

48. Thorstensson A, Arvidson A: Trunk muscle strength and low back pain. Scand J Rehabil Med 14:69–75, 1982.

49. Estlander AM, Mellin G, Vanharanta H, et al.: Effects and follow-up of a multimodal treatment program including intensive physical training for low back pain patients. Scand J Rehabil Med 23:97–102, 1991.

50. Jarvikoski A, Mellin G, Estlander AM, et al.: Outcome of two multimodal back treatment programs with and without intensive physical training. J Spinal Disord 6:93–98, 1993.

50a. Faas A, van Eijk JT, Chavannes AW, et al.: A randomized trial of exercise therapy in patients with acute low back pain: efficacy on sickness absence. Spine 15:941–947, 1995.

51. Ready AE, Boreskie SL, Law SA, et al.: Fitness and lifestyle parameters fail to predict back injuries in nurses. Can J Appl Physiol 18:80–90, 1993.

52. Mostardi RA, Noe DA, Kovacik MW, et al.: Isokinetic lifting strength and occupational injury: a prospective study. Spine 17:189–193, 1992.

53. Rainville J, Ahern DK, Phalen L, et al.: The association of pain with physical activities in chronic low back pain. Spine 17:1060–1064, 1992.

54. Bigos SJ, Battie MC, Spengler DM, et al.: A longitudinal, prospective study of industrial back injury. Clin Orthop 279:21–34, 1992.

55. Waddell G, Somerville D, Henderson I, et al.: Objective clinical evaluation of physical impairment in chronic low back pain. Spine 17: 617–628, 1992.
56. Biering-Sorensen F: Physical measurements as risk indicators for low-back trouble over a one-year period. Spine 9:107–116, 1984.
56a. Silman AJ, Ferry S, Papageorgiou AC, et al.: Number of children as a risk factor for low back pain in men and women. Arthritis Rheum 38:1232–1235, 1995.
57. Hadler NM: Industrial rheumatology: clinical investigations into the influence of pattern of usage on the pattern of regional musculoskeletal disease. Arthritis Rheum 20:1019–1025, 1977.
58. Hayne CR: Ergonomics and back pain. Physiotherapy 70:9–13, 1984.
59. Manning DP, Shannon HS: Slipping accidents causing low-back pain in a gearbox factory. Spine 6:70–72, 1981.
60. Grandjean E, Hunting W, Pidermann M: VDT workstation design: preferred settings and their effects. Human Factors 25:161–175, 1983.
61. Weinstein SM, Scheer SJ: Industrial rehabilitation medicine. 2. Assessment of the problem, pathology, and risk factors for disability. Arch Phys Med Rehabil 73:S360–S365, 1992.
62. Dolan P, Adams MA, Hutton WC: Commonly adopted postures and their effect on the lumbar spine. Spine 13:197–201, 1988.
63. Magora A: Investigation of the relation between low back pain and occupation. Indus Med Surg 412:5–9, 1972.
64. Magnusson M, Granqvist M, Jonson R, et al.: The loads on the lumbar spine during work at an assembly line. Spine 15:774–779, 1990.
65. Svensson HO, Andersson GBJ: Low-back pain in 40 to 47-year-old men: work history and work environment factors. Spine 8:272–276, 1983.
66. Hoehler FK, Tobis JS: Psychological factors in the treatment of back pain by spinal manipulation. Br J Rheumatol 22:206–212, 1983.
67. Harkapaa K: Psychosocial factors as predictors for early retirement in patients with chronic low back pain. J Psychosom Res 36:553–559, 1992.
68. Bigos SJ, Battie MC, Spengler DM, et al.: A prospective study of work perceptions and psychosocial factors affecting the report of back injury. Spine 16:1–6, 1991.
69. Linton SJ, Warg LE: Attributions (beliefs) and job satisfaction associated with back pain in an industrial setting. Percept Mot Skills 76(1): 51–62, 1993.
70. Bigos SJ, Battie MC, Fisher LD: Methodology for evaluating predictive factors for the report of back injury. Spine 16(6):669–670, 1991.
71. Millard RW, Jones RH: Construct validity of practical questionnaires for assessing disability of low-back pain. Spine 16(7):835–838, 1991.
72. Swimmer GI, Robinson ME, Geisser ME: Relationship of MMPI cluster type, pain coping strategy, and treatment outcome. Clin J Pain 8: 131–137, 1992.
73. Deyo RA, Tsui-Wu YJ: Functional disability due to back pain. Arthritis Rheum 30:1247–1253, 1987.
74. Jacobsson L, Lindgarde F, Manthorpe R, Ohlsson K: Effect of education, occupation, and some lifestyle factors on common rheumatic complaints in a Swedish group aged 50–70 years. Ann Rheum Dis 51(7):835–843, 1992.
75. Volinn E, Van Koevering D, Loeser JD: Back sprain in industry: the role of socioeconomic factors in chronicity. Spine 16(5):542–548, 1991.
76. Jamison R, Matt, DA, Parris WCV: Treatment outcome in low back pain patients: do compensation benefits make a difference? Orthop Rev 17(12):1210–1215, 1988.
77. Frymoyer JW, Pope MH, Costanza MC, et al.: Epidemiologic studies of low-back pain. Spine 5:419–423, 1980.
78. Boshuizen HC, Verbeek JH, Broersen JP, et al.: Do smokers get more back pain? Spine 18: 35–40, 1993.
79. Holm S, Nachemson A: Nutrition of the intervertebral disc: acute effects of cigarette smoking. An experimental animal study. Int J Microcirc Clin Exp 3:406, 1984.
80. Ernst E: Smoking, a cause of back trouble? Br J Rheumatol 32:239–242, 1993.
81. Deyo RA, Bass JE: Lifestyle and low-back pain: the influence of smoking and obesity. Spine 14:501–506, 1989.
82. Dillane JB, Fry J, Kalton G: Acute back syndrome: a study from general practice. Br Med J 2:82–84, 1966.
83. Simons DG, Travell JG: Myofascial origins of low back pain. 1. Principles of diagnosis and treatment. Postgrad Med 73(2):66–108, 1983.
84. Bywaters EGL: Tendinitis and bursitis. Clin Rheum Dis 5:883–927, 1979.
85. Fairbank JCT, Obrien JP: The iliac crest syndrome: a treatable cause of low-back pain. Spine 8:220–224, 1983.
86. Blomberg S, Svardsuud K, Tibblin G: Manual therapy with steroid injections in low back pain. Scand J Prim Health Care 11:83–90, 1993.
86a. Blomberg S, Hallin G, Gran K, et al.: Manual therapy with steroid injections: a new approach to treatment of low back pain. Spine 19:569–577, 1994.
87. Vleeming A, Mooney V, Snijders C, et al., eds.: Low back pain and its relation to the sacroiliac joint. Rotterdam, the Netherlands: ECO, 1992.
88. Bernard TN, Kirkaldy-Willis WH: Recognizing specific characteristics of nonspecific low back pain. Clin Orthop 217:266–280, 1987.
89. Hallin RP: Sciatic pain and the piriformis muscle. Postgrad Med 74(2):69–72, 1983.
90. Sheon RP: Providing cost-effective care for low back stiffness and pain. J Musculoskel Med 8(1):57–81, 1991.

91. Leavitt F: Evaluation of psychological distur-bance in low back pain using verbal pain mea-surement. Intern Med Specialist 4:43–49, 1983.

92. Capra P, Mayer TG, Gatchel R: Adding psycho-logical scales to your back pain assessment. J Musculoskel Med 2:41–52, 1985.

93. Deyo RA, Walsh NE, Schoenfeld LS, Rama-murthy S: Studies of the modified somatic per-ceptions questionnaire (mspq) in patients with back pain: psychometric and predictive proper-ties. Spine 14(5):507–510, 1989.

94. Roberts N, Bennett S, Smith R: Psychological factors associated with disability in arthritis. J Psychosom Res 30(2):223–231, 1986.

95. Barnes D, Smith D, Gatchel RJ, Mayer TG: Psychosocioeconomic predictors of treatment success/failure in chronic low-back pain patients. Spine 14(4):427–430, 1989.

96. Crown S: Psychological aspects of low back pain. Rheumatol Rehabil 17:114–122, 1978.

97. Uden A, Astrom M, Bergenudd H.: Pain draw-ings in chronic back pain. Spine 13:389–393, 1988.

98. Kolar E, Hartz A, Roumm A, et al.: Factors associated with severity of symptoms in patients with chronic unexplained muscular aching. Ann Rheum Dis 48:317–321, 1989.

99. Chadwick PR: Examination, assessment, and treatment of the lumbar spine. Physiotherapy 70:2–7, 1984.

100. Selby DK: Conservative care of nonspecific low back pain. Orthop Clin North Am 13:427–437, 1982.

100a. Parker H, Wood PL, Main CJ: The use of the pain drawing as a screening measure to predict psychological distress in chronic low back pain. Spine 15:236–243, 1995.

101. Mann NH, Brown MD, Enger I: Expert perfor-mance in low-back disorder recognition using patient pain drawings. J Spinal Disord 5(3):254–259, 1992.

102. MacNab I: Backache. Baltimore: Williams & Wilkins, 1977.

102a. Liu AC, Byrne E: Cost of care for ambulatory patients with low back pain. J Fam Pract 40:449–455, 1995.

102b. Roach KE, Brown M, Ricker E, et al.: The use of patient symptoms to screen for serious back problems. J Orthop Sports Phys Ther 21:2–6, 1995.

103. Troup JDG: Research methods on predicting occupational low-back pain. Spine 16:671, 1991.

104. Mooney V: Evaluating low back disorders in the primary care office. J Musculoskel Med 1:16–26, 1984.

105. Hall H: Examination of the patient with low back pain. Bull Rheum Dis 33:1–8, 1983.

106. van der Hoogen HMM, Koes BW, van Eijk JTM, et al.: On the accuracy of history, physical examination, and erythrocyte sedimentation rate in diagnosing low back pain in general practice. Spine 20:318–327, 1995.

107. Clark WL, Haldeman S, Johnson P, et al.: Back impairment and disability determination: another attempt at objective, reliable rating. Spine 13(3):332–341, 1988.

108. Sullivan MD, Loeser JD: The diagnosis of dis-ability: treating and rating disability in a pain clinic. Arch Intern Med 152:1829–1835, 1992.

109. Main CJ, Wood PL, Hollis S, et al.: The distress and risk assessment method: a simple patient classification to identify distress and evaluate the risk of poor outcome. Spine 17(1):42–52, 1992.

110. Calin A: Back pain: mechanical or inflamma-tory? Am Fam Phys 20:97–100, 1979.

110a. Katz JN, Dalgas M, Stucki G, et al.: Degenera-tive lumbar spinal stenosis: diagnostic value of the history and physical examination. Arthritis Rheum 38:1236–1241, 1995.

111. Currey HLF, Greenwood RM, Lloyd GG, Mur-ray RS: A prospective study of low back pain. Rheumatol Rehabil 18:94–101, 1979.

112. Blower PW: Neurologic patterns in unilateral sciatica. Spine 6:175–179, 1981.

113. Nelson MA, Allen P, Clamp SE, et al.: Reliabil-ity and reproducibility of clinical findings in low-back pain. Spine 4:97–101, 1979.

114. Rothenberg, RJ: Rheumatic disease aspects of leg length inequality. Sem Arthritis Rheum 17(3):196–205, 1988.

115. Brown MD: Diagnosis of pain syndromes of the spine. Orthop Clin North Am 6:233–248, 1975.

116. Deyo RA, Rainville J, Kent DL: What can the history and physical examination tell us about low back pain? JAMA 268(6):760–765, 1992.

117. Hultman G, Saraste H, Ohlsen H: Anthropome-try, spinal canal width, and flexibility of the spine and hamstring muscles in 45–55-year-old men with and without low back pain. J Spinal Disord 5(3):245–253, 1992.

118. ARA Glossary Committee: Dictionary of rheu-matic diseases. Vol 1. Signs and symptoms. New York: American Rheumatism Association, Con-tact Associates, 1982.

119. McRae IF, Wright V: Measurement of back movement. Ann Rheum Dis 28:584–589, 1969.

120. Merritt JL, McLean TJ, Erickson RP, et al.: Measurement of trunk flexibility in normal sub-jects: reproducibility of three clinical methods. Mayo Clin Proc 61:192–197, 1986.

121. Goto I, Nagasaka H, Kuroiwa Y: Rigid spine syndrome. J Neurol Neurosurg Psychiatry 42:276–279, 1979.

122. Miller SA, Mayer T, Cox R, Gatchel RJ: Relia-bility problems associated with the modified Schober technique for true lumbar flexion mea-surement. Spine 17(3):345–348, 1992.

123. Russek AS: Biomechanical and physiological basis for ambulatory treatment of low back pain. Orthop Rev 5:21–31, 1976.

124. Nice DA, Riddle DL, Lamb RL, et al.: Intertester reliability of judgments of the presence of trigger points in patients with low back pain. Arch Phys Med Rehabil 73:893–898, 1992.

125. McCombe PF, Fracs JC, Fairbank T, et al.: Reproducibility of physical signs in low-back pain. Spine 14(7):908–918, 1989.

125a. Njoo KH, van der Does E: The occurrence and inter-rater reliability of myofascial trigger points in the quatratus lumborum and gluteus medius: a prospective study in non-specific low back pain patients and controls in general practice. Pain 58:317–323, 1994.

126. Pederson OF, Petersen R, Staffeldt ES: Back pain and isometric back muscle strength of workers in a Danish factory. Scand J Rehabil Med 7:125–128, 1975.

127. Singewald ML: Sacroiliac lipomata: an often unrecognized cause of low back pain. Johns Hopkins Med J 118:492–498, 1966.

128. Ries E: Episacroiliac lipoma. Am J Obstet Gynecol 34:490–494, 1937.

129. Pace JB, Henning C: Episacroiliac lipoma. Am Fam Phys 6:70–73, 1972.

130. Matthews JA: Backache. Br Med J 1: 432–434, 1977.

131. Troup JDG, Martin JW, Lloyd DCEF: Back pain in industry: a prospective survey. Spine 6:61–69, 1981.

132. Shiqing X, Quanzhi Z, Dehao F: Significance of the straight-leg-raising test in the diagnosis and clinical evaluation of lower lumbar intervertebral-disc protrusion. J Bone Joint Surg 69A(4): 517–522, 1987.

133. Pheasant HC: The problem back. Curr Pract Orthop Surg 7:89–115, 1977.

134. Felsenthal G, Reischer MA: Asymmetric hamstring reflexes indicative of L5 radicular lesions. Arch Phys Med Rehabil 63:377–378, 1982.

135. Kopp JR: Examining the patient with low back pain efficiently. J Musculoskel Med 1:11–17, 1984.

136. Hadler NM: A rheumatologist's view of the back. J Occup Med 24:283–285, 1982.

137. Hadler NM: Legal ramifications of the medical definition of back disease. Ann Intern Med 89:992–999, 1978.

138. Lehmann TR, Brand RA: Disability in the patient with low back pain. Orthop Clin North Am 13:559–568, 1982.

139. Scavone JG, Latshaw RF, Rohrer GV: Use of lumbar spine films. JAMA 246:1105–1108, 1981.

140. Lawrence JS, Bremner JM, Bier F: Osteoarthrosis: prevalence in the population and relationship between symptoms and x-ray changes. Ann Rheum Dis 25:1–24, 1966.

141. Lawrence JS: Disc degeneration: its frequency and relationship to symptoms. Ann Rheum Dis 28:121–138, 1969.

142. Granda JL, Wertheimer TM, Salas JM, et al.: X-ray changes in the lumbar spine. (Abstract #248) Arthritis Rheum 25(4) [Suppl], 1982.

143. Frymoyer JW, Newberg A, Pope MH, et al.: Spine radiographs in patients with low back pain. J Bone Joint Surg 66A:1048–1055, 1984.

144. Pening L, Wilmink JT, van Woerden HH: Inability to prove instability; critical appraisal of clinical-radiological flexion-extension studies in lumbar disc degeneration. Diagn Imag Clin 53:186–192, 1984.

145. Dupuis PR, Young-Hing K, Cassidy JD, Kirkaldy-Willis WH: Radiologic diagnosis of degenerative lumbar spinal instability. Spine 10:262–279, 1985.

146. Raskin SP: Introduction to computed tomography of the lumbar spine. Orthopedics 3: 1011–1023, 1980.

147. Jackson DW: Low back pain in young athletes: evaluation of stress reaction and discogenic problems. Am J Sports Med 7:364–366, 1979.

148. Alarcon GS, Ball GV, Blackburn WE, et al.: The value of CT scan in the evaluation of inflammatory back pain. (Abstract #52) Arthritis Rheum 28(4) [Suppl], 1985.

149. Wiesel SW, Sourmas N, Feffer HL, et al.: Nonspecific back pain. Spine 9:549–552, 1984.

150. Bell GR, Rothman RH, Booth RE: A study of cat. II. Comparison of metrizamide myelography and CAT in diagnosis of herniated lumbar disc and spinal stenosis. Spine 9:552–557, 1984.

151. Modic MT, Pavlicek W, Weinstein MA, et al.: Magnetic resonance imaging of intervertebral disk disease. Radiology 152:103–111, 1984.

152. Jensen MC, Brant-Zawadzki, Obuchowski N, et al.: Magnetic resonance imaging of the lumbar spine in people without back pain. N Engl J Med 331:69–73, 1994.

153. Janssen ME, Bertrand SL, Joe C, et al.: Lumbar herniated disc disease: comparison of MRI, myelography, and post-myelography CT scan with surgical findings. Orthopedics 17:121–127, 1994.

154. Lynch MC, Taylor JF: Facet joint injection for low back pain. J Bone Joint Surg 68B:138–141, 1986.

155. Dory MA: Arthrography of the lumbar facet joints. Radiology 140:23–27, 1981.

156. Murphy WA: The facet syndrome. Radiology 151:533, 1984.

157. Porter RW, Wicks M, Ottewell D: Measurement of the spinal canal by diagnostic ultrasound. J Bone Joint Surg 60B:481–484, 1978.

158. Abraham EA: Thermography: uses and abuses. Contemp Orthop 8:95–99, 1984.

159. Hochschuler SH: Diagnostic studies in clinical practice. Orthop Clin North Am 14:517–526, 1983.

160. Cherkin DC, Deyo RA, Wheeler K, et al.: Physician variation in diagnostic testing for low back pain. Arthritis Rheum 37:15–22, 1994.

161. Bywaters EGL: Viewpoint, mobility with rigidity: a view of the spine. Ann Rheum Dis 41: 210–214, 1982.

162. Terry AF, DeYoung R: Hip disease mimicking low back disorders. Orthop Rev 8:95–104, 1979.

163. Sternbach,RA, Murphy RW, Akeson WH, Wolf SR: Chronic low-back pain: the "low-back loser." Postgrad Med 53:135–138, 1973.

164. Connolly JF, Dehaven KE, Mooney V: Changing approaches to back pain, fractures, pediatrics. J Musculoskel Med 8:14–18, 1993.

165. Gill TM, Feinstein AR: A critical appraisal of the quality of Quality of Life measurements. JAMA 272:619–626, 1994.

166. Lawrence VA, Tugwell P, Gafni A, et al.: Acute low back pain and economics of therapy: the iterative loop approach. J Clin Epidemiol 45(3): 301–311, 1992.

167. Korff MV, Barlow W, Cherkin D, et al.: Effects of practice style in managing back pain. Ann Intern Med 121:187–195, 1994.

168. Malmivaara A, Hakkinen U, Aro T, et al.: The treatment of acute low back pain: bed rest, exercises, or ordinary activity? N Engl J Med 332: 351–355, 1995.

169. Beaumont G: The use of psychotropic drugs in other painful conditions. J Int Med Res 4(2) [Suppl]:56–57, 1976.

170. Basmajian JV: Acute back pain and spasm: a controlled multicenter trial of combined analgesic and antispasm agents. Spine 14(4):438–439, 1989.

171. Maigne R: Orthopedic medicine: a new approach to vertebral manipulations. Springfield, IL: Charles C Thomas, 1972.

172. Doran DML, Newell DJ: Manipulation in treatment of low back pain: a multicentre study. Br Med J 2:161–164, 1975.

173. Swezey RL: The modern thrust of manipulation and traction therapy. Sem Rheum Dis 12: 321–331, 1983.

174. Saunders HD: Use of spinal traction in the treatment of neck and back conditions. Clin Orthop Res 179:31–38, 1983.

175. Firman GJ, Goldstein MS: The future of chiropractic: a psychosocial view. N Engl J Med 293:639–642, 1975.

176. Glover JR, Morris JG, Khosla T: Back pain: a randomized clinical trial of rotational manipulation of the trunk. Br J Ind Med 31:59–64, 1974.

177. Kane RL, Leymaster C, Olsen D, et al.: Manipulating the patient: a comparison of the effectiveness of physician and chiropractic care. Lancet 1:1333–1336, 1974.

178. Godfrey CM, Morgan PP, Schatzker J: A randomized trial of manipulation for low-back pain in a medical setting. Spine 9:301–304, 1984.

179. Jayson MIV, Sims-Williams H, Young S, et al.: Mobilization and manipulation for low-back pain. Spine 6:409–416, 1981.

180. Greenland S, Reisbord LS, Haldeman S, et al.: Controlled clinical trials of manipulation: a review and a proposal. J Occup Med 22:670–676, 1980.

181. Hoehler FK, Tovis JS, Buerger AA: Spinal manipulation for low back pain. JAMA 245: 1835–1838, 1981.

182. Haldeman S: Spinal manipulative therapy. Clin Orthop Related Res 179:62–70, 1983.

183. Koes BW, Bouter LM, van Mameren H, et al.: The effectiveness of manual therapy, physiotherapy, and treatment by the general practitioner for nonspecific back and neck complaints. Spine 17(1):28–35, 1992.

184. Koes BW, Bouter LM, van Mameren H, et al.: Randomised clinical trial of manipulative therapy and physiotherapy for persistent back and neck complaints: results of one year follow up. Br Med J 304(6827):601–605, 1992.

185. Jarvis KB, Phillips RB, Morris EK: Cost per case comparison of back injury claims of chiropractic versus medical management for conditions with identical diagnostic codes. J Occup Med 33(8):847–852, 1991.

186. Shekelle PG, Adams AH, Chassin MR, et al.: Spinal manipulation for low-back pain. Ann Intern Med 117:590–598, 1992.

187. Anderson R, Meeker WC, Wirick BE, et al.: A meta-analysis of clinical trials of spinal manipulation. J Manipul Physiol Therap 15(3): 181–194, 1992.

188. Hadler NM, Curtis P, Gillings DB, Stinnett S: A benefit of spinal manipulation as adjunctive therapy for acute low-back pain: a stratified controlled trial. Spine 12(7):703–706, 1987.

189. Ottenbacher K, Difabio RP: Efficacy of spinal manipulation/mobilization therapy. Spine 10(9): 833–837, 1985.

190. Khalil TM, Asfour SS, Martinez LM, et al.: Stretching in the rehabilitation of low-back pain patients. Spine 17(3):311–317, 1992.

191. Waddell G: A new clinical model for the treatment of low-back pain. Spine 12(7):632–644, 1987.

191a. Meade TW, Dyer S, Browne W, et al.: Randomised comparison of chiropractic and hospital outpatient management for low back pain: results from extended followup. Br Med J 311: 349–351, 1995.

191b. Carey TS, Garrett J, Jackman A, et al.: The outcomes and costs of care for acute low back pain among patients seen by primary care practitioners, chiropractors, and orthopedic surgeons. The North Carolina Back Pain Project. N Engl J Med 333: 913–917, 1995.

192. Saal JA, Saal, JS: Nonoperative treatment of herniated lumbar intervertebral disc with radiculopathy. Spine 14(4):431–437, 1989.

192a. Cutler RB, Fishbain DA, Rosomoff HL, et al.: Does nonsurgical pain center treatment of chronic pain return patients to work? Spine 19:643–652, 1994.

193. Deyo RA, Loeser JD, Bigos SJ: Herniated lumbar intervertebral disk. Ann Intern Med 112(8): 598–604, 1990.

194. Cole H, ed.: Diagnostic and Therapeutic Technology Assessment (DATTA). JAMA 264(11): 1469–1472, 1990.

195. Muralikuttan KP, Hamilton A, Kernohan WG, et al.: Chemonucleolysis and disk surgery for lumbar disk herniation. Spine 17:381–387, 1992.

196. Javid MJ, Norby EJ, Ford LT, et al.: Safety and efficacy of chymopapain (Chymodiactin) in herniated nucleus pulposus with sciatica. JAMA 249:2489–2494, 1983.

197. Crawshaw C, Frazer AM, Merriam WF, et al.: A comparison of surgery and chemonucleolysis in the treatment of sciatica: a prospective randomized trial. Spine 9:195–199, 1984.

198. McCullock JA: Chemonucleolysis for relief of sciatica due to a herniated intervertebral disc. Can Med Assoc J 124:879–882, 1981.

199. Waring EM, Weisz GM, Bailey SI: Predictive factors in the treatment of low back pain by surgical intervention. In: Bonica JJ, Albe-Fessard DG, eds. Advances in pain research and therapy. Vol 1. New York: Raven Press, 1976.

200. Finneson BE: Modulating effect of secondary gain on the low back pain syndrome. In: Bonica JJ, Albe-Fessard DG, eds. Advances in pain research and therapy. Vol 1. New York: Raven Press, 1976.

201. Mayer TG, Gatchel RJ, Kishino N, et al.: A prospective short-term study of chronic low back pain patients utilizing novel objective functional measurement. Pain 25:53–68, 1986.

202. Mayer TG: Rehabilitation of the patient with spinal pain. Orthop Clin North Am 14(3): 623–637, 1983.

203. Tollison CD, Kriegel ML, Satterthwaite JR: Comprehensive pain center treatment of low back workers' compensation injuries. Orthop Rev 18(10):1115–1125, 1989.

204. Von Korff M, Deyo RA, Cherkin D, Barlow W: Back Pain in primary care: outcomes at 1 year. Spine 18(7):855–862, 1993.

205. Fordyce WE, Roberts A, Sternbach RA: The behavioral management of chronic pain: a response to critics. Pain 22:113–125, 1984.

206. Beals RK, Hickman NW: Industrial injuries of the back and extremities. J Bone Joint Surg 54A:1593–1611, 1972.

206a. Newton-John TR, Spense SH, Schotte D: Cognitive-behavioural therapy versus EMG biofeedback in the treatment of chronic low back pain. Behav Res Ther 33:691–697, 1995.

207. Keegan JJ: Alterations of the lumbar curve related to posture and seating. J Bone Joint Surg 35A:589–603, 1953.

208. Berquist-Ullman M, Larsson US: Acute low back pain in industry: a controlled prospective study with special reference to therapy and confounding factors. Acta Orthop Scand 170: 1–117, 1977.

209. Wosk J, Voloshin AS: Low back pain: conservative treatment with artificial shock absorbers. Arch Phys Med Rehabil 66:145–148, 1985.

210. White AH, White LA, Maltmille WA: Back school and other conservative approaches to low back pain. St. Louis: CV Mosby, 1983.

210a. White AH: The back school of the future. Occup Med: 7(1):179–182, 1992.

211. Zachrisson MF: The back school. Spine 6:104–106, 1981.

212. Simmons JW, Dennisz MD, Rath D: The back school, a total back management program. Orthopedics 7:1453–1456, 1984.

213. Versloot JM, Roszeman A, van Son AM, van Akkerveeken PF: The cost-effectiveness of a back school program in industry: a longitudinal controlled field study. Spine 17(1):22–27, 1992.

214. Shi L: A cost-benefit analysis of a California county's back injury prevention program. Public Health Rep 108(2):204–211, 1993.

215. deJong RH: Central pain mechanisms. JAMA 239:2784, 1978.

216. Pheasant H, Bursk A, Goldfarb J, et al.: Amitriptyline and chronic low-back pain. Spine 8:552–557, 1983.

217. Matheson LN, Ogden LD, Violette K, Schultz K: Work hardening: occupational therapy in industrial rehabilitation. Am J Occup Therapy 39: 314–321, 1985.

218. Steindler A, Luck JV: Differential diagnosis of pain low in the back: allocation of the source of pain by the procaine hydrochloride method. JAMA 110:106–113, 1938.

219. Hameroff SR, Crago BR, Blitt CD, et al.: Comparison of bupivacaine, etidocaine, and saline for trigger-point therapy. Anesthesia Analgesia 60:752–755, 1981.

220. Hendler N, Fink H, Long D: Myofascial syndrome: response to trigger-point injections. Psychosomatics 24:993–999, 1983.

221. Brown BR: Myofascial and musculoskeletal pain. Int Anesth Clin 21:139–151, 1983.

222. Collee G, Dijkmans BA, Vandenbroucke JP, Cats A: Iliac crest pain syndrome in low back pain: a double-blind, randomized study of local injection therapy. J Rheumatol 18(7): 1060–1063, 1991.

223. Breneman JC: The herniated disc syndrome. J Occup Med 11:475–479, 1969.

224. Dilke TFW, Burry HC, Grahame R: Extradural corticosteroid injection in management of lumbar nerve root compression. Br Med J 2:635–637, 1973.

225. Garvey TA, Marks MR, Wiesel SW: A prospective, randomized, double-blind evaluation of trigger-point injection therapy for low-back pain. Spine 14(9):962–964, 1989.

226. Bourne IHJ: Treatment of backache with local injections. Practitioner 222:708–711, 1979.

227. Sonne M, Christensen K, Hansen SE, Jensen EM: Injection of steroids and local anesthetics as therapy for low-back pain. Scand J Rheumatol 14:343–354, 1985.

228. Moran R, O'Connell D, Walsh MG: The diagnostic value of facet joint injections. Spine 13(12):1407–1410, 1988.

229. Helbig T, Lee CK: The lumbar facet syndrome. Spine 13(1):4, 1988.
230. Carette S, Marcoux S, Truchon R, et al.: A controlled trial of corticosteroid injections into facet joints for chronic low back pain. N Engl J Med 325(14):1002–1007, 1991.
231. Lilius G, Harilainen A, Laasonen EM, Myllynen P: Chronic unilateral low-back pain: predictors of outcome of facet joint injections. Spine 15(8): 780–782, 1990.
232. Lilius G, Laasonen EM, Myllynen P, et al.: Lumbar facet joint syndrome: a randomised clinical trial. J Bone Joint Surg 71B(4): 681–684, 1989.
233. Murtaugh FR: Computed tomography and fluoroscopy guided anesthesia and steroid injection in facet syndrome. Spine 13(6):686–689, 1988.
234. Vollertsen RS, Nobrega FT, Michet CJ, et al.: Economic outcome under medicare prospective payment at a tertiary-care institution: the effects of demographic, clinical, and logistic factors on duration of hospital stay and part A charges for medical back problems (DRG 243). Mayo Clin Proc 63:583–591, 1988.
235. Bush D, Hillier S: A controlled study of caudal epidural injections of triamcinolone plus procaine for the management of intractable sciatica. Spine 16(5):572–575, 1991.
236. Warfield CA, Crews DA: Work status and response to epidural steroid injection. J Occup Med 29(4):315–316, 1987.
237. Wallace G, Solove GJ: Epidural steroid therapy for low back pain. Postgrad Med 78:213–218, 1985.
238. Simmons JW, McMillin JN, Emery SF, Kimmich SJ: Intradiscal steroids: a prospective double-blind clinical trial. Spine 17(6):S172–S175, 1992.
239. Reed JW, Harvey JC: Rehabilitating the chronically ill: a method for evaluating the functional capacity of ambulatory patients. Geriatrics 19:87–103, 1964.
240. Richardson RR, Arbit J, Siqueira EB, et al.: Transcutaneous electrical neurostimulation in functional pain. Spine 6:185–188, 1981.
241. Deyo RA, Walsh NE, Martin DC, et al.: A controlled trial of transcutaneous electrical nerve stimulation (TENS) and exercise for chronic low back pain. N Engl J Med 322(23):1627–1634, 1990.
242. Murphy TM: Subjective and objective followup assessment of acupuncture therapy without suggestion in 100 chronic pain patients. In: Bonica JJ, Albe-Fessard DG, eds. Advances in pain research and therapy. Vol 1. New York: Raven Press, 1976.
243. Mendelson G, Selwood TS, Kranz H, et al.: Acupuncture treatment of chronic back pain: a double-blind placebo-controlled trial. Am J Med 74:49–55, 1983.
244. Wiltse LLL: Common problems of the lumbar spine: degenerative spondylolisthesis and spinal stenosis. JCE Orthop 7:17–30, 1979.
245. Cuckler JM, Bernini PA, Wiesel SW, et al.: The use of epidural steroids in the treatment of lumbar radicular pain. J Bone Joint Surg 67A:63–66, 1985.
246. Stanton-Hicks M: Therapeutic caudal or epidural block for lower back or sciatic pain (Letter). JAMA 243:369–370, 1980.
247. Tarlov E: Therapeutic caudal or epidural block for lower back or sciatic pain (Letter). JAMA 243:369, 1980.
248. Oudenhoven RC: The role of laminectomy, facet rhizotomy, and epidural steroids. Spine 2: 145–147, 1979.
249. Gottlieb H, Strite LC, Koller R, et al.: Comprehensive rehabilitation of patients having chronic low back pain. Arch Phys Med Rehabil 58:101–108, 1977.
250. Hubbard JH: Chronic pain of spinal origin: rationales for treatment. In: Rothman RH, Simeone FA, eds. The back. Philadelphia: WB Saunders, 1982.
251. Cairns D, Thomas L, Mooney V, Pace JB: A comprehensive treatment approach to chronic low back pain. Pain 2:301–308, 1976.
252. Newman RI, Seres JL, Yospe LP, et al.: Multidisciplinary treatment of chronic pain: longterm follow-up of low-back pain patients. Pain 4:283–292, 1978.
253. Reiter RC, Gambone JC: Nongynecologic somatic pathology in women with chronic pelvic pain and negative laparoscopy. J Reprod Med 36(4):253–259, 1991.
254. Vickers RJ, May AE: Long-term backache after extradural or general anaesthesia for manual removal of placenta: preliminary report. Br J Anaesth 70(2):214–215, 1993.
255. MacArthur C, Lewis M: Investigation of longterm problems after obstetric epidural anaesthesia. Br Med J 304(6837):1279–1282, 1992.
256. Blaschke JA: Clinical characteristics of osteitis condensans ilii (Abstract). Paper presented to VI Pan-American Congress on Rheumatic Diseases, June 16–21, 1974.
257. Singal DP, deBosset P, Gordon DA, et al.: HLA antigens in osteitis condensans ilii and ankylosing spondylitis. J Rheumatol 4(3) [Suppl]: 105–108, 1977.
258. Arturi AS, Marcos JC, Maldonado-Cocca JA, et al.: Osteitis condensans ilii in apatite crystal deposition disease. Arthritis Rheum 26: 567–569, 1983.
259. Samellas W, Finkelstein P: Osteitis pubis: its surgical treatment. J Urol 87(4):553–555, 1962.
260. Scott DL, Eastmond CJ, Wright V: A comparative radiological study of the pubic symphysis in rheumatic disorders. Ann Rheum Dis 38: 529–534, 1979.
261. O'Duffy JD: Increasing evidence suggests polymyalgia rheumatica is not a muscle disease. Wellcome Trends in Rheumatology 1:1–2, 1979.

262. Barnes WC, Malament M: Osteitis pubis. Surg Gynecol Obstet 117:277–284, 1963.

263. Grace JN, Sim FH, Shives TC: Wedge resection of the symphysis pubis for the treatment of osteitis pubis. J Bone Joint Surg 71A(3):358–364, 1989.

264. Wiley JJ: Traumatic osteitis pubis: the gracilis syndrome. Am J Sport Med 11:360–363, 1983.

264a. Ashby EC: Chronic obscure groin pain is commonly caused by enthesopathy: "tenniis elbow of the groin." Br J Surg 81:1632–1634, 1994.

265. Thiele GH: Coccygodynia and pain in the superior gluteal region and down the back of the thigh: causation by tonic spasm of the levator ani, coccygeus, and piriformis muscles and relief by massage of these muscles. JAMA 109:1271–1275, 1941.

266. Sinaki M, Merritt JL, Stillwell GK: Tension myalgia of the pelvic floor. Mayo Clin Proc 52:717–722, 1977.

267. Traycoff RB, Crayton H, Dodson R: Sacrococcygeal pain syndromes: diagnosis and treatment. Orthopedics 12(10):1373–1377, 1989.

268. Johnson PH: Coccygodynia. J Arkansas Med Soc 77:421–424, 1981.

268a. Wray CC, Easom S, Hoskinson J: Coccydynia: aetiology and treatment. J Bone Joint Surg 73B:335–338, 1991.

269. Sohn N, Weinstein MA, Robbins RD: The levator syndrome and its treatment with high-voltage electrogalvanic stimulation. Am J Surg 144:580–582, 1982.

270. Nicosia FJ, Abcarian H: Levator syndrome: a treatment that works. Dis Colon Rectum 28:406–408, 1985.

271. Swartout R, Compere EL: Ischio-gluteal bursitis. JAMA 227:551–552, 1974.

272. Robinson DR: Piriformis syndrome in relation to sciatic pain. Am J Surg 73:355–358, 1947.

273. Pace JB, Nagle D: Piriform syndrome. Western J Med 124:435–439, 1976.

274. Jankiewicz JJ, Hennrikus WL, Houkom JA: The appearance of the piriformis muscle syndrome in computed tomography and magnetic resonance imaging. Clin Orthop 262:205–209, 1991.

275. Papadopoulos SM, McGillicuddy JE, Albers JW: Unusual cause of "piriformis muscle syndrome." Arch Neurol 47:1144–1146, 1990.

276. Vandertop WP, Bosma NJ: The piriformis syndrome. J Bone Joint Surg 73A(7):1095–1097, 1991.

277. DeValera E, Raftery H: Lower abdominal and pelvic pain in women. In: Bonica JJ, Albe-Fessard DG, eds. Advances in pain research and therapy. Vol 1. New York: Raven Press, 1976.

278. Applegate WV: Abdominal cutaneous nerve entrapment syndrome. Am Fam Physician 8:132–133, 1973.

279. Slocumb JC: Neurological factors in chronic pelvic pain: trigger points and the abdominal pelvic pain syndrome. Am J Obstet Gynecol 149(5):536–543, 1984.

280. Kleiner JB, Donaldson WF III, Curd JG, Thorne RP: Extraspinal causes of lumbosacral radiculopathy. J Bone Joint Surg 73A(6):817–821, 1991.

281. Hameroff SR, Carlson GL, Brown BR: Ilioinguinal pain syndrome. Pain 10:253–257, 1981.

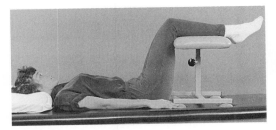

Exercise 5.A. Acute Rest Position

The 90/90 position, in which both hips and knees are flexed to 90 degrees each, can be used several times daily for pain relief.

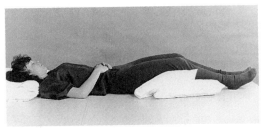

Exercise 5.B. Supine Rest Position

Management of chronic low back pain includes proper sleeping and resting positions as demonstrated here. An alternative side-lying position can be found in the Introduction, Figure I.3(b).

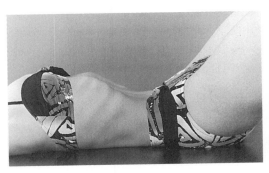

Exercise 5.C. Posterior Pelvic Tilt

A basic maneuver in back rehabilitation. The abdominal and gluteal muscles are contracted to flatten the lumbar spine. This position is held 5–10 seconds and can be repeated frequently.

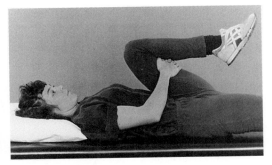

Exercise 5.D. Single Knee-to-Chest

This exercise is well tolerated during the early phase of a back rehabilitation program. Stretching of the low back muscles and fascia is obtained with this mobilizing procedure. The subject pulls one knee toward the chest and holds this position 5–10 seconds, doing 6–10 repetitions twice daily.

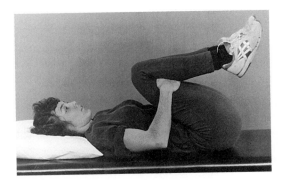

Exercise 5.E. Double Knee-to-Chest

In the double knee-to-chest exercise, the knees are drawn toward the chest and returned to the starting position one at a time. The subject holds the double knee stretch 5–10 seconds, doing 6–10 repetitions twice daily.

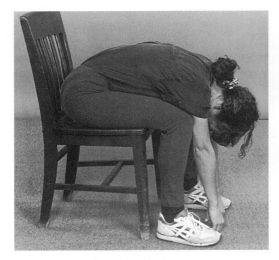

Exercise 5.F. Sitting Chest-to-Knees

This exercise, performed while seated on a chair, is an alternative method for those who do not perceive a stretching sensation in the low back during the standard knee-to-chest exercises (perhaps due to hypermobility of the hips). Each stretch is held 5–10 seconds, with 6–10 repetitions twice daily.

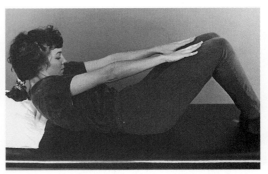

Exercise 5.G. Abdominal Curl

This abdominal strengthening exercise is properly performed with the knees bent and the subject raising the trunk no more than 6 inches from the surface. This contracts the abdominal muscles without bringing the psoas muscle into play. Exhale during the curl up.

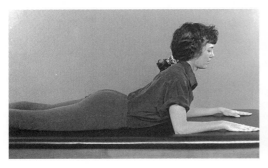

Exercise 5.H. Elbow Prop

This exercise is performed during the early phase of progression in a back extension program. Hold 30–60 seconds as tolerated.

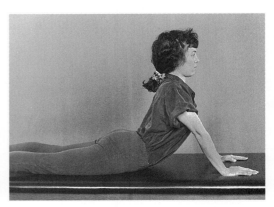

Exercise 5.I. Prone Push-up into Lumbar Extension

Press the top half of the body up with the arms, keeping the elbows straight. Legs and pelvis are kept against floor. Hold 30–60 seconds.

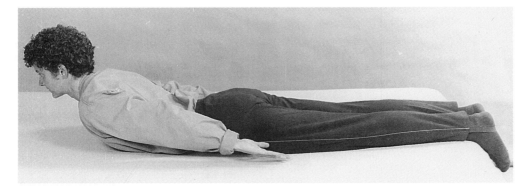

Exercise 5.J. Prone Lumbar Extension

Using the back (spinal erector) muscles, lift the upper body from the surface. Strengthening is emphasized in this antigravity position. Hold 10–30 seconds.

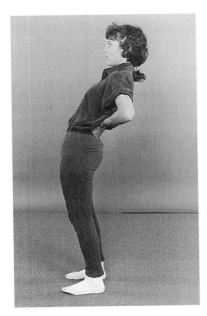

Exercise 5.K. Standing Lumbar Extension

A useful technique for postural correction. Subjects should be encouraged to perform this exercise frequently, especially after being in a flexed posture for a period of time.

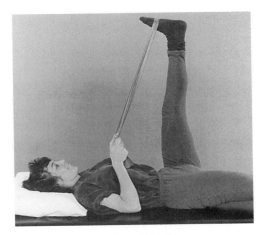

Exercise 5.L. Straight Leg Stretching

Tightness in the hamstring, gastrocnemius, and soleus muscles and in the Achilles tendon may be stretched progressively using a 5-foot length of Theraband or rope looped across the ball of the foot as illustrated. The straight leg is pulled gradually toward the maximum tolerated upright position and held for 30–60 seconds during which further stretching may be accomplished. Do not allow the knee to bend during the maneuver.

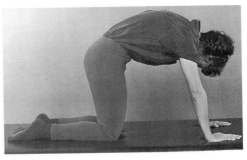

Exercise 5.N. Back Flexibility Exercises

5.N (a). Assume a hands-and-knees posture as illustrated. Tuck the chin to the chest and arch the back. Keep the elbows straight and do not rock back and forth. Hold 5 seconds.

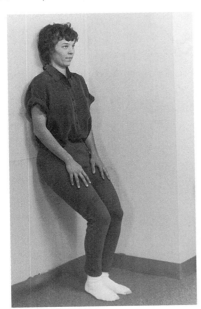

Exercise 5.M. Wall Slide

Stand against the wall with the feet approximately 6 inches out from the wall. Flatten the lower spine against the wall and gently slide down the wall by bending the knees. Gradually progress the hold in this position from 5–30 seconds. This exercise effectively strengthens thigh muscles and aids in postural alignment.

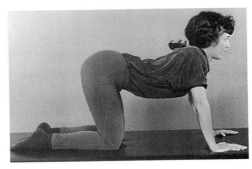

5.N (b). After arching the back, raise the head and let the back sag. Again, keep the elbows straight and do not rock back and forth. Hold 5 seconds.

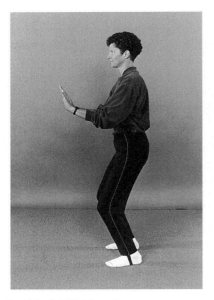

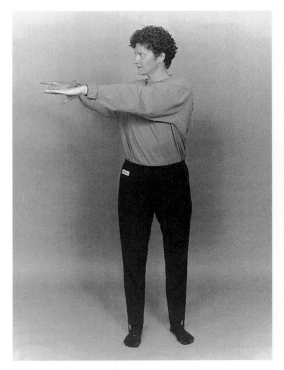

Exercise 5.O. Tai Chi Squat

This shallow knee bend is isolated from the slow, sequential patterns of Tai Chi. The position strengthens the thigh muscles and emphasizes postural alignment. Keep the knees positioned behind the great toes.

Exercise 5.P. Trunk Rotation

Stand with the feet a comfortable distance apart. Holding the arms out straight at shoulder height, rotate the upper body to one side as illustrated. Hold 5 seconds. Reverse to the opposite side. There are multiple variations to this exercise, including in sitting and supine positions as well as standing.

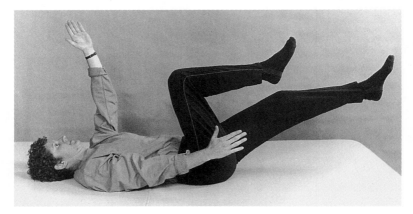

Exercise 5.Q. Supine Lumbar Stabilization

Holding a neutral or stable pelvic position, alternate opposite leg and arm movements for progressively longer time.

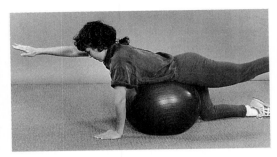

Exercise 5.R. A therapeutic ball provides challenge and interest to a back program.

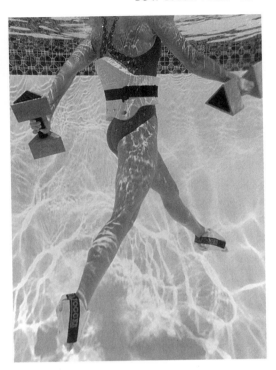

Exercise 5.S. Aquatic Exercise

Aquatic exercise is well suited for many soft tissue conditions. The Aquajogger is an example of available flotation equipment. See Appendix E for the source of this device.

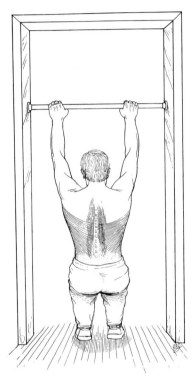

Exercise 5.T. Chinning Bar Exercise

Grasping a chinning bar placed in a doorway, the subject ''relaxes'' into a sitting position. The weight of the lower body stretches the musculature and soft tissues about the lumbar spine. The subject should spend a minute or two repetitively holding this position as long as grasping permits.

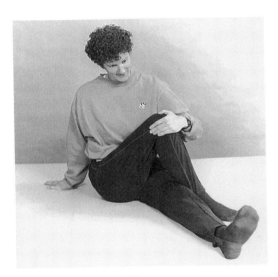

Exercise 5.U. Piriformis Stretch

In a sitting position, cross the right leg over the left, placing the right foot at the outer left knee. Place the left hand on the outer right knee. Using the left hand, pull the right knee across the midline toward the left. Stretching should be felt at the right buttock and outer thigh. Hold 10–30 seconds.

6: Lower Limb Disorders

Lower limb pain and disability may be intrinsic, referred from other structures, or part of a systemic disease. Most problems occur in association with movement and result from trauma. Often, a subtle structural fault can predispose an individual to a sports-related or other injury.

We have used the term ''cumulative movement disorders'' because it reflects the etiologic relationship of the disorder to improper or excessive movement patterns. Thus, tendinitis, bursitis, stress fractures, compartment syndromes, and plantar fasciitis fall into this designation.

The conditions described here usually occur as a degeneration of tissue in response to excessive or improper movement or excessive strain. The pathology is described more fully in Chapter 1.

The spectrum of lower extremity injury is changing. Children have suffered more severe and more frequent injuries in the last decade due to the greater popularity of soccer, skateboarding, and gymnastics. Injury to tendons and apophyses are being seen with greater frequency; growth and maturation may constitute additional risk factors for injury (1).

Other factors that can contribute to recurrent or perplexing lower limb distress include osteoporosis in women who participate in long-distance running, spondylarthritis and enthesitis of lower limb structures, improper footwear, moving from a home with wood flooring to one with a slab foundation, prolonged standing on concrete floors, and structural disorders such as joint laxity or malalignment of the lower limbs.

Psychosocial factors are important in the persistence of lower limb pain. Health care professionals should search for a history of troubled relationships, workplace politics, depression, drug dependency, particularly alcohol in the elderly, and/or issues related to compensation.

The lower limb performs its task with a remarkably complex series of movements during movement on various surfaces and when climbing or pivoting. For example, the knee must provide sliding, gliding, rotating, and bending functions. Knee movement includes the ''screw home'' mechanism: as the knee extends or straightens from the bent position, the tibia rotates externally and the femur rotates internally. This rotation mechanism requires joint stability, particularly during running. The menisci, while not completely understood, appear to act both as shock absorbers and as stabilizers to help rotational stability (2). At least a dozen bursae are situated in the knee region; several of them communicate with the joint itself (Fig. 6.1).

PREVENTION MEASURES

Proper shoes should provide support and comfort (proper fit) for the weightbearing foot,

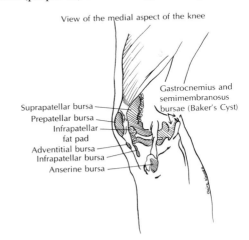

View of the medial aspect of the knee

Suprapatellar bursa
Prepatellar bursa
Infrapatellar fat pad
Adventitial bursa
Infrapatellar bursa
Anserine bursa
Gastrocnemius and semimembranosus bursae (Baker's Cyst)

Figure 6.1. Bursae of the knee region. The suprapatellar, prepatellar, infrapatellar, and adventitial bursae lie anteriorly. The anserine bursa and the sartorius bursa (not shown) are located on the medial aspect. Posteriorly, the large popliteal (Baker's) cyst may originate from the gastrocnemius or semimembranosus bursa.

with room for the toes to extend fully and to broaden out during weightbearing. Proper fit should be determined by having foot size measured while standing. Cushion soles should be used if walking or working on concrete.

Improper shoes can cause or exacerbate lower limb disorders, including hallux valgus, hammer toes, hard corns, and plantar keratoses. Leather soles were meant to be used on wood floors; newer microcellular foam shock absorbing material used in most exercise and walking shoes is preferred for walking and standing on concrete.

The shoe industry has come a long way toward meeting contemporary lifestyles, and price is no longer relevant as a guide to proper fit and style. The running or jogging shoe, the walking shoe, and many offshoots and variations of these, must be considered when living in the concrete world of condominiums, shopping malls, and places of work (Fig. 6.2). Seeing the fashion-conscious urban woman walking to work in running shoes, carrying a bag with her dress shoes, is proof of the acceptance and intelligent use of contemporary shoes. Unfortunately, men in the business world continue to demand the narrow-toed, leather-soled shoe to "fit in" with their peers. Lower limb pain is common among male bankers, male insurance executives, and businessmen who continue to use these shoes in their concrete or terrazzo-floored workplace areas. Adapting shoes to the patient can be a valuable contribution to the comprehensive treatment of rheumatic diseases of the lower limb and foot.

Conditioning exercise can prevent injury. In a study of 10 frail, institutionalized men 90 years and older, high-intensity strength training for 8 weeks resulted in an average of 174% strength gain, 9% gain in muscle mass, and 48% gain in tandem gait speed. Falling episodes with resulting injury were sharply reduced in frequency (5). Thus, strength training can be a helpful preventive measure for reducing frequency of falls.

DIFFERENTIAL DIAGNOSIS

The conditions described in this chapter are regional local disorders. However, pain in the region can also arise from systemic or multifo-

cal disease, such as herniation of a lumbar disc, Paget's disease, migratory osteolysis, inflammatory rheumatic diseases, panniculitis, occult sepsis, or neoplastic disorders (6–8).

Lower limb pain is frequently attributed to osteoarthritis. This diagnosis must not be taken for granted as the only cause for pain. When roentgenographic evidence of osteoarthritis has been noted, these changes may have little to do with the patient's symptoms. A soft tissue problem which may coexist can be easily diagnosed and treated, thus avoiding more complex procedures. Among patients referred for symptomatic osteoarthritis of the knee, up to 60% had pain arising in soft tissues; knee surgery was not indicated and conservative measures directed at the specific sites were effective (3, 4). Up to 60% of the patients with knee pain had anserine bursitis (4).

HISTORY AND PHYSICAL EXAMINATION

The art of history taking is an acquired skill. Often, the history and physical examination provide information that limits the diagnostic possibilities and suggests appropriate treatment and prevention strategies. Pain and symptom location will determine much of the focused history and physical examination (see also Appendix A). The anatomy of the lower limb may be reviewed in Plates X–XIII.

The Hip and Thigh Region

Rule out intrinsic disease of the bony skeleton. Pain arising from either the spine or hip will be aggravated by movement and by bearing weight, and usually a limp will be noted. Often the patient does not mention a limp; the patient must be asked or observed.

Always ask the patient to point to the area of pain. Do not be misled by the patient describing sacroiliac and ischiogluteal pain as "hip pain." Pain may be located at a distance from the actual source. For example, compression of the L4 nerve root is a common cause for hip and upper thigh pain.

Intrinsic hip disease, such as osteoarthritis of the hip, may refer pain to the ipsilateral buttock or groin, or to the medial knee region. Hip

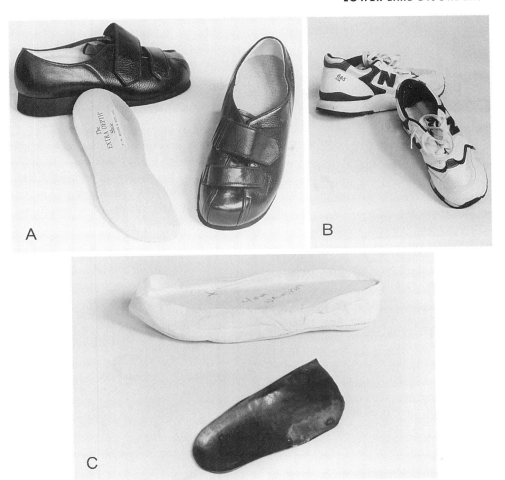

Figure 6.2. A. The extra-depth shoe. Often prescribed with the additional feature of the enlarged toe box, this shoe is helpful for patients with metatarsal and metatarsophalangeal joint difficulties, hammer toe, and rheumatoid or other inflammatory arthritides with forefoot deformity. If required, the molded soft plastic insert may be provided additionally. Occupational therapists, orthopaedists, or podiatrists are skilled in making the mold. **B.** A running shoe has microcellular foam and a rigid forefoot. These are important differences from other sport shoes. **C.** Orthoses can be used for a variety of purposes: to correct a leg length discrepancy; to correct foot/floor contact as in pronation/supination disorders; and to redistribute weightbearing patterns. Orthoses may be obtained over the counter or may be custom made.

fracture in the elderly is not uncommon and can be missed; the aged patient may forget the traumatic incident. Any elderly person with an abnormal and painful gait should be examined for a hip fracture as a cause of symptoms. Suggestive features include pain on the instant of weightbearing and pain during examination for passive range of hip motion. Deep tenderness over the pubic ramus should suggest fracture of this structure. Pain may be referred to the inner thigh. Hip or pelvis fracture may not be visible at first roentgenographic study, but will usually be evident at subsequent roentgen-ographic examination (9). Scintigraphy may be helpful as well.

Herniation of the nucleus pulposus and other causes for L4 nerve entrapment may present with hip pain or pain and paresthesia from below the lower buttock crease to below the knee, accompanied by weakness, and aggravated by cough, sneeze, or strain at defecation.

Pseudosciatica, which lacks the symptoms of weakness and aggravation by cough, sneeze, or strain at defecation, points to a likely soft tissue disturbance such as trochanteric bursitis, myofascial gluteus pain, or the piriformis syndrome.

Buttock claudication and leg paresthesia after walking one or two blocks suggests *spinal stenosis* as a likely problem.

When you suspect hip disease, do not be misled by a normal lumbar spine roentgenographic report; the hips are often not visible unless a view of the pelvis was specifically requested.

Entrapment neuropathies are characterized by intermittent symptoms, lancinating pain, and aggravation by a particular motion. (Refer to the list of critical features in Table 6.1.)

The fascia lata and its component, the iliotibial tract or band, are important sites of soft tissue injury and can cause frustrating chronic leg pain (see Anatomic Plates X and XI). The fascia lata is a thickened deep fascia of the lateral thigh. Superiorly the fascia lata attaches to the anterior superior iliac spine, the inguinal ligament, the body of the pubic bone, the ischial tuberosity, the sacrotuberous ligament, the sacrum, and the iliac crest. The iliotibial tract is a conjoint aponeurosis of the fascia lata and the gluteus maximus muscle. The iliotibial tract inserts on the anterolateral aspect of the tibia. When contracted, it exerts a pull upon the hip, resulting in flexion and abduction; it can also cause the ''snapping hip syndrome'' (discussed below).

Tendinitis of the gluteus medius and gluteus minimus muscles at their insertion also causes lateral hip pain. Distinction from trochanteric bursitis is difficult and is probably unnecessary, as treatment is the same for both. Knowledge of the location of the superficial and deep trochanteric bursae, the iliopectineal bursa, and the origin and points of potential injury or entrapment of the various superficial peripheral nerves of this region allows the examiner to palpate for trigger points and sites of nerve entrapment, and to reproduce the pain that results from disturbances of these soft tissue structures.

PHYSICAL EXAMINATION

Physical examination begins with observing the patient arising from the chair, standing, and walking (bare legs, if possible). Observe the range of spinal movement in flexion, extension, rotation, and side-bending; if movement appears limited, measure chest expansion to detect a spondyloarthropathy. Rotational disturbances of the lower limb (e.g., malrotation of the femur or tibia) can be detected by suspending a weight on the end of a string located at the level of the anterior iliac crest; the patient stands with the feet together, and the weight should touch the second toe.

The following degrees of hip movement are considered normal (Fig. 6.3):
Flexion: 120–135 degrees
Abduction in extension: 35–40 degrees
Abduction in flexion: 70–75 degrees
Adduction (crossing leg): 25–30 degrees
Internal rotation in extension or flexion: 45 degrees
External rotation in extension or flexion: 45 degrees
Hip extension: 20–30 degrees
The examiner should measure leg length after determining the patient's ability to straighten the knees fully. With the leg drawn straight and the patient lying flat on his/her back, the true leg length can be measured from the anterior superior iliac spine to the medial malleolus of each ankle. Normal individuals may have as much as a 1-cm discrepancy without symptoms. Pelvic rotations can cause apparent leg length discrepancies. ''Apparent'' (or functional) limb length disparity is determined by measuring the distance from the umbilicus to each medial malleolus. An examination of the abdomen, back, and groin and a careful neurologic examination appropriate to the clinical presentation should be performed.

SPECIAL MANEUVERS OR OTHER TESTS

Testing for *Trendelenburg's sign* is important for the detection of involvement of the hip stabilizers (gluteus medius, gluteus minimus).

TABLE 6.1 CRITICAL FEATURES FOR THE LOWER LIMB

1. Fever and chills or weight loss
2. Lymphadenopathy
3. Constant and progressive pain
4. Buckling, locking, or giving way
5. Pain or paresthesia at night
6. Limb claudication or bruit
7. Any visible swelling, warmth, or discoloration
8. Joint instability or positive stress tests during passive examination
9. Weakness or atrophy or reflex change
10. Compartment symptoms: pain, paresthesia, pulseless paralysis

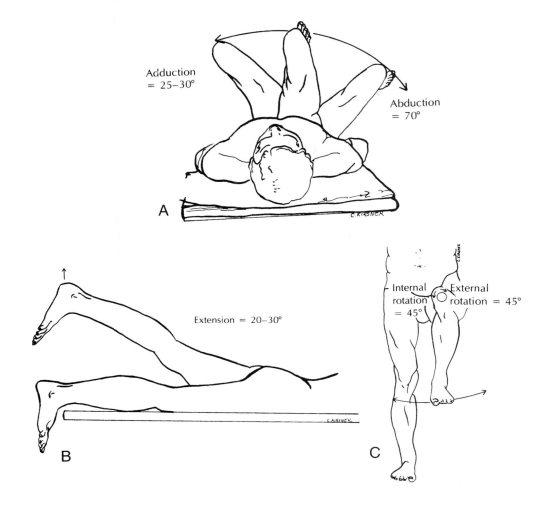

Figure 6.3. Examination for range of movement of the hip. This ball-and-socket joint provides: **A.** Adduction, abduction, and flexion; **B.** Extension; and **C.** Internal and external rotation. These illustrations demonstrate some of the methods for the determination of these movements.

The examination consists of having the patient stand with his/her back to the examiner. A point is marked on each of the posterior iliac spines. The patient then stands on one foot and raises the other; the side supporting the body's weight is the side being tested. If the pelvis falls toward the side not bearing weight, the test is positive (Trendelenburg's sign) and suggests muscle disease affecting the abductors or the stabilizers of the hip, congenital dislocation of the hip, coxa vara, Legg-Calvé-Perthes disease (avascular necrosis of the femoral head), or abnormalities in the proximal femoral epiphysis.

Patrick's test, which Patrick mnemonically named the *fabere sign* to describe the maneuver (*f*lexion, *ab*duction, *e*xternal *r*otation, and *e*xten-

sion—though the latter is usually omitted), is a physical examination maneuver to detect intrinsic disease in the hip. With the patient supine, the foot of the involved extremity is placed on the opposite knee. The examiner then presses the knee and thigh downward; pain results if intrinsic hip disease is present (Fig. 6.4).

Erichsen's sign: The examiner provides compression across the iliac bones; if pain occurs, the test is suggestive of sacroiliac joint inflammation rather than hip disease.

Ober's test (for contracture of the iliotibial tract): The patient lies with the affected side up and the opposite side down; the uppermost leg (symptomatic side) is drawn backward into

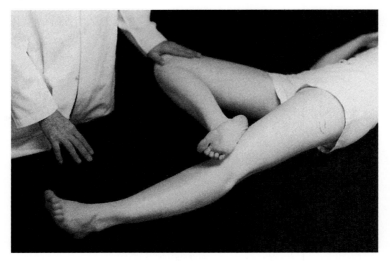

Figure 6.4. The Patrick or fabere test. If pain results when the examiner presses the knee and thigh downward, then intrinsic hip disease should be suspected.

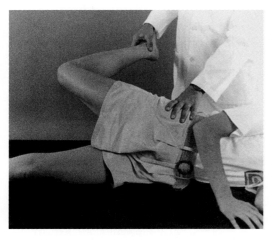

Figure 6.5. The Ober test. This test is useful for determining the presence of a contracture of the iliotibial tract or tightness in the hip flexor musculature.

posterior extension by the examiner and then bent at the knee (Fig. 6.5). The Ober test is positive if, after the examiner lets go of the involved thigh, the knee does not drop to the table. Failure of the leg to fall suggests a contracture of the iliotibial tract. The Ober test also reproduces pain resulting from hip flexor muscle contractures. The pain presents at the lower anterior thigh and knee.

The Knee Region

When the history is that of disabling knee pain, the physician must consider the age of the

patient, any preceding injury, and the pain pattern. In addition, the mode of onset, the localization of pain, and any associated phenomena of locking, clicking, catching, buckling, swelling, or loss of motion should be noted. Features suggesting the need for more detailed evaluation and consultation are listed in Table 6.1.

A careful history searching for improper use or calisthenic exercise is important. (Refer to Table 6.2 on joint protection for the lower limb.)

Intermittent "giving way" (buckling) or locking, followed by a period of recovery, may result from a torn meniscus, intraarticular loose bodies, plicae, cruciate ligament inadequacy, patellofemoral instability, hypertrophy of the infrapatellar fat pad, or intraarticular tumors of the knee. These disorders collectively are termed "internal derangements of the knee." Early recognition of an internal derangement of the knee, followed by appropriate therapy, may relieve symptoms and prevent secondary osteoarthritis. Warmth and swelling in association with a persistent locked knee are signs of serious internal derangement; surgical consultation should be sought.

Asking the patient to point to the area of maximum pain, or having the patient indicate whether the pain is anterior, posterior, medial, or lateral, assists the clinician in diagnosis. However, referred pain from another knee compartment is not uncommon.

TABLE 6.2 JOINT PROTECTION FOR THE LOWER EXTREMITY

Do not carry a large wallet in a back pocket. Check for pressure placed on the pelvic bones by a wallet, tight belt, or constricting jeans that can squeeze nerves in the pelvis or groin.
Always bend at the knees, not at the waist.
Wear cushion-soled shoes when standing or walking on concrete.

KNEE

Strengthen the thigh muscles (quadriceps/hamstrings) to protect the knee.
If stair climbing causes or increases knee pain, limit the activity and strengthen the thigh muscles until the pain subsides.
Knee pain can be caused by foot disorders: evaluate the entire lower leg when investigating knee pain.
Avoid deep knee bending—use reacher tools for assistance.
During prolonged sitting, straighten the knees or stand up at least every 30 minutes to relieve pressure and stretch tight muscles.
Short, brisk walks will increase leg circulation and exercise muscles.
Buy shoes with proper heels and check them often for signs of wear.
Use the thigh muscles to rise from a chair—it provides good exercise.
Use a mechanic's or milker's stool when working on the floor or on the ground. Sit with the legs apart and reach forward to perform tasks such as gardening or scrubbing floors.
If you must work on hands and knees, use protective knee pads.
Consider raised or container gardening to reduce stress and effort.
Stationary biking provides safe, low-impact exercise. Adjust the seat height so that the knees are slightly bent at the low point of the down-stroke and no more than 90 degrees flexed on the up-stroke. Increase resistance gradually.
Perform a regular stretching program for the muscles of the upper and lower leg. Tight muscles can contribute to knee problems.

Sports

Treat knee injuries promptly with RICE techniques. If pain and instability persist, seek medical attention.
Adjust bicycle seats as described above.
Engage in exercise and sports activities on a regular basis rather than occasional weekend participation. Include warm-up and cool-down activities as well as appropriate stretching in your routine.
Modify or avoid knee-twisting dance steps or exercises.

ANKLE AND FOOT

Choose footwear with comfort, support, and utility in mind.
Do not wear shoes that cause pain or fatigue. Get professional advice when necessary.
Loose-jointed persons should be especially careful to protect the ankles and feet. Sprains and strains can increase instability.
Orthoses can provide needed support and positioning assistance. Consult an experienced professional regarding the choice of an orthosis, whether having it custom-made or obtaining it over-the-counter.
Maintain appropriate weight to reduce stress on feet and ankles.
Running shoes, walking shoes, or aerobics shoes are more supportive and comfortable to the flexible or arthritic foot.
Use a metatarsal pad or bar to relieve pressure or pain at the forefoot.
If you must stand or walk on concrete (even if it is carpeted), select shoes with shock-absorbing soles.
Treat ankle sprains promptly with RICE techniques. Seek medical advice if swelling and pain do not subside.

Sports

Use footwear that is especially designed for the sport you are playing.
Run on dirt or track surfaces—avoid running on concrete or asphalt.
Use orthoses in sport shoes as well as in everyday shoes.

- Pain at the medial joint line is seen with injury to the medial collateral ligament, disease of the medial joint compartment, anserine bursitis, or an internal derangement
- Pain posterior to the knee joint may result from a shortened hamstring, a popliteal cyst, or tendinitis
- Pain at the lateral aspect of the knee joint may represent bursitis adjacent to the head of the fibula, arthritis, or internal derangement of the lateral compartment of the knee
- Pain anterior to the knee joint is strongly suggestive of patellofemoral disturbances or derangements of the quadriceps mechanism

Although pain location is helpful, referred pain from a distant etiological site may be pres-

TABLE 6.3 CAUSES FOR KNEE PAIN

I. Anterior Knee Symptoms
    Patellofemoral pain syndrome (younger patient without significant disorder)
    Patellofemoral osteoarthritis (older patient)
    Overload syndromes (osteochondral injuries in runners, athletes)
    Malalignment (tracking) syndromes (with genu valgus or rotation abnormalities of the limb; quadriceps dysplasia; patellar dislocation; fracture)
    Other patellar disorders (patella alta, odd facet syndrome, chondromalacia, osteochondritis)
    Cruciate ligament injury
    Synovial disorders (plicae, inflammatory arthritis, villonodular synovitis)
    Prepatellar neuritis, bursitis
    Reflex sympathetic dystrophy

II. Medial Knee Pain
    Ligamentous injuries (joint laxity, hypermobility syndrome, trauma)
    Anserine bursitis
    Meniscus lesions
    Medial plica syndrome
    Synovitis (arthritis)
    Referred pain from the hip
    Osteonecrosis

III. Lateral Knee Pain
    Fibular bursitis
    Meniscus injury
    Collateral ligament injury
    Iliotibial band friction syndrome
    Fascia lata fasciitis
    Pseudosciatica

IV. Posterior Knee Pain
    Tendinitis
    Capsulitis
    Bursitis
    Synovitis
    Peroneal nerve injury
    Vascular lesions
    Popliteal cyst

ent and confuse the diagnosis. Burning, throbbing, or other neuritis-like symptoms may result from reflex sympathetic dystrophy in the knee region (10), or from a prepatellar neuralgia (11). Refer to Table 6.3 on causes of knee pain, and Table 6.4, a decision chart for the lower limb.

Sports and industrial knee injuries may result in part from underlying foot, ankle, leg, or hip problems. Question the patient regarding recent changes in lower extremity function and activity, particularly new exercise patterns. Syndromes that result from excessive cumulative movement are particularly important and common. If not recognized, the aggravation will only be repeated, leading to dissatisfaction with outcomes by both physician and patient. For example, middle-aged men might be advised to use stair climbing as exercise for cardiac conditioning and find themselves with patellofemoral pain. Stair-climber exercise machines may also cause new knee pain. Patients often will not volunteer this information regarding new activities; it has to be elicited. Runners who overtrain with mileage in excess of 20 miles per week commonly develop knee ailments. Cycling, hockey, basketball, soccer, and downhill skiing may stress the collateral ligaments. Refer also to Table 6.2 on joint protection for the lower limb.

PHYSICAL EXAMINATION

A careful examination includes evaluation of the appearance of the extremity when the patient is lying, rising, standing, and walking. The common maneuvers of knee examination are described here, though more specialized examination techniques can be found in the article by Hughston et al., "Classification of Knee Ligament Instabilities" (12).

While the patient is standing with feet slightly apart and parallel (pointing directly forward), the clinician may note congenital abnormalities of alignment and joint mobility:

- Genu recurvatum (hyperextension or excessive backward knee joint mobility), patella alta (a high-riding patella).
- Abnormal patellar alignment, viewed in relation to the tibial tubercle. From the frontal aspect, the patellae may both point away from the midline, denoting lateral patellar subluxation ("grasshopper eye patellae"); this often occurs in association with chondromalacia patellae (13).
- Femoral anteversion (external rotational malalignment) with inwardly pointing patellae may also predispose to patellofemoral subluxation (14).
- Genu varum (bowleg) or genu valgum (knock-knee). The terms varus and valgus, through common usage, imply inward or outward deviation of the foreleg from the midline, respectively. However, discussions in the literature have emphasized that these commonly used terms are inaccurate and inadequate (15). Accordingly, it is usually best to add additional descriptions

TABLE 6.4 DECISION CHART LOWER LIMB

Problem	Action	Other Actions

A. Lateral Hip Pain
  Not acute, no limp
  Painful when lying on
    side
  Normal hip motion
B. Lateral Hip Pain
  Limp, weakness
  Neurologic findings
    positive or suspicious
  No visible swelling
  Pain with use
  No numbness/tingling
C. Tendinitis
  Pain on passive
    stretching
  Pain on active
    movement
D. Bursitis
  Night pain
    Point tenderness
E. Anterior Hip Pain
  Morning stiffness
  Limited motion
  No neurologic findings
	Physical examination
	Conservative care
	Assess how activities at work
	  and home/play are done
	Advise regarding correction of
	  aggravating factors
	Exercise
	Medications—NSAIDs, ASA,
	  acetaminophen, muscle
	  relaxants
	Local injection of crystalline
	  steroid and local
	  anesthetic mixture
	Roentgenograms in older
	  patients
	Electrodiagnostic studies as
	  appropriate
	
	+ Advise about position while
	  sleeping
	
	→ ± Ultrasound or CT Scan
		If conservative care not
		  effective, reexamine
		  patient, order
		  roetgenograms, CT scan,
		  workup for inflammatory
		  disease
		Consultation with orthopaedic
		  surgeon, physiatrist

F. Acute Hip Pain
  Older patient
  Limp, limited motion
	→ Immediate roentgenographic
	  examination	

G. Anterior Knee Pain
  Diffuse pain not acute
  Gait normal
  Interferes with sleep
  Normal motion
Patellofemoral pain
Medial or lateral pain and
  locking or buckling
H. Bursitis, Knee Region
  Swelling and stiffness
  Night pain
	Physical examination
	Conservative care
	Assess how activities at work
	  and home/play are done
	Advise regarding correction of
	  aggravating factors
	Exercise, may require rest
	Medications—NSAIDs, ASA,
	  acetaminophen
	Local injection of steroid and
	  local anesthetic mixture
	Roentgenogram when
	  appropriate
	Advise about sports and
	  training
	Advise about supportive shoes
	+ Advise about sleep position
	+ Synovial fluid analysis for
	  crystals, Gram stain, sugar
		Orthopaedic consultation
		
		Arthroscopy/Arthrography
		  Bracing
		  Rest/Crutches
		    ↓
		Scintigraphy, ultrasonography
		Systemic workup for
		  inflammation
		
		    ↓
		Consultation:
		  Orthopaedist
		  Rheumatologist
		
		→ Orthopaedic consultation

I. Posterior Knee Pain	→ + Aspirate Baker's Cyst	

J. Posterior Heel Pain
  Increased pain on
    dorsiflexion
K. Plantar Heel Pain
L. Ankle Pain and/or
  Instability
M. Midfoot Pain
N. Tendinitis
  Swelling and tenderness
  Pain on passive
    stretching of tendon
  Pain on active ankle
    movement
	Physical examination
	Conservative care
	Assess how activities at work
	  and home/play are done
	Advise regarding correction of
	  aggravating factors
	Medications—NSAIDs, ASA
	Local injection of steroid and
	  local anesthetic mix
	Exercises, stretching
	Shoes—support, orthoses,
	  cushioning
	Roentgenograms as
	  appropriate
	+ Rest, ankle support, RICE
		Bone scan for fatigue fracture
		Tests for systemic inflammatory
		  disease
		Stress roentgenograms of the
		  ankle
		Weightbearing foot
		  roentgenograms
		Rheumatology, orthopaedic,
		  podiatry, or other
		  consultation
		
		→ MRI and workup for inflam-
		  matory rheumatic disease

(continued)

TABLE 6.4 DECISION CHART LOWER LIMB (continued)

Problem	Action	Other Actions
O. Metatarsalgia Without Paresthesia	Shoes, orthoses, and exercise as appropriate	
P. Metatarsalgia With Paresthesia	+ Test for diabetes, vascular insufficiency, nerve entrapment	
Q. Plantar Pain Without Paresthesia	+ Examine for joint laxity, flatfoot, tight and tender plantar fascia	
R. Plantar Pain and Paresthesia Nocturnal aggravation	Shoes with long counter, inject plantar fascia + Test for tarsal tunnel syndrome, inject tarsal tunnel	
Danger Signs Color change or warmth Swelling Lymphadenopathy Paresthesia Increasing pain with weightbearing Claudication Neurologic findings Positive stress tests Atrophy	Comprehensive examination and treatment Vascular, neurologic, endocrine studies or consultation	→ Immediate appropriate action, consultation

(e.g., bowleg, knock-knee) when defining changes related to these anatomic deviations.

Genu valgum may also predispose to lateral patellar dislocation or displacement. Prepatellar bursitis, synovitis with suprapatellar fullness, or a Baker's cyst may be apparent by observation while the patient is standing.

Observe the patient walking toward and away from you with legs uncovered. The feet may point away 30 degrees from the midline. Pes planus (flatfoot) may give rise to knee region discomfort and should be noted.

The patient should be observed while rising from a seated position without the use of hands for assistance; this is a simple test for the integrity and strength of the quadriceps extensor mechanism, but may also suggest knee disorders located in the patellofemoral region, or primary muscle disease. Inspection and palpation of the knee may reveal a relatively painless chronic granular cellulitis in the patellar region, as seen in coal miners (the "beat knee") (16). Chronic prepatellar bursal thickening occurs in relation to certain occupations involving kneeling, such as carpet laying (Fig. 6.6).

Lateral patellar displacement or subluxation may be observed as the seated patient straightens the knee and the patella moves outward

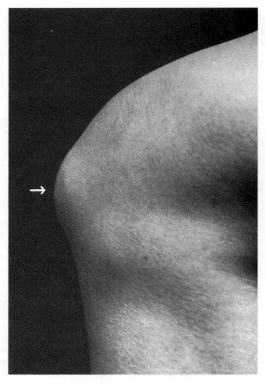

Figure 6.6. Prepatellar bursitis. The bursitis is visible and palpable superficial to the patella.

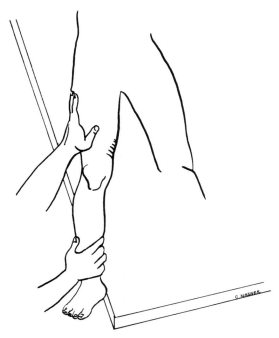

Figure 6.7. The valgus stress test. When the examiner attempts to deviate the knee into a valgus position with the knee extended, the integrity of both the posterior cruciate and the medial collateral ligaments is tested; repeating the maneuver with the knee bent tests the collateral ligament alone.

instead of straight upward, often called the "J sign." Excessive tightness in the lateral patellar retinaculum may be noted. The laterally tilted patella should be manually correctable when the patient is lying supine. Also, the patella should be displaceable medially about 1 cm from its resting position when the knee is flexed to 30 degrees. If not, the lateral patellar retinaculum is abnormally tight, and stretching exercise is suggested (17).

The joint capsule is supported on each side by complex medial and lateral collateral ligament systems (12), and inadequacy of these structures may result in excessive side-to-side motion of the joint.

SPECIAL KNEE JOINT MANEUVERS

The collateral ligament stress tests are performed with the patient supine. The examiner first tests the involved leg with the knee in full extension (Fig. 6.7), and then repeats the test with the knee flexed 30 degrees. Grasping the involved leg, the examiner attempts to deviate

the foreleg away from the midline inwardly and outwardly (varus and valgus, respectively). Performing the maneuver with the knee extended tests the integrity of both the posterior cruciate and the collateral ligaments; repeating the maneuver with the knee bent tests the collateral ligaments alone. The examiner observes for opening or widening of the medial or lateral joint compartment. Stress tests may be misleading if reflex spasm from pain prevents relaxation during the examination.

Cruciate ligament insufficiency is associated with excessive anteroposterior motion. If there is any suggestion of instability, stress testing is important to help define the problem. Posttraumatic ligamentous instability that is not treated may lead to quadriceps femoris muscle atrophy, which complicates the clinical presentation.

Tests of knee motion are highly dependent on examiner experience. Studies of knee motion performed by experienced orthopaedists in cadaveric knees (18), in nine injured patients with one control (19), and in 85 anesthetized patients (20), compared the Lachman test, the pivot shift tests, and the anterior drawer sign for specificity and sensitivity. All three studies revealed intra- and interobserver variation and unreliability, and all three emphasize the need for more objectively derived findings, although the Lachman test and the pivot shift tests were found to be helpful when positive. The tests lack standardized reporting, however; the development of standardized instrumented teaching models, it is hoped, will improve interexaminer clinical test reproducibility (18–20).

The anterior drawer sign, more helpful in chronic knee instability than in the acute setting (20), is performed with the patient supine, the hip flexed 45 degrees, and the patient's head supported on a pillow; otherwise, should the patient arise to look forward, the hamstring muscles may become tense. The involved knee is flexed approximately 80–90 degrees, and the foot is stabilized by the examiner's sitting on it. The hamstrings should be relaxed. The tibia is gently pulled and pushed straight in and out, anteriorly and posteriorly, back and forth. The maneuver should be performed separately with the foot in the straight-forward or neutral position, then with the foot rotated internally,

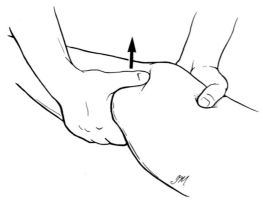

Figure 6.8. The Lachman test. The knee is flexed 20 degrees; the proximal tibia is grasped and moved forward while the femur is held with the other hand. (From Steinberg GG et al., Ramaurti's orthopaedics in primary care. 2nd ed. Baltimore: Williams & Wilkins, 1992)

and lastly with the foot rotated externally. Both legs should be examined for comparison. Excessive anterior motion (more than 5 mm) supports a diagnosis of insufficiency of the anterior cruciate ligament or of the medial portion of the joint capsule (12).

The Lachman test is performed with the patient supine, with the involved extremity on the side of the examiner. The injured knee is compared with the uninjured knee. With the patient's knee in 10–20 degrees of flexion, the femur is stabilized with one hand. The other hand applies forward pressure to the posteromedial aspect of the proximal tibia in an attempt to displace it anteriorly. Any subluxation in the injured knee as compared to the uninjured knee demonstrates a positive Lachman test and insufficiency of the anterior cruciate ligament (20) (Fig. 6.8).

The pivot shift test is a test of anterolateral rotatory instability and tests subluxation of a loaded knee joint. The knee is placed in 10–20 degrees of flexion and torque is applied to the tibia by rotating it internally and applying valgus stress to the knee joint. If there is anterior subluxation of the lateral tibial plateau underneath the femoral condyle, then the test is positive, indicating insufficiency of the anterior cruciate ligament. The knee reduces spontaneously with flexion to 40 degrees, which causes the iliotibial tract to tighten, reducing the subluxated tibia (20) (Fig. 6.9).

The posterior drawer sign is determined passively by observing whether the tibia is displaced posteriorly while the patient is resting in the

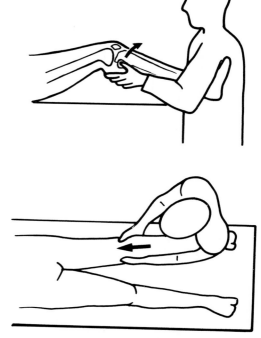

Figure 6.9. The Pivot shift test. The ankle and leg are held under the axilla. The leg is abducted and the knee extended. The hands are under the proximal tibia applying gentle anterior and internal rotation force. The tibia will subluxate forward and, as pressure is applied in line with the leg, the tibia will flex and reduce. (From Steinberg GG et al., eds. Ramamurti's orthopaedics in primary care. 2nd ed. Baltimore: Williams & Wilkins, 1992.)

same position as described for the anterior drawer sign. The examiner then grasps the tibia and attempts to displace it further posteriorly. A positive posterior drawer sign indicates insufficiency of the posterior cruciate ligament (21) (Fig. 6.10). Tenderness along the joint line is assessed by performing the maneuver with the patient's knee flexed 90 degrees.

Perkin's test for patellofemoral pain syndrome: Pain may be reproduced by patellofemoral compression with the knee flexed or straight as the patella is pushed from side to side. The examiner must avoid squeezing the synovium during the examination.

Fairbank's apprehension sign for lateral patellar subluxation is performed by placing the knee in 30 degrees of flexion and applying lateral pressure against the medial aspect of the patella. This causes patient apprehension.

Assessing whether full extension of the knee can be obtained is an important test for internal

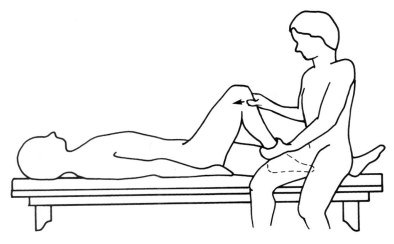

Figure 6.10. The posterior drawer test. With the knee at 90 degrees of flexion, push back on the tibia to see whether there is increased motion or sag compared with the other leg. (From Steinberg GG et al., eds. Ramamurti's orthopaedics in primary care. 2nd ed. Baltimore: Williams & Wilkins, 1992.)

derangement problems. With the patient supine, the examiner grasps the patient's knee just above the patella with one hand and, if possible, gently pushes the knee into extension. At the same time the examiner grasps the patient's great toe and tries to extend the leg. With this maneuver, even small side-to-side differences can be detected (22).

Loose bodies (''joint mice'') may cause symptoms similar to those of a torn meniscus, including sensations of locking, grating, giving way, and swelling of the knee. The loose body may represent a chondral or osteochondral fragment, meniscus material, or a sequestered fragment from an osteochondritis dissecans lesion (23). Radiographic evidence may not be apparent if the fragment is of cartilaginous origin or is hidden in the posterior compartment. Occasionally, a loose body may be the first sign of synovial chondromatosis. Periodic giving way or locking, without apparent injury, strongly suggests the presence of a loose body.

The McMurray test for meniscus damage is performed by acutely flexing the symptomatic knee of the supine patient, so that the heel of the involved extremity approximates the buttock. The examiner then grasps the ankle and rotates the tibia medially and then laterally while straightening it into extension. A palpable or auditory click on rotation represents a positive test (Fig. 6.11).

The Apley grinding maneuver is performed with the patient prone. The knee is flexed 80–90 degrees, and the examiner then presses

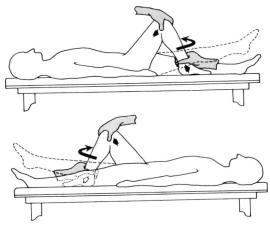

Figure 6.11. McMurray's test. (From Steinberg GG et al., eds. Ramamurti's orthopaedics in primary care. 2nd ed. Baltimore: Williams & Wilkins, 1992.)

down upon the foot and foreleg while rotating them. Pain, clicking, or locking comprise a positive Apley grinding maneuver. This usually indicates a derangement of the meniscus or articular surface rather than of the ligament complex (Fig. 6.12).

Tests for meniscal pathology are also highly examiner dependent and individually are insensitive; but when performed collectively, their value increases. In a study comparing the McMurray click test, the Apley grinding maneuver, pain on forced flexion of the knee, presence of joint line tenderness, and presence of a block to extension with findings at arthroscopy in 161 knees, the authors conclude that joint line tenderness, a positive McMurray test,

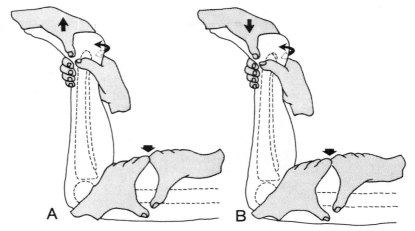

Figure 6.12. Apley's test. **A.** Pain is compatible with ligament injury. **B.** Pain is compatible with meniscus injury. (From Steinberg GG et al., eds. Ramamurti's orthopaedics in primary care. 2nd ed. Baltimore: Williams & Wilkins, 1992.)

and presence of a block to extension were together best for predicting arthroscopic findings. The Apley grinding maneuver was least helpful (22).

Sometimes a patient provides a history of the knee "giving way" but stress tests reveal only slight or no abnormal motion. In such patients a diagnosis of hypermobility syndrome with disuse quadriceps femoris muscle weakness should be considered; signs of joint laxity elsewhere in the musculoskeletal system should be sought (24, 25). Similar symptoms may result from patellofemoral disturbances (refer to the section "Patellofemoral Derangements" below).

The Ankle and Foot Region

Foot complaints must be assessed in a logical sequence in order to determine local versus systemic causes, or traumatic, genetic, or acquired disturbances. The quality of pain should help to distinguish neuropathic types of discomfort (burning, tingling) from the more common deep aching symptoms of tissue strain or injury. When symptoms are intermittent rather than persistent, further inquiry should include the type of flooring in the home or at the workplace, any recent change in occupation that might require prolonged standing, or whether recent recovery from a protracted illness has occurred. New activities such as jogging, racquetball, or other activities with foot

impact should be discussed (refer to Table 6.2 on joint protection).

PHYSICAL EXAMINATION

Inspection of the foot while the patient is seated includes noting skin color, hair distribution on the foot and foreleg, presence of a normal arch, forefoot width, and the presence of calluses and other dermatologic features. Next, with the patient standing, the physician looks for spinal curvatures, pelvic tilt, femoral or tibial torsion, patellae rotating away from the midline, and the direction of the weightbearing foot. The flatfoot is accompanied by pronation, a tilting outward of the foot, and valgus deviation of the heel. This can be seen best by inspecting the foot from behind the standing patient. From the frontal view, a line carried from the midpoint of the patella down the anterior spine of the lower tibia should project forward through the web between the second and third toes.

While the patient is standing, the physician should look for toe deformities, particularly hallux valgus, metatarsus primus varus of the first toe (the first metatarsus is shortened and deviated to the midline, and the toe is rotated slightly medially as noted by the slant of the toenail), and for evidence of toe crowding.

With the patient lying supine the examiner should next determine the rigidity or softness of the plantar fascia. This is performed by grasping the toes and dorsiflexing them with one hand while palpating the plantar aspect of

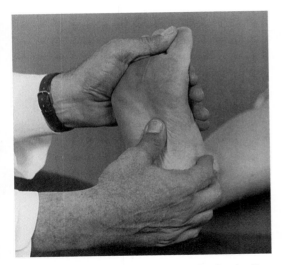

Figure 6.13. Examination of the plantar fascia. The toes are drawn into extension, thus tensing the bands of the plantar fascia. Palpation reveals points of induration and tenderness. The two feet should be compared.

the foot, particularly the bands compressing the plantar fascia. Only by examining many normal feet can the physician become familiar with the pathologic tightly bound plantar fascia (Fig. 6.13). A tear of the plantar fascia should be suspected if the banded fascia is not palpable. The assessment of the circulation and neurologic status of the foot should complete the examination.

Cost-effective care must begin with a comprehensive appropriate history and physical examination. Only then can efficient further diagnosis and care be rendered. *If the initial patient encounter has no critical signs, begin symptomatic treatment, provide an expected outcome, and have the patient return within a reasonable time; if symptoms persist, proceed with laboratory or radiologic procedures.*

CUMULATIVE MOVEMENT DISORDERS

Contemporary lifestyles include much more body movement at all ages. Health clubs have become popular. Working out, participating in sports, the resurgence of crafts, and longer hours at work result in more frequent and more persistent lower limb pain and dysfunction.

The Hip and Groin Area

Constant groin pain can result from other articular and nonarticular causes. Recurrent groin strain is common among hockey and soccer players. Injury to the pubis with resultant osteitis pubis should be considered (26). Other causes for groin pain include conditions of the femoral triangle such as abscesses, hernias, cellulitis, hematomas, lipomas, aneurysm, femoral vein thrombosis, and tumors. Patients with persistent pain in this region require appropriate laboratory and radiologic examinations. Radiographic examination should include the spine and both hips for appropriate evaluation. Use of magnetic resonance imaging and radionuclide scans of this region can be helpful, particularly in the injured youth (27). An erythrocyte sedimentation rate determination, a complete blood count, a urinalysis, a rectal examination, and a stool examination for occult blood are essential in patients with any persistent pelvic or hip region pain. A careful vaginal pelvic examination should be performed by the clinician experienced in this examination. The pelvic ligaments are uncommon sites of origin for low pelvic pain in females, and the degree of tenderness is a subjective determination. Prostate infection can refer pain into the groin and bilateral medial thighs along the adductor tendons.

Snapping Hip: An actual dislocation of the hip is painful, whereas the snapping hip is a painless annoying noise (28). The snapping hip often results from a taut iliotibial tract slipping over the greater trochanter. Other causes for snapping hip include the iliopsoas tendon jumping across the iliopectineal or iliopubic eminence (29), the gluteus maximus sliding across the greater trochanter, and generalized joint laxity. Arthrography under fluoroscopy, with special attention to the iliopsoas tendon during hip motion, may be necessary for diagnosis. In our experience the iliotibial tract is most often the culprit, and treatment for this etiology usually provides benefit, thus averting the need for expensive diagnostic tests. Treatment consists of stretching the iliotibial tract for a few moments twice daily (Table 6.5, Exercises 6.A and 6.B). Usually within a period of weeks the snapping diminishes. Stretching exercise for the iliotibial tract can be done in the side-lying position, as in Exercise 6.A, using both the

TABLE 6.5 LOWER LIMB EXERCISES

Condition	Exercise/Physical Measure	Exercise Number
Intrinsic hip disease	Hip Pendulum	6.C
Snapping hip	IT Band Stretch—Side-lying	6.A(a,b)
	IT Band Stretch—Standing	6.B
	Hip Pendulum	6.C
Fascia lata fasciitis	IT Band Stretch—Side-lying	6.A(a,b)
	IT Band Stretch—Standing	6.B
	Hip Pendulum	6.C
Hamstring injuries	Posterior Leg Stretch—Wall	6.H
	Posterior Leg Stretch—Doorway	6.I
	Supine Leg Stretch	6.K
Semimembranosus insertion	Posterior Leg Stretch—Wall	6.H
	Posterior Leg Stretch—Doorway	6.I
	Supine Leg Stretch	6.K
Quad muscle/tendon disruption	Resistive Quad Strengthening	6.E, 6.F, 6.G
	Hip Flexor Stretch	6.D
Quad disuse atrophy	Resistive Quad Strengthening	6.E, 6.F, 6.G
Myofascial knee pain	Hip Flexor Stretch	6.D(a,b)
PF pain syndrome	Resistive Quad Strengthening (cautiously graded)	6.E, 6.F, 6.G
Popliteal tendinitis (tennis leg)	Posterior Leg Stretch—Wall	6.H
	Posterior Leg Stretch—Doorway	6.I
	Supine Leg Stretch	6.K
Plantar fasciitis	Calf–Plantar Fascia Stretch—Theraband (sitting)	6.J
	Toe Curls	6.M(a,b)
	Foot-Ankle Circles	6.L
Running injuries (general)	Resistive Quad Strengthening	6.E, 6.F, 6.G
	Calf–Plantar Fascia Stretch (sitting)	6.J
	Posterior Leg Stretch—Wall	6.H
	Posterior Leg Stretch—Doorway	6.I
	Supine Leg Stretch	6.K
Myofascial leg pain	Posterior Leg Stretch—Wall	6.H
	Posterior Leg Stretch—Doorway	6.I
	Supine Leg Stretch	6.K
Ankle sprains	Foot-Ankle Circles	6.L
Ankle tendinitis	Foot-Ankle Circles	6.L
	Calf–Plantar Fascia Stretch (sitting)	6.J
Achilles disorder	Posterior Leg Stretch—Wall	6.H
	Posterior Leg Stretch—Doorway	6.I
	Calf–Plantar Fascia Stretch (sitting)	6.J
Plantar fasciitis	Toe Curls	6.M(a,b)
	Calf–Plantar Fascia Stretch (sitting)	6.J
	Toe Towel Curls	6.N
	Foot-Ankle Circles	6.L
Metatarsalgia	Toe Curls	6.M(a,b)
	Toe Towel Curls	6.N
Osgood-Schlatter disease	*Cautious* Resistive Quad Strengthening	6.F, 6.G
Leg cramps	Posterior Leg Stretch—Wall	6.H
	Calf–Plantar Fascia Stretch (sitting)	6.J
Restless legs	Posterior Leg Stretch—Doorway	6.H
	Calf–Plantar Fascia Stretch (sitting)	6.J
Inflammatory ankle capsulitis	Foot-Ankle Circles	6.L
Flexible flatfeet	Toe Curls	6.M(a,b)
	Toe Towel Curls	6.N
	Foot-Ankle Circles	6.L

front and rear stretching positions. The standing position for iliotibial tract stretching (Exercise 6.B) is recommended for the more agile patient with good balance. The "hip pendulum" exercise (Exercise 6.C) is also recommended to stretch and lengthen the hip capsule tissues and to relax the muscles surrounding the hip.

"Internal snapping hip" is a painful snapping hip located in the anterior groin region (30). The symptoms occur during movement when extending the hip from a flexed, abducted, and externally rotated position. Iliopsoas bursography combined with cineradiography can demonstrate a sudden jerking movement of the iliopsoas tendon between the anterior inferior iliac spine and the iliopectineal eminence at the time of induced pain on movement. Surgery to lengthen the iliopsoas tendon may be necessary (30).

Fascia Lata Fasciitis: Symptoms may result from inflammation or tightness of the fascia lata due to overuse or disuse. The patient may describe vague discomfort upon arising in the morning and after prolonged walking. Initially, symptoms may be relieved by walking, only to be aggravated by further, prolonged walking. The discomfort is a dull ache over the low back and lateral hip and thigh region radiating down the lateral thigh to the lateral knee region. Physical examination requires positioning the patient on the examining table with the involved hip uppermost. A weight (ranging from 3 to 5 pounds depending on tolerance) is applied to the ankle. The patient should flex the hip to a degree that allows a pulling sensation to be felt along the lateral compartment of the thigh (Fig. 6.14). The weighted straight leg draws the fascia lata taut. In slender individuals we have seen dimpling along the fascia resulting from adhesions (Fig. 6.15). The dimpling or tenderness to palpation may be detected in the region of the trochanteric bursa, 2 inches below the trochanter, and then along the crevice between the anterior and posterior muscle compartments of the lateral thigh. These areas should be marked for later injection. Tenderness should be sought as high as the gluteus medius and as low as 2 to 3 inches below the fibular head.

In our experience, patients with fascia lata pain of 3 months' duration or longer will often have relief of symptoms with injection of a

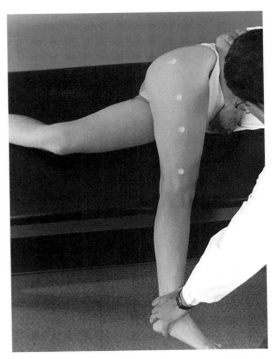

Figure 6.14. Method of examination for taut iliotibial tract or fascia lata fasciitis.

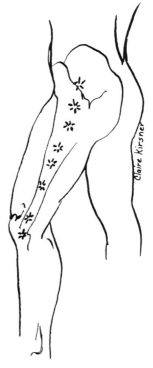

Figure 6.15. Sites of tenderness or adhesions along the fascia lata.

corticosteroid–local anesthetic mixture into the involved symptomatic sites in the fascia lata, with the fascia stretched by having the patient assume the position described for the examination (Fig. 6.14). To perform intralesional injections, prepare the area with soap and alcohol. Draw up to 80 mg methylprednisolone acetate sterile aqueous suspension (or other equivalent corticosteroid suspension) with an equal amount of lidocaine hydrochloride 1%. The mixture will flocculate within the syringe. Using the shortest needle that can reach the required depth, use the needle as a probe. When the lesion is reached, pain is usually perceived. Inject 20 mg corticosteroid or less per lesion, and no more than 80 mg in total. Have the patient apply ice for 10 to 20 minutes after the injection. Injection should not be repeated within 6 to 8 weeks. Refer to Fig. 6.15 for usual sites of injection.

Persistent thigh pain should lead to suspicion of an L4–L5 herniated disc with referred pain to the lateral hip area. Also, meralgia paresthetica (below) can cause similar distress.

The patient with fascia lata fasciitis should also begin a regimen of stretching the fascia lata in which the patient assumes the same position as that described for the examination; at home, the patient lies on the edge of a bed with a weight (ranging from 3 to 5 pounds, depending on tolerance) applied to the ankle. The patient should flex the hip to a degree that generates a pulling sensation along the lateral compartment of the thigh (Exercise 6.A). Instruction in the exercises described for Snapping Hip should also be provided (refer to Table 6.5 and indicated exercises). Manual techniques such as trigger/tender point pressure and myofascial release can relieve specific areas of pain and promote flexibility. Strengthening and stretching exercises to the gluteus medius and lateral thigh muscles will restore length and flexibility to tissues. However, exercise must be carefully progressed in intensity, duration, and number of repetitions in order to avoid overuse or strain. Posture assessment should address pelvic and lower limb positions in standing and walking, and gait assessment can identify a wide-based pattern that may lead to, or have been caused by, lateral thigh tissue shortening.

Bursitis in the Hip Area: Of the 18 or more bursae in the hip region, the most important are the trochanteric, iliopectineal, and ischiogluteal bursae. *Ischiogluteal bursitis* is discussed in Chapter 5 (see section "Ischial (Ischiogluteal) Bursitis").

Trochanteric Bursitis: The deep trochanteric bursa lies between the tendon of the gluteus maximus and the posterolateral prominence of the greater trochanter (31). A more superficial bursa directly over the greater trochanter may also become inflamed and tender.

Characteristic night pain of bursitis may be added to that which is secondary to osteoarthritis of the hip. Point tenderness over the trochanteric bursa with pain reproduction is strong evidence of the presence of bursitis. This point of tenderness usually lies approximately 1 inch posterior and superior to the greater trochanter, and is located about 3 inches deep to the skin. Obesity, compression injury, or other minor local trauma may be aggravating factors. The act of arising from a position of lumbar spine flexion (back bent forward) while the knees are kept straight requires a lever action of the glutei and is perhaps the most common cause for gluteal strain, which in turn may predispose to trochanteric bursitis. Such patients must learn to bend their knees before bending their backs. Treatment consists of injecting the trochanteric bursa with a local anesthetic–corticosteroid agent (Fig. 6.16), sleeping with a small pillow under the involved buttock to keep the body weight shifted off of the bursa, and stretching the gluteal muscles utilizing knee-to-chest exercises (Exercises 5.D and 5.E). Some patients describe relief by lying with the involved hip on a strategically placed tennis ball, so that the pressure of the ball relieves the pain.

The need for repeated injections of the hip should lead to consideration of other diagnoses, aggravating factors, or additional consultation. Repeated injections can result in osteonecrosis (32). Surgical excision of the bursa is rarely necessary (33).

Iliopectineal and Iliopsoas Bursitis: The iliopectineal bursa lies between the iliopsoas muscle and the iliopectineal eminence. Posteriorly it lies lateral to the femoral vessels and overlies the capsule of the hip. The iliopsoas bursa lies medially in Scarpa's triangle (the femoral tri-

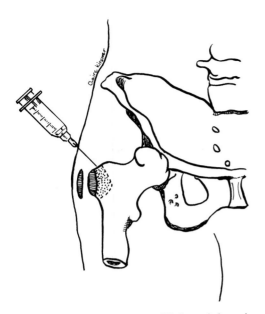

Figure 6.16. Superficial (adventitial) and deep trochanteric bursitis. After localizing the points of maximum tenderness by deep palpation, a 1½- to 4-inch needle is used as a probe; the points of maximum tenderness are determined, and aliquots of a corticosteroid–local anesthetic are injected into each site.

angle). Bursitis in the anterior hip region (rare in our experience) causes pain in the anterior pelvis, groin, and thigh region. The iliopectineal bursa often communicates with the hip joint, and bursitis may result from intrinsic joint disease. Diagnosis and progress can be demonstrated by MR imaging. Plain radiographic examination may be normal (33a). Careful aspiration and injection of the bursa with a corticosteroid–local anesthetic mixture probably is best performed by a rheumatologist or orthopaedist. Persistence of symptoms may indicate surgical intervention and excision of the bursa (34).

Hamstring Injuries: Overstretching during sport or exercise can injure the hamstring group of muscles at their origin or insertion. Onset of pain is often sudden, and may impair walking. Deep tenderness in the region of the ischium or proximal thigh posteriorly is suggestive.

Hamstring injuries are common in runners. The ''pulled hamstring'' injury is aggravated during the runner's long stride, during the concentric contraction of the muscle. Tenderness can be detected at the origin or insertion of the

muscle. Ice, heat, and temporary cessation or decrease of the offending physical exercise or reduction in a training program should be the first order of treatment, followed by graded stretching exercises. These measures should provide relief; however, recovery may require up to 6 weeks of treatment before full activity can be resumed. Recurrent hamstring injuries may be related to an underlying lumbar spine abnormality, including spondylolisthesis, stress lesion, or herniation of the nucleus pulposus (L4-L5) (35).

Rehabilitation of hamstring function begins with appropriate rest or cessation of the aggravating exercise, ice, and gentle movement. Once the acute pain and spasm have diminished, exercise can include more aggressive stretching and strengthening (36) (refer to Table 6.5 for exercises). Hamstring stretching exercises such the posterior leg stretches described in Exercises 6.H and 6.I can be effectively done in a home program, as can be the leg stretch/mobilize activity with a Theraband (Exercise 6.K). Hamstring strengthening exercises should be done with eccentric (shortening) and concentric (lengthening) contractions and at slow and fast speeds in order to prepare for functional needs.

The Semimembranosus Insertion Syndrome: Chronic persistent pain is noted at the medial aspect of the knee joint, increased by exercise, walking, descending stairs, and squatting. Palpation, performed with the leg extended, reveals tenderness of the tensed lowest part of the hamstring muscles; sharp pain is elicited by finger pressure over the attachment of the semimembranosus tendon to the posteromedial aspect of the medial tibial condyle, 1–2 cm below the medial joint line, and pain is accentuated by passive rotation of the knee bent 90 degrees in the prone position (37). Although the patients in one series had symptoms for an average duration of 2 years before treatment, 90% responded to injection into the insertion of the semimembranosus tendon at the bony tubercle attachment site. The author used 30 mg triamcinolone mixed with lidocaine hydrochloride (37). Immediately following the injection the pain should subside, allowing painless walking, bending, and descending stairs. Other measures include rest, stretching (Table 6.5, Exercises 6.H, 6.I, and 6.K), nonsteroidal antiinflammatory drugs (NSAIDs), and transcutaneous nerve stimulation. When conservative measures fail, scintigraphy is indicated. Findings of increased uptake at the posteromedial corner of the tibia are characteristic. Nevertheless, arthroscopy may be advisable in order to rule out other intrinsic knee derangements. Surgical treatment consists of tendon exploration, drilling of the insertion site, and tendon transfer (38).

Chronic Compartment Compression Syndromes in the Thigh: Compartment syndromes result from increased tissue pressure within a closed muscle compartment, compromising local circulation and neuromuscular function. They occur in association with limb trauma, drug and alcohol abuse, limb surgery, limb ischemia, and physical exertion. Clinical features include (*a*) tense compartment envelope, (*b*) severe pain in excess of that clinically expected for the specific condition, (*c*) pain on passive stretch of the muscles in the compartment, (*d*) muscle weakness within the compartment, and (*e*) altered sensation in the distribution of the nerves coursing through the compartment (39). Chronic compartment syndrome locations in the hip area can occur in the gluteal muscles or in the quadriceps femoris muscle. Direct measurement of the compartment pressure using a wick catheter is diagnostic. Nonsurgical treatment includes eliminating any external compression, maintaining local arterial pressures, and preserving peripheral nerve function. Surgery to decompress and debride nonviable tissue may be required and should not be delayed if pain is persistent.

The Knee Region

The knee joint performs a complex series of movements and suffers from degenerative processes that begin by age 15. Nevertheless, many athletes maintain good knee function into late age. Others who ignore pain and strength training may suffer debilitating persistent disability from sport activities and improperly attended injuries in their youth.

The Plica Syndrome: Folds, pleats, bands, or shelves of synovium are normally present in the knee joint; the term ''plica'' is used to describe these synovial remnants (40). The most common remnant is the medial suprapatel-

lar plica originating beneath the quadriceps tendon and extending to the medial wall of the joint. Also common is the infrapatellar plica, which is attached to the intercondylar notch and runs distally to the infrapatellar fat pad. Synovitis or hemorrhage involving a plica can accompany osteochondral fractures, anterior cruciate ligament tears, peripheral tears of the meniscus, or partial capsule tears. The original injury may resolve, but a thickened plica may persist. Also, plica thickening may occur in association with loose bodies, subluxating patellae, and systemic inflammatory processes (41). Knee joint synovitis, plica thickening, pain, and effusion often follow dashboard injuries or a blunt or twisting trauma in contact sports. Many cases arise from overuse. Additional features, similar to those of internal derangement, include a sensation of the joint giving way. Pain and tenderness occur over the medial joint line. As the flexed knee is extended, the plica can be palpated as it rolls over the medial femoral condyle, depending on the plica thickness. In some cases, a palpable patellar snap may occur during physical examination. When the plica is palpable, injection with a corticosteroid and local anesthetic may suffice. Rovere and Adair reported in a study of competitive athletes that 73% (22/31) had complete relief with injection of the plica and knee, using a local anesthetic combined with a long-acting corticosteroid (Aristocort). When a bupivacaine alone was used initially, only transient relief occurred (42).

Definitive diagnosis is based on demonstrating the plica(e) by arthroscopy or pneumoarthrography. Conservative treatment with hamstring/posterior leg stretching (Table 6.5, Exercises 6.H and 6.K), rest, ice or heat, and antiinflammatory agents is helpful in some patients (43); in others the plica can be released or excised during arthroscopy (41, 44, 45), but some patients require arthrotomy and partial synovectomy.

Pellegrini-Stieda Syndrome: Following knee strain, an occasional patient notes progressively worsening pain at the medial joint line, and knee joint flexion becomes restricted. Presumably a soft tissue injury in the region of the medial tibial collateral ligament is followed by calcification in this area with permanent obstruction to knee joint motion. Similar medial joint calcification has been reported in the ankle and elbow joint regions. If present, synovitis is usually transient. Palpable indurated swelling in the soft tissues about the medial femoral condyle, restriction of knee joint flexion, and evidence of calcification on roentgenographic films of the knee joint are noted. Adult males are most commonly affected. The calcification appears 3 to 4 weeks following injury, and has the appearance of a narrow, elongated, amorphous shadow adjacent to the medial aspect of the femoral condyle (Fig. 6.17). Similar calcification may be seen in asymptomatic patients as well. Pain gradually disappears over a period of months or years. Surgical excision of the calcification may be considered if symptoms persist.

Iliotibial Band Friction Syndrome: The iliotibial tract or band is a thickened part of the fascia lata that inserts over the lateral tibial

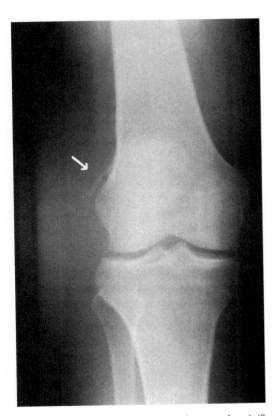

Figure 6.17. Pellegrini-Stieda syndrome of calcification in the region of the medial or lateral collateral ligament. This narrow elongated amorphous shadow adjacent to the femoral condyle may occur in patients with or without symptoms. (Courtesy of Toledo Hospital.)

condyle. Patients with this syndrome present with pain in the region of the lateral knee joint following vigorous running or hiking. Use of worn-out shoes or shoes with insufficient cushioning can predispose long-distance runners to iliotibial band syndrome (46). These patients develop a painful limp and experience point tenderness over the lateral femoral condyle. Friction is thought to provoke the inflammation. Pain is accentuated by having the patient support all of his weight on the affected leg with the knee bent 30 to 40 degrees. Furthermore, a palpable ''creak'' during flexion and extension of the knee is noted, having the consistency of rubbing over a wet balloon (47). Synovial effusion or excessive lateral joint motion does not occur. NSAIDs and joint rest are helpful. Local corticosteroid injection into the point of insertion may be attempted, if necessary. In a series of 100 long-distance runners with this affliction, rest and reduction of the training program and a single steroid injection resulted in relief in 30 patients; 21 patients required two injections, and eight required three injections. Five patients required surgery. Others required total rest from running for 4 to 6 weeks (48). Surgical treatment consists of a limited resection of a small triangular piece at the posterior part of the iliotibial tract covering the lateral femoral condyle (49).

Knee problems in runners are often secondary to abnormal foot-to-ground contact, flatfeet, or high arches. Stretching exercises for the plantar fascia (Exercise 6.J), flexibility exercises to mobilize the toes (Exercises 6.M and 6.N), proper shoes, and if necessary, an orthotic insert consisting of leather with a molded plastic insert are usually beneficial.

Quadriceps Muscle and Tendon Disruption: In young athletes the extensor quadriceps mechanism consists of strong tendons, so that rupture generally involves the muscle mass. In older persons rupture usually occurs at the tendinous portion. The injury generally occurs during forced knee joint flexion with a contracted quadriceps femoris muscle. Swelling occurs above the patella, and the patient notes various degrees of loss of extension activity of the knee joint. With complete rupture, at any age, immediate surgical repair is recommended. Occasionally a partial muscle rupture occurs with less severe trauma. In such patients, acute pain, swelling, and hemorrhage occur, but knee extension is possible. These patients are treated by immobilization in extension, followed by gentle manual techniques and carefully progressed exercise. It is critical to mobilize the connective tissues with myofascial techniques. Exercise should begin with isometric quadriceps contractions (quad sets), progressing to short-arc quadriceps strengthening (Exercise 6.G), then to more aggressive strengthening with resistive quadriceps activities (Exercises 6.E and 6.F). Hip flexor and iliotibial tract stretching should be included in the program to address any shortening of the quadriceps mechanism (Exercises 6.D and 6.A). These techniques can all be done in the home setting after appropriate instruction has been provided. Persons who require higher performance from the quadriceps mechanism for exercise or daily activities can utilize the more technologically advanced exercise equipment such as isokinetic machines. Aquatic exercise programs can be designed specifically for rehabilitation of quadriceps function.

Disuse Atrophy: This is one of the most common disorders leading to knee joint instability. It occurs secondary to other knee joint disturbances, including rheumatoid arthritis and osteoarthritis, and it is associated with reflex inhibition of the quadriceps mechanism. Often disuse quadriceps femoris muscle atrophy is associated with the chronic use of the hands to assist in the act of rising from the seated position. Middle-aged and elderly persons should be advised to use their thighs, not their hands, when rising from a chair. Hands should be placed forward on the thighs for assistance. This prophylactic advice may prevent a significant number of chronic painful joint disabilities. Raising the chair up on a 2.5-inch wooden platform, raising the cushion in the chair with a folded blanket, or using a high-backed executive desk chair that can be height-adjusted may be necessary for elderly persons with complex or chronic degenerative illness who cannot strengthen weak legs. Often a trivial self-limited knee joint disturbance becomes a major disability because of disuse quadriceps atrophy or myofascial pain. By providing higher seating for taller individuals, less hip and leg effort will be needed in arising from the chair.

Myofascial Knee Pain: Myofascial knee pain may occur after prolonged sitting. Pain may occur throughout the anterior knee region, is worse when first arising from sitting, and then disappears during walking. Activities such as prolonged driving, playing bingo or cards, or recovery from illness may result in shortening of the hip flexors and the vastus intermedius muscle. Examination reveals a tender (trigger) point (Fig. 6.18) when performing the Ober test, in which the hip is extended and the knee flexed (Fig. 6.5). Hip flexor and iliotibial tract stretching are helpful in patients with a taut vastus intermedius (myofascial knee pain) (Table 6.5, Exercises 6.D and 6.A).

Resistive or isometric quadriceps exercise may be performed by patients at any age in the comfort of their home, and does not require frequent physical therapy supervision once the exercise program is established (Exercises 6.E, 6.F, and 6.G).

Acute Calcific Quadriceps Tendinitis: Pain in the region of the suprapatellar pouch may

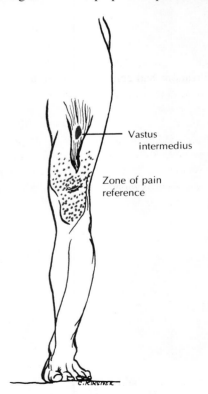

Vastus intermedius

Zone of pain reference

Figure 6.18. A myofascial trigger point in the region of the insertion of the vastus intermedius muscle may cause pain in the anterior lower leg and knee region.

be associated with calcification in the region of the quadriceps tendon, particularly at the superior pole of the patella. These radiographic findings (anterosuperior patellar whiskers) may also be seen in asymptomatic patients; when associated with chronic knee pain, however, such patients frequently have evidence of degenerative joint disease (50). Accordingly, the calcification may be an asymptomatic coincidental finding. The possibility that calcific quadriceps tendinitis is related to calcific tendinitis in other joint areas as a general metabolic disturbance has been suggested (50).

Calcific Tendinitis of the Vastus Lateralis Muscle: This may present with a painful, indurated mass in the posterior thigh region. Findings on conventional roentgenography or computed tomography are diagnostic (51). Although surgical excision is the usual treatment, Steidl and Ditmar have described treatment with oral magnesium lactate (3 g/day first month, 1.5 g/day thereafter) and injection of the lesion with MgSO$_4$ (10–20 mL of 10% MgSO$_4$) daily for 1 week, then every other day for the second week, then 2–3 times per week under local anesthesia. Seventy-five percent of 80 patients treated for spontaneous or traumatic soft tissue calcifications had complete improvement (52).

Prepatellar Calcification: Prepatellar swelling and pain in association with repeated kneeling (as in prayer) can give rise to acute inflammation and calcification of the prepatellar soft tissues. In a study reporting this disorder, synovial fluid was found not to reveal crystals. Hydroxyapatite deposition disease was suspected as the cause (53).

PATELLOFEMORAL DERANGEMENTS

Patellar region pain results from a number of complex problems, most of which respond well to nonsurgical treatment. The disorders described here often are symptomatic only because of injury or misuse, and although mild structural disturbances may coexist, symptoms often respond to treatment with restoration of stability to the limb. (Refer to Table 6.3, on causes for knee pain.)

Etiology. These patellofemoral disturbances are often associated with conditions that result in a change in the angle of pull of the patellar ligament. Such disturbances include internal femoral torsion with a lateral deviation of the quadriceps femoris muscle, other malrotations of the tibia or femur, alteration or imbalances of the quadriceps femoris muscle, abnormal position or tightness of the iliotibial tract, idiopathic tightness of the vastus lateralis muscle due to rapid distal femoral growth, or malformation in the posterior surface of the patella or femoral condyles. Also, patellofemoral compression syndrome with tightness of the lateral capsule and patellofemoral ligament can coexist (53–55).

Symptoms may also result from chronic trauma, such as repeated scrubbing of floors on hands and knees or devout kneeling in prayer. Joint laxity and the hypermobility syndrome have been noted as predisposing disorders. Quadriceps flaccidity and relative elongation of the patellar ligament may allow a high-riding patella (patella alta). Degenerative pathologic findings of cartilage softening and fissuring are frequently noted, though there is often a lack of correlation between pathologic findings and symptoms.

Painful knee injury or strain with resulting quadriceps femoris muscle inhibition may lead to loss of quadriceps power, endurance, and mass, and to quadriceps excursion. Patella baja, a low-lying patella, with a visible sag in the extensor mechanism, may result. Knee instability and giving way occurs (55).

The Patellofemoral Pain Syndrome: This syndrome is characterized by pain and crepitation in the region of the patella during activities that require knee flexion under load conditions, such as stair climbing. Joint swelling may be seen; symptoms are often intermittent (56). Primary idiopathic adolescent chondromalacia, posttraumatic adolescent chondromalacia, "patellofemoral syndrome of adolescents and young adults," and "adult chondromalacia with secondary degenerative joint disease" are various terms for a group of disorders with similar symptoms.

Underlying etiologic disturbances include malalignment of the quadriceps with lateral patellar subluxation, an abnormal medial patellar facet (57), patella alta, and the hypermobility syndrome. Ectopic patella and/or compressive arthropathy in any plane may occur in the adolescent; pain is greatly aggravated by athletic activity and prolonged deep flexion of the knee.

Findings of joint mobility, Q angle measurement, genu valgum, and anteversion were not found to be different in a study of athletes with and without anterior knee pain (58). In another study, signs of patellofemoral subluxation were reported in 500 patients. The more common findings included dysplastic vastus medialis muscle (91%); a high patella (68%); tight patellofemoral ligaments (68%); Fairbank's sign (66%), or hypertrophied vastus lateralis muscle and tenderness (59).

Imaging studies also reveal no correlation of the severity of patellar subluxation to outcome or indications for surgery (60, 61). Chondromalacia of the patella is a prominent associated finding in patellofemoral pain. The exact relationship of patellofemoral crepitation to the presence of pain is debatable (50, 56, 62, 63). The cost of MRI and arthroscopy is a major deterrent to their use; arthroscopy has the added risks of an invasive procedure and anesthesia. MRI at present is not very sensitive to the early articular cartilage lesions. Significant cartilage lesions observed by arthroscopy were often missed on MRI.

Bergenudd et al. (64) found psychosocial factors important in middle-aged persons when the patient had limited education, a boring or physically demanding job, and had previous meniscectomy surgery.

The "cinema sign" refers to patellofemoral pain following prolonged sitting with knees in flexion, relieved by subsequent knee extension. Similarly, patellofemoral pain may follow prolonged sitting when traveling.

Physical findings suggestive of the patellofemoral pain syndrome include the reproduction of pain when the examiner presses the patella against the femur during knee motion, or the detection of tenderness over the medial articulating surface of the patella. Patellofemoral crepitation during knee flexion and extension is usually palpable (57). The Perkin's test (described above) will usually be helpful.

The young adult or teenager with patellofemoral pain should be examined for lateral patellar displacement (dislocation or subluxation) during knee flexion and extension.

Lateral Patellar Subluxation can be detected by having the patient seated and the examiner's index finger and thumb positioned on the lateral and medial upper borders of the patient's patella. The examiner observes and palpates for lateral patellar displacement as the flexed knee is extended; this finding is commonly seen in patients with hypermobility syndrome. Fairbank's apprehension sign (described above) is another helpful maneuver.

"Grasshopper eye patellae" refers to the condition in which the patellae point outward from the midline, suggesting the appearance of grasshopper's eyes when viewed from the front. This condition is correlated with malrotation of the limbs, lateral patellar subluxation, and chondromalacia.

Hoffa's Disease: This eponym refers to hypertrophy of the infrapatellar fat pad in young persons after mild injury or in association with patellar subluxation (59). The infrapatellar fat pad may then become impinged between the femur and tibia when the flexed knee is suddenly extended. Pain is localized and occurs during weightbearing knee activity. Symptoms simulate internal knee derangements, but locking does not occur. Physical examination reveals swelling on either side of the infrapatellar ligament and sometimes quadriceps atrophy; the general appearance may be that of a double hump, the camelback sign of Hughston. Hypertrophy of the infrapatellar fat pad may be recurrent as a premenstrual syndrome.

Infrapatellar Tendinitis: This disorder is common in persons with lateral patellar displacement or malrotations of the tibia or fibula (2). Infrapatellar pain or crepitation may result from jumping in athletic endeavors ("Jumper's knee"). Other sports that can result in patellar tendinitis include volleyball, soccer, and bicycling. Most patients respond to conservative measures (65) (see "Management" section, below). Infrapatellar bursitis causes similar discomfort in the infrapatellar region.

Anterior leg pain and a sensation of swelling lateral and inferior to the tibial tubercle can result from a contracted or tight hamstring muscle. In any case, the pain is not articular. The anterior leg pain is reproduced during the straight-leg-raising test as the leg is forced straight upward. Pain is relieved by exercises that stretch the hamstring muscles (Exercise 6.K).

Rupture of the infrapatellar tendon may occur singly or symmetrically from trauma or sport activity. Swelling, a proximally displaced patellar dislocation, and a palpable defect at the inferior pole of the patella will be notable (66). Surgical repair should be followed with graded exercises. (Refer also to the section "Laboratory, Radiographic Findings, and other Imaging Technologies" below.)

Arthroscopy for more definitive diagnosis is indicated if conservative measures fail to provide symptomatic relief in 3 to 6 months (63). Thermography was found to suggest quadriceps femoris muscle imbalance in one study of 30 athletes with patellofemoral pain; all responded to physical therapy and exercise (67).

MANAGEMENT OF PATELLOFEMORAL DERANGEMENTS

Conservative measures that are helpful for patellofemoral derangements include:

- Aspirin or other NSAIDs for pain.
- Restriction of competitive activities or overuse, weight reduction for obese patients, and an exercise regimen to lengthen (stretch) and balance the hip and thigh muscles.
- Exercises should include isometric quadriceps strengthening and short-arc quadriceps strengthening in which the lower leg moves through the last 30 degrees of extension against the maximum weight that can be moved without pain at least 10 times. Exercises must be performed without pain in the patellar area. (Refer to Table 6.5 and Exercises 6.D through 6.G, whichever is best tolerated.)
- Bracing, ranging from an elastic support and a lateral felt pad, a popular and widely available elastic splint with a patellar cutout that positions the patella, to a customized dynamic patellar brace, are often helpful and may enhance the results of exercise (67a).
- Self-mobilization of the tissues surrounding the patella in which the patient grasps the patella between the thumb and index finger and moves it side to side and up and down, applying gentle stretching in the direction away from tightness. The

patient should be instructed to do this several times daily.

- Improper or worn shoes can contribute to patellar pain. Check the patient's athletic shoes and suggest changes as necessary. A shoe that controls heel position can affect knee pain. Simple orthotic devices can also relieve discomfort. (Refer also to the section "Outcome and Additional Suggestions for Patellofemoral Pain Syndrome" below.)

Disturbances of the infrapatellar fat pad, infrapatellar ligament, and the infrapatellar bursa usually respond to rest followed by graded resistance quadriceps femoris muscle exercise; relief usually requires many weeks of exercise done at home on a regular basis. Injecting the infrapatellar fat pad with a local anesthetic–corticosteroid mixture is helpful if swelling has persisted after 4 to 6 weeks of joint protection. The injection is administered from a lateral approach after careful skin preparation; the needle should rest well away from the tendon (Fig. 6.19). With a 1-inch No. 23 needle, a mixture of 1 mL 1% procaine or lidocaine hydrochloride and 20 mg triamcinolone may be injected in two aliquots into the medial and lateral borders of the fat pad. *The tendon must not be penetrated, as this may*

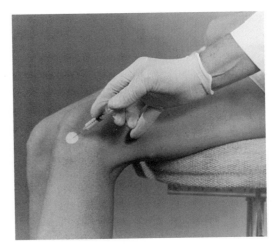

Figure 6.19. Injection for Hoffa's disease if the fat pad has become significantly large and disturbing to gait. The needle should be directed into the fat pad well away from the infrapatellar tendon. Furthermore, patients receiving such an injection must be warned to limit stressful activities or stair climbing for several weeks in order to avoid tendon disruption.

promote future tendon rupture. These patients rarely require more than one injection. *Athletes or persons who must kneel repeatedly should not be given a local corticosteroid injection* (68). In all cases, patients should be advised to avoid knee overuse for 10 to 14 days due to possible tendon weakening secondary to the steroid effect.

Management of patellofemoral pain syndrome also requires recognition and prevention of aggravating factors, such as improper kneeling, working on the hands and knees excessively, and prolonged sitting. Exercise equipment may aggravate the symptoms and require modification. For example, bicycle seat height may be adjusted to change the downstroke knee angle if cycling is painful. Step machines, stair climbing, and trampoline use may have to be replaced with less severe patella-loading exercise. Aquatic programs can be designed to accomplish the same goals while relieving mechanical stress. (Refer to Table 6.2 and Chapter 8.)

OUTCOME AND ADDITIONAL SUGGESTIONS FOR PATELLOFEMORAL PAIN SYNDROME

Whitelaw et al. report that 68% had good results with conservative therapy at 16 months' follow-up in 85 patients (69). In another series of 100 patients graded according to arthroscopic findings and followed for 2 years, conservative measures and isometric exercises resulted in complete recovery in 100% of those with no demonstrable intraarticular abnormality and in 75% of those with only patellar cartilage fibrillation. However, in the small group with fibrillation of both the patella and the femur, conservative measures often failed and surgical care was required (70).

Adolescents with patellofemoral pain syndrome (chondromalacia patellae) frequently have spontaneous improvement without residual disturbance (3, 56, 57). As mentioned earlier, the key to managing patellar disturbances is to maintain a strong quadriceps mechanism with normal alignment. Special braces are available and include the patellar stabilization brace for lateral patellar dislocation and bracing for patellar tendinitis, knee hyperextension, rotation abnormalities, and joint laxity (59, 71). Orthopaedic consultation would be wise when considering special braces for young athletes.

In patients whose symptoms are resistant to conservative programs, surgical intervention may be indicated. Arthroscopic surgery may have to be directed toward the underlying basic abnormality. Procedures include proximal realignment with fascial transfer, tendon slings, quadricepsplasty, lateral release, distal realignment, and combinations. Chondral defects may require patellar shaving, drilling, and rarely, patellectomy (21, 72). In experienced hands, up to 75% of patients for whom exercise and bracing therapy have been ineffective can achieve stable joints after arthroscopic surgery (73–75). Open surgical procedures may be required. Other corrections may have to be directed toward more general problems, such as joint laxity, genu valgum, or tibial torsion.

OTHER KNEE DERANGEMENTS

In addition to patellofemoral disorders and plicae, other derangements, including meniscus tears, loose bodies (joint mice), synovial lesions, extrasynovial lesions, and ligament disruption following trauma, are common causes for weightbearing symptoms. Locking, buckling, or a sense of the limb's giving way occur. Often, when trying to get out of a car, the patient cannot straighten the leg until after some jiggling and shaking of the limb. Physical examination maneuvers to assess ligament and menisci stability were discussed at the beginning of this chapter.

LABORATORY, RADIOGRAPHIC FINDINGS, AND OTHER IMAGING TECHNOLOGIES

Inflammatory connective tissue disease is rarely associated with these patellar and internal derangements. Therefore, tests of inflammation tend to produce normal results. Radiographic examination should include the tangential patellofemoral roentgenographic techniques (skyline, Hughston views) that best demonstrate the patellar facets and lateral patellar deviation. Radiographic findings unfortunately may add little to the diagnosis. In a study in which 71 patients operated upon for patellofemoral disturbances were compared with 97 others operated upon for meniscectomy, radiographic findings were found to be poorly correlated with operative findings (76). Nevertheless, in the older patient, osteoarthritis, osteonecrosis, fracture, tumor, or rheumatoid arthritis may be seen and defined. Athletes may develop osteochondritis of the patella or femur.

Patella alta can be measured on the lateral roentgenogram; the lengths of the patella and patellar tendon should be equal. If the tendon length exceeds the patella length by 10%, patella alta can be diagnosed (77). Others believe that patella alta is a rare finding and not relevant in the young athlete (78).

Bone scan for stress fractures, osteonecrosis, or reflex sympathetic dystrophy is sometimes indicated, depending upon clinical presentation. Magnetic resonance imaging is the most definitive test. However, the findings must be correlated with clinical features. Imaging is operator dependent and the clinician must have confidence in the report. Ultrasound imaging of the patellar tendon may be helpful only if performed by an experienced operator. It is the least expensive of the imaging technologies (79).

Imaging technologies have many pitfalls when used to examine the knee. Many normal subjects are found to have significantly abnormal imaging findings of the knee; and when arthroscopic findings are compared with MRI findings, the MRI accuracy is found to be highly operator-dependent (80). Pitfalls to MRI for evaluation of the knee include insensitivity of MRI for patellofemoral disturbances and the presence of loose bodies. A high rate of false-negative MRI findings in the knee is also problematic (81). In a study of 64 *asymptomatic* subjects, Kornich et al. report increasing occurrence of meniscal abnormalities with aging. Thus grade 1 and grade 2 changes were seen in all decades; grade 3 (tears) were common in subjects over 50 years of age; and 55% of persons in their 70s had grade 3 lesions (82). Presence of a bursa of the popliteus tendon can simulate a tear of the posterior horn of the lateral meniscus, and the course of the transverse geniculate ligament can simulate a tear of the anterior horn of the lateral meniscus (83). MRI is more useful for popliteal region disorders (84, 85).

MANAGEMENT OF INTERNAL KNEE DERANGEMENTS

Often a therapeutic trial of conservative care—assuming that a careful physical examination has excluded critical features (Table 6.1)—will result in benefit and obviate the need for elaborate studies.

Functional knee braces should reduce or eliminate functional instability following ligamentous injury. Braces should be comfortable and should not predispose to repeat injury (86). Prescription for bracing of the athlete should be undertaken only by those with expertise in the field of sports medicine. If symptoms persist, then further assessment with referral to an orthopaedist skilled in arthroscopic examination and treatment is justified.

ARTHROSCOPIC TREATMENT OF KNEE DERANGEMENTS

Arthroscopic examination and treatment have made remarkable progress over the years. Compared to MRI findings, arthroscopy is more reliable for cartilage lesions (87–89). Today, arthroscopic diagnosis and treatment is preferable to open surgical exploration and treatment; however, the operator must have experience and good judgment (90–93). Complications include damage to the articular cartilage, hemarthrosis, infection, herniation of a fat pad, thrombophlebitis, granuloma formation, instrument breakage, neurovascular injury, and development of a fistula (94, 95). Arthroscopic diagnosis and management of disorders of menisci are now widely accepted and allow remarkably prompt recovery. *Partial tears of the cruciate ligaments* may result in locking. These can also be diagnosed and graded by arthroscopy (96).

BURSITIS ABOUT THE KNEE

At least 12 bursae regularly occur in the knee region: the suprapatellar, prepatellar, infrapatellar, and an adventitious cutaneous bursa lie in the anterior knee region; the gastrocnemius and semimembranosus bursae are located in the posterior region and often give rise to a popliteal (Baker's) cyst; the sartorius and anserine bursae lie medially; three bursae lie adjacent to the fibular collateral ligament (97) and the popliteus tendon in the lateral region of the knee (98–100) (Fig. 6.1). Not to be forgotten is the ''no name–no fame'' bursa of Stuttle (101), located at the front edge of the anterior fibers of the medial (tibial) collateral ligament.

Bursitis is characterized by pain at specific sites, aggravated by motion, and at times worse at night. Point tenderness is present over the involved bursa; active motion may or may not be limited. Inspection may immediately reveal a swollen prepatellar bursa. Prepatellar bursitis may be a chronic condition secondary to certain occupations, such as coal mining, farming, carpet laying, scrubbing floors on the hands and knees; or it may be secondary to similar activities performed by overconscientious housekeepers (100). The "no name–no fame" bursa may be palpable during knee flexion when the examiner feels a small, tender, rounded nodule jumping onto the leading edge of the medial collateral ligament (101). Another bursa, the adventitious cutaneous bursa, may be palpable as a swelling over the tibial tuberosity. Popliteal bursitis is discussed under the commonly used term "Baker's cyst" below.

Anserine Bursitis: Anserine bursitis should be suspected when pain occurs in the medial knee region. It is often bilateral, and it may accompany panniculitis in obese postmenopausal females (99). Osteoarthritis is often present and may predispose to bursitis. Pain originating in the medial collateral ligament may also coexist. Pain of both anserine bursitis and medial collateral ligament disease is worse with activity. Pain at night is more characteristic of anserine bursitis. Occasionally, the anserine bursa is distended with fluid and presents as a firm cystic mass on the anteromedial aspect of the knee region, 4 to 5 cm below the medial joint line. Ultrasonography can demonstrate the cystic nature of the mass (102).

Bursitis about the knee often occurs in females. Pes planus may be a predisposing cause for bursitis in the medial knee region (101). The suprapatellar bursa and the posterior bursae often communicate with the knee joint. Swelling of these "pouches" often reflects synovial swelling due to inflammatory arthritis or internal derangement of the true knee joint; the most common cause is rheumatoid arthritis. None of the bursae in the medial or lateral knee regions communicates with the synovial cavity, and therefore inflammatory joint disease rarely is related to inflammation of these bursae (99).

Panniculitis: Women with large fat panniculi overlying the medial knee joint may present with pain that is worse at night; this nocturnal pain should alert the physician to the presence of panniculitis or an anserine bursitis deep to the panniculus. Whether pressure from the panniculus is significant in the cause of anserine bursitis is unknown. (Refer to the section "Management" below.)

Prepatellar bursitis, though usually secondary to pressure phenomena, may also result from infection. Aspiration of prepatellar bursa fluid for a white blood cell count and differential, Gram stain, sugar, culture and sensitivity determination, and crystal identification are diagnostically indicated. In acute knee bursitis of local origin, tests for systemic inflammation produce normal results.

Radiographic examination is seldom abnormal but may reveal osteoarthritis consistent with age. Calcific tendinitis and bursal calcification may rarely be seen. Chondrocalcinosis with pseudogout syndrome may occur in elderly patients with bursitis, but the findings are likely coincidental. Ultrasonography can be helpful in unusual cases. Contrast arthrography (pneumoarthrography) for the diagnosis of some types of knee pain may be required, but the procedure is probably best considered only after orthopaedic consultation when diagnosis is difficult. The choice between arthroscopy and arthrography depends upon the experience of the available personnel. Both are operator dependent procedures. Subtle disorders of the popliteus bursa evident on arthrography may be observed and can suggest tears of the lateral meniscus, discoid menisci, adhesive capsulitis, and anatomic variants (103). Arthroscopy is not without risk, as has been mentioned. Use of MRI is noninvasive but is operator dependent; sensitivity and specificity and correlation to clinical features are problematic in the knee region.

Differential Diagnosis: Diagnosing acute bursitis is seldom a problem. Swelling in the region of the bursa may also result from tumors of the bursae, including osteochondromatosis, villonodular synovitis, xanthomatosis, and synovioma.

A patient with osteonecrosis of the femur may present with medial compartment knee pain that is constant (day and night). Radiographic features may be normal. Radionuclide imaging with strontium-85 or technetium-99 reveals a localized increased area of uptake in the involved femoral condyle (104).

Management: Nonseptic bursitis about the knee responds readily to reduction in local pressure and local corticosteroid–anesthetic injection (99) (Fig. 6.20). The injection is administered after careful skin preparation. With the needle used as a probe, points of maximum tenderness should be injected. A 2-inch No. 22 or No. 23 needle is usually sufficient. A mixture of 1 mL 1% procaine or lidocaine hydrochloride and 20–40 mg methylprednisolone is injected. These patients rarely require more than one injection. If the prepatellar bursa is distended with fluid, use a No. 16 needle to aspirate the fluid before injecting the bursa.

Patients with bursitis in the medial aspect of the knee should sleep with a small cushion placed between the thighs so that the opposite knee does not rest upon the medial aspect of the involved knee. Use of kneeling pads is important for miners, carpet layers, and others whose daily activities expose them to prepatellar bursitis.

Bursitis about the head of the fibula presents with pain over the head of the fibula on movement. A twisting injury is thought to cause compression of the bursa. Treatment consists of injecting the deep subcutaneous tender area just inferior to the head of the fibula as described above. A spiral knee support to stabilize rotation of the fibula is helpful as well.

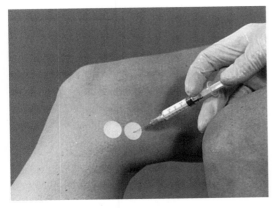

Figure 6.20. Injection of the medial collateral ligament or the anserine bursa. Tenderness in the medial region of the knee may result from one or both structures.

Septic bursitis requires the use of parenteral antibiotics and immobilization. Aspiration and open drainage may be required. Ho and Su report the advantage of using antibiotic therapy for 5 days after documented sterile cultures. Although they report oral antibiotic use for some cases of olecranon bursitis, patients of patellar bursitis in their series were treated with intravenous antibiotics, with cure in all cases (105). Recurrence of infection should lead to consideration of total bursal excision during the quiescent phase of the disease. An arthroscopic technique for bursectomy has been described (106).

Outcome and Additional Suggestions: Chronic bursitis about the knee is rarely encountered; it is limited mostly to the prepatellar bursa (100). Gout, rheumatoid arthritis, and villonodular synovitis are differential diagnostic entities that should be considered in patients with persistent bursitis. As noted, surgical excision may be indicated in chronic bursitis (100).

POPLITEAL CYST (BAKER'S CYST)

Swelling in the posterior aspect of the knee (in the popliteal fossa) may occur in children and adults. In children, the cyst is usually congenital and usually disappears spontaneously after a prolonged period of observation; surgery is rarely indicated (107, 108). In adults, a Baker's cyst is usually secondary to underlying disease of the knee joint, such as internal derangement, osteoarthritis, or rheumatoid arthritis. The patient frequently presents with aching discomfort in the popliteal region, leg, and calf. The discomfort is aggravated by walking, and often relieved by rest. Frequently the patient reports the presence of an egg-shaped mass behind the knee (Fig. 6.21).

When a Baker's cyst is suspected but not certain after physical examination, have the patient hold the leg extended as in Exercise 6.K; this results in a more readily palpable cyst. Needle aspiration of the Baker's cyst reveals fluid ranging from jelly-like consistency or cholesterol-laden fluid to acute inflammatory fluid, depending on the presence of underlying inflammatory disease in the knee joint. A large-bore (No. 15) needle may be required for aspiration.

Rupture of a Baker cyst occasionally occurs acutely before the physician has been consulted.

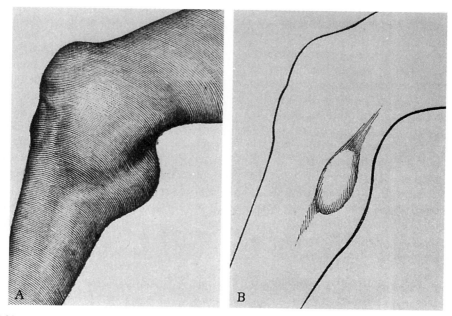

Figure 6.21. Popliteal (Baker's cyst) bursitis. (Reprinted from the original report by W. M. Baker. Saint Bartholomew's Hospital Reports, London, 1877.)

This may occur with any activity but is especially common during repetitive squatting movements, such as those performed while taking inventory or restocking in a store. Patients with a ruptured Baker's cyst present with features suggestive of thrombophlebitis. They may have minimal or no synovitis in the knee, the cyst is often no longer palpable, and swelling, heat, and diffuse tenderness of the calf and posterior foreleg are evident.

Patients sometimes demonstrate evidence of both popliteal cyst formation, with or without rupture, and thrombophlebitis. This combined process results when prolonged pressure from the cyst has led to venous stasis.

A Homan's sign (pain on passive dorsiflexion of the foot), suggestive of phlebitis, may be positive. At this point it is apparent that the diagnosis may be uncertain, and the differential between a ruptured popliteal cyst and acute phlebitis is an important consideration. In those patients in whom the diagnosis is unclear, studies should be performed to exclude phlebitis. Ultrasound examination or MRI may be warranted if diagnosis is unclear (109). Contrast pneumoarthrography reveals evidence of rupture with extravasation of dye into the calf. In comparing ultrasonography with arthrography, Gompels and Darlington found that the

ultrasound technique missed three cysts and gave three false-positive results in their 48 cases (109). The noninvasive nature of the procedure is a distinct advantage, but we would prefer arthrography when a ruptured cyst is suspected.

Magnetic resonance imaging may be the most sensitive diagnostic test (85). A single section through the calf may discriminate between pseudophlebitis and phlebitis (110). Unfortunately, when treatment method was compared with the investigations that had been carried out, Soriano and Catoggio noted that test results were often ignored and the patients were treated for phlebitis with anticoagulation despite a negative venogram (111). Nevertheless, they propose early use of arthrography and a venogram.

Although these procedures are diagnostically confirmatory, they are not always essential if clinical findings are characteristic. In our experience, when the Baker's cyst is due to inflammatory joint disease, local treatment as described below is almost always without risk. In that situation, then, studies are probably not necessary unless swelling and tenderness do not rapidly improve. Certainly, within a week, signs and symptoms should be resolved.

In patients in whom the diagnosis of a ruptured cyst has been made, management consists of treatment with bed rest, heat, and elevation. Introduction of local steroids into the joint that has an effusion may be helpful. NSAIDs may also be of assistance. After symptoms have begun to show significant improvement, ambulation can slowly be increased.

Management of an uncomplicated Baker's cyst includes aspiration of the contents of the cyst (and of the knee if synovitis is present), and instillation of a corticosteroid-anesthetic mixture (40 mg methylprednisolone or equivalent mixed with 1 mL 1% lidocaine hydrochloride) into the cyst and joint cavity. A mild pressure bandage applied to the posterior popliteal region is helpful, as are isometric quadriceps and gentle lengthening exercises for the hamstring and calf muscles (Table 6.5). Weightbearing should be minimized for several days or weeks.

The need for surgical excision of the cyst depends on recurrences and the presence of primary disease within the knee joint. Cyst excision without therapy directed to the primary knee disease is usually associated with cyst recurrence. This results from fluid transmission through the one-way valve in the communication between the knee and cyst. The fluid accumulates in the bursa and cannot flow back into the knee. The bursa gradually descends into the calf and may rupture and produce further local inflammation. Proper care of the underlying knee joint arthritis or internal derangement is essential.

POPLITEAL REGION TENDINITIS

Tenosynovitis of the popliteal tendon or hamstring may cause pain in the posterior or posterolateral aspects of the knee. Tenderness to palpation with the knee bent 90 degrees may be found, and straight leg raising reveals marked tightness in the involved muscles (112). If conservative management fails or pain limits exercising, then corticosteroid-anesthetic injections into points of tenderness within the muscle often provide prompt relief. Injection of the tendons behind the knee should be avoided unless performed by someone with experience, as this area is hazardous for soft tissue injection. Hamstring and posterior leg

stretching exercises (Exercises 6.H through 6.K, whichever is best tolerated) performed twice daily are helpful (37). Whenever a steroid injection has been performed near a tendon, the patient should be cautioned against overuse because of the risk of rupture.

Tendon Disruptions: Patients may suffer from a partial rupture of one of the calf muscles. Symptoms commonly are due to a tear of the plantaris muscle or the medial head of the gastrocnemius, but may also result from a partial rupture of any of the other muscles of the popliteal and calf region. The term "tennis leg" has been given to this symptom complex.

The patient often perceives a "snap" followed by a sudden burning in the calf; the leg gives way and the patient finds himself on the ground. Examination reveals pain aggravated by passive dorsiflexion of the ankle. Treatment of the partial tear is protective, with the use of adhesive strapping to immobilize the ankle in plantarflexion and to limit weightbearing; the use of heat, massage, and gentle exercises (initially) are helpful. Exercises should progress to include more active strengthening and lengthening. Limited activity for 3 to 4 weeks is usually required.

Spontaneous *rupture of the posterior tibialis tendon* results in pain, tenderness, and swelling behind and below the medial malleolus with loss of foot stability. Often a tenosynovitis characterized by slight swelling behind and beneath the medial malleolus has been present for some time. Lower leg pain after walking is noted.

Running Injuries

Long-distance runners may have complaints that result from the accumulated impact loading of long-distance running (113–115). Often these problems are related to biomechanical overuse in patients with minor structural disorders. Malalignments with mechanical disadvantages, muscle contractures, and use of untrained muscles may lead to biomechanical failure (114). Physical examination of the runner should include examination of the alignment of the entire lower extremities. The physician should note limb length, range of movement, configuration of the weightbearing foot and heel, and forefoot alignment. The heel should be aligned parallel to the longitudinal axis of the distal tibia when viewed posteriorly. The plane of the metatarsal heads should be perpendicular to the heel (113).

A bursitis at the insertion of the tendo Achillis may also occur in athletes and requires a change in the heel counter of the athlete's shoe. When an Achilles tendinitis coexists, the heel should be elevated ¼ to ½ inch with heel padding. Local steroid injections should be avoided due to the risk of tendon rupture.

SHIN SPLINTS AND COMPARTMENT SYNDROMES

The leg has four fascial compartments, each enclosed in a constricting fascia (116):

1. The anterior tibial compartment contains the tibialis anterior and the extensor hallucis longus muscles
2. The deep posterior compartment contains the tibialis posterior muscle, the flexor digitorum longus, and the flexor hallucis longus
3. The lateral compartment contains the fibularis (peroneus) longus and fibularis (peroneus) brevis muscles
4. The superficial posterior compartment contains the soleus muscle and the two heads of the gastrocnemius muscle

The foot contains at least nine compartments in addition (117), which may be important in crush injuries to the foot (118, 119).

''*Shin splints syndrome*'' is a descriptive term that has been applied to a symptom complex of pain and discomfort in the lower leg after repetitive overuse, such as in running, jogging, or walking. Discomfort emanates from the lower half of the posteromedial border of the tibia, the anterior tibial compartment, the tibia itself, or the interosseous membrane region of the foreleg.

Other terms, including ''*medial tibial stress syndrome,*'' ''*posterior tibial tendinitis,*'' and ''*anterior (or medial) shin splints,*'' are in current use to describe exertional shin pain more precisely (116).

The symptoms are a dull ache followed by a gradually worsening pain, which is at first relieved by rest, and later becomes continuous. Accompanying foreleg pain, numbness, or loss of sensation over the fourth toe may be noted.

The pain and discomfort in the leg are associated with repetitive motion such as running or aerobic dance, particularly on a hard surface, or with forcible, excessive use of foot flexors. Usually the pain is confined to the anterior portion of the leg, but the site of involvement may be more diffuse. Tenderness can usually be elicited over symptomatic sites. Mild swelling and induration may occur at the site of tenderness. Sensory or motor nerve deficits suggest a compartment syndrome rather than shin splints (116).

Stress fractures, periostitis, tears of musculotendinous structures, or definite ischemic compartment syndromes are important alternative diagnostic considerations. Fracture and vascular claudication must also be considered in the differential diagnosis of severe shin splints syndrome (120–122). If pain is out of proportion to the clinical findings, an intermittent or complete ischemic compartment syndrome should be excluded.

A *compartment syndrome* results from any increased tissue pressure within an anatomic space that compromises the circulation to the compartment (120, 123, 124). It requires a constricting envelope (a constricting fascia or cast) and an increased volume (blood, swelling). Ischemic compartment syndromes that must be distinguished from shin splints include those due to involvement in the anterior tibial compartment (121). Symptoms related to these ischemic syndromes often begin 10 to 12 hours after unaccustomed exercise, or in association with serious trauma; aching pain in the compartment region is noted.

Increased pain in the anterior compartment following passive flexion of the toes is an early sign. *Pain, pallor, and pulseless paralysis* are late hallmarks of the serious ischemic post-traumatic compartment syndromes. Chronic compartment syndrome differs from shin splints in the failure of rest to provide relief from pain. The only effective treatment is surgical compartment release (125).

Elevated compartment pressure is a confirmatory diagnostic finding for a compartment syndrome. Using a catheter inserted into the suspected compartment, pre- and postexercise compartment pressures can be determined (126–128). Similarly, the central plantar compartment pressure can be determined if a compartment syndrome in the foot is suspected (129, 130). Pre-and postexertion magnetic resonance imaging, using a radiopharmaceutical agent (methoxy isobutyl isonitrile) has been used to demonstrate and document the location of a chronic compartment syndrome when features are not typical (131).

Plantar fasciitis (discussed later in more detail) is another common overload injury to the attachment of the plantar fascia at the inferior aspect of the calcaneus. Excessive pronation, a flat or cavus foot, a tight Achilles tendon, and the type and degree of wear of the shoes may predispose the runner to plantar fasciitis (132, 133). Using Cybex peak torque and other measurements in a study of three groups of runners with and without plantar fasciitis, Kibler et al. (134) documented strength and flexibility deficits in the musculature of the posterior calf and foot in the affected runners. Though the study's validity would be greater had it been conducted in a prospective protocol, it does suggest that training and stretching may prevent plantar fasciitis in runners.

Most running injuries are due to training errors and the accumulation of excessive mileage; excessive repetitive movement may not be tolerated by the subtle anatomic deformities often found in these individuals (135). Shin splints and knee problems such as chondromalacia patellae and iliotibial tract tendinitis may occur.

Treatment includes having the runner decrease weekly mileage, avoid hard-surface running, change the running stride, stretch the hamstring and calf muscles (Exercises 6.H through 5.K, whichever is best tolerated), strengthen the quadriceps femoris muscles (Exercises 6.E, 6.F, or 6.G, whichever is best tolerated), and use shoes with waffle soles and orthoses when indicated, with alteration of the heel counter (113, 114). Manual techniques such as massage, myofascial release, and pressure applied to trigger/tender points have been helpful in our experience.

Stress fractures resulting from athletic competition or jogging must be recognized early in order to prevent more serious injury. Such fractures may occur in the spine, pelvis, femur, tibia, fibula, calcaneus, or metatarsal bones. Pain may be referred to sites distant from the fracture. The etiology is thought to be bone

"fatigue." Female runners over the age of 30 tend to fracture the inferior ramus of the pubis; high school track or cross-country runners tend to fracture the distal fibula (136). Tenderness and pain is well localized and usually persists several weeks, and swelling without redness may be present. Treatment measures include rest, substitution of sports such as swimming, strengthening exercises, gentler training, and monitored return to running. Orthoses are of uncertain value but there are many positive anecdotal reports of benefit.

Management of Running Injuries: RICE is an acronym for the usual care of running injuries: rest, ice, compression of injured tissue, and elevation. Leg elevation and application of ice packs for 15 minutes at a time are initial treatment measures. Stretching (lengthening) followed by strengthening exercises directed to the musculature of the involved site of the leg are helpful. If the injury is recurrent, assess pelvic, spinal, and lower extremity structure and alignment for imbalances.

Shoes and orthoses have improved greatly in recent years (and since the previous edition of this text). But first and foremost is a proper shoe fit, and recognition of excessive shoe wear. The foot often widens with age and shoe size should be reexamined at each time of purchase. Width should be determined while standing. Women in particular should be sure that the heel provides adequate support, as the female heel is much narrower than that of the male. Orthoses can be helpful in runners with excessive pronation, leg length discrepancy, patellofemoral disorders, plantar fasciitis, Achilles tendinitis, and shin splints. In one study, most runners were found to prefer a flexible orthosis (137). Some practitioners suggest a semiflexible orthosis (138) (Table 6.6; refer also to Table 6.2 on joint protection).

Outcome and Additional Suggestions for Running Injuries: Brief rest usually allows the pain to subside, at which time activity may be resumed. Local tenderness should no longer be palpable. Symptoms of recurrent or persistent pain require exclusion of a true compartment syndrome (121). A stress fracture may be difficult to distinguish from shin splints; bone scans, positive in the presence of stress fracture, are diagnostically helpful. Triple-phase bone scanning can discriminate periostitis from

TABLE 6.6 COMMON SHOE MODIFICATIONS

Problem Area	Possible Shoe Modification
Great toe	Broad toe box, shoe cutout around bunion, vinyl patch to enlarg box, thicker or more rigid sole, broad external rocker bar, felt and plastic cap.
Other toes	"X" incision above toe, wider shoe size, metartarsal pads, and e. depth shoes
Metatarsal area	Pads, excavation of innersole beneath lesion, "closed cell" foam pad (Spenco), molded flexible insert with "open cell" foam (Plastizote), short external metatarsal bar (1 inch wide), longer external rocker bar, vinyl covering to widen toe box, and ante placed heel.
Plantar region of midfoot, flexible flatfoot, plantar fasciitis	Long-counter shoe, Thomas heel, scaphoid pad, flexible arch sup cutout under heel spur, scaphoid pad, 3/16-inch foam medial c insert, and wedging of the medial sole.
Dorsal midfoot	Strips of foam rubber cemented to inner tongue to lift tongue off lesion, and elastic shoe laces.
Heel	Heel lift, heel pad, cutout heel pad, excavation of innersole ben heel spur or lesion, plastic heel cup, and "V" incision into rim counter.

stress fracture. Scintigraphy and MR imaging may identify abnormality within a few days, while roentgenography often only reveals the late changes of stress fracture (115, 136, 139).

Ankle Injury and Sprains

The ankle is probably the most commonly injured joint in athletics. Arthritis of the ankle, however, is fortunately uncommon. Imaging technology has enhanced our knowledge of the ankle and can distinguish among many soft tissue injuries and problems (140–142). The cost of magnetic resonance imaging is a significant deterrent to its use; however, when pain and disability are prolonged or perplexing, MRI of the ankle should be considered.

Ligament Sprain: The most common problem of the soft tissue supporting structures of the ankle joint are sprains. The ligamentous structures of the medial side of the ankle are less commonly injured than those of the lateral side. Sprains may be subclassified into three types: type 1 is a mild stretching of the ligament with the fibers still intact; type 2 is a more severe injury with partial disruption of the fibers of the ligaments; and type 3 is a complete disruption of the ligament. The more severe sprains should be referred to an orthopaedic surgeon.

The lateral ligaments, comprising the anterior talofibular ligament, the posterior talofi-

bular ligament, and the calcaneofibular ligament are most commonly involved in ankle sprain. Usually the patient notes pain associated with an inverted ankle and has a sensation of the ankle's "giving way."

Syndesmotic sprains (high ankle sprain) may involve the anterior tibiofibular ligament, the posterior tibiofibular ligament, and the interosseous membrane. These ligaments are critical to ankle stability, and syndesmotic ligament injuries contribute to chronic ankle instability. Injury probably results from an external rotational force. A squeeze test, consisting of compression of the fibula against the tibia at the mid-calf level, will elicit pain near the ankle when the syndesmosis has been injured (143). These injuries require more prolonged treatment, and they are more likely to result in recurrent ankle sprain and formation of heterotopic ossification (144–146).

Pain is increased upon forced ankle inversion. The examiner can palpate for tenderness and often determine which portion of the ligament is involved. The medial (deltoid) ligament can also suffer sprain; gentle eversion accentuates this pain. Swelling, local tenderness, and ecchymosis may occur, and weight-bearing becomes painful.

Stress tests include the anterior drawer test in which excessive anterior displacement of the foot on the tibia is detectable (more than 3 mm) and graded from 1+ to 3+ excessive movement; the talar tilt test for excessive ankle inversion, also graded from 1 + to 3 + ; and the squeeze test for syndesmotic injury (144, 147).

Management of type 1 sprain includes immediate application of cold with compression, elevation, and rest for the first 24 to 48 hours. In most cases, radiographic examination to exclude bony injury should be carried out (148). Special radiographic procedures, including arthrography and stress roentgenograms and imaging, should be left to the orthopaedist (148–150). In mild injury, when the edema subsides, adhesive strapping or elastic support should be applied and continued until symptoms subside. *Chronic instability of the ankle joint* often results from the additive damage of multiple "turned ankles"; therefore, proper care of the acute injury is essential. Athletic injuries to the ankle may appear to be trivial, but are important in the context of the athlete's future endeavors. Prevention of further injury includes ankle strapping to limit inversion or eversion, use of elastic ankle supports, and shoes with rigid toe boxes and firm soles. Air or gel stirrup braces, laced supports with malleable metal stays, and lightweight plastic posterior leg splints have been advocated for some ankle problems. The foot should not be held in a plantarflexed position. Refer also to the decision chart in Table 6.4.

Following recovery from injury, the athlete may progress from walking to jogging, and then to running in figure-eights, with gradually tighter circles and broken patterns in order to test the stability of the ankle before competitive activity is resumed. Initial exercises should include foot-ankle circles with emphasis on movement toward the area of sprain to strengthen those muscles (Exercise 6.L). Balance retraining and activities to improve kinesthetic awareness of the injured ankle may be necessary (see Chapter 8). The rehabilitation exercise program should be carried out over several weeks to provide protection against further injury. Incomplete rehabilitation can lead to the "weak ankle" problem. The patient should be referred to physicians who have expertise in this area if the injured joint has not improved within 2 to 3 weeks, or if there is any question about the degree of sprain.

Tendinitis: Inflammation and degeneration of a tendon sheath (some prefer the terms peritendinitis and tendinosis, respectively) at the ankle may result from repetitive activity or unaccustomed extraordinary work. Other causes include improper footwear resulting in injury, particularly to the extensor hallucis longus or to the Achilles tendon. Eleven muscles have tendons crossing the ankle. The shoe vamp may impinge upon the tendons of the dorsum of the ankle and forefoot, and local heat, redness, and tenderness may result. Severe or repeated traumatic tenosynovitis may result in cicatrization and require surgical excision of the tendon sheath.

A chronic nonspecific tendinitis may affect several tendons at the ankle, similar to that seen in de Quervain's tenosynovitis at the wrist (151). Tenosynovitis involving the tibialis anterior, tibialis posterior, extensor digitorum longus, or fibularis (peroneal) tendons at the ankle may occur where the tendons become angulated at the ankle; friction can then cause inflammation of the tendon sheath. A bulbous swelling that occurs distally to areas of constriction is helpful in demonstrating points of constriction. Histologic examination of the tendon sheath demonstrates nonspecific inflammation. Occasionally rheumatoid arthritis, spondylarthritis, and rarely, oxalosis, xanthomas, or giant cell tumors are found. Tuberculosis is an uncommon cause for tendinitis in this region.

Physical examination often reveals a tubular swelling of the tendon sheath, tenderness, pain on passive stretching of the tendon, pain on active ankle movement, and normal palpation of the ankle joint. Comparison with the uninvolved side is helpful.

Herniation of the anterior tibialis muscle may present with a painful nodule in the anterolateral lower foreleg; such nodules are more evident during weightbearing (152).

Posterior tibial tendinitis and dysfunction presents with pain and swelling over the medial ankle and longitudinal arch. If not treated, longstanding inflammation can lead to tendon disruption and progressive flatfoot deformity. If antiinflammatory agents do not provide adequate relief, tendon sheath injection and, if necessary, casting for a short time followed by use of an orthosis are helpful. Surgical intervention is sometimes necessary (153).

Radiographic abnormalities in tendinitis are usually absent, although new bone formation over the posterior aspect of the medial malleolus can occur. Complete rupture of the posterior tibial tendon may be suspected if a sag of the naviculocuneiform joint or mild subluxation of the talonavicular joint is evident. Magnetic resonance imaging can often provide definitive information. Tenography may be helpful for planning surgical treatment, particularly when stenosing tenosynovitis is suspected (154).

Treatment of tendinitis includes partial immobilization of the ankle with bandaging or an elastic ankle support and, at home, physical therapy with exercises. Simple exercises to maintain range of motion and strength, including the foot-ankle circles (Exercise 6.L), can be done several times daily with increasing repetitions and intensity as healing progresses. Stretching and lengthening of the calf muscles and plantar fascia (Exercise 6.J) should begin gently and be continued as activity increases. Massage (deep friction) of the involved tendon/tendon sheath is recommended to improve tissue flexibility. Sometimes complete immobilization in a cast is helpful. NSAIDs or tendon sheath injection with a corticosteroid-anesthetic mixture may be tried.

When injecting a tendon sheath, keep the needle parallel to the tendon in order to minimize the risk of injecting steroid into the tendon itself. Do not repeat injections around the ankle or foot region, as tendon rupture may result; one injection usually will suffice (155).

Excision of the tendon sheath for diagnosis and treatment is rarely necessary. Persistent symptoms in a 20–30-year-old should raise suspicion of a tarsal coalition. This fusion of two or more tarsal bones may give rise to vague foot pain after use or prolonged standing, and fibularis (peroneal) muscle spasm is common. Roentgenographic examination with attention to this possible etiology should be considered (156).

Tendon Dislocation: The fibularis (peroneus) longus and brevis tendons are the most commonly dislocated leg tendons. They may become taut and may dislocate, and the patient may experience an audible painless snapping sensation in the tendon(s). Such dislocation occurs in older children and, because walking is not affected, it may go unrecognized. The dislocated tendon(s) may be seen lying over the lateral malleolus. The patient notes the leg or ankle giving way if the fibularis longus muscle goes into spasm with abduction and plantarflexion of the foot (157). Occasionally the dislocation may result from trauma; more often it results from a congenital shallowness of the tendon groove located on the posterior surface of the lateral malleolus. Usually spontaneous reduction occurs; if not, active reduction may be required. After reducing the dislocation, treatment includes immobilization with a cast for 5 to 8 weeks, which usually results in permanent benefit. Exercise to restore strength and length of immobilized tissues (as described above) is essential following a period of immobilization. Occasionally, surgical intervention to reconstruct the sheath or to deepen the groove is necessary.

Disorders of the Achilles Tendon Region: A tight Achilles tendon may result from disuse, from complex factors associated with growth, or more often as a problem occurring in women who wear high-heeled shoes; persons who wear boots with high heels are also at risk. The patient presents with pain over the heel; dorsiflexion of the ankle increases the pain and tenderness. Gentle progressive stretching and lengthening exercises to the lower leg muscles are helpful (Exercises 6.H, 6.I, or 6.J, whichever is best tolerated). As tissues lengthen and pain resolves, the patient should obtain shoes with appropriate heels and use the higher heeled shoes only for special occasions. However, transition to low-heeled shoes should be gradual. Deep friction massage to the involved tendon may provide relief of pain and facilitate stretching. Achilles tendinitis in runners may respond to use of viscoelastic or other heel inserts to cushion and raise the heel.

Calcific tendinitis of the Achilles tendon produces swelling and often redness along the lower 5 cm of the tendon. Calcification may be evident in the tendon sheath on roentgenogram. Ultrasonographic study of the Achilles tendon is sometimes of value for diagnosis (158). A history of previous episodes of bursitis at the shoulder, hip, or wrist may indicate more general calcium apatite deposition disease.

Gout rarely strikes the posterior heel region, but rheumatoid arthritis will involve the Achilles tendon on occasion. Treatment with NSAIDs is helpful; the condition may require several weeks of medication. Recurrent episodes may be prevented with colchicine 0.6 mg two times a day. Achilles tendinitis may present as a feature in association with diffuse idiopathic skeletal hyperostosis (DISH) (158a).

Bursitis: may involve bursae that lie superficial and deep to the tendon near its insertion onto the calcaneus. *Neither the deep bursa nor the tendon sheath should be injected because of the possibility of tendon rupture as a result of steroid-induced atrophy.* Oral NSAIDs are helpful. Bursography of the retrocalcaneal bursa has been described (159), but an MRI is noninvasive and may provide added detail to the retrocalcaneal region. Also, retrocalcaneal stress fracture can be difficult to distinguish from bursitis. Scintigraphy would be useful to help in diagnosis. Chronic bursitis due to inflammatory rheumatic disease can be diagnosed by aspiration of bursal fluid to be analyzed for inflammation, indicated by the presence of inflammatory cells and a poor mucin clot test (160).

Rupture of the Achilles Tendon may occur after abrupt calf muscle contraction. Usually the patient is a male over 30 years of age who sporadically engages in sports and does not do a regular leg conditioning program. The patient may note an audible snap, followed by pain in the calf as if struck with a baseball. The patient may then be unable to stand up on his toes. The Thompson test may be performed for further evidence of rupture of the Achilles tendon. The patient kneels on a chair with the feet hanging over the edge; when the examiner squeezes the calf muscle on the normal side, the foot responds with plantar flexion; when this maneuver is performed on the side with a ruptured Achilles tendon, there is no foot response. Orthopaedic consultation for immobilization or surgical repair is necessary. Extensive exercise rehabilitation is necessary before return to sports, and continued conditioning to the lower leg is advised. Ultrasonic identification of subcutaneous rupture has been reported in a small study of 12 patients (161). Magnetic resonance imaging is useful if the severity of the tendinitis is in doubt (162).

"Pump bumps" are visible, firm, nodular soft tissue lesions at the lower end of the tendo Achillis. They are commonly associated with wearing high-heeled pumps or loafers. The bump may be an exostosis of the superior tuberosity of the calcaneus or may appear as a hatchet-shaped calcaneus with a prominent posterosuperior margin (163, 164). They are often bilateral and asymptomatic. Occasionally an overlying bursa becomes inflamed. Symptomatic pump bumps are often the result of wearing closely contoured heel counters (163). The pump bump may also be associated with an adventitial bursitis located at the posterior surface of the calcaneus, lateral or medial to the Achilles tendon. Ill-fitting shoes may cause another adventitial bursitis, "last bursitis," located lateral to the heel (165).

Haglund's Syndrome: A prominent enlarged bony posterior calcaneal tubercle sometimes causes compression of soft tissue and pain. A retrocalcaneal bursitis may result. Nonoperative treatment includes a well-fitted heel cup, a laced or strapped shoe that reduces heel counter friction, heel padding to raise the heel, and, if a bursitis is present and persistent, a "V" cutout heel counter to decompress the bursa; incising the heel counter with a deep "V" will provide less friction. A local injection of a corticosteroid agent into the bursa should only be undertaken rarely, if ever, because this can induce rupture of the Achilles tendon. Surgical excision should be considered if the exostosis is large and symptoms persist (166).

Rheumatoid nodules in this region usually can be distinguished from pump bumps: the former occur 1 or 2 inches above the point of attachment of the tendon to the calcaneus, while pump bumps are farther down, at the superior border of the calcaneus. Treatment includes use of shoes that fit without pressure areas, such as soft sandals or laced shoes; protective padding or a plastic heel cup; a heel lift; and, rarely, a corticosteroid injection into the adventitial superficial bursa (160). Conservative therapy is usually helpful; if not, resection of the posterior prominence of the calcaneus may be necessary (Table 6.4).

Tenosynovitis and bursitis near the heel are usually acute self-limited disorders. However, if chronic and accompanied by the wearing of boots, the condition is known as "Winter's heel" or "Haglund's disease."

To relieve compression of the heel counter for these disorders, have a "V" cut out from the counter of the shoe. Obviously, an old pair of shoes should be used for the first trial. Heel pads or molded heel cups are helpful (167) after tenderness has diminished.

Adhesive Capsulitis of the Ankle: An adhesive capsulitis may follow an intraarticular fracture or other severe injury. Persistent pain and limitation of motion develop. Arthrography is a useful diagnostic test. During arthrography a decreased capacity of the joint is evident. Ankle joint injection with a corticosteroid into the ankle and aggressive physical therapy may restore ankle motion (168). Physical therapy techniques should include the use of heat, cold, or electrotherapeutic modalities; progressive and extensive exercise to strengthen, stretch, and lengthen the lower leg muscles (Table 6.5, Exercises 6.H through 6.K, whichever is best tolerated, and 6.L and 6.N); manual techniques by an experienced physical therapist to improve tissue flexibility and the alignment of bony structures; and fabrication of orthotic devices as necessary for gait retraining.

Plantar Heel Pain

The following conditions cause heel disturbance or pain: periostitis of the calcaneus, piezogenic papules, apophysitis, neoplasms, calcaneal spurs, and plantar fasciitis (169, 170). Referred pain to the heel may result from disease of the subtalar joint or from sciatic nerve impingement.

Calcaneal periostitis may result from trauma, Reiter's disease, ankylosing spondylitis, psoriatic arthritis, or rheumatoid arthritis (170). The resulting painful heel may have to be raised 1 to 2 cm with a heel lift for relief.

Calcaneal spurs develop on the plantar tuberosity and extend across the entire width of the calcaneus. The apex is embedded in the plantar fascia. Pain occurs if the apex is angled downward by depression of the long arch. In the past, an acutely painful heel spur was thought to be a manifestation of gonorrhea. More recent studies have demonstrated it to be due to other diseases, such as ankylosing

spondylitis, Reiter's syndrome, or rheumatoid arthritis.

Heel spurs are more often asymptomatic, rarely causing pain themselves. When symptomatic, another mechanical etiology is usually responsible. Plantar fasciitis is a likely cause of heel pain with or without spur formation. Use of shoes with cushion soles or crepe soles, cut out heels, heel inversion, or arch supports that reduce the forces acting upon the plantar aponeurosis are helpful. A local corticosteroid injection into the point of maximum tenderness is usually helpful (171, 172). Repeated injections may cause heel pad atrophy (155). Some patients with persistent and recurrent heel pain have a gait disturbance with excessive heel strike; in these cases symptoms can often be altered with simple awareness of the phenomenon.

Painful heel pad syndrome in marathon runners and others is thought to result from disruption of the fibrous septa that compartmentalize the fat in the heel pad. The pain is localized to the heel pad; the plantar fascia is not tender, and pain is not accentuated as the examiner dorsiflexes the toes. Insertion of heel cups is helpful (173). "Plastizote" that is individually molded to the patient's heel has proved very helpful (174). Rarely, an osteocartilaginous nodule may be detected within the heel pad. Surgical excision may be necessary (175).

Piezogenic papules, herniations of fat that occur as painful papules at the medial inferior border of the heel, may be noted only upon weightbearing and are an uncommon cause of painful heels. Weight reduction, use of felt padding, and cushion-soled or crepe-soled shoes may provide relief (176). We have noted these in asymptomatic patients as well.

Apophysitis in children may result in heel pain, often following a change of shoe or increased sports activity. Tenderness at the posterior aspect of the heel and radiographic features of a fluffy, moth-eaten, flattened, and fragmented apophysis are seen. Treatment includes using a sponge-heel elevation, elastic strapping, and avoiding of vigorous running (169).

"Black heel" is a black or bluish-black plaque that usually develops on the heel of the foot. The lesion is oval or circular and may develop on the posterior or posterolateral plan-

tar surfaces of one or both heels. It results from a shearing force during sports that causes intracutaneous bleeding. The lesion is painless, most common in adolescents or young adults, and requires no treatment (177).

Plantar Fasciitis is one of the most common causes of foot pain. Heel spurs often coexist and may represent a secondary response to an inflammatory reaction. The deep plantar fascia (plantar aponeurosis) is a thick, pearly-white tissue with longitudinal fibers intimately attached to the skin. The central portion is thickest and attaches to the medial process of the tuberosity of the calcaneus; distally it divides into five slips, one for each toe.

Symptoms include pain in the plantar region of the foot, made worse when initiating walking. A hallmark for diagnosis is local tenderness. Point tenderness along the longitudinal bands of the plantar fascia is best determined by bimanual examination. The examiner dorsiflexes the patient's toes with one hand, pulling the plantar fascia taut, and then palpates with an index finger along the fascia from the heel to the forefoot (Fig. 6.13). Points of discrete tenderness can be elicited and may be marked for possible later local anesthetic–corticosteroid injection. The patient should be examined for inflammatory arthritis, the hypermobility syndrome, tarsal tunnel syndrome, neuropathy, or pes planus with valgus heel deformity. The condition may be indistinguishable from anterior calcaneal bursitis, tenosynovitis of the flexor hallucis longus, and medial calcaneal nerve injury (178).

Etiology. Strain of the plantar fascia often follows jumping or prolonged standing or occurs in association with obesity and flatfeet (171, 179), and a relation to heel spurs has been frequently noted (171). In one sizable study of plantar fasciitis (171), diagnoses of rheumatoid arthritis, gout, or ankylosing spondylitis were made at the time of the initial examination in 10% of the patients. Subsequently, another 5% developed rheumatoid arthritis or gout. In total, then, systemic rheumatic diseases occurred in 15% of the patients. Plantar fasciitis in association with obesity and pes planus was more common. Over half of the patients had plantar spurs, but the presence or absence of plantar spurs had no relationship to outcome. Reiter's syndrome may present

with plantar pain; a soft, fluffy calcification in the region of the insertion of the plantar fascia is characteristic. Plantar fasciitis is common among ballet dancers and those performing dance aerobic exercise. Plantar fascia strain and minute avulsions are more common in dancers with an inelastic arch. Fatigue fracture of the metatarsals must be ruled out in these patients (180).

Patients with fibromyalgia frequently report foot pain with symptoms similar to plantar fasciitis. The symptoms may interfere with systemic exercise programs used in fibromyalgia treatment such as aerobic walking or pool programs. Treatment of the foot symptoms may be necessary in order to enable the patient to continue the exercise program.

Heel spurs probably are just a further development associated with plantar fasciitis (181). Plantar pain may also result from use of fluoride for treatment of osteoporosis (182). Plantar fasciitis was reported in five patients in association with nutritional osteomalacia. The five reported women were all Asian vegetarians (183).

Laboratory and Roentgenographic Examination. Unless systemic disease is also present, tests for inflammation are normal. Radiographic examination will delineate pressure spurs that are usually unrelated to symptoms or outcome. Tumors, fractures, periostitis, and the fluffy bone change characteristic of Reiter's syndrome and other spondyloarthropathies, Lofgren's syndrome, and sarcoidosis are to be considered in differential diagnosis and are further reasons for obtaining roentgenograms. Imaging with technetium scintigraphy (183a) or with MRI (183b) may be helpful in localizing the inflammation if the process is resistant to management.

Management. Treatment of obesity, symptomatic flatfeet, and systemic inflammation is undertaken when the respective conditions are present. Athletic shoes, arch-supporting shoes, particularly with a long counter, or shoes with inserted orthoses with foam-rubber raised arches and rubber or tub heels, are helpful. Often shoes with rigid shanks and cushion or crepe soles are helpful. Initially the patient may not tolerate wearing the arch-supporting shoes all day. The patient can carry along an older pair of shoes when leaving the house, and after several hours may switch from the new shoes to the old ones. Molded ankle-foot orthoses used as night splints may be helpful (184, 184a). Commercial night foot splints are available as well (Fig. 6.22).

Wearing slippers or going barefoot may result in recurrence. Patients who work or reside in buildings with concrete floors should use cushion-soled or crepe-soled shoes.

Heel cups may be helpful. Leather or rubber longitudinal arches may be added in ³⁄₁₆–¼-inch thicknesses. Local strapping of the plantar arch and midfoot may also be temporarily helpful. A soft, moldable, flexible orthosis that can be shaped to the foot while it is held in position of correction may be helpful if structural deformities are also present. Foot orthoses remain controversial, and there are considerable variations in prescribing habits of podiatrists, orthopaedists, and prosthetists. Viscoelastic insoles are now widely available and in a wide variety. A controlled study of their use for back pain supports the view that viscoelastic inserts do modify weightbearing back pain (185). Orthotic devices may be fabricated from viscoelastic materials, closed-cell thermoplastic foam, closed-cell nitrogen bubbles, polyurethane foam, or felt (186).

NSAIDs may be helpful, but prolonged use should be reserved for patients with systemic inflammation.

Ultrasound therapy with or without corticosteroid creme may be used for relief of pain. Ice massage, deep friction massage to fascial tenderness, and strengthening and lengthening exercises for the calf and intrinsic foot muscles are additional recommended physical measures (Table 6.5, Exercises 6.J, 6.L, 6.M, and 6.N). Patients can also be taught to mobilize and stretch the plantar fascia by rolling the bare foot over a hard cylindrical bottle, rolling pin, or dumbbell while sitting in a chair.

In resistant cases, the points of tenderness along the plantar fascia may be injected with a mixture of corticosteroid and local anesthetic (1 mL 1% lidocaine hydrochloride and 20–40 mg methylprednisolone or equivalent). A 1-inch No. 23 or No. 25 needle is inserted ¼ to ½ inch deep into the plantar fascia for deposition of the mixture (no more than 40 mg methylprednisolone or equivalent for each foot). In the injection of multiple sites, injections should begin distally and move toward the heel (Fig. 6.23). Repeated injections may cause heel pad atrophy (155). Plantar fascia rupture may also follow corticosteroid injection (186a). This rare complication presents with dorsal and lateral foot pain and palpable diminution in the tension of the plantar fascia on the involved side. Resolution is slow and treatment is supportive.

Outcome and Additional Suggestions. If patients adhere to the therapeutic program by wearing proper shoes for correction of associated structural foot disorders, benefit often occurs after several weeks to several months in the majority of patients. In our experience, surgical intervention is rarely needed. Furey reported that only 2% of patients with plantar

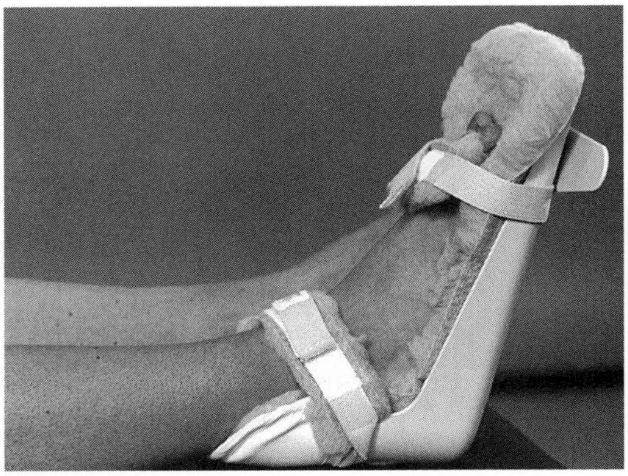

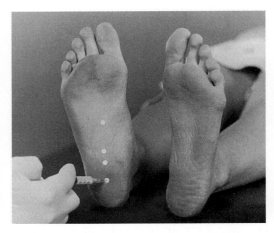

Figure 6.22. A resting padded foot splint such as the one pictured here may be helpful for symptoms of plantar fasciitis.

Figure 6.23. Injection technique for the painful heel and plantar fasciitis. Alternatively these sites are approached from a lateral direction.

fasciitis required a Steindler stripping procedure (stripping of the plantar fascia) (171). Surgical intervention in massively obese patients with persistent symptoms may be justified if all other efforts fail (187). A more recent report of surgical experience at Mayo Clinic consisted of only 16 operations in a 12-year study period. Operation was performed after conservative measures failed. Duration of symptoms prior to operation ranged from 5 to 50 months. The procedures undertaken included heel spur resection in two patients, calcaneal drilling in four, Steindler stripping in two, and division of the nerve to the abductor digiti minimi muscle in one. All had, in addition, division of the central component of the plantar fascia (plantar fasciotomy). After 4 to 15 years, 10 of 14 patients available for follow-up had little pain, three patients had a discernible limp, and results were considered poor in 4 patients. Eleven of the 14 had footwear limitations or used orthoses (188).

Runners and dancers with persistent symptoms and a demonstrable exostosis on roentgenographic examination will usually benefit from excision of a portion of the plantar fascia and removal of the spur (189) (refer also to the decision chart in Table 6.4).

Midfoot Disorders and Injuries

Following an inversion injury, a ligamentous sprain of the calcaneocuboid joint often occurs. Pain, swelling, and tenderness over the lateral border of the foot are noted. For treatment, the midfoot should be taped or wrapped with an elastic bandage or gelocast; recovery generally follows 24 to 48 hours of rest.

Tendinitis of the superficial extensor tendons of the foot commonly results from tight shoe lacing or from ridges on the tongue of the shoe. Frequently, point tenderness and pain follow the use of a new pair of work shoes; swelling is uncommon. To relieve the pressure, a lipstick mark is applied to the point of maximum tenderness, and the shoe is replaced and laced; after removing the shoe, the lipstick mark will appear on the undersurface of the tongue of the shoe. A strip of adhesive-backed foam rubber ⅜ to ½ inch wide should be positioned on the undersurface of the tongue at each side of the lipstick mark, thus providing a gap over the point of tenderness. Use of elastic shoe laces may also be helpful.

A painful hard spur or fibroma on the dorsal aspect of the first tarsometatarsal joint in adults or children may result from tight-fitting shoes.

Metatarsalgia

Although *Morton's neuroma* is a common cause for forefoot pain, many other conditions occur in this region and must be distinguished. The disorders described here are *not* acute in onset, and although they may suggest mild gouty symptoms, they are not as abruptly painful as acute gout.

Disturbances of the metatarsal region may result from congenital structural abnormalities of the foot, weakness of intrinsic foot muscles, arthritis, or trauma. Upon weightbearing, the ''metatarsal arch'' normally flattens and is therefore not a functioning arch. The metatarsal arch created by the transverse metatarsal ligament and the abductor hallucis longus is further supported during push-off by the intrinsic toe flexors, which help to elevate the three central metatarsals.

If a deformity of the first metatarsal is present, the axis of weightbearing may shift to the second metatarsal, with resultant strain upon the normal function of the metatarsal ligaments and musculature. The most common of these deformities is probably metatarsus primus varus, in which the great toe is rotated on its longitudinal axis so that the toenail points medially. Metatarsal pain in the plantar region of the first metatarsophalangeal joint may result from a hallux valgus deformity, hallux rigidus (degenerative joint disease), or arthritis of a sesamoid articulation. The second metatarsal bone is tightly fixed between the three cuneiform bones and is therefore relatively immobile. The region under the second metatarsal head is easily aggravated by wearing high-heeled shoes, by weakness of the intrinsic foot muscles, or by contracture of the flexor tendons. Congenital ligamentous laxity, particularly if associated with obesity, also may result in metatarsalgia during prolonged standing and may result in a splay foot (150), with the development of plantar calluses under the second metatarsal head.

A properly fitted shoe with a broad toe box, a metatarsal pad, or a metatarsal bar placed behind the metatarsal heads is helpful. Rocker soles can relieve and redistribute metatarsal pressure during the push-off phase of gait. Weight reduction is essential in obese patients. Calluses can be softened with 20% salicylic acid and collodion; the application is removed after 2 or 3 days with warm soaking. Toe flexion and extension exercises may also be helpful (Exercises 6.M and 6.N).

The use of an anterior heel, "earth shoe," running shoe, soft insoles such as Spenco or Plastizote (190), or comma-shaped inserts are additional methods for relieving weightbearing from the metatarsal region (Table 6.6 and Figs. 6.24, 6.25, and 6.26). An extended steel shank inserted between the outsole and midsole of a shoe can minimize motion at the metatarsophalangeal joints of the first and second toes (191). Combining soft Plastizote, micropore rubber, cork, and a viscoelastic polymer at pressure points can be utilized (191).

Metatarsal bars may be straight or curved along the inferior surface. The short rocker bar (¼ inch thick), the most commonly prescribed type, is placed externally behind the metatarsal heads (192) (Fig. 6.26). The metatarsal bar may have a forward curve if the patient has this configuration of the metatarsal heads. A "horseshoe" bar may be used if there is a painful plantar callus. If the metatarsal bar is malpositioned it may aggravate pain and require revision. When positioned properly, symptoms are usually promptly improved.

Plastizote insoles are self-molding but may require an extra-depth shoe with an enlarged toe box (Fig. 6.2A). The simple metatarsal foam rubber pad, approximately ³⁄₁₆ inch thick, is widely available. The patient can mark the painful area of the foot with lipstick, stand in the shoe, and then place the pad just behind the lipstick mark. Occasionally the pad requires a concave forward edge to accommodate a particularly painful metatarsophalangeal joint. Obviously, the shoe must hold the foot securely and prevent forward slipping. This requires a strap or lacing. The sole should be firm but not rigid, and cushion or crepe soles are helpful (190).

Metatarsalgia of traumatic origin may result from prolonged walking or jumping that results in a sprain of the intermetatarsal ligaments. Dancers may suffer a stress fracture of a sesamoid bone (193). Swelling may or may not be present.

An intermetatarsal bursitis from tight, narrow shoes may also occur (194). With aging, the metatarsal arch flattens, the metatarsal heads become broader, and the metatarsal heads often impinge upon the bursa. The resulting bursitis gives rise to symptoms similar to a

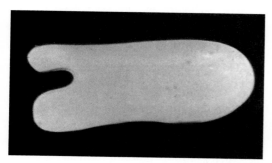

Figure 6.24. A total contact orthosis for relief of first or second metatarsal pain often associated with bunion. The felt or other material is fabricated with increased thickness proximal to the painful second metatarsal head. (From McCarty DJ, Koopman WJ, eds. Arthritis and allied conditions. 12th ed. Philadelphia: Lea & Febiger, 1993.)

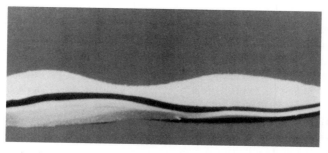

Figure 6.25. A total contact orthosis made with various grades of polyethylene foam (Plastizote). The device depicted here includes a middle layer of shear-relieving micropore rubber. (From McCarty DJ, Koopman WJ, eds. Arthritis and allied conditions. 12th ed. Philadelphia: Lea & Febiger, 1993.)

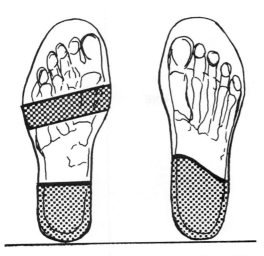

Figure 6.26. *Left,* An external metatarsal bar distributes weight posterior to the metatarsal region. When standing, the patient should be certain the bar has been placed behind the metatarsophalangeal joints; if it does not, the bar should be removed and reattached in the proper location. The bar should be placed on both shoes to allow normal balance. A bar may also be inserted into the sole of a running shoe. *Right,* The Thomas heel provides support for patients with symptomatic pes planus, valgus heel deformity, or plantar fascia strain.

Morton's neuroma (194). Pain due to a bursitis tends to occur quickly upon initiating walking or standing; pain due to a neuroma usually occurs after walking for longer duration, or else while driving or sitting. The pain due to a neuroma subsides with removal of the shoe. Bursitis should be considered if pain can be accentuated by compressing the metatarsal tissue about 1 inch proximal to the web space between the metatarsal heads. Sometimes thumbnail pressure is necessary. Visible swelling is rare. Nevertheless, either condition may respond to conservative measures. Treatment with antiinflammatory agents or local intralesional local anesthetic–corticosteroid injection, along with better fitting shoes, will usually provide relief. A rocker bar can be beneficial. Surgical intervention is not often necessary (195).

Technique for Local Injection. Determine the site of tenderness between the metatarsal heads. A ¾-inch No. 25 needle can be used with a mixture of 10 mg methylprednisolone and 0.5–1 mL local anesthetic. Inject between the metatarsal heads to a depth of about ⅓ to ½ inch. In cases in which more than one interspace is tender, inject these also.

Sprain of the first metatarsophalangeal joint can incapacitate an athlete; tenderness in the great toe region is aggravated by running, though less so by walking; roentgenograms are normal. The adolescent, when engaged in sports, may suffer a stress fracture at the base of the fifth metatarsal, presenting with a painful prominence on the lateral side of the foot. Treatment of the stress fracture includes relief from weightbearing, and if symptoms persist a cast may be necessary (196).

Occasionally children suffer a painful disturbance beneath the first metatarsophalangeal joint. In the past this disorder was thought to be due to sesamoiditis, but it probably represents a bursitis associated with physical trauma.

Stress (March) Fracture: A nondisplaced fracture that occurs just proximal to the metatarsal head is often a fatigue fracture. Although frequently seen in military personnel, particularly in new recruits after their first long march, this condition is also seen frequently in people after prolonged shopping, in joggers, in other overuse syndromes, and in persons with a short first metatarsal (193, 196). The second or third metatarsal shaft is most commonly fractured. These stress fractures rarely occur before age 12 (196). The patient notes tenderness and diffuse forefoot pain accompanied by swelling on the dorsal surface of the metatarsal region. Slight erythema may be present. The onset is subacute and never reaches the intensity of gout. Radiographic evidence of a fracture may be present only after several weeks (Fig. 6.27). A bone callus usually appears by 3 to 4 weeks and confirms the diagnosis. Imaging with a technetium bone scan may be helpful if the diagnosis is in doubt. The use of crutches and a fracture shoe (carried by most orthopaedic supply pharmacies) usually provides prompt pain relief. A molded arch support, snug elastic wrapping, short walking cast, or support with a simple external short metatarsal rocker bar usually provides good results if a fracture shoe is not helpful.

ENTRAPMENT NEUROPATHIES OF THE LOWER LIMB

Symptoms of intermittent numbness, tingling, and a sensation of swelling suggest an entrap-

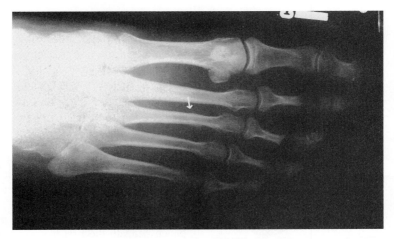

Figure 6.27. Fatigue (march) fracture. Pain and swelling in the mid-metatarsal region on the dorsal aspect of the foot in a middle-aged patient is suggestive of a fatigue fracture. Roentgenographic films 2 weeks following the pain should be scrutinized carefully for evidence of fracture and callus *(arrow).*

ment neuropathy. Lower limb neuropathies result from a diverse group of disorders and activities.

Occupation risk factors for entrapment neuropathy are not uncommon as causes for entrapment neuropathies. For example, peroneal palsy, or foot-drop syndrome, may result from occupations requiring crouching, squatting, or kneeling such as in the work of agriculturists, miners, and shoe salesmen; peroneal palsy has even been reported in a baseball catcher (197). Increased pressure at the popliteal fossa may occur in persons who tilt back in chairs; this may result in a posterior tibial nerve injury. Symptoms similar to those of the *tarsal tunnel syndrome* may occur. The tarsal tunnel syndrome itself may result from the use of shoes with improper arch support. Strain of the posterior tibialis muscle due to pes planus may provoke a tendinitis within the tunnel and secondarily compress the nerve. On the other hand, unnecessary arch supports themselves may induce the syndrome (197). Kneeling with the toes flexed inside tight shoes may cause interdigital nerve injury during such work as that of electricians or of carpet layers. People who need to work close to the floor should either use a small stool or develop sufficient range of motion so that they can squat with flat feet (Oriental style).

Obturator Nerve Entrapment: Following a pelvic fracture, osteitis pubis, or development of an obturator hernia, the patient notes groin area pain and paresthesia that travels down the inner aspect of the thigh; these symptoms are aggravated during passive or active hip motion. Local nerve block is necessary to establish the diagnosis and is often therapeutic.

Meralgia Paresthetica: Entrapment of the lateral femoral cutaneous nerve is a frequent entrapment neuropathy of the thigh region. Intermittent paresthesia, hypesthesia, or hyperesthesia over the upper anterolateral thigh occur (Fig. 6.28). Symptoms are often aggravated by hyperextending the hip. The entrapment usually occurs at the anterior superior iliac spine where the nerve passes through the lateral end of the inguinal ligament or adjacent iliac fascia (198). The nerve also perforates the sartorius muscle and exits through a canal in the fascia lata. Entrapment may also occur within the spinal canal in association with spinal stenosis (199), in intervertebral foramina, or in the retroperitoneal region. Trauma, a pelvic tilt resulting from a short limb, prolonged sitting with crossed legs, improperly placed lap belts while driving, tight jeans or corset, or increased abdominal girth with bulging fat or with pregnancy may be causative. If necessary for diagnostic or other reasons, electrodiagnostic study may be helpful. The use of 8-cm strip electrodes was found to provide definitive neurophysiological evidence in 12 of 13 reported patients (199a).

Around one-half of patients are helped by ice applications to reduce swelling of the nerve

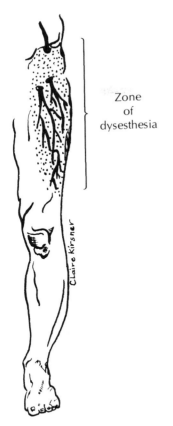

Zone
of
dysesthesia

Claire Kirsner

Figure 6.28. Entrapment of the lateral femoral cutaneous nerve (meralgia paresthetica). The nerve is frequently impinged at the anterosuperior iliac spine; dysesthesias are noted over the upper anterior lateral thigh.

at the site of entrapment, applied three times daily for 20 to 30 minutes; NSAIDs for 7 to 10 days; and restricted aggravating activity (200). If symptoms persist, infiltration with local anesthetic–corticosteroid agents into the site of nerve exit at the inguinal ligament and into the region of dysesthesia can provide benefit for others (200). A ¾-inch or longer No. 25 needle can be used with small amounts of a mixture of 40 mg methylprednisolone and 5–10 mL of a local anesthetic; injecting aliquots every inch or so throughout the area is usually helpful. No more than 40 mg of steroid is necessary. Some believe that the steroid reduces nerve swelling distal to the site of entrapment. Repeated injections are occasionally necessary. Also helpful is avoiding contact pressure in the region of the inguinal ligament, weight normalization, and if necessary, use of a heel-

lift for a short limb. Padding the seat belt with a towel-wrap may be helpful. In one study, only 24 of 277 patients required surgical decompression (200). Manual techniques to relieve tender points and improve tissue flexibility in the groin and thigh may be helpful. Electrotherapies such as interferential current may provide pain relief.

Sciatic Pseudoradiculopathy: A symptom complex simulating radiculopathy (pseudoradiculopathy) may result from trochanteric bursitis; relief of the sciatica-like pain occurs following injection of the trochanteric bursa (201). Sometimes hip capsule stretching such as the hip pendulum exercise is of additional help (Exercise 6.C). As mentioned earlier, this affliction often results from improper bending with the knees straight.

The sciatic nerve may be involved in disease entities beyond the pelvis. Constricting myofascial bands in the posterior thigh have been described (202). Nerve entrapment by heterotopic ossifications have been reported (203). Localization by CT scan and resection are recommended.

Traumatic Prepatellar Neuralgia: This type of neuralgia follows trauma to the anterior patella and may be preceded by transient prepatellar swelling. After a few weeks, exquisite tenderness occurs over the medial outer border of the patella at the site of emergence of the neurovascular bundle; even slight stroking is exquisitely painful. Treatment with a local anesthetic or corticosteroid injection into the point of maximum tenderness is usually helpful (11). Local application of capsaicin cream may be helpful.

Saphenous Nerve Entrapment: Entrapment of the saphenous nerve usually occurs within the adductor (Hunter's) canal and results in medial knee pain, dysesthesia, and hypesthesia in the distribution of the nerve. The diagnosis is made by localization using local anesthesia injected at the point of maximum tenderness, about 10 cm proximal to the medial epicondyle of the femur. Swelling of the anserine bursa may also impinge the nerve. The pain often is misdiagnosed as a stress fracture (204).

Compression Neuropathy of the Common Peroneal Nerve: Foot-drop with inability to dorsiflex the foot often results from peroneal nerve compression due to crossing the leg,

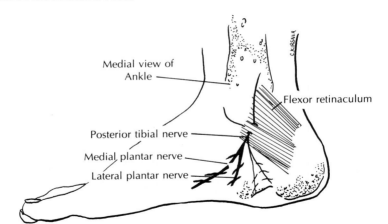

Figure 6.29. Tarsal tunnel. The posterior tibial nerve is often trapped beneath the flexor retinaculum on the medial side of the ankle. Entrapment may also include the two branches, the medial and lateral plantar nerves.

hanging the leg over a constricting rigid object, or from direct trauma. A tight boot or cast may also result in sensory or motor peroneal nerve loss, and a partial or complete foot-drop. Nerve conduction measurement can localize the site of entrapment. A posterior foot-drop splint may be required for many months following injury.

ENTRAPMENT NEUROPATHIES AT THE ANKLE AND FOOT

With the increased use of high boots with high heels and with the popularity of activities such as jogging, entrapment neuropathies of the foot and ankle are being seen more often. When the patient complains of burning paresthesia day and night, this disorder should be suspected. However, that history is often not volunteered and must be sought. Any nocturnal foot symptoms and foot pain that radiates out to the toes should suggest an entrapment neuropathy (205, 206).

Tarsal Tunnel Syndrome: This syndrome refers to an entrapment neuropathy of the posterior tibial nerve as it passes through the tunnel beneath the flexor retinaculum on the medial side of the ankle (207). Beneath this retinaculum (or laciniate ligament) (208) lies a tunnel containing the tendons of the flexor digitorum longus and flexor hallucis longus muscles, the vascular bundle, the posterior tibial nerve, and the medial and lateral plantar nerves (Fig. 6.29).

Most commonly the patient presents with aching, burning, numbness, and tingling involving the plantar surface of the foot, the distal foot, the toes, and occasionally the heel. The pain may also radiate up to the calf or higher (209). The discomfort is often nocturnal and may be worse after standing; the discomfort sometimes leads to removal of the shoe even while driving. Physical examination seldom reveals swelling or atrophy. Sensory nerve loss is variable and often is not found. The Hoffman-Tinel test, in which the nerve is tapped with a finger or reflex hammer, is often positive at the flexor retinaculum posterior and inferior to the medial malleolus. For a complete examination, tapping must be performed over the entire course of the posterior tibial nerve or one of its branches. Occasionally, firm rolling pressure across the nerve may be required to reproduce the symptoms. A tourniquet applied just above the ankle may reproduce the symptoms by creating venous engorgement of the tarsal tunnel.

A tenosynovitis of one or more of the tendons can cause compression neuropathy within the tarsal tunnel. Causes include injury, rheumatoid arthritis or other sources of inflammation, and tumors (210). Perhaps the most common cause for a tarsal tunnel syndrome is a fracture or dislocation involving the talus, calcaneus, or medial malleolus (208). Previous involvement of a *carpal tunnel* has been described in patients who later develop a tarsal tunnel syndrome (211).

Most often the tarsal tunnel syndrome occurs in the absence of inflammatory rheumatic disease, but if other features are suggestive, an erythrocyte sedimentation rate determination and tests for rheumatic disease, including rheumatoid factor and antinuclear factor, should be performed. Diabetic neuropathy may cause similar symptoms unrelated to tarsal tunnel involvement.

Histopathologic study reveals preferential loss of large axons in fascicles at the periphery in comparison to fascicles in the center of the posterior tibial nerve. The changes differ from those associated with ischemia of the lower limb (212).

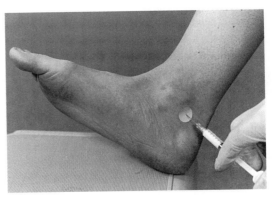

Figure 6.30. Sites for injection of the tarsal tunnel or posterior tibialis tendinitis on the medial aspect of the ankle. A 1-inch No. 23 needle should be used and the medication instilled in a fan-like pattern.

Diagnosis of tarsal tunnel syndrome may be confirmed by electrodiagnostic tests. Tibial nerve conduction velocity normally is 49.9 ± 5.1 milliseconds, and latency from the malleolus to the abductor hallucis muscle normally is 4.4 ± 0.9 milliseconds. Prolonged latency in excess of 6.1 milliseconds for the medial plantar nerve and 6.7 milliseconds for the lateral plantar nerve is indicative of disease (208, 213, 214); however, normal values do not exclude the syndrome (214).

Magnetic resonance imaging is excellent for discerning the contents of the tarsal tunnel and other soft tissue compartments of the ankle (106, 215, 216). But the procedure is most cost-effective if used after conservative measures have been tried. If no recent injury has occurred and symptoms are not disabling, conservative measures should precede imaging or electrodiagnostic tests.

Nonoperative treatment includes use of proper shoes, arch supports when indicated, ensuring proper gait and stride, orthoses if significant pronation is present, and NSAIDs. Perhaps the best diagnostic test is response to a corticosteroid–local anesthetic injection into the region of the tarsal tunnel, with relief confirming the presence of the syndrome.

In most persistent cases a corticosteroid–local anesthetic mixture injected once or twice into the region inferior and posterior to the medial malleolus and injected in a fan-like pattern provides relief (Fig. 6.30). Inject 20 mg methylprednisolone mixed with 1% procaine or lidocaine hydrochloride, taking care not to inject the nerve. Some practitioners report only a 30% response and recommend decompression surgery (209). However, the value of decompression surgery itself has been questioned; in one large study only 44% benefited from surgery. The authors suggest that surgery be restricted to patients who have an associated lesion near or within the tarsal tunnel (217). It may be that surgical intervention is most often required when the tarsal tunnel syndrome follows fracture or dislocation or when imaging reveals a space-occupying lesion. Takakura et al. recommend surgery no later than 10 months after onset of symptoms; results were poor in those with longer symptom duration. In this latter study the majority of operated patients had a space-occupying lesion (218).

If symptoms persist, local or systemic underlying disorders causing a tarsal tunnel or similar symptomatic syndromes must be considered. These include vascular disease with venous stasis, diabetes mellitus with neuropathy, rheumatoid arthritis, myxedema, pregnancy, and amyloidosis (213).

Children may develop the tarsal tunnel syndrome but symptoms differ from those of adults in that night pain is less common; the involvement is unilateral rather than bilateral; the symptoms more likely are burning pain in the sole of the foot while walking, or recurrent spontaneous sudden sharp pain in the foot. Paresthesias in the sole of the foot result when the nerve is percussed behind the medial malleolus. In one series, all patients involved were girls between the ages of 9 and 15. Trauma was unlikely as a cause. Often the child walked with the affected foot in supination, allowing only the lateral border of the sole to contact the ground (219).

Anterior Tarsal Tunnel Syndrome: In this syndrome the deep peroneal nerve is entrapped beneath the inferior extensor retinaculum at the anterior aspect of the tarsal tunnel, giving rise to paresthesias on the dorsum of the foot and often in the great toe. The discomfort is increased at night. Relief following local infiltration with corticosteroids, along with an avoidance of boots, high-heeled shoes, or tight lacing is helpful and confirms the diagnosis (220). When the entrapment follows a crush injury, surgical decompression is often necessary (221).

Plantar Nerve Entrapment: Forced overpronation or pressure associated with a hallux rigidus, tenosynovitis, or venous engorgement of the posterior tibial veins may compress the plantar nerve on the medial aspect of the foot below the calcaneonavicular ligament. The patient may present with a painful heel as well as numbness or tingling across the sole of the foot. Correction of abnormal foot mechanics with a medial shoe wedge, a scaphoid pad, or molded soft flexible inserts should provide relief. A local anesthetic–corticosteroid injection at the site of compression may help those with persistent symptoms.

Interdigital Plantar Neuroma (Morton's Neuroma): Entrapment neuropathy with or without an associated plantar neuroma often develops between the third and fourth toes on the plantar surface. This involves the anastomoses of the medial and lateral plantar nerves. Pain radiates forward from the metatarsal heads to the third and fourth toes. Similar involvement of other interdigital plantar nerves may occur. This neuropathy, commonly called *Morton's neuroma,* has features of hyperesthesia of the toes, numbness and tingling, and aching and burning in the distal forefoot. It is aggravated by walking on hard surfaces and wearing tight or high-heeled shoes. The pain frequently persists for some time after cessation of weightbearing.

Physical examination reveals tenderness in the plantar aspect of the distal foot over the third and fourth metatarsals; compressing the forefoot reproduces the symptoms. The tenderness is occasionally aggravated by direct pressure to the plantar aspect of the third and fourth

metatarsophalangeal joints. There should be a concomitant sensation of burning distally.

Possible causes include excessive mobility of the fourth metatarsal, nerve impingement between flattened metatarsal heads, or compression of the nerve as it is angulated over the transverse tarsal ligament. Chronic compression leads to neuroma formation.

Similar signs and symptoms may occur from an *intermetatarsal bursitis* rather than a neuroma. The neurovascular bundle lies close to the bursa (194).

Conservative treatment requires decreasing stresses at the metatarsal heads with the use of a metatarsal support, metatarsal bar, or a comma-shaped metatarsal shoe insert. Although symptoms are unilateral in 85% of cases, external appliances should be placed on both shoes so that the patient walks evenly. A broad-toed shoe that allows spreading of the metatarsal heads or an extra-depth shoe (Fig. 6.2A) is helpful. Intermetatarsal bursitis may cause similar symptoms. A local anesthetic–corticosteroid injection into the site of compression may be beneficial. Surgical removal of the neuroma and nerve may be required in patients who are resistant to nonoperative therapy (191).

Joplin's Neuroma: Perineural fibrosis of the proper plantar digital nerve may follow a bunionectomy or trauma to the first metatarsophalangeal joint. This results in pain and paresthesia at the plantar aspect of the first metatarsophalangeal joint of the great toe. A Hoffman-Tinel test may be positive beneath the first metatarsophalangeal joint. Relief occurs with foot rest or removal of the shoe. Surgical excision of the nerve may be necessary.

OTHER LOWER LIMB DISORDERS

Soft Tissue Calcifications: Heterotopic ossification and myositis ossificans or calcific tendinitis may result from trauma or may occur in association with calcium apatite deposition disease (CADD), which may result from metabolic derangements or, more commonly, may be idiopathic. Ectopic calcification of the hip may follow hip joint replacement, particularly in patients with ankylosing spondylitis. Large calcifications may cause nerve entrapment. Heterotopic ossifications also may result from spinal cord trauma (222). Calcific tendinitis may affect the hip or Achilles tendon regions. Long-term use of isotretinoin and etretinate, synthetic retinoids used for cystic acne, has been associated with tendon and ligament calcification (223).

Presentation depends upon type and prior medical history or history of trauma. CADD-associated disease has a gout-like presentation with acute onset of erythema and swelling of the involved tendon. When heterotopic ossification occurs following surgery, the presentation may be of soft tissue swelling, pseudophlebitis, or entrapment neuropathy (222, 224). Imaging with triple-phase bone scan or CT scan may be necessary for diagnosis if plain roentgenography is not helpful.

Treatment modalities with antiinflammatory agents, etidronate, radiation therapy, and surgical excision have been used (222). Colchicine may be used for prevention of CADD-associated attacks of calcific tendinitis. Diltiazem in a dosage of 240 mg/day was successful in treating calcinosis associated with CREST syndrome (calcinosis, Raynaud's phenomenon, esophageal dysfunction, sclerodactyly, and telangiectasia) and in tumor calcinosis. The authors suggest that the increased influx of calcium into affected cells is normalized by the drug (225).

Adiposis Dolorosa (Dercum's Disease): Medial knee pain in women with fat knees is common after menopause. Often anserine bursitis is coexistent. When squeezing the fat panniculi results in pain reproduction, knee arthritis is unlikely to be the main contributing factor. Thus radiographic changes of osteoarthritis of the knee may not be relevant and could lead to other inappropriate treatment. Treatment consists of local injection of a corticosteroid (40 mg methylprednisolone or equivalent) and local anesthetic into the point of maximum tenderness and is usually helpful. Some advocate liposuction treatment, but this is more invasive and carries risks (226).

Osgood-Schlatter Disease: Patients with this disease, usually boys during periods of rapid growth, have pain, tenderness, and soft tissue swelling about the tibial tubercle just below the patella. Pain occurs when climbing stairs, kneeling, or kicking in association with quadriceps femoris muscle contraction. The discomfort and swelling usually cease before or by the age of 18. The etiology is thought to be traumatic and may result from avulsion of the tibial tubercle during adolescence. However, Rosenberg et al. report CT scan and MRI findings of *tendinitis* in 28 patients, in many of whom distended infrapatellar bursa were also revealed; after recovery the tendinitis partially disappeared. An ossicle was seen in only nine of the 28 cases (227). In three patients the ossicle remained nonunited despite relief of symptoms. Accordingly, these authors argue that in most cases "Osgood-Schlatter syndrome" represents an insult to the tendon and bursa rather than an avulsion fracture.

Plain radiographic findings may include swelling of the patellar ligament, fragmentation of the tibial tubercle, soft tissue swelling, avulsion of an ossification center, or avascular necrosis.

Treatment includes the use of a cylinder cast for several weeks, avoidance of contact sports, and maintenance of quadriceps femoris muscle strength with cautious use of isometric exercise. The initial strengthening program should use moderate to maximum contraction for 5 to 30 repetitions, each of 10–30 seconds' duration. In later phases of rehabilitation, quadriceps exercise can progress to using the resistance of a Theraband or weights, working first in the short 30-degree arc and later in the full arc (Exercises 6.E, 6.F, and 6.G). The result is a prominent tubercle that is usually painless. In one study, 116 of 142 patients recovered within 1 year with conservative measures. In those who did not, surgical intervention consisted of excision of a portion of the surface of the tibial tuberosity and multiple perforation with a thin drill point (228).

Growing Pains: The term "growing pains," attributed to Deschamps in the early 19th century (229), is in fact a misnomer, as the most common age of occurrence is not at a time of rapid growth. These pains usually occur around age 8 and disappear by age 12 (230). The discomfort is described as an intermittent annoying pain or ache, usually localized to the muscles of the legs and thighs, associated with a feeling of restlessness. These pains do not occur in joint areas and are often bilateral (229); they often awaken the child from sleep.

The etiology of the problem remains elusive. Theories of developmental or postural causes, as well as of a relationship with severity of activity or emotional stress, have all been discarded (231). A family history of rheumatic pain was found in over half of the children with growing pains, compared to 10% in a control group. Children with only nocturnal pain often had relatives with only nocturnal pain, whereas children with diurnal pain had a strong family history of diurnal pain (230).

The differential diagnosis of recurrent pain in the lower limbs in children and adolescents includes trauma, occult infection, avascular necrosis of bone, vascular disturbances, congenital structural disorders, tumors, connective tissue diseases, and the soft tissue rheumatic pain disorders. Benign causes of leg pain are usually bilateral, whereas most of the serious disorders with leg pain are unilateral.

Treatment for children with these benign leg pains is empiric. If the leg muscles are tight, gentle hamstring muscle stretching exercises may be beneficial. These should also be done as a warm-up before competitive sports. Leg pains may be relieved by movement such as walking about the room. A hot tub bath, leg elevation, and leg massage are additional helpful measures. The discomfort may be accentuated by running or other strenuous play activities. When myofascial trigger points have been found, ice massage and manual techniques might help (232).

Infrequently the clinician sees a child or adolescent with leg pain without any distinguishing features; psychogenic factors may have to be considered (230, 233). The clinician should then look for the following:

1. Death of a parent or separation from a significant other person
2. Marital discord between parents
3. Family history or similar complaints of pain in parents or siblings
4. Difficulty in school with academic subjects, teachers, or peers

When an emotionally charged situation has been discovered, therapeutic intervention must focus on the psychosocial disorder as well as on its resulting symptoms. With removal of the emotionally charged situation, the pain or dysfunction state often improves (233).

Leg Cramps: Cramps that involve the legs and feet are probably more common than physicians realize. Patients often do not mention the complaint unless asked. Benign nocturnal leg and foot aches and cramps may be related to exertion and often awaken the patient. Physical findings are usually normal.

Symptoms must be differentiated from pain of intermittent claudication, which occurs during limb use and is relieved by rest. Night cramps occur in all decades of life.

Structural disorders, including flatfeet, genu recurvatum, hypermobility syndrome, prolonged sitting, and inappropriate leg position during sedentary activity predispose to leg cramp. Diuretics, beta-agonists, beta-blockers with intrinsic sympathomimetic activity, inadequate ingestion of water, excessive sweating without salt replacement, hypocalcemia, low serum magnesium, and motor neuron disease are additional causes of cramp (234–236).

A history of working on a concrete floor, or having moved to a home built on a cement slab foundation (even with floor coverings) may be correlated with the occurrence of leg cramps. Wearing thick cushion-soled shoes is often helpful in such situations. Symptoms frequently recur in clusters. Sedentary persons may prevent nocturnal leg cramp by riding a stationary bicycle for a few minutes before retiring. Stretching exercises should be done in the weightbearing position, such as in posterior leg stretching illustrated in Exercises 6.H and 6.I (237). Position should be held 20 seconds, repeated three times in succession, four times a day for 1 week, and then twice a day thereafter. In many cases, these stretching exercises may prevent leg cramps. Use of a hot shower, warm tub bath, or ice massage may be helpful for some. (Judicious imbibing of brandy is a time-honored remedy.) Regular aquatic exercise for conditioning and stretching is helpful to many.

Quinine sulfate given at bedtime may be helpful in preventing recurrences. This agent is administered daily at bedtime until the patient has been free of night cramps for several days. Therapy is then discontinued and reinstituted when a new cluster of cramps recurs. In patients allergic to quinine, or who fail to respond, a trial of diphenhydramine (Benadryl) 12.5–50 mg may be of value. Other medications recommended for night cramps include vitamin E (238), meprobamate and other simple muscle relaxants, and verapamil (120 mg at bedtime) (237–240). Chloroquine phosphate at 250 mg daily for 2 or 3 weeks was reported to be effective within 1 to 3 weeks. Thereafter, 250–500 mg given once a week provided preventive benefit (241). We have also used hydroxychloroquine sulfate 200 mg daily for 2 weeks, then once a week, with good results. Patients with cramps may benefit from increased hydration as well.

If a structural disorder or muscle contraction is found, muscle stretching or strengthening exercises to the posterior leg and plantar fascia (Exercises 6.H and 6.J), and use of long-countered shoes and other proper footgear may be of value. If a cramp occurs, walking or leg-jiggling followed by leg elevation may be helpful.

The postphlebitic syndrome has a presentation of gradual onset of aching calf pain and dependent edema, a sensation of fullness in the calf, worsening with prolonged standing and walking, and relieved by rest and elevation. The presentation may mimic acute deep vein thrombosis. The pathogenesis probably reflects venous hypertension (242).

Restless Leg Syndrome (Ekbom syndrome): Painless, spontaneous, continuous leg movements are often of psychogenic origin, but may also accompany organic disease states. Hypoglycemia, hyperglycemia, hypothyroidism, neuropathies, spinal stenosis, uremia, anemia, and caffeinism have been associated with the syndrome (234, 243, 244). If accompanied by expressions of exquisite pain, they may be of hysterical origin. The use of low-dose tricyclic antidepressant medication and leg stretching exercises have been helpful for some (240). Other recommended treatment includes propranolol 40–120 mg or more (245); carbamazepine 100 mg or more at bedtime with gradually increasing dosage (246); or clonazepam 0.5–4.0 mg, with dosage increased by 1 mg per week, one hour before bedtime (247). For severely distressed patients, we have found higher doses of diazepam (20–50 mg) helpful when used for brief intervals. Levodopa in a titrated dosage (50–100 mg at bedtime) is recommended for elderly patients (248). Stretching exercises for the posterior leg muscles

should be performed before retiring (Exercises 6.H and 6.J). If symptoms persist, sclerotherapy for coexisting venous insufficiency may be helpful. Kanter (248a) has reported that 98% of 113 patients treated had initial benefit, and 72% maintained the benefit after 2 years. Doppler study may be indicated to identify patients who might benefit.

Night Starts: Although not limited to the leg, sudden jerking contractures of the limbs that occur shortly after falling asleep are common. They awaken the patient, and the severity of the jerky movement is frightening. They seldom recur after falling back to sleep. No definite cause is known. The condition is self-limited, and treatment is reassurance of the benign and temporary nature of the disturbance. Occasionally both night starts and restless leg syndrome coexist with severe emotional disturbance. Diazepam, up to 20 mg at bedtime, is often helpful.

Reflex Sympathetic Dystrophy: As described previously in Chapter 3, throbbing, burning, aching pain following trauma suggests reflex sympathetic dystrophy (RSD). The lower limb is less commonly involved, but when it occurs, diagnosis may be difficult. The pain quality is suggestive of the diagnosis if throbbing or burning occur. The limb is often discolored with dependent rubor or cyanotic mottling noted about the entire foot and lower foreleg. The skin is cool, and hyperhidrosis may be present. Diffuse swelling throughout the ankle and forefoot can occur.

Less commonly involved are the perineum (249) and knee regions (250). Severe knee pain following arthroscopy or trauma should suggest RSD. Relief with a sympathetic block can be used to confirm the diagnosis of RSD of the knee (251). Radiographic evidence of spotty osteoporosis is suggestive but not diagnostic. Bone scan results are variable with either decreased or increased uptake. A short course of prednisone, beginning with doses of 20–30 mg daily, may be beneficial. Patients in whom steroids are contraindicated or ineffective may benefit from a series of lumbar sympathetic blocks. Sympathetic drugs such as guanethidine 10 mg three times a day, or phenoxybenzamine 10 mg three times a day, are less consistently effective. Use of a transcutaneous electrical nerve stimulation (TENS) unit may provide symptomatic benefit, particularly in children (252, 253). Multiple physical and psychosocial interventions may be necessary. Topical doxepin and capsaicin cream is under investigation. Weightbearing is essential for recovery, and ambulation activities should be encouraged even when pain is present. Graded rehabilitation activities should be conducted under the guidance of an experienced physical therapist and should include desensitization, progressive weightbearing, muscle strengthening, stretching and lengthening, and balance retraining. If necessary, Bier blocks, described in Chapter 3, should be utilized before considering sympathectomy.

Nodules: Pseudorheumatoid nodules occur in the pretibial region in infants and children. No articular abnormalities are seen, and the nodule is painless. No treatment is necessary.

Surfer's nodules also may occur in the pretibial foreleg region. They result from activities in which the foreleg and the hyperextended ankle are brought in contact with a hard surface. Recurrent bumping from a surf board is a known cause. The lesions may resemble rheumatoid nodules. Avoiding surface contact is curative. Similar nodules can occur on children's forefeet if they repeatedly sit on their legs with their feet in plantarflexion and in contact with hardwood floors. Similarly, ''painter's bosses'' are nodules where the foreleg strikes the rungs of a ladder (255).

Differential diagnosis includes panniculitis due to infectious agents (tuberculosis, histoplasmosis) (256); erythema nodosum; sarcoidosis; streptococcal infections; peripheral manifestation of inflammatory bowel disease, occult neoplasm; and primary bone tumors of the foreleg.

Inflammatory fasciitis with swelling and redness of the lateral borders of the feet may result from local infection (usually unilateral) or may be part of systemic inflammatory diseases (usually bilateral). Nonseptic inflammatory diseases include eosinophilic fasciitis, Reiter's syndrome and other spondylarthritides, Kimura's disease (angiolymphoid hyperplasia) (in Asians), trichinosis, sarcoidosis, Löffler's syndrome, and vasculitis (257).

Adhesive Capsulitis of the Hip and Ankle: Adhesive capsulitis of the hip with painless limitation of movement has been reported in association with juvenile diabetes. The elastic tissue appears contracted (258). Treatment with physical therapy and possibly manipulation can be helpful.

An adhesive capsulitis of the ankle may follow an intraarticular fracture or other severe injury. Persistent pain and limitation of motion develop. Arthrography is a useful diagnostic test, revealing a decreased capacity of the joint. Instillation of a corticosteroid into the ankle and aggressive physical therapy may restore ankle motion (168). Physical therapy techniques should include the use of heat, cold, or electrotherapeutic modalities, progressive and extensive exercise to strengthen, stretch, and lengthen lower leg muscles (Exercises 6.H through 6.K, whichever is best tolerated, and 6.L and 6.N), manual techniques by an experienced physical therapist to improve tissue flexibility and align bony structures, and fabrication of orthotic devices as necessary for gait retraining.

Flexible Flatfeet: There are nearly as many terms for flatfeet as there are orthopaedists writing about flatfeet. The flexible type is the most common and important type (178). Blacks and Native Americans normally have flatfeet, yet they are not necessarily a precursor of painful feet. Asymptomatic persons with flatfeet should be left alone. Flatfeet, however, do require more intrinsic foot muscle contraction with each step of walking (259); nevertheless, the degree of flatness or pronation bears no correlation with future foot pain.

The flexible flatfoot, by definition, appears normal before it strikes the ground and bears weight; the arch flattens upon weightbearing. Symptoms, when present, include excessive muscular fatigue and aching and intolerance to prolonged walking or standing. In some patients walking improves symptoms. Symptoms often develop following foot injuries, illness, or a change in work habits that includes prolonged standing.

Physical examination reveals a normal arch at rest and loss of the longitudinal arch upon weightbearing, increased prominence of the navicular bone and the head of the talus, or an exostosis on the medial aspect of the foot. The calcaneus is everted (valgus position) as shown in Figure 6.31.

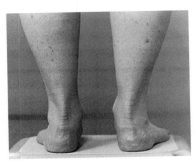

Figure 6.31. Pes planus (flatfeet) with eversion of the heels is best viewed posteriorly. Examination for pes planus should be part of the examination of any patient with a rheumatologic complaint in the lower extremity.

The determination that the foot (subtalar joint) can be inverted is essential in order to demonstrate the presence of a flexible rather than a rigid flatfoot. Tenderness may also be noted over the navicular bone, the inferior calcaneonavicular ligament, or the sole of the foot. While walking, the flatfooted patient raises the heel and toe together rather than using a heel-to-toe gait and demonstrates a splay-foot with the toes turned outward. This results from an attempt to prevent strain on the tarsal or metatarsal ligaments. The patient's gait has no ''spring'' to it. The shoe wears down more on the medial side of the sole than on the lateral sides. A corn on the fifth toe is further evidence of altered weightbearing. If the flatfoot is not evident from the frontal view, then it should become evident from a posterior view. In the rigid flatfoot, the arch is flat both at rest and upon weightbearing. The anterior and posterior tibial tendons and plantar muscles become stretched, and the tendo Achillis may become shortened. Painful reflex spasm of the fibularis (peroneal) muscles can result from a rigid flatfoot (259). The forefoot swings outward and the foot becomes rotated externally in relation to the leg. Occasionally, edema of the dorsum of the foot and tenderness over the medial aspect of the foot occur.

Etiology. The infant is born flatfooted and acquires an arch after a year or so of ambulation. The symptomatic flexible flatfoot may result from general hypermobility and a failure of postural muscle function to maintain the arch. In any event, it is probably not a result of improper footwear. Of patients with flatfeet,

70% have an inherited predisposition to flatfeet.

Laboratory and Radiologic Examination. Flatfeet may be a late manifestation of any inflammatory rheumatic disease, other features of which should be manifest at the time of examination. When confronted with a rigid flatfoot, special roentgenographic techniques are required to demonstrate bony bridging due to inflammatory or congenital defects of the tarsal region. CT scan or MRI provide definitive information.

Management. The most important rule in this section is: *''Do not treat asymptomatic flatfeet with a rigid arch support.''*

- Basic to the treatment of the symptomatic flatfoot is to move the center of gravity of the foot more to the outside of the foot and to remove points of pressure that are causing symptoms. This can be accomplished by the use of a firm heel counter and a tight, well-fitted instep with a low heel or a Thomas heel and a gradual shoe correction.
- Do not be hasty and order an expensive plastic rigid molded insert. Most patients require only a firm long-countered oxford shoe, and only a few require an insert.
- The examiner must determine whether the foot can be inverted, and if so an arch support can be tried. Such a support should not be rigid and should seldom exceed 1/8 inch of rise in the longitudinal arch. Felt-type padding is not a permanent insert, as it packs down over time. However, it is inexpensive and can be used in the shorter term to determine whether an insert will provide relief. If so, a permanent type should be prescribed for relief of pressure.
- The Thomas heel for the symptomatic flatfoot should provide a varus tilt to the heel in order to put the ankle in a more vertical alignment. The Thomas heel can extend to the midpart of the navicular bone so that it intersects the longitudinal axis of the fibula (Fig. 6.26).
- The shank of the shoe should remain flexible unless an appliance is being added to the shoe or if a hallux rigidus coexists.
- Only after failure of proper shoes without orthoses, followed by a trial of flexible

leather orthoses, should moldable soft plastic orthoses be considered. More often the latter inserts are used to treat structural foot disorders, such as forefoot or hindfoot varus, or valgus deformities. In general, the molded insert is not necessary in patients suffering from flexible flatfeet.

- Recognition of aggravating symptomatic factors such as work on concrete floors, prolonged standing, obesity, or coexisting plantar fasciitis is essential for effective management.
- Grasping exercises for intrinsic foot muscles and mobilizing exercises that plantarflex the foot and invert the ankle are helpful (Exercises 6.L, 6.M, 6.N). Crinkling newspaper with the feet on the floor and ankle rotation performed with the foot constantly cupped, first clockwise, then counterclockwise, may help in maintaining mobility in the involved soft tissues.

Outcome and Additional Suggestions. In our experience, patients with flexible flatfeet have self-limited episodes of pain brought about by prolonged weightbearing in improper shoes, excessive weight gain, carrying heavy objects, or moving to a home or workplace with a concrete floor. Often such episodes of pain are due to plantar fasciitis rather than flatfeet per se. Patients with chronic foot pain must be examined for the systemic disorders mentioned in association with plantar fasciitis. If symptoms have persisted despite conscientious use of proper foot gear and no other underlying cause has been found, the clinician should carefully reexamine the entire lower extremity and lumbar spine for evidence of other disorders, such as peripheral neuropathy, gout, and lumbar disc disease.

TOE DISORDERS

Bunions: The term "bunion" refers to soft tissue swelling over the first metatarsophalangeal joint. It is often mistakenly used to describe all disorders that enlarge the first metatarsophalangeal joint. Several of the more common disorders of this joint region as well as disorders affecting the other toes are discussed here.

Hallux Valgus Deformity: The patient with this common foot deformity presents with medial deviation of the head of the first metatarsal bone and lateral deviation of the great toe, often accompanied by a painful soft adventitial bursa. Because of this disorder, the second toe is forced dorsally and may develop into a hammer toe. Displacement of a sesamoid bone is often associated with this deformity. The condition occurs more commonly in cultures where shoes are worn, and in females. Generally the large toe is rotated so that the nail faces medially. The bursa overlying the medial bony prominence may become secondarily infected or acutely inflamed from the pressure of ill-fitting shoes. The patient often sees the physician not because of pain, but rather because of the inability to wear "dress shoes." (Refer to Table 6.6, on common shoe modifications.)

Hallux Rigidus: Progressive loss of motion of the great toe joint is associated with arthritis of the first metatarsophalangeal joint. This condition may follow hallux valgus deformity or trauma, or may be associated with pes planus, the pronated foot, or metatarsus varus primus deformity (260). Hallux rigidus is usually more disabling than hallux valgus deformity.

Treatment of hallux valgus without rigidus includes the use of shoes with an enlarged toe portion, the use of a felt ring, or the use of a plastic cap. Occasionally we have had a shoemaker remove the dorsal portion of the shoe and replace it with a wide, roomy vinyl covering. An extended metal shank can be added. Additional measures include pads of felt or rubber behind the first metatarsophalangeal joint, or arch supports with lateral and medial flanges to fit over medial and lateral bunions. High-heeled or soft flexible shoes are not well tolerated.

Surgical intervention should be performed only for symptoms and not for cosmetic reasons.

If the bursa over a hallux valgus deformity is swollen and tender, measures to keep the shoe covering from rubbing against it are imperative. In summer months the use of an open sandal may be helpful. When a shoe must be worn, the vamp should be cut with a linear slit through the lining just above the sole and over the bunion (261). We have found it advantageous for patients to cut a wide half-circle throughout the medial portion of an old laced shoe. This allows support for the hind foot, provides a rigid sole for the forefoot, and reduces friction across the medial surface of the first metatarsophalangeal joint.

In addition to these measures, treatment of hallux rigidus requires the use of a thick and rigid shoe sole (262). The clinician may also try a long rocker bar to add rigidity to the sole (192). On occasion, a local anesthetic–corticosteroid injection into the region of a dorsal exostosis at the first metatarsophalangeal joint line is helpful. Stretching the toe downward for a moment or so, morning and evening, has also been helpful. Joint fusion, debridement, arthroplasty, or other surgical procedures may be necessary.

Hammer Toe Deformity: This disorder is usually acquired as a result of pressure from hallux valgus or from tight shoes, or it may be congenital. It is usually a bilateral deformity with the second toe nearly always involved. The toe is flexed at the proximal interphalangeal (PIP) joint and the tip of the toe points downward; thus the middle and distal phalanges of the second toe are flexed on the proximal phalanges. A painful bursa and callus often form over the dorsal aspect of the flexed proximal interphalangeal joint. The toe tip becomes broadened and thick. An "X" incision in the shoe vamp over the pressure point is helpful (261). When keratoses are also present, surgical correction is often necessary. In children with congenital hammer toe, treatment is best handled with adhesive strapping and the use of shoes with an adequate depth of toe box.

None of these toe disorders results in soft tissue swelling of the toe. When swelling occurs, sepsis (felon or whitlow), systemic rheumatic disease (e.g., rheumatoid arthritis, psoriatic arthritis), and other disease entities (e.g., gout, tumors) should be considered.

Table 6.6 (above) presents possible shoe modifications for various foot problems. Combinations of these modifications may be indicated depending upon careful assessment of the individual problem. Information for moldable plastics or extra-depth shoes may be obtained from the following sources:

AliMed, 138 Prince Street, Boston, Massachusetts 02113

P. W. Minor & Son Inc., Batavia, New York 14020

Alden Shoe Company, Taunton Street, Middleborough, Massachusetts 02346

REFERENCES

1. Micheli LF, Fehlandt AF: Overuse injuries to tendons and apophyses in children and adolescents. Clin Sports Med 11(4):713–726, 1992.
2. Grossman RB, Nicholas JA: Common disorders of the knee. Orthop Clin North Am 8:619–640, 1977.
3. Trayoff R, Trapp R: Extra-articular pain syndrome: frequency of osteoarthritis of the knees and effect on responsiveness to intra-articular corticosteroids. (Abstract #246) Arthritis Rheum 25(4) [Suppl], 1982.
4. Larsson L, Baum J: The syndrome of anserine bursitis: an overlooked diagnosis. Arthritis Rheum 28:1062–1065, 1985.
5. Fiatarone MA, Marks EC, Ryan MD, et al.: High-intensity strength training in nonagenarians. JAMA 263:3029–3034, 1990.
6. Benson R, Fowler PD: Treatment of Weber-Christian disease. Br Med J 2:615–616, 1964.
7. Swezey RL: Transient osteoporosis of the hip, foot, and knee. Arthritis Rheum 13:858–868, 1970.
8. Duncan H, Frame B, Frost HM, Arnstein AR: Migratory osteolysis of the lower extremities. Ann Intern Med 66:1165–1173, 1967.
9. Aaron JE, Gallagher JC, Anderson J, et al.: Frequency of osteomalacia and osteoporosis in fractures of the proximal femur. Lancet 1:229–233, 1974.
10. Kim HJ, Kozin F, Johnson RP, Hines R: Reflex sympathetic dystrophy syndrome of the knee following meniscectomy. Arthritis Rheum 22: 177–181, 1979.
11. Gordon GC: Traumatic prepatellar neuralgia. J Bone Joint Surg 34B:41–44, 1952.
12. Hughston JC, Andrews JR, Cross MJ, Moschi A: Classification of knee ligament instabilities. J Bone Joint Surg 58A:159–172, 1976.
13. Dehaven KE, Dolan WA, Mayer PJ: Chondromalacia patellae and the painful knee. Am Fam Physician 21:117–124, 1980.
14. Cooke TDV, Chir B, Price N, et al.: The inwardly pointing knee: an unrecognized problem of external rotational malalignment. Clin Orthop 260: 56–60, 1990.
15. Houston CS, Swischuk LE: Varus and valgus—no wonder they are confused. N Engl J Med 302:471–472, 1980.

16. Sharrard WJ: Aetiology and pathology of beat knee. Br J Ind Med 20:24–31, 1963.

17. Post WR, Fulkerson JP: Anterior knee pain: a symptom, not a diagnosis. Bull Rheum Dis 42(2):5–7, 1993.

18. Noyes FR, Cummings JF, Grood ES, et al.: The diagnosis of knee motion limits, subluxations, and ligament injury. Am J Sports Med 19(2): 163–171, 1991.

19. Daniel DM: Assessing the limits of knee motion. Am J Sports Med 19(2):139–147, 1991.

20. Katz JW, Fingeroth RJ: The diagnostic accuracy of ruptures of the anterior cruciate ligament comparing the Lachman test, the anterior drawer sign, and the pivot shift test in acute and chronic knee injuries. Am J Sports Med 14(1):88–91, 1986.

21. Kennedy JC, Roth JH, Walker DM: Posterior cruciate ligament injuries. Orthop Digest 7: 19–31, 1979.

22. Fowler PJ, Lubliner JA: The predictive value of five clinical signs in the evaluation of meniscal pathology. Arthroscopy 5(3):184–186, 1989.

23. Zeman SC, Nielsen MW: Osteochondritis dissecans of the knee. Orthop Rev 7:101–112, 1978.

24. Kirk JA, Ansell BM, Bywaters EGL: The hypermobility syndrome: musculoskeletal complaints associated with generalized joint hypermobility. Ann Rheum Dis 26:419–425, 1967.

25. Howorth BM: General relaxation of the ligaments. Clin Orthop 30:133–143, 1963.

26. Muckle DS: Associated factors in recurrent groin and hamstring injuries. Br J Sports Med 15: 37–39, 1982.

27. Gitschlag KF, Sandler MA, Madraso BL, Hricak H, Eyler WR: Disease in the femoral triangle: sonographic appearance. AJR 139:515–519, 1982.

28. Carter C, Wilkinson J: Persistent joint laxity and congenital dislocation of the hip. J Bone Joint Surg 46B:40–45, 1964.

29. Lyons JC, Peterson LFA: The snapping iliopsoas tendon. Mayo Clin Proc 59:327–329, 1984.

30. Jacobson T, Allen WC: Surgical correction of the snapping iliopsoas tendon. Am J Sports Med 18(5):470–474, 1990.

31. Swezey RL, Spiegel TM: Evaluation and treatment of local musculoskeletal disorders in elderly patients. Geriatrics 34:56–75, 1979.

32. Roseff R, Canoso JJ: Femoral osteonecrosis following soft tissue corticosteroid infiltration. Am J Med 77:1119–1120. 1984.

33. Brooker AF Jr: The surgical approach to refractory trochanteric bursitis. Johns Hopkins Med J 145:98–100, 1979.

33a. Flanagan FL, Sant S, Coughlan RJ, et al.: Symptomatic enlarged iliopsoas bursae in the presence of a normal plain hip radiograph. Br J Rheumatol 34:365–369, 1995.

34. Toohey AK, LaSalle TL, Martinez S, Polisson RP: Iliopsoas bursitis: clinical features, radiographic findings, and disease associations. Semin Arthritis Rheum 20(1):41–47, 1990.

35. Muckle DS: Recurrent hamstring injuries as an expression of lumbar stress syndromes. J Orthop Rheumatol 3:75–82, 1990.

36. Leach RE: Running injuries of the knee. Orthopedics 5:1358–1378, 1982.

37. Weiser HI: Semimembranosus insertion syndrome: a treatable and frequent cause of persistent knee pain. Arch Phys Med Rehabil 60:317–319, 1979.

38. Ray JM, Clancy WG Jr, Lemon RA: Semimembranosus tendinitis: an overlooked cause of medial knee pain. Am J Sports Med 16:347–351, 1988.

39. Nakano KK: Peripheral nerve entrapments, repetitive strain disorder, and occupation-related syndromes. Curr Opin Rheumatol 2:253–269, 1990.

40. Hardaker WT, Whipple TL, Bassett FH: Diagnosis and treatment of the plica syndrome of the knee. J Bone Joint Surg 62A:221–225, 1980.

41. Blatz DJ, Fleming R, McCarroll J: Suprapatellar plica: a study of their occurrence and role in internal derangement of the knee in active duty personnel. Orthopedics 4(2):181–184, 1981.

42. Rovere GD, Adair DM: Medial synovial shelf plica syndrome: treatment by intraplical steroid injection. Am J Sports Med 13(6):382–386, 1985.

43. Whipple TL, Hardaker WT: Symptomatic plica and shelf syndromes in the knee. Orthop Review 14:61–64, 1985.

44. Reid GD, Glasgow M, Gordon DA, Wright TA: Pathological plicae of the knee mistaken for arthritis. J Rheumatol 7:573–576, 1980.

45. Munsinger U, Ruckstuhl J, Scherrer H, Gschwend N: Internal derangement of the knee joint due to pathologic synovial folds: the mediopatellar plica syndrome. Clin Orthop 155:59–64, 1981.

46. Barber FA, Sutker AN: Iliotibial band syndrome. Sports Med 14(2):144–148, 1992.

47. Renne JW: The iliotibial band friction syndrome. J Bone Joint Surg 57A:1110–1111, 1975.

48. Noble CA: Iliotibial band friction syndrome in runners. Am J Sports Med 8:232–234, 1980.

49. Martens M, Libbrecht P, Burssens A: Surgical treatment of the iliotibial band friction syndrome. Am J Sports Med 17(5):651–654, 1990.

50. Trujeque L, Spohn P, Bankhurst A, et al.: Patellar whiskers and acute calcific quadriceps tendinitis in a general hospital population. Arthritis Rheum 20:1409–1412, 1977.

51. Ramon FA, Degryse HR, DeSchepper AM, Van Marck EA: Calcific tendinitis of the vastus lateralis muscle. Int Skeletal Soc 20: 21–23, 1991.

52. Steidl S, Ditmar R: Soft tissue calcification treated with local and oral magnesium therapy. Magnesium Research 3(2):113–119, 1990.

53. Stevens MP, Sack KE: Prepatellar calcifications from repeated kneeling. N Engl J Med 321(3): 194, 1989.

54. Yates C, Grana WA: Patellofemoral pain: a prospective study. Orthopedics 9:663–666, 1986.

55. Johnson RP: Lateral facet syndrome of the patella. Clin Orthop 238:148–158, 1989.

56. Abernethy PJ, Townsend PR, Rose RM, Radin EL: Is chondromalacia patellae a separate clinical entity? J Bone Joint Surg 608:205–210, 1978.

57. Goodfellow J, Hungerford DS, Woods C: Patello-femoral joint mechanics and pathology. J Bone Joint Surg 58B:291–299, 1976.

58. Fairbank JCT, Pynsent PB, van Poortvliet JA, Phillips H: Mechanical factors in the incidence of knee pain in adolescents and young adults. J Bone Joint Surg 66B:685–693, 1984.

59. Henry JH: Conservative treatment of patello-femoral subluxation. Clin Sports Med 8(2): 261–278, 1989.

60. Inoue M, Shino K, Hirose H, et al.: Subluxation of the patella: computed tomography analysis of patellofemoral congruence. J Bone Joint Surg 70:1331–1337, 1988.

61. Shellock FG, Mink JH, Deutsch AL, Fox JM: Patellar tracking abnormalities: clinical experience with kinematic MR imaging in 130 patients. Radiology 172:799–804, 1989.

62. Insall J: Current concepts review: patella pain. J Bone Joint Surg 64:147–152, 1982.

63. Radin EL: Chondromalacia of the patella. Bull Rheum Dis 34:1–6, 1984.

64. Bergenudd H, Nilsson B, Lindgarde F: Knee pain in middle age and its relationship to occupational work load and psychosocial factors. Clin Orthop 245:210–215, 1989.

65. Martens M, Wouters P, Burssens A, Mulier JC: Patellar tendinitis: pathology and results of treatment. Acta Orthop Scand 53:445–450, 1982.

66. Podesta L, Sherman MF, Bonamo JR: Bilateral simultaneous rupture of the infrapatellar tendon in a recreational athlete. Am J Sports Med 19(3): 325–327, 1991.

67. Devereaux MD, Lachmann SM, Thomas DP, et al.: Thermographic diagnosis in athletes with patellofemoral arthralgia. J Bone Joint Surg 68B: 42–44, 1986.

67a. Cerny K: Vastus media oblique/vastus lateralis muscle activity ratios for selected exercises in persons with and without patellofemoral pain syndrome. Phys Ther 75:672–683, 1995.

68. Ismail AM, Balakrishnan R, Rajakumar MK: Rupture of patellar ligament after steroid infiltration: report of a case. J Bone Joint Surg 51B: 503–505, 1969.

69. Whitelaw GP, Rullo DJ, Markowitz HD, et al.: A conservative approach to anterior knee pain. Clin Orthop 246:234–237, 1989.

70. Wissinger HA: Chondromalacia patella: a non-operative treatment program. Orthopedics 5: 315–316, 1982.

71. Malone T, Blackburn TA, Wallace LA: Knee rehabilitation. Phys Ther 60:1602–1610, 1980.

72. Grana WA, O'Donoghue DH: Patellar-tendon transfer by the slot-block method for recurrent subluxation and dislocation of the patella. J Bone Joint Surg 59A:736–741, 1977.

73. Williams PH, Trzil KP: Management of meralgia paresthetica. J Neurosurg 74:76–80, 1991.

74. Fabbriciani C, Schiavone PA, Delcogliano A: Arthroscopic lateral release useful for selected patellofemoral conditions. Arthroscopy 8: 531–536, 1992.

75. Aglietti P, Pisaneschi A, Buzzi R, et al.: Arthroscopic lateral release for patellar pain or instability. Arthroscopy 5(3): 176–183, 1989.

76. Perrild C, Hejgaard N, Rosenklint A: Chondromalacia patellae. Acta Orthop Scand 53: 131–134, 1982.

77. Worrell RV: the diagnosis of disorders of the patellofemoral joint. Orthop Review 10:73–76, 1981.

78. Radin EL: Anterior knee pain, the need for a specific diagnosis: stop calling it chondromalacia! Orthop Review 14:33–39, 1985.

79. Davies SG, Baudouin CJ, King JB, Perry JD: Ultrasound, computed tomography, and magnetic resonance imaging in patellar tendinitis. Clin Radiol 43:52–56, 1991.

80. Speer KP, Spritzer CE, Goldner JL, Garrett WE: Magnetic resonance imaging of traumatic knee articular cartilage injuries. Am J Sports Med 19(4):396–402, 1991.

81. Kriegsman J: Negative MRI findings in knee injury: clinical implications. Contemp Orthop 22(5):549–555, 1991.

82. Kornick J, Trefelner E, McCarthy S, et al.: Meniscal abnormalities in the asymptomatic population at MR imaging. Radiology 177(2):463–465, 1990.

83. Watanabe AT, Carter BC, Teitelbaum GP, Bradley WG: Common pitfalls in magnetic resonance imaging of the knee. J Bone Joint Surg 71A(6): 857–862, 1989.

84. Soudry M, Lanir A, Angel D, et al.: Anatomy of the normal knee as seen by magnetic resonance imaging. J Bone Joint Surg 68:117–120, 1986.

85. Hull RG, Rennie JN, Eastmond CJ, et al.: Nuclear magnetic resonance (NMR) tomographic imaging for popliteal cysts in rheumatoid arthritis. Ann Rheum Dis 43:56–59, 1984.

86. Ott JW, Clancy WG Jr: Functional knee braces. Orthopedics 16(2):171–176, 1993.

87. Bassett LW, Jaswinder SG, Seeger LL: Magnetic resonance imaging of knee trauma. Skeletal Radiol 19:401–405, 1990.

88. Fisher SP, Fox JM, Del Pizzo W, et al.: Accuracy of diagnoses from magnetic resonance imaging of the knee. J Bone Joint Surg 73A(1):2–10, 1991.

89. Kelly MA, Flock TJ, Kimmel JA, et al.: MR imaging of the knee: clarification of its role. Arthroscopy 7(1):78–85, 1991.

90. Johnson LL: Impact of diagnostic arthroscopy on the clinical judgement of an experienced arthroscopist. Clin Orthop 167:75–83, 1982.

91. Sprague NF III: Arthroscopic surgery: degenerative and traumatic flap tears of the meniscus. Contemp Orthop 9:23–46, 1984.

92. Pettrone FA: Meniscectomy: arthrotomy versus arthroscopy. Am J Sports Med 10:355–359, 1982.

93. Seale KS, Haynes DW, Nelson CL: The effect of meniscectomy on knee stability. (Abstract #42) Arthritis Rheum 25(4) [Suppl], 1982.

94. Hadied AM: An unusual complication of arthroscopy: a fistula between the knee and the prepatellar bursa. J Bone Joint Surg 66A:624, 1984.

95. Lindenbaum BL: Complications of knee joint arthroscopy. Clin Orthop 160:158, 1981.

96. Monaco BR, Noble HB, Bachman DC: Incomplete tears of the anterior cruciate ligament and knee locking. JAMA 247:1582–1584, 1982.

97. Hendryson IE: Bursitis in the region of the fibular collateral ligament. J Bone Joint Surg 28: 446–450, 1946.

98. Moschcowitz E: Bursitis of sartorius bursa: an undescribed malady simulating chronic arthritis. JAMA 109:1362–1364, 1937.

99. Brookler MI, Mongan WS: Relief for the pain of anserina bursitis in the arthritic knee. Cal Med 119:8–10, 1973.

100. Quale FB, Robinson MP: An operation for chronic prepatellar bursitis. J Bone Joint Surg 58B:504–506, 1976.

101. Stuttle FL: The no-name and no-fame bursa. Clin Orthop 15:197–199, 1959.

102. Voorneveld C, Arenson AM, Fam AG: Anserine bursal distention: diagnosis by ultrasonography and computed tomography. Arthritis Rheum 32(10):1335–1337, 1989.

103. Pavlov H, Goldman AB: The popliteus bursa: an indicator of subtle pathology. Am J Rheumatol 134:313–321, 1980.

104. Lotke PA, Ecker ML, Alavi A: Painful knees in older patients. J Bone Joint Surg 59A: 617–621, 1977.

105. Ho G Jr, Su EY: Antibiotic therapy of septic bursitis: its implication in the treatment of septic arthritis. Arthritis Rheum 24:905–911, 1981.

106. Kerr R, Frey C: MR imaging in tarsal tunnel syndrome. J Comput Assist Tomogr 15(2): 280–286, 1991.

107. Dinham JM: Popliteal cysts in children: the case against surgery. J Bone Joint Surg 57B:69–71, 1975.

108. Wigley RD: Popliteal cysts: variations on a theme of Baker. Semin Arthritis Rheum 12: 1–10, 1982.

109. Gompels BM, Darlington LG: Evaluation of popliteal cysts and painful calves with ultrasonography: comparison with arthrography. Ann Rheum Dis 41:355–359, 1982.

110. Vaughan BJ: CT of swollen legs. Clin Radiol 41:24–30, 1990.

111. Soriano ER, Catoggio LJ: Baker's cysts, pseudothrombophlebitis, pesudo-pseudothrombophlebitis: where do we stand? Clin Exp Rheumatol 8:107–112, 1990.

112. Halperin N, Axer A: Semimembranosus tenosynovitis. Orthop Rev 9:72–75, 1980.

113. James SJ, Bates BT, Osternig LR: Injuries to runners. Am J Sports Med 6:40–50, 1978.

114. Baugher WH, Balady GJ, Warren RF, Marshall JL: Injuries of the musculoskeletal system in runners. Contemp Orthop 1:46–54, 1979.

115. Brady DM: Running injuries. Clinical Symposium (CIBA) 32(4):2–36, 1980.

116. Moore MP: Shin splints: diagnosis, management, prevention. Postgrad Med 83(1):199–210, 1988.

117. Manoli A II, Weber TG: Fasciotomy of the foot: an anatomical study with special reference to release of the calcaneal compartment. Foot Ankle 10(5):267–275, 1990.

118. Fakhhouri AJ, Manoli A II: Acute foot compartment syndromes. J Orthop Trauma 6:223–228, 1992.

119. Myerson MS: Management of compartment syndromes of the foot. Clin Orthop 271: 239–248, 1991.

120. Matsen FA: Compartmental syndromes. N Engl J Med 300:1210–1211, 1979.

121. Matsen FA: Compartmental syndromes. Hosp Pract 15:113–117, 1980.

122. Detmer DE, Sharpe K, Sufit RL, Girdley FM: Chronic compartment syndrome: diagnosis, management, and outcomes. Am Orthop Soc Sports Med 13:162–170, 1985.

123. Mubarak SJ, Hargens AR, Owen CA, et al.: The wick catheter technique for measurement of intramuscular pressure. J Bone Joint Surg 58: 1016–1019, 1976.

124. Mubarak SJ, Owen CA: Double-incision fasciotomy of the leg for decompression in compartment syndromes. J Bone Joint Surg 59: 184–187, 1977.

125. Turnipseed W, Detmer DE, Girdley F: Chronic compartment syndrome: an unusual cause for claudication. Ann Surg 210(4):557–563, 1989.

126. Pedowitz RA, Hargens AR, Mubarak SJ, Gershuni DH: Modified criteria for the objective diagnosis of chronic compartment syndrome of the leg. Am J Sports Med 18(1):35–40, 1990.

127. Wiley JP, Short WB, Wiseman DA, Miller SD: Ultrasound catheter placement for deep posterior compartment pressure measurements in chronic compartment syndrome. Am J Sports Med 18(1):74–79, 1990.

128. Black KP, Taylor DE: Current concepts in the treatment of common compartment syndromes in athletes. Sports Med 15(6):408–418, 1993.

129. Dayton P, Goldman FD, Barton E: Compartment pressure in the foot: analysis of normal values and measurement technique. J Am Podiatry Med Assoc 80(10):521–525, 1990.

130. Bartolomei FJ: Compartment syndrome of the dorsal aspect of the foot. J Am Podiatr Med Assoc 81(10):556–559, 1991.

131. Amendola A, Rorabeck CH, Vellett D, et al.: The use of magnetic resonance imaging in exertional compartment syndromes. Am J Sports Med 18(1):29–34, 1990.

132. Chandler TJ, Kibler WB: A biomechanical approach to the prevention, treatment, and reha-

bilitation of plantar fasciitis. Sports Med 15(5): 344–352, 1993.

133. Warren BL: Plantar fasciitis in runners: treatment and prevention. Sports Med 10(5): 338–345, 1990.

134. Kibler WB, Goldberg C, Chandler TJ: Functional biomechanical deficits in running athletes with plantar fasciitis. Am J Sports Med 19(1): 66–71, 1991.

135. Macera CA, Pate RR, Powell KE, et al.: Predicting lower-extremity injuries among habitual runners. Arch Intern Med 149:2565–2568, 1989.

136. Warren RF, Sullivan D: Stress fractures in athletes: recognizing the subtle signs. J Musculoskel Med 1(March):33–35, 1984.

137. Gross ML, Davlin LB, Evanski PM: Effectiveness of orthotic shoe inserts in the long-distance runner. Am J Sports Med 19(4):409–412, 1991.

138. Riegler HF: Orthotic devices for the foot. Orthop Rev 16(5):293–303, 1987.

139. Norfray JF, Schlachter L, Kernahan WT Jr, et al.: Early confirmation of stress fractures in joggers. JAMA 243:1647–1649, 1980.

140. Kier R, McCarthy S, Dietz MJ, Rudicel S: MR appearance of painful conditions of the ankle. Radiographics 11(3):401–414, 1991.

141. Sobel M, Bohne WH, Markisz JA: Cadaver correlation of peroneal tendon changes with magnetic resonance imaging. Foot Ankle 11(6): 384–388, 1991.

142. Cardone BW, Erickson SJ, Den Hartog BD, Carrera GF: MRI of injury to the lateral collateral ligamentous complex of the ankle. J Comput Assist Tomogr 17(1):102–107, 1993.

143. Hopkinson WJ, St Pierre P, Ryan JB, et al.: Syndesmosis sprains of the ankle. Foot Ankle 10:325–330, 1990.

144. Swain RA, Holt WS Jr: Ankle injuries: tips from sports medicine physicians. Postgrad Med 93(3):91–100, 1993.

145. Boytim MJ, Fischer DA, Neumann L: Syndesmotic ankle sprains. Am J Sports Med 19(3): 294–298, 1991.

146. Taylor DC, Englehardt DL, Bassett FH III: Syndesmosis sprains of the ankle: the influence of heterotopic ossification. Am J Sports Med 20(2):146–150, 1992.

147. Marder RA: Current methods for the evaluation of ankle ligament injuries. J Bone Joint Surg 76A:1103–1111, 1994.

148. Stanley KL: Ankle sprains are always more than "just a sprain." Postgrad Med 89(1):251–255, 1991.

149. Harrington KD: Degenerative arthritis of the ankle secondary to long-standing lateral ligament instability. J Bone Joint Surg 61: 354–361, 1979.

150. Cass JR, Morrey BF: Ankle instability: current concepts, diagnosis, and treatment. Mayo Clin Proc 59:165–170, 1984.

151. Parvin RW, Ford LT: Stenosing tenosynovitis of the common peroneal tendon sheath. J Bone Joint Surg 38A:1352–1357, 1956.

152. Harrington AC, Mellette JR Jr: Hernias of the anterior tibialis muscle: case report and review of the literature. J Am Acad Dermatol 16:123–124, 1994.

153. Supple KML, Hanft FR, Murphy BJ, et al.: Posterior tibial tendon dysfunction. Semin Arthritis Rheum 22:106–113, 1992.

154. Zivot ML, Pearl SH, Pupp GR, Pupp JB: Stenosing peroneal tenosynovitis. J Foot Surg 28(3): 220–224, 1989.

155. D'Ambrosia RD: Conservative management of metatarsal and heel pain in the adult foot. Orthopedics 10(1):137–142, 1987.

156. Sartoris DJ, Resnick DL: Tarsal coalition. Arthritis Rheum 28:331–338, 1985.

157. Maclellan GE, Vyvyan B: Management of pain beneath the heel and Achilles tendonitis with visco-elastic heel inserts. J Sports Med 165: 117–121, 1981.

158. O'Reilly MA, Massouh H: Pictorial review: the sonographic diagnosis of pathology in the Achilles tendon. Clin Radiol 48:202–206, 1993.

158a. Gerster JC: Achilles tendinitis as a severe clinical feature of diffuse idiopathic skeletal hyperostosis (Letter). J Rheumatol 22:1212–1214, 1995.

159. Frey C, Rosenberg Z, Shereff MJ, Kim H: The retrocalcaneal bursa: anatomy and bursography. Foot Ankle 13(4):203–207, 1992.

160. Canoso JJ, Wohlgethan JR, Newberg AH, Goldsmith MR: Aspiration of the retrocalcaneal bursa. Ann Rheum Dis 43:308–312, 1984.

161. Maffulli N, Dymond NP, Capasso G: Ultrasonographic findings in subcutaneous rupture of Achilles tendon. J Sports Med Phys Fitness 29(4):365–368, 1989.

162. Weinstabl R, Stiskal M, Heuhold A, et al.: Classifying calcaneal tendon injury according to MRI findings. J Bone Joint Surg 73B(4): 683–685, 1991.

163. Dickinson PH, Coutts MB, Woodward EP, Handler D: Tendo Achillis bursitis. J Bone Joint Surg 48:77–81, 1966.

164. Fiamengo SA, Warren RF, Marshall JL, et al.: Posterior heel pain associated with a calcaneal step and Achilles tendon calcification. Clin Orthop 167:203–211, 1982.

165. Layfer LF: "Last" bursitis: a cause of ankle pain. Arthritis Rheum 23:261, 1980.

166. Kleiger B: The posterior calcaneal tubercle impingement syndrome. Orthop Rev 17(5): 487–493, 1988.

167. Heneghan M, Pavlow H: The Haglund painful heel syndrome. Clin Orthop Rel Res 187: 228–234, 1984.

168. Goldman AB, Katz MC, Freiberger RH: Posttraumatic adhesive capsulitis of the ankle: arthrographic diagnosis. Am J Roentgenol 127: 585–588, 1976.

169. Sorrells RB: Heel pain. J Arkansas Med Soc 74:494–497, 1978.
170. Gerster JC, Saudan Y, Fallet GH: Talalgia: a review of 30 severe cases. J Rheumatol 5:210–216, 1978.
171. Furey JG: Plantar fasciitis: the painful heel syndrome. J Bone Joint Surg 57A:672–673, 1975.
172. Michetti ML, Jacobs SA: Calcaneal heel spurs: etiology, treatment, and a new surgical approach. J Foot Surg 22:234–239, 1983.
173. Katoh Y, Chao ETS, Morrey BF, Laughman RK: Objective technique for evaluating painful heel syndrome and its treatment. Foot Ankle 3:227–237, 1983.
174. Spiegl PV, Johnson KA: Heel pain syndrome: which treatments to choose? J Musculoskel Med 1:66–72, 1984.
175. Satku K, Pho RWH, Wee A, Path MRC: Painful heel syndrome: an unusual cause. J Bone Joint Surg 66A:607–609, 1984.
176. Shelley WB, Rawnsley HM: Painful feet due to herniation of fat. JAMA 205:308–309, 1968.
177. Siebert JS, Mann RA: Dermatology and disorders of the toenails. In: RA Mann, ed. DuVries' Surgery of the foot. 4th Ed. St Louis: CV Mosby, 1978.
178. Jahss MH: The abnormal plantigrade foot. Orthop Rev 8:31–34, 1978.
179. Dagnall JC, Calabro JJ: Chiropody (podiatry) and arthritis. Bull Rheum Dis 23:692, 695, 1972.
180. Fry RM: Dance and orthopaedics—each type has its special medical problems. Orthop Rev 12:49–56, 1983.
181. Campbell JW, Inman VT: Treatment of plantar fasciitis and calcaneal spurs with the UC-BL shoe insert. Clin Orthop 103:57–62, 1974.
182. Riggs BL, Hodgson SF, Hoffman DL, et al.: Treatment of primary osteoporosis with fluoride and calcium. JAMA 243:446–449, 1980.
183. Paice EW, Hoffbrand BI: Nutritional osteomalacia presenting with plantar fasciitis. J Bone Joint Surg 69B(1):38–40, 1987.
183a. Dasqupta B, Bowles J: Use of technetium scintigraphy to locate the steroid injection site in plantar fasciitis. (Abstract #581) Arthritis Rheum 38(9 Suppl):S250, 1995.
183b. Helie O, Dubayle P, Boyer B, Pharaboz C: Magnetic resonance imaging of lesions of the superficial plantar fasciitis. J Radiol 76:37–41, 1995.
184. Wapner KL, Sharkey PF: The use of night splints for treatment of recalcitrant plantar fasciitis. Foot Ankle 12(3):135–137, 1991.
184a. Ryan J: Use of posterior night splints in the treatment of plantar fasciitis. Am Fam Physician 52(3):891–898, 901–902, 1995.
185. Tooms RE, Griffin JW, Green S, Cagle K: Effect of viscoelastic insoles on pain. Orthopedics 10(8):1143–1147, 1987.
186. Bordelon RL: Practical guide to foot orthoses. J Musculoskel Med 6:71–87, 1989.

186a. Sellman JR: Plantar fascia rupture associated with corticosteroid injection. Foot Ankle 15:376–381, 1994.
187. Lester DK, Buchanan JR: Surgical treatment of plantar fasciitis. Clin Orthop 186:202–205, 1984.
188. Daly PJ, Kitaoka HB, Chao EYS: Plantar fasciotomy for intractable plantar fasciitis: clinical results and biomechanical evaluation. Foot Ankle 13(4):188–195, 1992.
189. Kahn C, Bishop JO, Tullow HSS: Plantar fascia release and heel spur excision via plantar route. Orthop Rev 4:69–72, 1985.
190. Miller WE: Nonoperative approach to foot problems. Orthop Rev 7:19–21, 1978.
191. Gould JS: Metatarsalgia. Orthop Clin North Am 20(4):553–562, 1989.
192. Milgram JE, Jacobson MA: Footgear: therapeutic modifications of sole and heel. Orthop Rev 7:57–62, 1978.
193. Epps CH: Fractures of the forepart and midpart of the adolescent foot. Orthop Rev 7:63–69, 1978.
194. Bossley CJ, Cairney PC: The intermetatarsophalangeal bursa: its significance in Morton's metatarsalgia. J Bone Joint Surg 62:184–187, 1980.
195. Greenfield J, Rea J, Illfeld FW: Morton's interdigital neuroma: indications for treatment by local injections versus surgery. Clin Orthop 185:142–145, 1984.
196. Gross RH: Foot pain in children. Pediatr Clin N Am 24:813–823, 1977.
197. Feldman RG, Goldman R, Keyserling WM: Peripheral nerve entrapment syndromes and ergonomic factors. Am J Ind Med 4:661–681, 1983.
198. Macnicol MF, Thompson WJ: Idiopathic meralgia paresthetica. Clin Orthop 254:270–274, 1990.
199. Guo-Xiang J, Wei Dong X, Ai-Hao W: Spinal stenosis with meralgia paraesthetica. J Bone Joint Surg 70B(2):272–273, 1988.
199a. Spevak MK, Prevec TS: A noninvasive method of neurography in meralgia paraesthetica. Muscle Nerve 18:601–605, 1995.
200. Williams RM, Dymond JB Jr: New outpatient treatment of recurrent patellar dislocations. Orthop Rev (21):1329–1332, 1992.
201. Swezey RL: Pseudo-radiculopathy in subacute trochanteric bursitis of the subgluteus maximus bursa. Arch Phys Med Rehabil 57:387–390, 1976.
202. Banerjee T, Hall CD: Sciatic entrapment neuropathy. J Neurosurg 45:216–217, 1976.
203. Brooke MM, Heard DL, deLateur BJ, et al.: Heterotopic ossification and peripheral nerve entrapment: early diagnosis and excision. Arch Phys Med Rehabil 72:425–429, 1991.
204. Hemler DE, Ward WK, Karstetter KW, Bryant PM: Saphenous nerve entrapment caused by pes anserine bursitis mimicking stress fracture of

the tibia. Arch Phys Med Rehabil 72: 336–337, 1991.

205. Kernohan J, Levack B, Wilson JN: Entrapment of the superficial peroneal nerve. J Bone Joint Surg 67B:60–61, 1985.

206. Lowdon IM: Superficial peroneal nerve entrapment: a case report. J Bone Joint Surg 67B: 58–59, 1985.

207. Keck C: The tarsal tunnel syndrome. J Bone Joint Surg 44:180–182, 1962.

208. Goodgold J, Kopell HP, Spielholz NI: The tarsal tunnel syndrome. N Engl J Med 273: 742–745, 1965.

209. Wilemon WK: Tarsal tunnel syndrome. Orthop Rev 8:111–118, 1979.

210. Janecki CJ, Dovberg JL: Tarsal tunnel syndrome caused by neurilemoma of the medial plantar nerve. J Bone Joint Surg 59:127–128, 1977.

211. McGill DA: Tarsal tunnel syndrome. Proc R Soc Med 57:23–24, 1964.

212. Mackinnon SE, Dellon AL, Daneshvar A: Tarsal tunnel syndrome: histopathologic examination of a human posterior tibial nerve. Contemp Orthop 9:43–48, 1984.

213. Gretter TE, Wilde AH: Pathogenesis, diagnosis, and treatment of the tarsal tunnel syndrome. Cleve Clin Q 37:23–29, 1970.

214. Fu R, DeLisa JA, Kraft GH: Motor nerve latencies through the tarsal tunnel in normal adult subjects. Arch Phys Med Rehabil 61: 243–248, 1980.

215. Zeiss J, Saddemi SR, Ebraheim NA: MR imaging of the peroneal tunnel. J Comput Assist Tomogr 13:840–844, 1989.

216. Zeiss J, Fenton P, Ebraheim N, Coombs RJ: Normal magnetic resonance anatomy of the tarsal tunnel. Foot Ankle 10(4):214–218, 1990.

217. Pfeiffer WH, Cracchiolo A: Clinical results after tarsal tunnel decompression. J Bone Joint Surg 76A:1222–1230, 1994.

218. Takakura Y, Kitada C, Sugimoto K, et al.: Tarsal tunnel syndrome: causes and results of operative treatment. J Bone Joint Surg 73B:125–128, 1991.

219. Albrektsson B, Rudhold A, Rudhold U: The tarsal tunnel syndrome in children. J Bone Joint Surg 64:215–217, 1982.

220. Gessini L, Jandolo B, Pietrangeli A: The anterior tarsal syndrome. J Bone Joint Surg 66A: 786–787, 1984.

221. Dellon AL: Deep peroneal nerve entrapment on the dorsum of the foot. Foot Ankle 11(2): 73–80, 1990.

222. Garland, D: A clinical perspective on common forms of acquired heterotopic ossification. Clin Orthop 263:13–29, 1991.

223. DiGiovanna JJ, Helfgott RK, Gerber LH, Peck GL: Extraspinal tendon and ligament calcification associated with long-term therapy with etretinate. N Engl J Med 315(19):1177–1182, 1986.

224. Yarkony GM, Lee MY, Green D, Roth EJ: Heterotopic ossification pseudophlebitis. Am J Med 87:342–344, 1989.

225. Farah MJ, Palmieri MA, Sebes JI, et al.: The effect of diltiazem on calcinosis in a patient with the CREST syndrome. Arthritis Rheum 33: 1287–1293, 1990.

226. De Silva M, Earley MJ: Liposuction in the treatment of juxta-articular adiposis dolorosa. Ann Rheum Dis 49:403–404, 1990.

227. Rosenberg ZS, Kawelblum M, Cheung YY, et al.: Osgood-Schlatter lesion: fracture or tendinitis? Scintigraphic, CT, and MR imaging features. Radiology 185(3):853–858, 1992.

228. Soren A, Fetto JF: Pathology, clinic, and treatment of Osgood-Schlatter Disease. Orthopedics 7:230–234, 1984.

229. Peterson HA: Leg aches. Pediatr Clin North Am 24:731–736, 1977.

230. Naish JM, Apley J: "Growing pains:" a clinical study of non-arthritic limb pains in children. Arch Dis Child 26:134–140, 1951.

231. Atar D, Lehman WB, Grant AD: Growing pains. Orthop Rev 20(2):133–136, 1991.

232. Bates T, Grunwald E: Myofascial pain in childhood. J Pediatr 53:198–209, 1958.

233. Caghan SB, McGrath MM, Morrow MG, Pittman LD: When adolescents complain of pain. Nurse Practit 3:19–22, 1978.

234. Whiteley AM: Cramps, stiffness, and restless legs. Practitioner 226:1085–1087, 1982.

235. McGee SR: Muscle cramps. Arch Intern Med 150:511–518, 1990.

236. Zimlichman R, Krauss S, Paran E: Muscle cramps induced by b-blockers with intrinsic sympathomimetic activity properties: a hint of a possible mechanism. Arch Intern Med 151:1021, 1991.

237. Daniell HW: Simple cure for nocturnal leg cramps. N Engl J Med 301:216, 1979.

238. Ayres S Jr, Mihan R: Nocturnal leg cramps (systremma). Southern Med J 67:1308–1312, 1974.

239. Baltodano N, Gallo BV, Weidler DJ: Verapamil vs quinine in recumbent nocturnal leg cramps in the elderly. Arch Intern Med 148: 1969–1970, 1988.

240. Lee HB: Cramp in the elderly. Br Med J 2:1259, 1976.

241. More on muscle cramps. Drug Therapeutics Bull 21:83–84, 1983.

242. Leclerc JR, Jay RM, Hull RD, et al.: Recurrent leg symptoms following deep vein thrombosis. Arch Intern Med 145:1867–1869, 1985.

243. Lutz EG: Restless legs, anxiety, and caffeinism. J Clin Psych 39:11–16, 1978.

244. LaBan MM, Viola SL, Femminineo AF, Taylor RS: Restless legs syndrome associated with diminished cardiopulmonary compliance and lumbar spinal stenosis: a motor concomitant of "Vesper's Curse." Arch Phys Med Rehabil 71:384–388, 1990.

245. Derom E, Elinck W, Buylaret W, Van Der Straeten N: Which beta-blocker for the restless leg? Lancet 1:857, 1984.

246. Telstad W, Sorensen O, Larsen S, Lillevold PE, et al.: Treatment of the restless legs syndrome with carbamazepine: double-blind study. Br Med J 288:444–447, 1984.

247. Montplasir J, Godbout R, Boghen D, et al.: Familial restless legs with periodic movements in sleep: electrophysiologic, biochemical, and pharmacologic study. Neurology 35:130–134, 1985.

248. von Scheele C, Kempi V: Long-term effect of dopaminergic drugs in restless legs: a 2-year follow-up. Arch Neurol 47:1223–1224, 1990.

248a. Kanter AH: The effect of slerotheraphy on restless legs syndrome. Dermatol Surg 21:328–332, 1995.

249. Olson WL Jr: Perineal reflex sympathetic dystrophy treated with bilateral lumbar sympathectomy. Ann Intern Med 113(8):633–634, 1990.

250. Ogilvie-Harris DJ, Roscoe M: Reflex sympathetic dystrophy of the knee. J Bone Joint Surg 69B(5):804–806, 1987.

251. Cooper DE, DeLee JC, Ramamurthy S: Reflex sympathetic dystrophy of the knee. J Bone Joint Surg 71A(3):365–369, 1989.

252. Wilder RT, Berde CB, Wolohan M, et al.: Reflex sympathetic dystrophy in children. J Bone Joint Surg 74A:910–919, 1992.

253. Wesdock KA, Stanton RP, Singsen BH: Reflex sympathetic dystrophy in children. Arthritis Care Res 4:32–37, 1991.

254. Moore TL, Doner RW, Zuckner J: Complement-fixing hidden rheumatoid factor in children with benign rheumatoid nodules. Arthritis Rheum 21:930–934, 1978.

255. Ehrlich GE: Painter's bosses. Arch Intern Med 116:776–777, 1965.

256. Pottage JC, Trenholme GM, Aronson IK, Harris AA: Panniculitis associated with histoplasmosis and alpha l-antitrypsin deficiency. Am J Med 75:150–153, 1983.

257. Spinner RJ, Ginsburg WW, Lie JT, et al.: Atypical eosinophilic fasciitis localized to the hands and feet: a report of four cases. J Rheumatol 19(7):1141–1146, 1992.

258. Dihlmann W, Hopker WW: Adhesive (retractile) capsulitis of the hip joint in diabetes mellitus: an x-ray histomorphological synopsis. ROFO Fortschr Geb Rontgenstr Neuen Bildgeb Verfahr 157:235–238, 1992.

259. Mann RA: Biomechanics of the foot and ankle. Orthop Rev 7:43–48, 1978.

260. Giannestras NJ: Principles of bunion surgery. Orthop Rev 7:83–86, 1978.

261. Jacobson MA: Simple footgear corrections useful in office emergencies. Orthop Rev 8:63–68, 1979.

262. Lipscomb PR: Nonsuppurative tenosynovitis and paratendinitis. Am Acad Orthop Surg, Instructional Course Lectures, Vol 7. Ann Arbor, 1950.

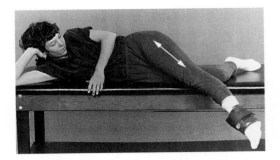

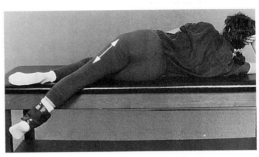

Exercise 6.A. Iliotibial Band Stretch—Side-lying

From a side-lying position, drop the leg on the affected side over the table or bed as indicated, first to the front and then to the rear, holding each position at least 30 seconds. The stretch should be felt on the side of the thigh. A 3–5-pound weight can be attached to the ankle to increase the stretch.

6.A (a). Front Position (anterior)

6.A (b). Rear Position (posterior)

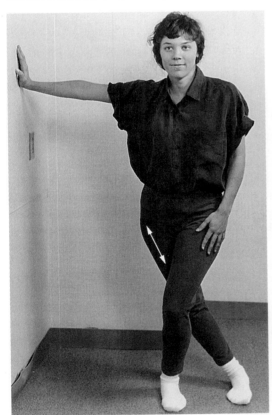

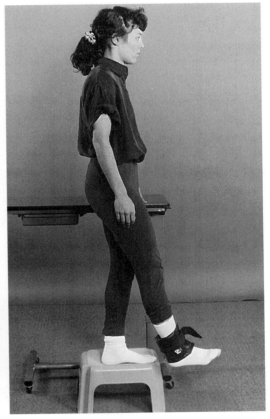

Exercise 6.B. Iliotibial Band Stretch—Standing

Standing sideways to the wall, support the body with the extended arm while dropping the hip on the affected side toward the wall. Stretch is felt along the outer thigh of the side next to the wall.

Exercise 6.C. Hip Pendulum

Stand on a stool or stair step so that the leg of the affected hip can swing free, holding a stable surface for balance. With a 2–5-pound weight attached to the ankle, swing the leg forward and backward, sideward, and in small circles. This movement provides gentle traction and stretching to the hip capsule and musculature, particularly the iliopsoas and gluteii muscles.

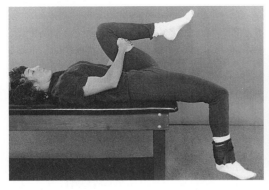

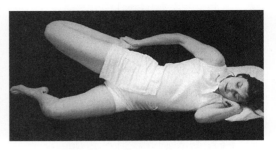

Exercise 6.D. Hip Flexor Stretch
6.D (a). Back-lying with the hips at the bottom edge of the bed, the leg on the side to be stretched is extended over the edge as the other knee is held bent as illustrated. The stretch should be felt in the front of the hip. A 2–4-pound weight may be attached to the ankle.

6.D (b). Side-lying hip flexor stretch. For those who are not so limber, a belt turned twice around the ankle can be used to pull the knee and thigh backward. Hold the stretched position for 20 seconds, performing three repetitions, twice daily.

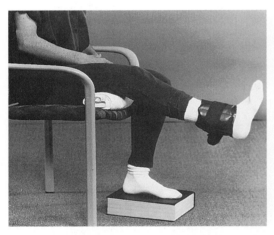

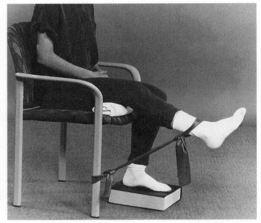

Exercise 6.E. Resistive Quad Strengthening, with Weight
Sit with a 2–10-pound weight attached to the leg to be strengthened. Lift the weight by slowly straightening the leg. Repeat 10 times per daily session, increasing the weight as possible.

Exercise 6.F. Resistive Quad Strengthening, with Theraband
The Theraband is attached to the chair as illustrated, then looped around the ankle of the leg to be strengthened. Slowly straighten the leg against the Theraband, 10 times per daily session.

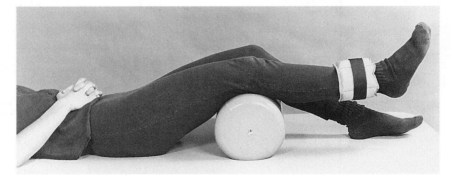

Exercise 6.G. Resistive Quad Strengthening, Back-lying, Short Arc
Back-lying with the knee supported and bent 30–45 degrees, a 2–10-pound weight on the ankle. Straighten the knee and hold the weight at the highest position 10 seconds, then slowly allow the knee to bend. Repeat 10 times per daily session.

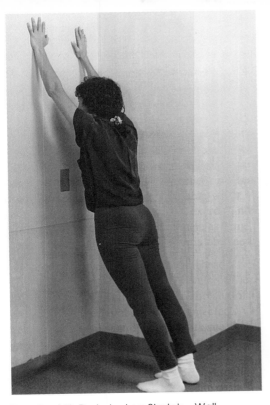

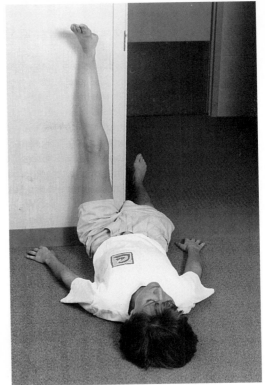

Exercise 6.H. Posterior Leg Stretch—Wall

Stand facing the wall, feet together and about 24" from the wall. With heels firmly on the floor and body aligned straight at hips and knees, lean forward to the wall, stretching the posterior leg tissues. Hold position 10–30 seconds, repeat five times per session, at least two sessions daily.

Exercise 6.I. Posterior Leg Stretch—Doorway

Back-lying in a doorway as illustrated, with the leg to be stretched up on the doorjamb with knee slightly bent and the other leg through the open doorway. Slowly straighten the bent knee to stretch the posterior leg tissues, and move the hips toward the doorjamb to increase the stretch. Hold the stretching position 10–30 seconds, relax the knee, repeat five times per daily session. The position can be held for as much as 3 minutes if doing so is comfortable.

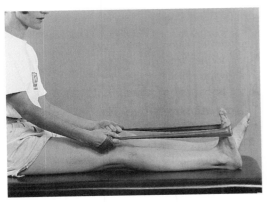

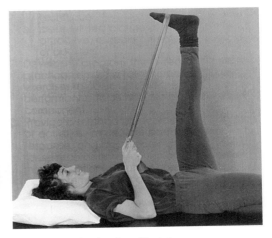

Exercise 6.J. Calf–Plantar Fascia Stretch—Theraband (sitting)

Sitting with knees extended, loop the Theraband around the foot of the leg to be stretched and pull the forefoot toward the knee. Hold the stretched position 10–30 seconds, repeat five times per session, two sessions per day. Pushing the foot against the Theraband may also be performed in order to activate/strengthen the plantarflexor muscles (mainly the gastrocnemius).

Exercise 6.K. Supine Leg Stretch

Back-lying with a Theraband or belt looped around the foot on the side to be stretched and the other knee bent with the foot flat. The straight leg is lifted and assisted with the Theraband/belt and the foot is flexed and extended against its resistance. Repeat five times per daily session.

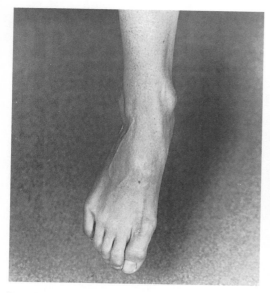

Exercise 6.L. Foot-Ankle Circles

Circle the foot at the ankle; move the foot as if drawing the letters of the alphabet; move the foot up and down by flexing and extending the ankle.

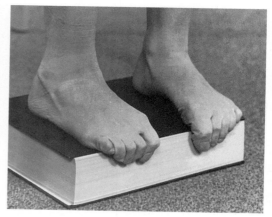

Exercise 6.M. Toe Curls

Alternate these movements so that toes curl and straighten. Perform these for 1–2 minutes twice daily.

6.M (a). Curl the toes.

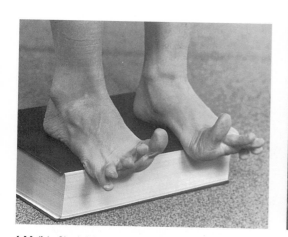

6.M (b). Straighten and spread the toes.

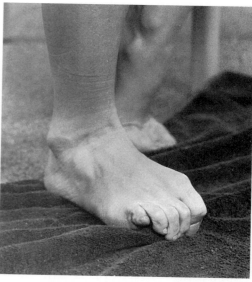

Exercise 6.N. Toe Towel Curls

Place a towel (or cloth or paper) on the floor. Grasp the towel with the toes and gather it with the toes.

7: Fibromyalgia and Other Generalized Soft Tissue Rheumatic Disorders

The criteria for fibromyalgia serve to distinguish fibromyalgia from the pain that is neurotically symbolic or that is a malingering pretense. *Fibromyalgia can coexist with other systemic disease; the compounded symptoms then may lead to more complex, inappropriate, and at times, hazardous medical or surgical treatment.*

Many systemic illnesses can affect the articular soft tissue structures; most of these can be specifically categorized. What is left for inclusion here are rheumatic symptom disorders including fibromyalgia, chronic fatigue syndrome, and somatization disorders. Unlike other symptom disorders, including vertigo or labyrinthitis, migraine, angina pectoris, temporomandibular myofascial pain syndrome, polymyalgia rheumatica, seasonal affective disorder, and depression, fibromyalgia lacks *specific therapy,* and treatment is therefore dependent upon the physician's current belief system.

FIBROMYALGIA

The term ''fibromyalgia'' is currently favored by most rheumatologists; others prefer the terms ''tension myalgia'' or ''generalized tendomyopathy.'' The terms ''fibromyositis'' and ''fibrositis'' have been discarded because inflammation has not been demonstrated in this syndrome. At present, *fibromyalgia* has become the official term of the American College of Rheumatology (1).

The term ''fibrositis'' was introduced by Gowers in 1904 (2) as a descriptive term that included ''traumatic fibrositis'' or ''cervical fibrositis.'' At first the term was used to imply any pain of muscular origin and was to some extent used interchangeably with fasciitis, myofibromyalgia, myofascitis, muscular rheumatism, and muscular strain (3). The involved tissues were thought to have suffered irritation, perhaps from overstretching.

Eosinophilic fasciitis and *polymyalgia rheumatica* are additional causes of widespread pain and disability and they are important in the differential diagnosis of this disease group.

Features

Fibromyalgia refers to a disorder with variable features that includes widespread aching and stiffness accompanied by localized sites of deep tenderness (tender points) at specific locations, and the absence of deep tenderness at other locations (Table 7.1). Ten control points are used by most examiners (Table 7.2). Sleep disturbance, fatigue, and chronicity are usual features (Table 7.3). Females are affected approximately nine times more often than males.

Fibromyalgia often begins in midlife, although persons of any age may become symptomatic. Fibromyalgia may follow a precipitating stressful life event such as a demotion at work, death of a loved one, divorce, another illness, or trauma.

Currently, the term fibromyalgia is reserved for a specific soft tissue pain syndrome with the following characteristics:

Widespread Aching and Stiffness: Soft tissue aching is widespread in broad regions of the cervical and lumbar spinal segments. The symptoms are aggravated by fatigue, tension, excessive work activity, immobilization, and chilling (4–7). Heat, massage, programmed activity, and vacations are helpful in symptom

TABLE 7.1 THE AMERICAN COLLEGE OF RHEUMATOLOGY CRITERIA FOR THE CLASSIFICATION OF FIBROMYALGIA

1. History of widespread pain.

   Definition. Pain is considered widespread when all of the following are present: pain in the left side of the body, pain in the right side of the body, pain above the waist, and pain below the waist. In addition, axial skeletal pain (cervical spine or anterior chest or thoracic spine or low back) must be present. In this definition, shoulder and buttock pain is considered as pain for each involved side. "Low back" pain is considered lower segment pain.

2. Pain in 11 of 18 tender point sites on digital palpation.

   Definition. Pain, on digital palpation, must be present in at least 11 of the following 18 tender point sites:

   Occiput: bilateral, at the suboccipital muscle insertions.

   Low cervical: bilateral, at the anterior aspects of the intertransverse spaces at C5–C7.

   Trapezius: bilateral, at the midpoint of the upper border.

   Supraspinatus: bilateral, at origins, above the scapula spine near the medial border.

   Second rib: bilateral, at the second costochondral junctions, just lateral to the junctions on upper surfaces.

   Lateral epicondyle: bilateral, 2 cm distal to the epicondyles.

   Gluteal: bilateral, in upper outer quadrants of buttocks in anterior fold of muscle.

   Greater trochanter: bilateral, posterior to the trochanteric prominence.

   Knee: bilateral, at the medial fat pad proximal to the joint line.

   Digital palpation should be performed with an approximate force of 4 kg.

   For a tender point to be considered "positive" the subject must state that the palpation was painful. "Tender" is not to be considered "painful."

For classification purposes, patients will be said to have fibromyalgia if both criteria are satisfied. Widespread pain must have been present for at least 3 months. The presence of a second clinical disorder does not exclude the diagnosis of fibromyalgia.

From Wolfe F, Smythe HA, Yunus MB, et al.: The American College of Rheumatology 1990 criteria for the classification of fibromyalgia. Arthritis Rheum 33:160–172, 1990.

TABLE 7.2 TEN CONTROL POINTS FOR FIBROMYALGIA EXAMINATION

Forehead, right and left
Distal dorsal forearm, right and left
Thumbnail, right and left
Third metatarsal ray, dorsum, right and left
Great toenail, right and left

TABLE 7.3 COMMONLY ASSOCIATED FEATURES (PERCENT OF PATIENTS WITH FEATURE)

Fatigue	(78)
Morning stiffness	(76)
Sleep disorder	(75)
Paresthesias	(67)
Headache	(54)
Anxiety	(44)
Irritable bowel	(35)

Also common are:

Menstrual and sexual dysfunction
Major depression
Raynaud's phenomenon
Sicca complex
Memory deficits
Menopause occurs earlier

From Wolf F, Smythe HA, Yunus MB, et al.: The American College of Rheumatology 1990 criteria for the classification of fibromyalgia. Arthritis Rheum 33:160–172, 1990.

relief. Although these symptoms may vary from day to day, they are nevertheless always present, and "normal" days are rare. Pain usually is bilateral and symmetric, although use may cause one side to be more tender than the other. Stiffness occurs more diffusely and is mainly in the trunk rather than in specific joint areas. (This differs from the pattern of morning stiffness in rheumatoid arthritis, in which stiffness is peripheral, in the limbs and maximally localized to joints.)

Tender Points: Tender points are reproducible areas of tenderness that occur in precise and predictable locations. Table 7.1 and Figure 7.1 indicate the 18 tender point locations identified in the American College of Rheumatology diagnostic criteria. The diagnosis depends upon a point count: 11 or more of the 18 points must be present. *Tender points are the essential feature of fibromyalgia.* Because patients with fibromyalgia are more tender generally, the tender point count is controlled with up to 10 control points that are used for discriminating fibromyalgia from other causes of generalized tenderness. If more than three control points are found, the diagnosis of fibromyalgia is tenuous.

These tender points are reproducible and have been validated (1, 8). The number of tender points is correlated with the severity of pain (9), and with increasing number of tender points the patient is more likely to have neck pain, skin fold tenderness, and headache (7, 10).

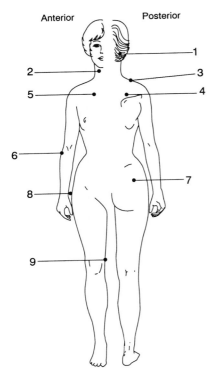

Figure 7.1. Locations of nine bilateral tender point sites for the American College of Rheumatology classification criteria for fibromyalgia.
1. Suboccipital muscle insertions
2. Cervical, at the anterior aspects of the inter-transverse spaces at C5–C7
3. Trapezius, at the midpoint of the upper border
4. Supraspinatus, at the origin, above the scapular spine near the medial border
5. Second rib, at the costochondral junction
6. Lateral epicondyle, 2 cm distal to the epicondyle
7. Gluteal, in upper outer quadrant of the buttock
8. Greater trochanter, just posterior to the trochanteric prominence
9. Knee, at the medial fat pad proximal to the joint line

(From McCarty DJ, Koopman WJ, eds. Arthritis and allied conditions. 12th ed. Philadelphia: Lea & Febiger, 1993.)

Examination technique for tender points: In fibromyalgia research, dolorimeter examination is conducted with 4 kg pressure applied to each tender point location. For clinical purposes, however, the pressure is applied in an amount sufficient to cause blanching of the examiner's thumbnail.

The tender point examination frequently begins by describing to the patient the examination to be undertaken as a method of discriminating between *pain* and *tenderness*. The midpoint of the patient's thigh might then be pressed with the examiner's thumb until the nail bed blanches; that is defined as *tenderness.*

The original fibromyalgia study *control points* were the dorsal distal third of the forearm, the thumbnail, and the midpoint of the dorsal right third metatarsal (1). Additional control locations often used are the lateral forehead, the styloid process, and the great toenail. Table 7.2 lists 10 common control points.

Control points should be interspersed with the others in the course of the examination. Do not assume bilaterality; both sides of the body should be examined for tender points.

The entire point count is the sum of the real points said to be painful rather than just tender. If more than three control points are described as painful, other causes for heightened sensitivity to pain should be considered. (Refer to the section ''Differential Diagnosis'' below.)

Hugh Smythe first suggested the use of a tender point count to help in diagnosing fibromyalgia (4). Controlled studies have shown that the presence of tender points will distinguish fibromyalgia from other disorders (1, 5, 6, 11, 12). When patients with established rheumatoid arthritis have more than four tender points, their pain and fatigue may be due to concomitant fibromyalgia. Wolfe et al. studied those rheumatoid patients with more than four tender points and found that these patients had features compatible with fibromyalgia; much of their symptomatology of morning stiffness and widespread aching and fatigue were thought to be the result of the fibromyalgia rather than of inflammation (12, 13).

Trigger points are different from *tender points* (14, 15). The term ''trigger points'' should be restricted to tender areas of muscle, usually unilateral, with characteristic zones of pain referral, in which the ''twitch response'' is observed following palpation. Trigger points and tender points are discussed in more detail in Chapter 1. Trigger points and regional pain disorders may coexist with fibromyalgia (Figs. 7.2A and 7.2B). The findings and definition of trigger points have been questioned because of a lack of interobserver validity (16, 17).

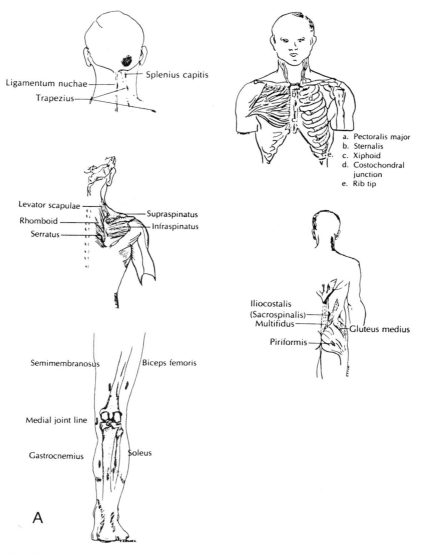

Figure 7.2. A. Pain (trigger) points.

Other Common Symptoms and Features

A review of systems often reveals a host of other symptoms. Many are suggestive of significant neurovascular and autonomic nervous system dysfunction (Table 7.3).

Arthralgia: Finger joint pain is common and may be the presenting complaint (18). When tested for joint tenderness, the periarticular tissues are often more tender than the joints. Strength is diminished; the resulting weakness often contributes to joint pain. When joint laxity is present, then the deconditioned state of

fibromyalgia may lead to more joint pain and disability (19).

Fatigue and Memory Complaints: These occur much more often as major complaints in fibromyalgia than in other rheumatic diseases or in control groups. Often patients wake up more tired than when they retired the night before (20).

Chronic fatigue syndrome and fibromyalgia share features of fatigue, widespread aching, and depression. As many as two-thirds of patients diagnosed with chronic fatigue syndrome have fibromyalgia (21). Features more characteristic of chronic fatigue syndrome

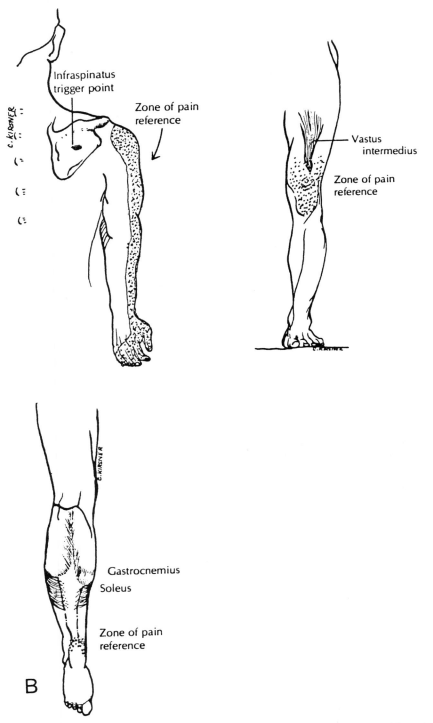

Figure 7.2. B. Pain (trigger) points and zones of reference. Upon palpating the pain (trigger) point, pain is produced at some distant point. This zone of reference is quite characteristic for each trigger point.

include preceding infection, sore throat, and painful lymph nodes. Because no single therapy has been highly effective for either condition, they are both thought by many physicians to be diagnostic labels for similar problems (22). Both disorders share responsiveness to low doses of serotonergic treatment (23). Many patients with multiple chemical sensitivity share similar features (24). Self-reporting of functional disability in patients with fibromyalgia is much worse than observed measurement of functional capacity (25).

Memory complaints include poor concentration, a loss of prompt recall, and often a sense of utter helplessness. When standardized tests are used, most patients have normal findings on these scales. Despite the patients' perceived helplessness many had a better outcome five years later (26).

Paresthesias: Paresthesias and the *sensation of swelling* of the hands and arms are common. Paresthesia of the lower extremities occurs commonly after prolonged sitting, or after performing any prolonged activity. Rings feel tight in the morning. *Visible swelling does not occur,* at least to the physician observer.

Sleep Disturbance: Although the patient may not mention suffering from sleep disturbance, the spouse often volunteers that the patient "moves all over the bed all night long." The patient may fall asleep promptly but then awakens frequently throughout the night. Characteristically, the patient feels more tired in the morning than when going to bed. Sleep is not restful. Sleep physiology is often disturbed (see below).

Raynaud's Phenomenon: Two color changes in the fingers and hands upon exposure to cold occurs three times more often in persons with fibromyalgia than in others. Objective studies, including the Nielsen test, digital photoplethysmography, and measurements of platelet α_2-adrenergic receptors, demonstrated significant abnormality in 40% of tested patients (27).

Sicca Complex: Dry eyes and mouth are also common complaints, and yet objective findings are lacking. Most complaining patients lack physical evidence of abnormality. Lip biopsy may identify a subset of patients who are negative for SSA(Ro) and SSB(La) antibodies but who have fibromyalgia, peripheral neuropathy, and many psychological complaints. In one study, ANA was positive in 66% of the patients (28).

Headache and Stress: Migraine headaches are often noted in the patient or in the patient's family. Patients with fibromyalgia were not found to be more anxious or to have enhanced pain perception when compared to a matched control group (29). However, when compared to patients with rheumatoid arthritis, fibromyalgia patients exhibited higher levels of psychological distress (30). When the clinical features of fibromyalgia and psychological status (MMPI testing) were analyzed by univariate and multivariate techniques, only pain severity was correlated with MMPI scores. The features of pain sites, number of tender points, fatigue, and poor sleep appear to be independent of psychologic status (31).

In a study in which fibromyalgia patients and their families were interviewed and examined for medical and psychiatric disorders using the Structured Clinical Interview for DSM-III-R (SCID), lifetime rates were found to be high for migraine, irritable bowel syndrome, chronic fatigue syndrome, major depression, and panic disorder. They were also found to have high rates of familial major mood disorder and much lower rates of narcolepsy, Tourette syndrome, obsessive-compulsive disorder, substance use disorders, schizophrenia, schizoaffective disorder, somatization disorder, eating disorders, and kleptomania (32). But fibromyalgia symptoms are not commonly correlated with psychological status (31). Depression, though more common in fibromyalgia, does not appear to cause the features of fibromyalgia.

Irritable Bowel Syndrome (IBS): IBS consists of abdominal pain and altered bowel habit with constipation, diarrhea, or both, and occurs in as many as 60% of patients with fibromyalgia (33). Conversely, in one report 65% of patients with IBS were found to have fibromyalgia (34). Stressful events commonly precipitate diarrhea.

Irritable Bladder Symptoms: Irritable bladder symptoms are common also. Urgency, daytime frequency, and retropubic pain may occur. Unpublished data suggest that interstitial cystitis may be related to fibromyalgia (35).

Other Physical Findings

Additional features that may occur include evidence of autonomic nervous system dysfunction with dermographism (36), cutis anserina ("goose skin"—contraction of the arrectores pilorum muscles, causing elevation of hair follicles) (3), cutis marmorata (a transitory purplish mottling of the skin), and excessive sweating (37). Skinfold tenderness with hyperesthesia over the upper scapular region may be noted. Following testing for skinfold tenderness performed by rolling the patient's skin in a gentle pinching fashion (above the supraspinatus and upper trapezius muscles), a marked hyperemia sometimes occurs.

Joint examination usually reveals normal range of active and passive motion. Some patients have reduced motion of the cervical spine. However, general musculoskeletal discomfort is evident. Grip testing is approached hesitantly and is carried out slowly but usually the patient demonstrates low normal levels of strength. When tested kinetically for strength these patients are often significantly deconditioned and have reduced endurance (38).

The patient often appears unhappy, seldom smiling, but is generally not overtly depressed and usually is forthright without much neurotic behavior.

Laboratory Findings

Unless fibromyalgia is overlaid upon another condition, all laboratory studies are normal, including complete blood counts, erythrocyte sedimentation rate, serum proteins, thyroid function measurement, muscle enzyme studies, and antinuclear and rheumatoid factor determinations.

Differential Diagnosis

About 6% of patients with symptoms of fibromyalgia will develop or have another rheumatic disease. In particular, fibromyalgia may coexist with rheumatoid arthritis or systemic lupus erythematosus (36). Widespread osteoarthritis, Forestier's disease (diffuse idiopathic skeletal hyperostosis, or DISH), ankylosing spondylitis, polymyositis, polymyalgia rheumatica, and vasculitis may cause similar complaints, but tender point counts never reach significant numbers unless fibromyalgia coexists. Other diagnoses that can give rise to symptoms of fibromyalgia include neuropathy, sarcoidosis, osteomalacia, systemic infections, paraneoplastic syndromes, hypothyroidism, hyperparathyroidism, inflammatory bowel disease, and anemias (20). Inflammatory myopathies have features of axial weakness (neck muscles and hip muscles) and pain is not prominent (Table 7.4).

When fibromyalgia coexists with other systemic disease, the compounded symptoms, if unrecognized as such, may lead to medical or surgical treatment disproportionate to the requirements of the primary systemic disease. If fibromyalgia is identified as a concomitant problem, therapy should be directed toward both disorders (39). For example, the addition of features of the fibromyalgia syndrome to the symptoms of patients suffering from rheumatoid arthritis or systemic lupus erythematosus often results in treatment with drugs far stronger than signs of inflammation would warrant. Following treatment of fibromyalgia, the dosages of antiinflammatory drugs or corticosteroids can be significantly reduced or even eliminated.

Sometimes symptoms similar to fibromyalgia are due to drug sensitivity. Drugs that might be incriminated include clofibrate, diuretics, cimetidine, lithium, cytotoxic drugs, alcohol, and amphetamines (40). Caffeine intoxication can contribute to sleep disorder and fibromyalgia.

Fibromyalgia is not synonymous with psychogenic rheumatism. It differs significantly from the latter by the presence, the location, and the constancy of tender points. The fibromyalgia patient often relates symptoms to changes in her *external* environment including

TABLE 7.4 CRITICAL FEATURES IN GENERALIZED SOFT TISSUE PAIN

1. Fever, sweats, weight loss
2. Lymphadenopathy, organomegaly
3. Raynaud's phenomenon
4. Neuropathy
5. Joint swelling or tenderness
6. Limitation of joint or spine motion
7. Bruits or diminished pulse
8. Any unexplained laboratory abnormality

weather, heat, cold, humidity, rest, or exercise. These external factors influence the patient's symptoms for better or for worse. Conversely, the patient with psychogenic rheumatism is at the mercy of changes in her *internal* environment; symptoms vary with mood, psyche, pleasure, excitement, mental distraction, worry, or fatigue. Diagnosis and treatment are problematic when a patient with fibromyalgia also has a marked neurosis.

The patient with psychogenic rheumatism frequently exhibits the "touch-me-not" reaction when a physical examination is performed (41). Such patients react excessively to the examiner's touch anywhere on the body. Therefore, both the control points and the real points are positive during the point-count examination.

Once diagnosed, the rate of hospitalization for patients with fibromyalgia is reduced significantly (42). The diagnosis itself may reduce anxiety and stress-related symptoms.

Epidemiology

Fibromyalgia is the third most common rheumatic disorder seen in some rheumatology practices (43, 44); as many as 5 million people might be afflicted in the U.S. (45).

The occurrence and the features of fibromyalgia sometimes vary from nation to nation. For example, using the 1990 American College of Rheumatology (ACR) criteria for fibromyalgia, fewer than 1% of inhabitants of eastern Denmark (6000 questioned, 1219 examined) satisfied criteria. Sleep disturbance was not common in the Danish subjects (46, 47). In other studies, prevalence rates range from 10.5% in Norwegian women (48); 3.2% in the U.S. (49), 3% in Germany (50), and 3.2% in a primitive African community (51). In the latter group widespread pain was noted in only 20% of subjects. Features in Japanese patients were similar to those in Caucasians (52).

Children experience fibromyalgia. In one study of 338 children aged 9–15 attending public school in Beersheba, Israel, fibromyalgia by 1990 ACR criteria was diagnosed in 21 (6%) children; and 17 of them had joint laxity (53). Others report fibromyalgia among children with chronic pain; the tender point count

readily differentiated patients with fibromyalgia from others (54, 55).

Podiatric patients should be screened for fibromyalgia. Harvey reports that among a podiatric practice of 355 patients, eight patients satisfied criteria for fibromyalgia. More importantly, of 35 patients with plantar heel and arch pain, seven had fibromyalgia. The foot complaints were bilateral in four patients. All had widespread aching and fatigue (56).

Etiology

Fibromyalgia appears to result from a central nervous system derangement. The peripheral tissues and tender points are likely secondary phenomena.

HISTOPATHOLOGIC FINDINGS

Histopathologic findings in the areas of muscle tenderness are reviewed in Chapter 1. In sum, no consistent and reproducible tissue findings are known. Findings in muscle consistent with ischemia and deconditioning have been reported (57).

DECONDITIONING

Deconditioning contributes significantly. Although patients may state that they always felt better when they could exercise, they often stopped exercising because exercise-induced pain became intolerable. Controlled studies of exhaustive physical exercise in fibromyalgia demonstrated not only lower mean maximum workload of fibromyalgia patients compared to control subjects, but also lower serum creatine kinase, myoglobin, cortisol, epinephrine, and norepinephrine levels than in control subjects. This suggests disturbed reactivity of the sympathetic nervous system (58). Oxygen uptake and utilization during muscular exercise did not differ in patients from controls, nor in relation to rate of exercise (59). Studies of dynamic muscular endurance (number of repeated knee extensions) revealed that fibromyalgia patients had significantly low voluntary muscular endurance compared to other patients with chronic regional pain disorders (60). Fibromyalgia patients have been found to display a phosphodiester resonance at a higher rate than control subjects when studied with phosphorus-31 nuclear magnetic resonance spectra, which suggested to the authors that the patients might have a sarcolemmal abnormality (61). If so, this might in turn result from hypoxia (62). Using similar MRI spectroscopy, Simms et al. found no difference in muscle energy metabolism between persons with fibromyalgia and sedentary controls (63).

The deconditioned patient may over time become disabled, with psychosocial problems aggravating the situation (64), leading potentially to high social costs (65).

TRAUMATIC AND STRESSFUL EVENTS

About one-fourth of patients with fibromyalgia relate the onset to a traumatic event. In a study in which patients with posttraumatic widespread musculoskeletal pain were compared with fibromyalgia patients, both groups were found to have an alpha EEG non–rapid eye movement sleep anomaly, suggesting a psychophysiologic arousal mechanism (see below) induced by trauma that becomes indistinguishable from fibromyalgia (66).

Similarly, fibromyalgia may follow an infectious insult such as Lyme disease (67, 68), cancer, or surgery (69). Fibromyalgia after *Parvovirus* infection has also been reported (70).

CENTRAL NERVOUS SYSTEM

The currently available evidence suggests that fibromyalgia is not a muscular disease but rather a response to central nervous system dysfunction, specifically in the area of pain transmission and modulation. Dry eyes, cold sensitivity, paresthesias, and sleep disturbances also suggest a central nervous system abnormality.

Moldofsky noted that non–rapid eye movement (non-REM) sleep was disturbed and contaminated by alpha rhythms in patients with the fibromyalgia syndrome (71). Furthermore, by depriving volunteers of non-REM sleep, the characteristic tender points were produced (71, 72). Some patients with fibromyalgia do not enter deep sleep (stage 4 sleep); they often feel that if they could keep moving and not stop, they would be better off. However, fatigue develops quickly. Others find this alpha-delta pattern less often in patients with fibromyalgia; also, other abnormal EEG patterns may be noted (73–76).

Sleep quality and its relation to pain, fatigue, and poor mood are well known. In fibromyalgia, poor sleep has been correlated with muscle aching and tender point count even after controlling for pain, depression, and disease severity (77). Sleep disturbance may result in diminished growth hormone needed for muscle tissue maintenance (78). Disturbed sleep also alters immune function, including pokeweed mitogen response and plasma interleukin 1 and interleukin 2 activity, but not cortisol diurnal pattern (79, 80). Alpha-delta sleep does not appear to be a marker for fibromyalgia, but it may contribute to illness in patients with fibromyalgia and chronic fatigue syndrome when major depression is not present (81).

The stress response and neuroendocrine linkage to the immune system are strongly supported by current research findings (82). Abnormalities within three broad areas are under intense investigation: pain transmission, biogenic amine abnormalities, and genetic factors, each of which is discussed below.

1. PAIN TRANSMISSION

After publication of David Reynolds's landmark paper in 1969 (83) demonstrating that electrical stimulation of the midbrain central gray area can cause analgesia, research began to focus on mediators of pain. A fine review of the history of this research has been published recently by Matucci-Cerinic (84).

Substance P, an undecapeptide discovered in 1931, is synthesized in the dorsal root ganglia and transported to central and peripheral nerve endings in the skin, blood vessels, joints, sympathetic ganglia and viscera. It is responsible for controlling vascular tone and in mediating nociceptive and neurogenic vasodilative responses, and it is a sensory neurotransmitter (84).

Several studies have reported results of substance P activity in the cerebrospinal fluid (CSF). In an uncontrolled study of 30 patients with fibromyalgia, Vaeroy et al. compared results to those of known normal standards using a radioimmunoassay procedure to measure immunoreactive substance P, and found significantly elevated levels of substance P (35.1 ± 2.7 fmol/mL, range 16.5–79.1 fmol/mL) compared to normal values (9.6 ± 3.2 fmol/

mL) (85). Russell et al. tested 32 patients and 30 controls and report a threefold elevation of substance P in fibromyalgia (86). The level of CSF substance P was not correlated with any particular clinical feature.

Russell speculates that other factors such as low CSF norepinephrine and other neuroendocrine abnormalities are necessary contributors to the widespread and varied nature of fibromyalgia. Substance P and somatostatin have also been demonstrably involved in functional gastrointestinal complaints (87).

Calcitonin gene related peptide (CGRP) is also found in sensory neurones that synthesize substance P. It also acts as a neurotransmitter and may be antagonistic to substance P. Its presence and significance in the CSF of patients with fibromyalgia is currently under investigation (85). Studies of other neuropeptides and endorphins in CSF have had mixed results (88–91). In the past, studies of plasma β-endorphin levels have not been conclusive (92, 93).

Hyperprolactinemia has been reported in fibromyalgia and is correlated with the number of tender points. Prolactin is also a factor in immune regulation (94).

2. BIOGENIC AMINE ABNORMALITIES

Plasma and urine catecholamines were measured by Yunus et al. in 30 patients with fibromyalgia matched with 30 control subjects. Plasma epinephrine, norepinephrine, and dopamine levels were not significantly different. Similarly, urine epinephrine, norepinephrine, and dopamine levels (ng/mg of creatinine) were not significantly different between patients and controls (95). These findings were corroborated by Crofford et al. in another controlled study. Findings included low 24-hour urinary free cortisol; normal peak and elevated trough plasma cortisol levels; decreased net integrated cortisol response to ovine corticotropin-releasing hormone; and lower neuropeptide Y compared to control subjects (96). On the other hand, CSF studies measuring 5-hydroxyindole acetic acid, 3-methoxy-4-hydroxyphenylethylene glycol, and homovanillic acid revealed lower levels of all three biogenic amines in 17 patients with fibromyalgia compared with 19 control subjects and with five patients with rheumatoid arthritis (97). In a cor-

ticotropin-releasing hormone test, fibromyalgia patients showed a markedly enhanced adrenocorticotropic hormone release compared to controls, suggesting a relative adrenal hyporesponsiveness (98).

The reported higher density of serotonin reuptake receptors on circulating platelets and lower levels of serum serotonin (99), tryptophan (100), and CSF serotonin suggests a likely explanation for the sympathetic nervous system–related symptoms of fibromyalgia as well as enhanced sensitivity to pain (97).

Serum levels of somatomedin C, a growth hormone peptide, is reported to be significantly lower in patients with fibromyalgia (n = 70) than in control subjects (n = 55). Bennett et al. suggested that disturbed sleep may disrupt growth hormone secretion and in turn alter normal muscle homeostasis (78). Many other studies have suggested an alteration in the immune systems of patients with fibromyalgia but most were not controlled. Others did not use the ACR criteria and point count to define fibromyalgia.

One report suggests reduced regional cerebral blood flow. In a controlled study of 19 patients with fibromyalgia using SPECT imaging of the caudate nucleus and injection with technetium-99m hexylmethylpropylene amineoxine (Tc-99m-HMPAO), Alexander et al. report unilateral and bilateral diminished flow in fibromyalgia patients compared with controls (101). The caudate nucleus is involved in pain transmission.

3. GENETIC FACTORS

No differences were found in class I and II HLA markers in persons with fibromyalgia compared with healthy controls (102). Family studies of patients with fibromyalgia suggest underlying genetic abnormality (103–105). In one study of 575 families, about two-thirds reported family clustering (105). This could provide a unifying concept. Thus, a genetically predisposed person, when exposed to a significant stressor, could have a cascade of neuroendocrine and biogenic amine disruptions. A circular effect among these might lead to perpetuation and persistence. Therapeutic intervention to alter the circular effect of these abnormalities awaits future research into the application of somatostatins and novel mediators of these abnormalities.

Management

Identification of 11 or more tender points and three or fewer control points is often a great moral victory for the patient. The clinician may now direct the patient away from a purely psychologic cause for the symptomatology.

A comprehensive program should be provided from the beginning. Treatment should follow the six-point management plan used for every other soft tissue disorder.

1. Each patient should have a complete, comprehensive examination to exclude coexisting disease. Widespread pain and fatigue of fibromyalgia can easily mask other illness.
2. Recognize psychosocial factors that may contribute. Also, attitudes and belief systems may be self-destructive. Work habits and hobbies should be altered as needed.
3. Explain the involvement of central nervous system factors. These include interactions of the sleep disorder, autonomic nervous system dysfunction, and muscle tightness.
4. Provide physical therapy and aerobic, stretching, and strengthening exercise interventions for conditioning and pain reduction. Deconditioning often results from fibromyalgia and then leads to disability.
5. Provide for pain reduction. In most patients, using intralesional injections to desensitize the points, ice massage, myofascial release massage, and behavior modification will help.
6. Outcome in fibromyalgia is never complete, and specific goals should be provided. These should be *achievable* goals, and might include reduction in pain and fatigue and improvement in strength, independence, attitude, and coping ability. In other words, the goal is not for the patient to feel perfect, but rather to regain control over his or her life.

Many patients with features of fibromyalgia have fewer than the required features for diagnosis. When the point count is less than 11 and there are fewer than four positive control points, and other reasons for widespread pain have been excluded, most patients will still benefit from this treatment plan.

Consider possible drug or alcohol abuse. Use a trial period of elimination of all dark beverages. Some decaffeinated beverages contain theophyllines that may aggravate sleep. Encourage proper sleep hygiene, including avoidance of stressful activity before sleep, use of relaxation tapes, mood alteration, reading, or imaging before sleep. If the patient is menopausal, consider hormone replacement therapy.

Treatment modalities include three broad areas, each of which is discussed below:

- Psychosocial Adjustment
- Physical Therapy (exercise and pain reduction techniques)
- Pharmacologic Interventions

PSYCHOSOCIAL ADJUSTMENT

The patient comes to the physician feeling threatened by the illness. Treatment should begin with reassurance, explanation, and relief from mechanical stress to the neck and low-back areas. A fibromyalgia pamphlet, available from the local chapter of the Arthritis Foundation, is helpful in patient education and understanding of disease consideration in treatment goals. Support groups exist as well. The Fibromyalgia Network has extensive patient literature and support:

Fibromyalgia Network
P.O. Box 31750
Tucson, AZ 85751-1750
Tel: (800) 853-2929
(520) 290-5508
Fax: (520) 290-5550

Also helpful is a member newsletter published by the Fibromyalgia Alliance of America (formerly the Fibromyalgia Association of Central Ohio) entitled ''Fibromyalgia Times'' (formerly ''The FMS Ohio Newsletter''). Membership is $25 per year.

Fibromyalgia Alliance of America
P.O. Box 21988
Columbus, OH 43221-0988
Tel: (614) 457-4222

Behavior modification should begin with reducing harmful habits such as smoking and/or substance abuse including alcohol and narcotics. Smoking can lead to tissue hypoxia and can delay strengthening and pain control (Table 7.5).

Some patients have caffeine intoxication that might contribute to symptoms. Caffeine enhances analgesic effects (106), but many patients ingest too much caffeine and aggravate sleep quality (107). Theophyllines, also found in dark beverages, can sometimes aggravate sleep. Encourage each patient to eliminate all but one cupful of dark beverages (the exception might be upon arising from sleep) for a 2-week trial. Those who are affected will note major improvement in sleep quality and muscle relaxation. In our experience, about 5 to 10% of patients are significantly affected.

Attitudinal changes should be discussed with the patient (108). The clinician should urge the patient to recognize perfectionist tendencies and impatience with activities of daily living, since these patients tend to complete a task no matter what the physical cost. These patients should be taught to pace physical activity, housekeeping, or hobbies.

Joint protection advice for the neck, back, and shoulder may be of value (see Chapter 8 and Appendix B). Harmful habits may not be apparent and may add a regional pain disorder to compound the problem. Information to assist in occupational problems is discussed in the Introduction.

TABLE 7.5 APPROACHES TO SELF-EFFICACY FOR FIBROMYALGIA

1. Perform an exercise program that suits your interests and ability. Must include aerobic exercise.
2. Healthy balanced diet, no caffeine, no heavy meals within 3 hours of bedtime. Stop smoking and alcohol ingestion.
3. Avoid aggravating habits and overuse by pacing activities and tasks.
4. Consistent sleep habit: try to go to bed and arise at the same time every day.
5. When medication for sleep is needed, take it with the evening meal to reduce hangover effect.
6. Get professional help and develop strategies to live with chronic pain.
7. Use coping strategies to manage stress.
8. Do not expect miracles. Set reachable goals within several months, not days or hours.

Interruption of employment can be a disaster. The patient should be kept both psychologically and physically active, keeping in mind the value of a job as a positive distraction. If fired or forced to resign because of failure to perform as a result of pain and exhaustion, these patients seldom return to full productive capacity.

The expertise of the Bureau of Vocational Rehabilitation may be utilized for evaluating the effect of chronic pain on job performance and the psychosocial makeup of the patient. We have had good results when the patient is brought into contact with a knowledgeable vocational counselor. Other resources include state Bureaus of Employment Services or guidance counselors at local colleges.

Ideally, work should not require prolonged sitting or standing. Rather, when possible, these patients should seek jobs that require variation in body positions. They seem to function better as secretaries, store managers, hostesses, or teachers, and less well as bookkeepers, accountants, and physicians!

If the patient has manifest deficiencies in coping skills, has unusual belief systems, exhibits persistent pain behavior, or has persistent or severe depression, consider referral to a skilled psychotherapist. Follow-up is then important to be certain the therapist is establishing the goal of self-efficacy early on (109, 110). Cognitive therapy and other behavior techniques are available. Resources for pain treatment and behavioralists include the Rehabilitation Accreditation Commission (using their former acronym, CARF) and the American Pain Society:

Rehabilitation Accreditation Commission (CARF)
4891 East Grant Road
Tucson, AZ 85712
Tel: (520) 325-1044

The American Pain Society
4700 Lake Avenue
Glenview, IL 60025
Tel: (708) 375-4700

PHYSICAL THERAPY

Many patients who arise from bed with a general sense of tightness in their muscles will benefit from a stretching exercises (Table 7.6).

Patients should pursue a physical fitness activity such as cardiovascular fitness training (111), swimming, roller skating, tennis, line dancing, or racquetball, depending on overall assessment. These activities tend to involve considerable muscular stretching as well as toning. Walking is generally not as helpful as more vigorous activities. Also, less helpful are the use of step machines and rowing machines because of the localized repetitive movements.

Often fibromyalgia patients have tight muscles that do not allow more than a few repetitions of exercise movement. One technique we find helpful is to begin with pool aerobic exercises or simply water walking for one half-hour. Alternatively, combining the use of a home exercise bicycle, cross-country ski machine, walking with weights, and a videotape-guided nonimpact aerobic exercise, with 1–5 minutes per modality, allows a full half-hour of exercise. The patient should increase the heart rate to 105–120 beats per minute. (Refer also to Table 7.6.)

Aquatic exercise programs are particularly effective in achieving aerobic conditioning when axial and posture muscles are weak. When necessary, use flotation devices, such as the AquaJogger (see Fig. 7.N).

Posture assessment and training are helpful in correcting alignment and body mechanics (Table 7.6). Movement education techniques such as the Feldenkrais method or the Alexander techniques can be helpful in restoring correct and efficient movement patterns (see below). Initial therapy should include proper sleep hygiene and positioning with support under the arch of the neck and the use of a firm mattress (see Fig. 7.P).

TABLE 7.6 EXERCISES FOR FIBROMYALGIA

Exercise	Figure Number
Stretching	7.B to 7.F
Posture Alignment	7.G
Myofascial release	7.I
Pressure point massage	7.J, 7.K
Tai Chi	7.L
Aerobic Exercise	7.M
Aquatic Therapy	7.N

Tension should be dealt with by rest, programmed exercise, and emotional escape. Stretching exercises should be included (Table 7.6). Breathing exercises promote better respiration, relaxation, and alignment. Biofeedback relaxation and learning to appreciate tension perception are often helpful (112).

Self-management strategies are essential, always encouraging the patient to be responsible for enacting and adhering to the program activities; avoid developing patient dependency on others.

Manual techniques such as massage, myofascial release, and pressure techniques for tender points can be helpful for short-term and long-term pain relief (Table 7.6). Massage can be provided in nonmedical settings by trained massage therapists at reasonable cost to the patient and may be of good cost-benefit ratio. Patients can learn self-treatment techniques for pressure therapy with aids such as tennis balls, frozen water balloons, and other devices such as the ''Theracane.''

Emphasize strategies to assist the patient in adhering to exercise and lifestyle programs over the long term. Many patients seem to have return of symptoms in 6-month cycles even if program activities have been carried out. Six-month ''tune-ups'' promote long-term adherence and provide a basis for outcome assessment. Keeping exercise logs, reminder phone calls, regular progress reports, and buddy systems are all good adherence aids.

When joint laxity coexists, therapeutic exercise is very important in order to prevent severe disability (113). Aquatherapy is a good place for such patients to begin fitness training. Pool aerobics, the Arthritis Foundation Aquatic program, and water walking can be used where available. Many motels and apartment complexes have indoor pools and offer their use to the public at a nominal charge.

PHARMACOLOGIC INTERVENTION

Narcotics do not play a role in the treatment of the fibromyalgia syndrome, and indeed they do not work. Similarly, oral corticosteroids and hypnotics are not helpful (114). Review other drugs being used by the patient for possible idiosyncratic reactions that can confound the problem. Diuretics, antihypertensives, eye medications, antihistamines, and, as mentioned, caffeine may impair progress by interrupting sleep (115). Codeine can cause widespread pain and sleep disorder as well.

Muscle Relaxants: Cyclobenzaprine (Flexeril) 5–40 mg/day has been helpful during flare-ups (116–118). Sometimes as little as ¼ tablet (2.5 mg) every other night is helpful, with higher dosages not adding to the response.

Other drugs that are useful include meprobamate, carisoprodol, and diazepam. These act to depress the brainstem activating systems and provide a sedative effect as well as acting centrally as skeletal muscle relaxants (119). Use the smallest doses possible. Patients should have a pill splitter, obtainable at the pharmacy, if needed. In those patients who require these agents for longer than a few weeks, rotation of the medications every few months may prevent the building of tolerance or habituation.

Psychotropic Agents: Fibromyalgia patients display high rates of concomitant disorders including migraine, irritable bowel syndrome, major depression, and panic disorder (32). Treatment with tricyclic antidepressants has been widely researched. Originally introduced because of favorable results on nocturnal sedation, amitriptyline (12.5–100 mg at bedtime) was one of the earliest reliable drugs used in the management of fibromyalgia (120–123). The observed deficiency in serotonin, when improved with tricyclic antidepressant therapy, was found to be correlated with clinical improvement (99). Occasionally amitriptyline hydrochloride will result in a stimulating rather than a sedative effect; patients should be warned that if this occurs, amitriptyline should be discontinued and another psychotropic agent should be tried. Doxepin hydrochloride is available as an elixir and may be more easily titrated. If morning "hangover" is a problem, the tricyclic might be taken after the evening meal. Other tricyclics can be tried; imipramine hydrochloride may be tried in patients with sensitivity to other tricyclics; desipramine hydrochloride may be less sedating. Trazodone hydrochloride is sometimes better tolerated by elderly patients.

Patients with concomitant major depression often respond to the serotonin reuptake inhibitors, including fluoxetine hydrochloride, sertraline hydrochloride, and paroxetine hydrochlo-

ride, usually taken upon arising from sleep. A tricyclic can be added if sleep is impaired. More studies need to be done in order to determine duration and choice of psychotropic agent.

Agents reportedly beneficial but not yet available in the U.S. include zopiclone, a piperazine derivative (124, 125) and S-adenosylmethionine. The latter agent has both antiinflammatory and antidepressant effects; patients with fibromyalgia receiving it experienced improvement in pain, fatigue, morning stiffness, and mood, but not in tender point score, muscle strength, or depression (126).

Many patients are resistant to using any medication, but they should be encouraged to try one or another of the agents mentioned. These agents can improve sleep, muscle tenderness, pain, and depression (127). Often, good management will depend on low dosages, trying various agents within the class of medication, and willingness to mix classes of agent. Thus, a tricyclic combined with a muscle relaxant at half the lowest usual dose may work for some patients. The drugs need not be taken permanently. Often, as exercise induces improvement, the drugs can be reduced to alternate day dosing and then eliminated.

Nonsteroidal antiinflammatory agents (NSAIDs) or analgesics alone are seldom of benefit. Ibuprofen combined with an anxiolytic, alprazolam, was found to be helpful both in a double-blind and in an open-label study (128). Other NSAIDs have given similar variable responses.

An antagonist to substance P, capsaicin, available for topical use is helpful for localized pain; oral preparations are under investigation (129–131). Doxepin cream (0.05%) is currently under investigation for covering larger body regions. The cream is currently available for generalized pruritus.

TENDER POINT INJECTION

Treatment by injecting tender points has many advocates but is controversial—and the literature is confusing as trigger points and tender points have often been confused. Our own experience is overwhelmingly favorable. Having used intralesional methylprednisolone and a local anesthetic for more than three decades in thousands of patients, we have found that the initial benefit is often dramatic and relieves much of the tightness and pain that prevents the performance of an exercise regimen. The benefit may not be perceived for 1 or 2 weeks following the injections (132, 133). Dependency must be avoided. To some extent, the injection rapidly desensitizes the tenderness, which allows the conditioning exercises to proceed more rapidly. If relief occurs, the patient then knows that the physician can provide significant help if flare-ups do not respond to noninvasive treatment.

Each tender point can be injected with 0.5–1 mL procaine/methylprednisolone mixture (not to exceed 40–60 mg steroid total dosage.) A 1-inch No. 23 needle is usually adequate except for use in the gluteus area, in which a 3.5-inch No. 20 spinal needle can be used. No controlled observations are available comparing the results of a corticosteroid-anesthetic injection to results obtained when a local anesthetic is used alone in fibromyalgia. Also, no data compare various corticosteroids and the various local anesthetics. However, as noted in Chapter 5, the addition of steroid was significantly more efficacious in the treatment of low back pain of myofascial origin. The steroid may be suspended in 1–5 mL of a local anesthetic. The mixture of methylprednisolone and lidocaine hydrochloride flocculates in the syringe; the mixture appears to provide a more prolonged effect but may be more painful. Ice applied to the area intermittently throughout the day, for 10 minutes at a time, is helpful. Triamcinolone may cause menstrual irregularity in young women, and steroid agents other than methylprednisolone may be useful, but we generally prefer the mixture of methylprednisolone and lidocaine hydrochloride. Tender point injections should be used as a means to working toward self-efficacy, and should be repeated only if pain persists despite exercise and other measures have been used. We would not repeat the injections in less than 2 or 3 months.

Alternatively, the tender points may be injected with procaine hydrochloride or bupivacaine alone, massaged with ice, or sprayed with Fluori-Methane while the involved muscle is stretched (134, 135).

DIET THERAPY

Vegetarian diet (136) and oral ingestion of L-tryptophan (137, 138) or phenylalanine (139) have been advocated. *No such therapy has withstood the test of time.* L-tryptophan has been associated with the *eosinophilia myalgia syndrome,* a severe reaction following ingestion of a contaminated supply of L-tryptophan, with myalgias, eosinophilia, and respiratory problems. The condition may be chronic, but no new cases have appeared since the offending agent was removed. Also, *eosinophilic fasciitis* was reported to result from L-tryptophan ingestion (140).

Magnesium has been advocated but has not been documented as helpful. One study suggested low levels of red blood cell magnesium concentration in patients with chronic fatigue syndrome (141), though this has been refuted (142). In another study on patients with fibromyalgia, red blood cell magnesium concentration was found to be normal (143). Patients requesting information about diet modification may be referred to the Fibromyalgia Network (address supplied above).

OUTCOME AND ADDITIONAL SUGGESTIONS

The patient should know at the outset that a multidisciplinary approach as outlined above will take several months before significant benefit is realized. Loss of all symptoms is unusual, and the longer the patient has suffered before entering treatment, the less favorable the outcome (133). It is wise for the clinician to inform the patient that during the first month the pain may actually seem worse. This can result from vigorous stretching, or simply from changes in the patient's routine. If the exercises are done with a gradual prolonged initiation of the stretching portion of each exercise, less irritation will occur.

In our experience, many fibromyalgia patients do obtain gratifying relief of symptoms. We have followed hundreds of these patients for many years; we remain amazed at their diligence in performing the exercise program twice daily, and often they no longer require drug therapy. A subgroup requires amitriptyline or cyclobenzaprine during stressful situations. Total cures are rare. After 4 years, 97% of one group of patients reported persistent symptoms and 85% still fulfilled diagnostic criteria (144). Thus true remission is rare, which is in sharp contrast to the results of rheumatoid arthritis and other connective tissue disease in which a significant minority have remissions. The young woman who develops fibromyalgia shortly after the establishment of a family has a less satisfactory outlook for remission than a similar patient with systemic lupus erythematosus or rheumatoid arthritis. Current research into neuroendocrine dysfunction may lead to more satisfactory solutions.

PSYCHOGENIC RHEUMATISM

The complaint "I hurt all over" or "The pain is so bad, you just don't know how bad it is!" will often put the clinician on the defensive— or else, provoke a massive diagnostic workup. Pain is a suffering of the body and mind (145) that can only be known to an individual in his or her consciousness (146). Like hunger, pain is an awareness-of-a-need state. It is a drain upon the physical, the emotional, and the economic resources of the patient (147).

What is called "psychogenic rheumatism" includes many manifestations of mental illness and exaggerated psychophysiologic responses to internal stress. These patients do not have the tenderness just in tender point areas; the tenderness is also exhibited in the control points, along with an exaggerated response to light touch.

The somatoform disorders include the following (45):

1. Somatization disorder (including classic hysteria)
2. Hypochondriasis
3. Conversion disorder (hysterical neurosis)
4. Psychogenic pain disorder (includes psychogenic rheumatism)

Wallace has described in addition a number of epidemics of pain attacks that he believes were forms of mass hysteria. These included epidemic fibromyalgia in British and American armed forces during World War II and epidemic neuromyasthenia during polio epidemics (45).

Psychogenic rheumatism often is regional or generalized pain so severe that the body cannot be touched—the "touch-me-not syn-

drome" (41). The scalp, face, trunk, and limbs may share the pain-to-touch equally. Tender points are not present. The patient usually can relate the onset to an emotionally charged situation. Whereas fibromyalgia has exacerbations brought on by the external milieu, psychogenic rheumatism is related to internal stress. The patient has an ache in the body when there is an ache in the mind. At other times, the patient feels just fine; often the patient will say, "Before this, I couldn't have felt better." That, too, differs from fibromyalgia, in that fibromyalgia symptoms rarely return completely to normal.

Other features of psychogenic rheumatism include (148):

1. Previous diagnosis of "arthritis"
2. Predominantly female
3. Have been seen by multiple physicians
4. Report "swelling" but no objective signs
5. Have great concern for family history of "arthritis"
6. Depressed, apprehensive, anxious
7. May have other rheumatic disease
8. Have normal laboratory tests
9. Pain in regions (e.g., whole left side of body)
10. Pain terms are bizarre (e.g., searing, pulsating, burning)
11. Location of pain changes, or becomes the "touch-me-not" response
12. May vigorously deny emotional factors
13. Refractory to medical and physical therapy
14. Often tearful, the symptoms are "so bad"

Conversion reactions are more impressive in focusing on a specific disability. In our experience, they usually involve the upper or lower limb, and can be confused with a reflex sympathetic dystrophy. Bone scans are helpful in differential diagnosis (see the section "Reflex Sympathetic Dystrophy" in Chapter 3). To complicate the problem further, reflex sympathetic dystrophy and conversion may both improve with the use of a transcutaneous electrical nerve stimulator! When confronted with an obvious conversion problem, consultation with an experienced psychiatrist is advisable.

Somatic delusions in schizophrenia are easily recognized if other delusions or hallucinations are brought out during the history.

Treatment often can be provided by the primary physician. With forthrightness from the beginning, the patient may be told that the heightened sensitivity to pain is a result of stress and can be improved. Stress management techniques include counseling, behavior or attitude modification, addressing lifestyle needs, and searching for new methods for self-efficacy. Many of the fibromyalgia strategies will be helpful.

THE CLENCHER SYNDROME

This disorder is easily missed and can lead to excessive testing and treatment. Jaw clenching and bruxism can result in neck pain and headache; fist clenching can lead to carpal tunnel syndrome, trigger finger, and other upper limb complaints; and rectal clenching can cause coccygodynia, low back pain, and perineal discomfort. Caffeine intoxication can contribute to the syndrome. In Chapter 3 we described a not uncommon example of a person who has a despicable job or supervisor, drives a half-hour to work all the while clenching teeth, fists, and rectum, arriving exhausted and possibly having generated symptoms of headache, carpal tunnel syndrome, and coccygodynia from the clenching.

Any repetitive movement might trigger a work-related ''injury'' in patients with the clencher syndrome. We see dozens of such patients presenting with one or more features. Just talking it out is good therapy. Sometimes caffeine intoxication is a factor. A 2-week trial of eliminating all dark beverages may be worthwhile.

THE HYPERMOBILITY SYNDROME

Minor structural skeletal disorders are common and are important causes for *regional* rheumatic pain and disability. Joint laxity (hypermobility) is the most common structural cause for more widespread soft tissue pain and disability. Joint laxity is practically never mentioned by the patient and must be sought by the examiner.

The diagnosis of the hypermobility syndrome is based upon finding three or more areas of joint laxity (149–151) (Table 7.7 and

TABLE 7.7 FEATURES OF THE BENIGN HYPERMOBILITY SYNDROME

A. History
1. Symmetrical joint pain and stiffness
2. Sensation of joint swelling of brief duration
3. Onset of joint symptoms after prolonged inactivity
4. Joint laxity in other family members
5. No other contributing illness or disease
B. Presence of three or more areas with joint laxity:
   Passive apposition of thumb to forearm
   Passive hyperextension of fingers
   Active hyperextension of elbow > 10 degrees
   Active hyperextension of knee > 10 degrees
   Ability to flex spine and place palms on the floor without bending knees

Fig. 7.3). Although more refined methods for measurement and diagnosis exist, this simple point count remains the preferred method for diagnosis (152). If a point is allowed for each side of the body, a total of nine possible points can occur; four to six points are usually found in symptomatic patients (153).

The diagnosis is difficult in children, who have greater joint laxity than adults (154). For older children, a goniometric quantitative measurement technique has been devised to assist in measurement and diagnosis (155).

Case Report: Norma T., a 26-year-old secretary, presented with the chief complaint of hand pain and swelling. She could no longer complete her typing and secretarial tasks because of pain and weakness when typing or writing for any length of time. The swelling, which was limited to her fingers, was characterized by a sensation, not by visible swelling. It was present upon arising from sleep, when she noted stiffness as well, which lasted about an hour. She did not have numbness or tingling. Her rings felt tight, and the fingers were stiff. The sensation occurred after any hand work such as typing, writing, or peeling vegetables, and it lasted 3 to 4 hours. She also noted pain and stiffness in the neck, hips, and knees. The problem began shortly after she returned to work after having been on medical leave to care for her new child. There was no family history of rheumatic disease. She had been athletic and participated in gymnastics in school, then joined an aerobics group until she became pregnant. Now she wanted to know if

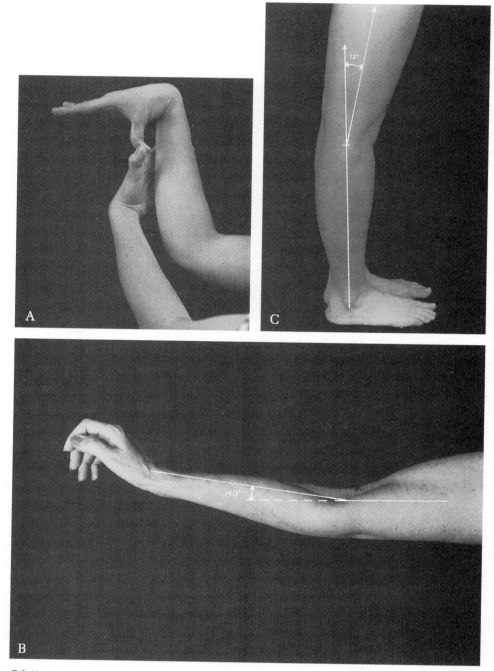

Figure 7.3. Hypermobility syndrome. **A.** Laxity of the wrist allows approximation of the thumb to the patient's ipsilateral forearm. **B.** Laxity of the elbow with greater than 10 degrees of joint extension. **C.** Laxity of the knee with greater than 10 degrees of joint extension.

arthritis would prevent her from returning to aerobics.

Physical examination revealed normal features on inspection. No skin hyperelasticity or striae were noted. A high arched palate was not present. General examination revealed no abnormalities. Joint palpation revealed no synovitis but the proximal interphalangeal joints

(PIP joints) were definitely tender. She did have flat feet. Joint range-of-motion examination revealed excessive mobility at the shoulder, elbow, wrist, thumb, and PIP joints. The latter revealed excessive side-to-side mobility. Laxity was also present at the hip, spine, and ankles. Roentgenograms of the hands and wrists and appropriate laboratory studies for inflammation were within normal limits.

In summary, the patient had a history of joint "swelling" that lasted for too brief a duration for inflammation, joint laxity in three or more joints, and no other features of underlying disease. These features constitute a syndrome known as the *benign hypermobility syndrome.*

The first known reference to joint laxity is attributed to Hippocrates, who, in the 4th century BC, described the Scythians as being "so-loose-limbed that they were unable to draw a bow-string or hurl a javelin" (156).

Joint laxity may result from more serious diseases of the connective tissues such as Marfan's syndrome, hyperlysinemia, osteogenesis imperfecta, pseudoxanthoma elasticum, homocystinuria, and Ehlers-Danlos syndrome as well as rheumatic fever, rheumatoid arthritis, acromegaly, and neurologic disease (Table 7.8). Furthermore, as an inherited disorder, joint laxity may occur in association with clubfoot and recurrent dislocations of hips, shoulders, or patellae. Toe deformities are commonly associated as well (157).

Joint laxity as an inherited cause for congenital joint dislocation has been reported many times in the past century (158). These are rare when compared to the much more common benign hypermobility syndrome, described by Kirk, Ansell, and Bywaters (159); they defined the hypermobility syndrome as generalized

TABLE 7.8 DISORDERS ASSOCIATED WITH JOINT LAXITY

Ehlers-Danlos syndrome	Acromegaly
	Acute rheumatic fever
Marfan's syndrome	Rheumatoid arthritis
Pseudoxanthoma elasticum	Poliomyelitis
	Tabes dorsalis
Osteogenesis imperfecta	Familial joint deformities
	Clubfoot
Myotonia congenita	Dislocation of shoulder, hip, patellae
Homocystinuria	Toe deformities
Hyperlysinemia	

From Sheon RP, Kirsner AB, Farber SJ, Finkel RI: The hypermobility syndrome. Postgrad Med 71:199–209, 1982.

joint laxity with musculoskeletal complaints in an otherwise normal person. Biro et al. emphasized similar features in children having juvenile arthritis (160). They and others (161–164) found that 5.7% (15 of 262) of children seen for a diagnosis of juvenile arthritis actually had the benign hypermobility syndrome, and only 3 of the 15 patients with inflammatory juvenile arthritis had coexisting joint laxity.

Thompson and colleagues noted joint laxity in 1.3% of high school athletes (165). Raskin and Lawless (166) reported results of a careful musculoskeletal examination of healthy medical students revealing 85 structural disorders among the 123 students. Of these, 22 had at least one lax joint and 14 others had three or more lax joints. Limited joint motion was detected in 33 students. Other studies suggest that 5% of children and 1% of adults have joint laxity. Joint laxity is more common in the right limb, in females, in blacks, and in children from families with higher socioeconomic status. Joint laxity is thus common and usually is not symptomatic. In an orthopaedic practice, Finsterbush and Pogrund noted that among 100 consecutive patients with joint laxity in three or more joint regions and without other discernible disease, 44% had generalized pain that was of long duration with acute exacerbations. In the remaining patients, pain in the knees or feet were common presenting complaints. They also noted that 65% of first-degree relatives (mostly mothers) had joint laxity (149).

Other extraarticular tissues and organs which rely on the tensile strength of normal collagen may be affected. The skin may be soft and develop striae. Mitral valve prolapse may be more common (153). Weakness in abdominal and pelvic floor support may occur. Bone fragility may lead to increased susceptibility to fracture, particularly stress fracture.

Our experience suggests that in a private rheumatology practice, benign hypermobility syndrome is as common as rheumatoid arthritis. But because joint laxity is so common in the general population, careful examination to exclude other more serious disease is essential (164). The marfanoid syndrome, with added features of Marfan's syndrome and Ehlers-Danlos syndrome including joint laxity, cardiac valvular lesions, symmetrical striae and a high arched palate, is occasionally seen (150, 167, 169). In our patients with joint laxity, a high arched palate, and striae, we have not seen any serious cardiac abnormalities. However, Grahame and colleagues (151) noted an increased frequency of mitral valve prolapse among their patients, though this has not been the experience of others (169).

As has been pointed out, these patients may have generalized or regional complaints. Many patients with hypermobility syndrome have additional features of fibromyalgia (113). The patients with both disorders may have axial pain of fibromyalgia and peripheral joint complaints of the hypermobility syndrome.

The significance of joint laxity in back pain also requires emphasis. Howes and Isdale (170) reported the "loose back" as a common and often unrecognized cause for backache among women. They reported that of 102 consecutive cases of "problem" back patients, musculoskeletal examination with careful attention for joint laxity revealed no cases of generalized joint laxity among the 59 male patients; all but 17 of the 59 males had disc or other skeletal lesions. Among the 17 males without a specific organic back disorder, three had one or more lax joints. Of the 43 female patients, 23 had local back derangements, but 20 had no discernible cause for backache. Whereas two women with a definable back condition also had joint laxity, 17 of the 20 without another cause for backache had joint laxity. This possible association of joint laxity with backache in women has also been recognized in several industrial centers in Europe (170).

Chondrocalcinosis and *precocious osteoarthritis* appear to have an increased association with joint laxity (163, 172).

Laboratory and Radiologic Examination. Tests for inflammation and rheumatoid factor are normal. Roentgenograms are usually normal, although in the older patient with hypermobility syndrome, they may reveal chondrocalcinosis or degenerative changes beyond those expected for age (163).

Management. Treatment consists of explanation, strengthening, joint protection, and symptomatic treatment medication (149, 157, 160). Upon reassuring the patient that serious crippling is not a consequence and that seden-

tary activity leads to decreased muscle tone and support for lax joints, most patients are receptive to a conditioning program. The use of individualized resistance exercise to forearm extensors, quadriceps, and abdominal muscles has been helpful (149).

The importance of proper body mechanics and the value of joint protection for this condition should be emphasized, as these measures are likely to reduce pain and disability. Patients should be warned to respect pain during repetitive activities. Those whose attitude is, "I'm going to finish this even if it kills me!" may cause cartilage injury due to joint laxity and overuse.

Patients should be taught to avoid arm hyperextension during sleep. Since these patients can assume unusual sitting, lying, and resting body positions, the physician should review each of these positions with the patient. In particular, these patients should not sit with knees tucked under or Indian style. Proper shoes should be recommended if pes planus is present. Refer to Appendix B for joint protection measures. Bracing is sometimes necessary for the knees. Referral to a physical therapist and occupational therapist may be very cost-effective. In severely deconditioned patients, or if fibromyalgia is also present, we find that aquatic exercises can be very helpful to begin reconditioning.

Outcome. Joint protection principles for hand use, lower limb joints, and the back are essential (153). Because the exercises may be required for several months until optimal strength is achieved, the patient should be told at the outset that exercise may seem to aggravate the problem or seem unhelpful for a month or longer. Use of NSAIDs for joint pain is therefore recommended (157, 160, 161, 171). Once exercises have provided improved strength, a lifelong sport or conditioning program should be strongly encouraged in order to maintain good muscle tone. When myofascial pain and spasm interfere with rehabilitation, an intralesional soft tissue corticosteroid injection can be helpful (153). In our experience, most patients, even older patients with premature osteoarthritis, respond reasonably well to a resistance exercise program. The younger the patient, we have found, the more complete has been the response to therapy.

Probably these patients should be told to avoid as much as possible occupations that require prolonged repetitive tasks as they grow older, in the hope of preventing premature osteoarthritis (172).

POLYMYALGIA RHEUMATICA

Widespread stiffness and aching of the shoulder girdle and/or the pelvic girdle are the usual complaints. The condition is rarely seen in persons younger than age 55. The onset is usually abrupt, and shoulder motion may rapidly become limited. The key distinction from fibromyalgia is the limitation of motion and a high erythrocyte sedimentation rate (173). A Westergren erythrocyte sedimentation rate determination is preferable to other methods because the longer tube provides the means for detecting a much greater range of abnormality than other methods. Bone scans may demonstrate uptake by the involved joints (174, 175).

Some physicians prefer to begin therapy with NSAIDs, but more common initial therapy is a 2-week trial with 10 mg prednisone to be taken as a single dose each morning. Dramatic relief in stiffness and pain and in range of shoulder movement is notable. The sedimentation rate will usually return toward normal by the end of 2 weeks. Persistent symptoms should lead to consideration of other diagnoses such as temporal arteritis (giant cell arteritis). About 6% of patients may have underlying rheumatoid arthritis or an occult neoplasm.

Temporal arteritis may present similarly. If any of the following *features of giant cell arteritis* are present, we recommend a temporal artery biopsy examination to exclude this diagnosis:

- Severe headache
- Dimming of vision, diplopia, blurred vision
- Jaw claudication
- Temporal artery swelling
- Scalp tenderness
- Eyeball pain
- Fever, anemia, neuropathy

In a temporal artery biopsy analysis, segments 0.3–1 cm or longer of the vessel are obtained, and the entire segment specially examined for arteritis. The biopsy may be done as an outpatient procedure. Some rheumatologists routinely recommend bilateral biopsy if frozen section studies of the initially examined vessel are normal. We find that 20% of patients with polymyalgia have abnormal biopsy results: 10% have frank giant cell arteritis, and 10% have less defined features of arteritis such as fibrosis and disruption of the internal elastic membrane. Although a therapeutic trial with 10 mg prednisone daily may provide dramatic articular symptomatic benefit, it may not be enough to prevent vascular occlusion if vasculitis is present. Blindness is a feared complication. When vasculitis is present, the prednisone dose should be high initially, between 40 and 80 mg daily. A prolonged steroid taper must be individualized. The patient usually will note significant symptomatic benefit after a few days of steroid therapy. If azotemia or urine sediment is present, other types of vasculitis should be considered, particularly when giant cells were not evident in the biopsy examination. Antineutrophil cytoplasmic antibodies (ANCAs) may suggest underlying Wegener's granulomatosis.

Other connective tissue disorders that have polymyalgia symptoms include rheumatoid arthritis, Sjögren's syndrome (176), systemic lupus erythematosus, vasculitis, polymyositis, paraneoplastic musculoskeletal syndromes, hypertrophic osteoarthropathy, Paget's disease, ankylosing spondylitis, calcium apatite deposition disease, and pseudogout. Older patients may have systemic infection presenting without fever and without localizing complaints. A blood culture should be considered if any suspicion exists (refer to Table 7.4 above on critical features of generalized soft tissue pain).

EOSINOPHILIC FASCIITIS

In eosinophilic fasciitis, usually pain, swelling, and tenderness followed by severe induration of the skin and subcutaneous tissue occur. The skin at first is erythematous and warm; later it becomes hyperpigmented and nodular. The extremities are the usual site of involvement. Circulating eosinophilia is regularly present. Biopsy examination reveals inflammation and fibrosis, frequently with eosinophils in the deep fascia. Immunoglobulin and complement is deposited in the subcutaneous fascia. Contractures and sclerodermatous skin changes or morphea may occur (177). Pulmonary fibrosis, autoimmune anemia, thrombocytopenia, Raynaud's phenomenon, Sjögren's syndrome, carpal tunnel syndrome, and myelofibrosis may occur (178, 179, 181). A wedge biopsy including skin and muscle should be examined. Treatment with low dose corticosteroids has been helpful in some cases (177, 179–181).

Systemic reactions to pollutants and contaminants may cause unusual presentations with soft tissue inflammation. Toxic oil syndrome, due to ingestion of adulterated oil, can similarly result in scleroderma, eosinophilia, neuropathy, myalgia, rash, and pulmonary edema (181).

Eosinophilia-myalgia syndrome following ingestion of contaminated L-tryptophan has been reported to present with eosinophilia, severe myalgia followed by edema, and cutaneous thickening. Some patients went on to develop eosinophilic fasciitis (182).

BORRELIAL FASCIITIS

Granter et al. describe *Borrelia burgdorferi* in tissue obtained from two patients with diffuse fasciitis and eosinophilia. Identification of the organism in deep fascia was possible using the modified Dieterle or Steiner technique or using rabbit polyclonal antibodies against the organism. For such cases, the authors recommend the term Borrelial fasciitis (183).

REFERENCES

1. Wolfe F, Smythe HA, Yunus MB, et al.: The American College Of Rheumatology 1990 criteria for the classification of fibromyalgia. Arthritis Rheum 33:160–172, 1990.
2. Gowers WR: Lumbago: its lessons and analogues. Br Med J 1:117–121, 1904.
3. Bonica JJ: Management of myofascial pain syndromes in general practice. JAMA 164: 732–738, 1957.
4. Smythe HA, Moldofsky H: Two contributions to understanding of the "fibrositis" syndrome. Bull Rheum Dis 28:928–931, 1977.
5. Campbell SM, Clark S, Tindall EA, Forehand ME, Bennett RM: Clinical characteristics of fibrositis. Arthritis Rheum 26:817–824, 1983.
6. Yunus MB, Masi AT: Juvenile primary fibromyalgia syndrome: a clinical study of 33 patients and matched normal controls. Arthritis Rheum 28:138–145, 1985.
7. Wolfe F, Sheon RP: When aching is generalized, consider fibrositis. Diagnosis (July):44–61, 1984.
8. Fischer AA: Pressure tolerance over muscles and bones in normal subjects. Arch Phys Med Rehabil 67:406–409, 1986.
9. Kolar E, Hartz A, Roumm A, et al.: Factors associated with severity of symptoms in patients with chronic unexplained muscular aching. Ann Rheum Dis 48:317–321, 1989.
10. Wolfe F: Tender points, trigger points, and the fibrositis syndrome. Clin Rheumatol Pract (Jan/Feb):36–38, 1984.
11. Yunus M, Masi AT, Colabro JJ, et al.: Primary fibromyalgia: clinical study of 50 patients with matched normal controls. Sem Arthritis Rheum 11:151–170, 1981.
12. Wolfe F, Cathey MA: The epidemiology of tender points: a prospective study of 1520 patients. J Rheumatol 12:1164–1168, 1985.
13. Wolfe F: Non-articular symptoms in fibrositis: rheumatoid arthritis, osteoarthritis, and arthralgia syndrome. (Abstract #E45) Arthritis Rheum 25(4) [Suppl], 1982.
14. Smythe H, Sheon RP: Fibrositis/fibromyalgia: a difference of opinion. Bull Rheum Dis 39(3): 1–8, 1990.
15. Sheon RP: Regional myofascial pain and the fibrositis syndrome (fibromyalgia). Comprehensive Ther 12:42–52, 1986.
16. Wolfe F, Simons DG, Fricton J, et al.: The fibromyalgia and myofascial pain syndromes: a preliminary study of tender points and trigger points in persons with fibromyalgia, myofascial pain syndrome, and no disease. J Rheumatol 19: 944–951, 1992.
17. McCombe PF, Fracs JC, Fairbank T, et al.: Reproducibility of physical signs in low-back pain. Spine 14(7):908–918, 1989.
18. Reilly PA, Littlejohn GO: Peripheral arthralgic presentation of fibrositis/fibromyalgia syndrome. J Rheumatol 19:281–283, 1992.
19. Goldman JA: Hypermobility and deconditioning: important links to fibromyalgia/fibrositis. Southern Med J 84:1192–1196, 1991.
20. Beethan WP Jr: Diagnosis and management of fibrositis syndrome and psychogenic rheumatism. Med Clin North Am 63:433–439, 1979.
21. Goldenberg DL, Simms RW, Geiger A, et al.: High frequency of fibromyalgia in patients with chronic fatigue seen in a primary care practice. Arthritis Rheum 33:381–387, 1990.

22. Goldenberg DL: Fibromyalgia, chronic fatigue, and myofascial pain syndromes. Curr Opin Rheumatol 4(2):247–257, 1992.
23. Goodnick PJ, Sandoval R: Psychotropic treatment of chronic fatigue syndrome and related disorders. J Clin Psychiatry 54(1):13–20, 1993.
24. Buchwald D, Garrity D: Comparison of patients with chronic fatigue syndrome, fibromyalgia, and multiple chemical sensitivities. Arch Intern Med 154:2049–2053, 1994.
25. Hidding A, vanSanten M, De Klerk E, et al.: Comparison between self-report measures and clinical observations of functional disability in ankylosing spondylitis, rheumatoid arthritis, and fibromyalgia. J Rheumatol 21:818–823, 1994.
26. Henriksson CM: Long-term effects of fibromyalgia on everyday life. Scand J Rheumatol 23:36–41, 1994.
27. Bennett RM, Clark SR, Campbell SM, et al.: Symptoms of Raynaud's syndrome in patients with fibromyalgia. Arthritis Rheum 34(3):264–269, 1991.
28. Small D: Clinical features of 256 patients with Sjögren's syndrome who are seronegative for antibodies to SSA(Ro) or SSB(La). (Abstract #26) Arthritis Rheum 36(9) [Suppl]:S43, 1993.
29. Clark SR, Forehand ME: Pain perception and anxiety with fibrositis. (Abstract #16) Arthritis Rheum 26(4) [Suppl], 1983.
30. Uveges JM, Parker JC, Smarr KL, et al.: Psychological symptoms in primary fibromyalgia syndrome: relationship to pain, life stress, and sleep disturbance. Arthritis Rheum 33(8):1279–1283, 1990.
31. Yunus M, Ahles TA, Aldag JC, Masi AT: Relationship of clinical features with psychological status in primary fibromyalgia. Arthritis Rheum 34(1):15–21, 1991.
32. Hudson JI, Goldenberg DL, Pope HG, Keck PE: Comorbidity of fibromyalgia with medical and psychiatric disorders. Am J Med 92:363–374, 1992.
33. Triadafidopoulos G, Simms RW, Goldenberg DL: Bowel dysfunction in fibromyalgia syndrome. Dig Dis Sci 36:59–64, 1991.
34. Veale D, Kavanagh G, Fielding JF, et al.: Primary fibromyalgia and the irritable bowel syndrome: different expressions of a common pathogenetic process. Br J Rheumatol 30:220–222, 1991.
35. Clauw DJ, Schmidt M, Radulovic D, et al.: The relationship between fibromyalgia and interstitial cystitis. (Abstract #1118) Arthritis Rheum 37(9) [Suppl]:S347, 1994.
36. Kraft GH, Johnson EW, LaBan MM: The fibrositis syndrome. Arch Phys Med Rehabil 49:155–162, 1968.
37. Travell J, Rinzler SH: The myofascial genesis of pain. Postgrad Med 11:425–434, 1952.
38. Bennett RM: Muscle physiology and cold reactivity in fibromyalgia syndrome. Rheum Dis Clin North Am 15:135–148, 1989.
39. Middleton GD, McFarlin JE, Lipsky PE: The prevalence and clinical impact of fibromyalgia in systemic lupus erythematosus. Arthritis Rheum 37:1181–1188, 1994.
40. Lane RJM, Mastaglia FL: Drug-induced myopathies in man. Lancet 2:562–566, 1978.
41. Hench PS, Boland EW: The management of chronic arthritis and other rheumatic diseases among soldiers of the United States Army: Ann Rheum Dis 5:106–114, 1946.
42. Cathey MA, Wolfe F, Kleinheksel SM, Hawley DJ: The socio-economic impact of fibrositis. (Abstract #B34) Arthritis Rheum 29(4) [Suppl], 1986.
43. Wolfe F, Cathey MA, Kleinheksel SM, Amos SP, et al.: Psychological status in primary fibrositis and fibrositis associated with rheumatoid arthritis. J Neurol Sci 58:73–78, 1983.
44. Reynolds MD: The definition of fibrositis. Arthritis Rheum 25:1506–1507, 1982.
45. Wallace DJ: Fibromyalgia: unusual historical aspects and new pathogenic insights. Mt Sinai J Med 51:121–134, 1984.
46. Prescott E, Kjoller M, Jacobsen S, et al.: Fibromyalgia in the adult Danish population: I. A prevalence study. Scand J Rheumatol 22(5):233–237, 1993.
47. Prescott E, Jacobsen S, Kjoller M, et al.: Fibromyalgia in the adult Danish population: II. A study of clinical features. Scand J Rheumatol 22(5):238–242, 1993.
48. Forseth KO, Gran JT: The prevalence of fibromyalgia among women aged 20–49 years in Arendal, Norway. Scand J Rheumatol 21:74–78, 1992.
49. Wolfe F, Ross K, Anderson J, et al.: The prevalence and characteristics of fibromyalgia in the general population. Arthritis Rheum 38:19–28, 1995.
50. Raspe H, Baumgartner C: The epidemiology of fibromyalgia syndrome in a German town. (Abstract) Scand J Rheumatol 94(Suppl):S38, 1992.
51. Lyddell C: The prevalence of fibromyalgia in a South African community. (Abstract) Scand J Rheumatol 94(Suppl):S143, 1992.
52. Nishikai M: Fibromyalgia in Japanese. J Rheumatol 19:110–114, 1992.
53. Gedalia A, Press J, Klein M, Buskila D: Joint hypermobility and fibromyalgia in schoolchildren. Ann Rheum Dis 52:494–496, 1993.
54. Buskila D, Press J, Gedalia A, et al.: Assessment of nonarticular tenderness and prevalence of fibromyalgia in children. J Rheumatol 20:368–370, 1993.
55. Malleson PN, Al-Matar M, Petty RE: Idiopathic musculoskeletal pain syndromes in children. J Rheumatol 19:1786–1789, 1992.
56. Harvey CK: Fibromyalgia. Part II: Prevalence in the podiatric patient population. J Am Podiatr Med Assoc 83(7):416–417, 1993.
57. Bennett RM: Fibromyalgia and the facts. Rheum Dis Clin North Am 19:45–59, 1993.

58. Van Denderen JC, Boersma JW, Zeinstra P, et al.: Physiological effects of exhaustive physical exercise in primary fibromyalgia (PFS): is PFS a disorder of neuroendocrine reactivity? Scand J Rheumatol 1992;21:35–37.

59. Sietsema KE, Cooper DM, Caro X, et al.: Oxygen uptake during exercise in patients with primary fibromyalgia syndrome. J Rheumatol 20: 860–865, 1993.

60. Jacobsen S, Danneskiold-Samsoe B: Dynamic muscular endurance in primary fibromyalgia compared with chronic myofascial pain syndrome. Arch Phys Med Rehabil 73(2): 170–173, 1992.

61. Jubrias SA, Bennett RM, Klug GA: Increased incidence of a resonance in the phosphodiester region of 31P nuclear magnetic resonance spectra in the skeletal muscle of fibromyalgia patients. Arthritis Rheum 37:801–807, 1994.

62. Wortmann RL: Searching for the cause of fibromyalgia: is there a defect in energy metabolism? (Editorial) Arthritis Rheum 37:790–793, 1994.

63. Simms RW, Roy SG, Hrovat M, et al.: Lack of association between fibromyalgia syndrome and abnormalities in muscle energy metabolism. Arthritis Rheum 37:794–800, 1994.

64. Reilly PA: Fibromyalgia in the workplace: a ''management'' problem. Ann Rheum Dis 52:249–251, 1992.

65. Bruusgaard D, Evensen AR, Bjerkedal T: Fibromyalgia. Scand J Soc Med 21(2):116–119, 1992.

66. Saskin P, Moldofsky H, Lue FA: Sleep and posttraumatic rheumatic pain modulation disorder (fibrositis syndrome). Psychosom Med 48(5): 319–323, 1986.

67. Dinerman H, Steere AC: Lyme disease associated with fibromyalgia. Ann Intern Med 117: 281–285, 1992.

68. Hsu VM, Patella SJ, Sigal LH: ''Chronic lyme disease'' as the incorrect diagnosis in patients with fibromyalgia. Arthritis Rheum 36(11): 1493–1500, 1993.

69. Greenfield S, Fitzcharles MA, Esdaile JM: Reactive fibromyalgia syndrome. Arthritis Rheum 35(6):678–681, 1992.

70. Leventhal LF, Naides SJ, Freundlich B: Fibromyalgia and Parvovirus infection. Arthritis Rheum 34:1319–1324, 1991.

71. Moldofsky H, Scarisbrick P, England R, et al.: Musculoskeletal symptoms and non-REM sleep disturbances in patients with ''fibrositis syndrome'' and healthy subjects. Psychosom Med 37:341–351, 1975.

72. Kirk JA, Ansell BM, Bywaters EGL: The hypermobility syndrome: musculoskeletal complaints associated with generalized joint hypermobility. Ann Rheum Dis 26:419–425, 1967.

73. Golden H, Weber SM, Bergen D: Sleep studies in patients with fibrositis syndrome. (Abstract #142) Arthritis Rheum 26(4) [Suppl], 1983.

74. McBroom P, Ware JC, Russell IJ: Sleep disturbances in primary and secondary fibromyalgia syndrome. Paper presented to the Nonarticular Rheumatism Study Group, American Rheumatism Association, Minneapolis, 1984.

75. Moldofsky H: Sleep and fibrositis syndrome. Rheum Clin North Am 15:91–103, 1989.

76. Horne JA, Shackel BS: Alpha-like activity in non-REM sleep and the fibromyalgia (fibrositis) syndrome. Electroencephalogr Clin Neurophysiol 79:271–276, 1991.

77. Hawley DJ, Wolfe F, Cathey MD: Pain and functional disability and psychological states: a 12-month study of severity in fibromyalgia. J Rheumatol 15:1551–1556, 1988.

78. Bennett RM, Clark SR, Campbell SM, et al.: Low levels of somatomedin C in patients with the fibromyalgia syndrome. Arthritis Rheum 35: 1113–1116, 1992.

79. Moldofsky H, Lue FA, Davidson JR, et al.: The effect of 64 hours of wakefulness on immune functions and plasma cortisol in humans. In: Horne J, ed. Sleep '88. Stuttgart and New York: Gustav Fischer Verlag, 1989:185–187.

80. Moldofsky H, Lue FA, Davidson JR, et al.: Effects of sleep deprivation on human immune functions. FASEB J 3:1972–1977, 1989.

81. Manu P, Lane TJ, Matthews DA, et al.: Alpha-delta sleep in patients with a chief complaint of chronic fatigue. Southern Med J 87:465–470, 1994.

82. Sternberg EM, Chrousos GP, Wilder RL, Gold PW: The stress response and the regulation of inflammatory disease. Ann Intern Med 117(10): 854–866, 1992.

83. Reynolds DV: Surgery in the rat during electrical analgesia induced by focal brain stimulation. Science 164:444–445, 1969.

84. Matucci-Cerinic M: Sensory neuropeptides and rheumatic diseases. Rheumatic Clin North Am 19:975–991, 1993.

85. Vaeroy H, Helle R, Forre O, et al.: Elevated CSF levels of substance P and high incidence of Raynaud phenomenon in patients with fibromyalgia: new features for diagnosis. Pain 32: 21–26, 1988.

86. Russell IJ, Orr MD, Littman B, et al.: Elevated cerebrospinal fluid levels of substance P in patients with the fibromyalgia syndrome. Arthritis Rheum 37:1593–1601, 1994.

87. Kaneko H, Mitsuma T, Uchida K, et al.: Immunoreactive-somatostatin, substance P, and calcitonin gene-related peptide concentrations of the human gastric mucosa in patients with nonulcer dyspepsia and peptic ulcer disease. Am J Gastroenterol 88(6):898–904, 1993.

88. Hyppa, MT, Alaranta H, Lahtela K, et al.: Neuropeptide converting enzyme activities in CSF of low back pain patients Pain 43:163–168, 1990.

89. Terenius L: Endorphins and modulation of pain. Adv Neurol 33:59–64, 1982.

90. Cleeland C, Schacham S, Dahl J, et al.: CSF B-endorphin and the severity of pain. Neurology 34:378–380, 1984.

91. Vaeroy H, Nyberg F, Terenius L: No evidence for endorphin deficiency in fibromyalgia following investigation of cerebrospinal fluid (CSF) dynorphin A and Met-enkephalin-Arg6-Phe7. Pain 46:139–143, 1991.

92. Hall S, Littlejohn GO, Jethwa J, Copolov D: Plasma beta-endorphin (BEP) levels in fibrositis. (Abstract #A6) Arthritis Rheum 26(4) [Suppl], 1983.

93. Yunus MB, Denko CW, Masi AT: Serum B-Endorphin in primary fibromyalgia syndrome. Paper presented to Nonarticular Rheumatism Study Group. Los Angeles, June 5, 1985.

94. Jara LJ, Lavelle C, Fraga A, et al.: Prolactin, immunoregulation, and autoimmune diseases. Semin Arthritis Rheum 20(5):273–284, 1991.

95. Yunus MB, Dailey JW, Aldag JC, et al.: Plasma and urinary catecholamines in primary fibromyalgia: a controlled study. J Rheumatol 19:95–97, 1992.

96. Crofford L, Pillemer SR, Kalogeras KT, et al.: Hypothalamic-pituitary-adrenal axis perturbations in patients with fibromyalgia. Arthritis Rheum 37:1583–1592, 1995.

97. Russell IJ, Vaeroy H, Javors M, et al.: Cerebrospinal fluid biogenic amine metabolites in fibromyalgia/fibrositis syndrome and rheumatoid arthritis. Arthritis Rheum 35:550–556, 1992.

98. Griep EN, Boersma JW, de Koet ER: Altered reactivity of the hypothalamic-pituitary-adrenal axis in the primary fibromyalgia syndrome. J Rheumatol 20:418–421, 1993.

99. Russell IJ, Bowden CL, Michalek JE, et al.: Platelet 3H-imipramine uptake receptor density and serum serotonin levels in patients with fibromyalgia/fibrositis syndrome. J Rheumatol 19: 104–109, 1992.

100. Yunus M, Dailey JW, Aldag JC, et al.: Plasma tryptophan and other amino acids in primary fibromyalgia: a controlled study. J Rheumatol 19:90–94, 1992.

101. Alexander RW, Mountz JM, Mountz JD, et al.: Spect imaging of caudate nucleus (cn) regional cerebral blood flow (rcbf): a sensitive physiological marker of fibromyalgia (fm). (Abstract) Arthritis Rheum 37(9) [Suppl]:346, 1994.

102. Horven S, Stiles TC, Holst A, et al.: HLA antigens in primary fibromyalgia syndrome. J Rheumatol 19:1269–1270, 1992.

103. Hudson JI, Hudson MS, Pliner LF, et al.: Fibromyalgia and major affective disorder: a controlled phenomenology and family history study. Am J Psychiatry 142:441–446, 1985.

104. Pellegrino MJ, Waylonis GW, Sommer A: Familial occurrence of primary fibromyalgia. Arch Phys Med Rehabil 70:61–63, 1989.

105. Stormorken H, Brosstad F: Fibromyalgia: family clustering and sensory urgency with early onset indicate genetic predisposition and thus a true disease (Letter). Scand J Rheumatol 21:207, 1992.

106. Sawynok J, Yaksh TL: Caffeine as an analgesic adjuvant: a review of pharmacology and mechanisms of action. Pharmacol Rev 45(1):43–85, 1993.

107. Strain EC, Mumford GK, Silverman K, et al.: Caffeine dependence syndrome. JAMA 272: 1043–1048, 1994.

108. Hester G, Grant AE, Russell IJ: Psychological evaluation and behavioral treatment of patients with fibrositis. (Abstract #E62) Arthritis Rheum 25(4) [Suppl], 1982.

109. Gonzalez VM, Goeppinger J, Lorig K: Four psychosocial theories and their application to patient education and clinical practice. Arthritis Care & Research 3(3):132–143, 1990.

110. Nielson WR, Walker C, McCain GA: Cognitive behavioral treatment of fibromyalgia syndrome: preliminary findings. J Rheumatol 19:98–103, 1992.

111. McCain GA, Bell D, Mai F, Zilly C: The effects of a double-blind supervised exercise program in the fibrositis/fibromyalgia syndrome (FS). (Abstract #D29) Arthritis Rheum 29(4) [Suppl], 1986.

112. Fowler RS Jr, Kraft GH: Tension perception in patients having pain associated with chronic muscle tension. Arch Phys Med Rehabil 55: 28–30, 1974.

113. Goldman JA: Hypermobility: the missing link to fibrositis. (Abstract #E62) Arthritis Rheum 25(4) [Suppl], 1986.

114. Clark S, Tindall E, Bennett R: A double-blind crossover study of prednisone in the treatment of fibrositis. (Abstract #D1) Arthritis Rheum 27(4) [Suppl], 1984.

115. Eichner ER: Ergolytic drugs in medicine and sports. Am J Med 94:205–211, 1993.

116. Campbell SM, Gatter RA, Clark S, Bennett RM: A double-blind study of cyclobenzaprine versus placebo in patients with fibrositis. (Abstract #D3) Arthritis Rheum 28(4) [Suppl], 1985.

117. Brown BR Jr, Womble J: Cyclobenzaprine in intractable pain syndromes with muscle spasm. JAMA 240:1151–1152, 1978.

118. Reynolds WJ, Moldofsky H, Saskin P, Lue FA: The effects of cyclobenzaprine on sleep physiology and symptoms in patients with fibromyalgia. J Rheumatol 18:452–454, 1991.

119. Domino EF: Centrally acting skeletal-muscle relaxants. Arch Phys Med Rehabil 55: 369–373, 1974.

120. Carette S, McCain GA, Bell DA, Fam AG: Evaluation of amitriptyline in primary fibrositis. Arthritis Rheum 29:655–659, 1986.

121. Jaeschke R, Adachi J, Guyatt G, et al.: Clinical usefulness of amitriptyline in fibromyalgia: the results of 23 N-of-1 randomized controlled trials. J Rheumatol 18:447–451, 1991.

122. Santandrea S, Montrone F, Sarzi-Puttini P, et al.: A double-blind crossover study of two cyclobenzaprine regimens in primary fibromyalgia syndrome. J Int Med Res 21(2):74–80, 1993.

123. Carette S, Bell MJ, Reynolds WJ, et al.: Comparison of amitriptyline, cyclobenzaprine, and placebo in the treatment of fibromyalgia: a randomized, double-blind clinical trial. Arthritis Rheum 1:32–40, 1994.

124. Gronblad M, Nykanen J, Konttinen Y, et al.: Effect of zopiclone on sleep quality, morning stiffness, widespread tenderness and pain, and general discomfort in primary fibromyalgia patients: a double-blind randomized trial. Clin Rheumatol 12(2):186–191, 1993.

125. Drewes AM, Andreasen A, Jennum P, Nielsen KD: Zopiclone in the treatment of sleep abnormalities in fibromyalgia. Scand J Rheumatol 20(4):288–293, 1991.

126. Jacobsen S, Danneskiold-Samsoe B, Andersen RB: Oral S-adenosylmethionine in primary fibromyalgia: double-blind clinical evaluation. Scand J Rheumatol 20:294–302, 1991.

127. Rummans TA: Nonopioid agents for treatment of acute and subacute pain. Mayo Clin Proc 69:481–490, 1994.

128. Russell IJ, Fletcher EM, Michalek JE, et al.: Treatment of primary fibrositis/fibromyalgia syndrome with ibuprofen and alprazolam: a double-blind, placebo-controlled study. Arthritis Rheum 34(5):552–560, 1991.

129. Snider RM, Constantine JW, Lowe JA: A potent nonpeptide antagonist of the substance P (NK1) receptor. Science 251:435–439, 1991.

130. Kolasinski SL, Haines KA, Siegel EL, et al.: Neuropeptides and inflammation: a somatostatin analog as a selective antagonist of neutrophil activation by substance P. Arthritis Rheum 35(4): 369–375, 1992.

131. Henry JL: Substance P and inflammatory pain: potential of substance P antagonists as analgesics. AAS Inflammatory Disease Therapy 41: 5–87, 1993.

132. Travell J: Myofascial trigger points: clinical view. In: Bonica JJ, Albe-Fessard DG, eds. Advances in Pain Research and Therapy. Vol. 1. New York: Raven Press, 1976.

133. Kraft GH, Johnson EW, LaBan MM: The fibrositis syndrome. Arch Phys Med Rehabil 49: 155–162, 1968.

134. Travell JG, Simons DG: Myofascial pain and dysfunction: the trigger point manual. Baltimore: Williams & Wilkins, 1983.

135. Rubin D: Myofascial trigger point syndromes: an approach to management. Arch Phys Med Rehabil 62:107–110, 1981.

136. Hostmark AT, Lystad E, Vellar OD, et al.: Reduced plasma fibrinogen, serum peroxides, lipids, and apolipoproteins after a 3-week vegetarian diet. Plant Foods for Human Nutrition 43: 55–61, 1993.

137. Hedaya RJ: Pharmacokinetic factors in the clinical use of tryptophan. J Clin Psychopharmacol 4(6):347–348, 1984.

138. Seltzer S, Stock R, Marcus R, Jackson E: Alteration of human pain thresholds by nutritional manipulation and L-tryptophan supplementation. Pain 13:385–393, 1982.

139. Mitchell MJ, Daines GE, Thomas BL: Effect of L-tryptophan and phenylalanine on burning pain threshold. Phys Ther 67:203–205, 1987.

140. Cotsarelis G, Werth V: Tryptophan-induced eosinophilic fasciitis. J Am Acad Dermatol 23(5-1):938–941, 1990.

141. Cox IM, Campbell MJ, Dowson D: Red blood cell magnesium and chronic fatigue syndrome. Lancet 337:757–760, 1991.

142. Durlach J: Chronic fatigue syndrome and chronic primary magnesium deficiency. (Commentary) Magnesium Res 5:68, 1992.

143. Prescott E, Norrgard J, Rothol Pedersen L, et al.: Fibromyalgia and Magnesia. Scand J Rheumatol 21:206, 1992.

144. Ledingham J, Doherty S, Doherty M: Primary fibromyalgia syndrome: an outcome study. Br J Rheumatol 32:139–142, 1993.

145. The New American Webster Handy College Dictionary. New York: New American Library, 1972.

146. Merskey H: Psychiatric aspects of the control of pain. In: Bonica JJ, Albe-Fessard DG, eds. Advances in Pain Research and Therapy. Vol. 1. New York: Raven Press, 1976.

147. Bonica JJ: Neurophysiologic and pathologic aspects of acute and chronic pain. Arch Surg 112:750–761, 1977.

148. Kaplan H: Fibrositis and psychogenic rheumatism. Arthron 3:3–7, 1984.

149. Finsterbush A, Pogrund H: The hypermobility syndrome: musculoskeletal complaints in 100 consecutive cases of generalized joint hypermobility. Clin Orthop Research 168:124–127, 1982.

150. Walker BA, Beighton PH, Murdock LJ: The Marfanoid hypermobility syndrome. Ann Intern Med 71:349–352, 1969.

151. Grahame R, Edwards JC, Pitcher D, Gabel A, Harvey W: A clinical and echocardiographic study of patients with hypermobility syndrome. Ann Rheum Dis 40:541–546, 1981.

152. Wolfe F: Clinical, laboratory, and radiographic assessments. Curr Opin Rheumatol 5: 138–145, 1993.

153. Beighton PB, Grahame R, Bird HA: Hypermobility of joints. 2nd ed. Berlin, Heidelberg, and New York: Springer, 1989.

154. Gedalia A, Person DA, Giannini EH, Brewer EJ: Joint hypermobility in juvenile episodic arthritis/arthralgia. Paper presented to the Central Region Interim Meeting, American Rheumatism Association, Chicago, 1984.

155. Fairbank JCT, Pynsent PB, Phillips H: Quantitative measurements of joint mobility in adolescents. Ann Rheum Dis 43:288–294, 1984.

156. Grahame, R: Joint hypermobility: clinical aspects. Proc Roy Soc Med 64:32–34, 1971.

157. Sheon RP, Kirsner AB, Farber SJ, Finkel RI: The hypermobility syndrome. Postgrad Med 71:199–209, 1982.

158. Finkelstein H: Joint hypotonia: with congenital and familial manifestations. New York Med J 104:942–944, 1916.

159. Kirk JA, Ansell BM, Bywaters EGL: The hypermobility syndrome: musculoskeletal complaints associated with generalized joint hypermobility. Ann Rheum Dis 26:419–425, 1967.

160. Biro F, Gewanter HL, Baum J: The benign hypermobility syndrome in pediatrics. (Abstract #E33) Arthritis Rheum 25(4) [Suppl], 1982.

161. Beighton PH, Horan ET: Dominant inheritance in familial generalized articular hypermobility. J Bone Joint Surg 52B:145–147, 1970.

162. Key JA: Hypermobility of joints as a sex linked hereditary characteristic. JAMA 88: 1710–1712, 1927.

163. Bird HA, Tribe CR, Bacon PA: Joint hypermobility leading to osteoarthrosis and chondrocalcinosis. Ann Rheum Dis 37:203–211, 1978.

164. James JIP, Wynne-Davies R: Genetic factors in orthopaedics. In: Apley AG, ed. Recent advances in orthopaedics. London: J & A Churchill, 1969.

165. Thompson TR, Andrish JT, Bergfeld JA: A prospective study of preparticipation sports examinations of 2670 young athletes: method and results. Cleve Clin Q 49:225–233, 1982.

166. Raskin RJ, Lawless OJ: Articular and soft tissue abnormalities in a "normal" population. J Rheumatol 9:284–288, 1982.

167. Goodman RM, Wooley CF, Frazier RL, Covault L: Ehlers-Danlos syndrome occurring together with the Marfan syndrome. N Engl J Med 273:514–519, 1963.

168. Cotton DJ, Brandt KD: Cardiovascular abnormalities in the marfanoid hypermobility syndrome. Arthritis Rheum 19:763–768, 1976.

169. Jessee EF, Owen DJ Jr, Sagar KB: The benign hypermobile joint syndrome. Arthritis Rheum 23:1053–1056, 1980.

170. Howes RG, Isdale IC: The loose back: an unrecognized syndrome. Rheum Phys Med 11: 72–77, 1971.

171. Sheon RP: Joint laxity and the hypermobility syndrome. Arthron (Fall):3–16, 1984.

172. Rowatt-Brown A, Rose BS: Familial precocious polyarticular osteoarthrosis of chondrodysplastic type. NZ Med J 65:449–461, 1966.

173. Hunder GG, Hazleman BL: Giant cell arteritis and polymyalgia rheumatica. In: Kelley WN, et al., eds. Textbook of Rheumatology. 2nd ed. Philadelphia: WB Saunders, 1985.

174. O'Duffy JD: Increasing evidence suggests PMR is not a muscle disease. Wellcome Trends in Rheumatology 1:1–2, 1979.

175. Chou CT, Schumacher HR: Clinical and pathologic studies of synovitis in polymyalgia rheumatica. Arthritis Rheum 27:1107–1117, 1984.

176. Bennett RM: Fibrositis: does it exist and can it be treated? J Musculoskel Med 1:57–72, 1984.

177. Shulman LE: Diffuse fascitis with hypergammaglobulinemia and eosinophilia: a new syndrome. J Rheum (Suppl):82, 1974.

178. Medsger TA Jr: Systemic sclerosis (scleroderma), eosinophilic fasciitis, and calcinosis. In: McCarty DJ, ed. Arthritis and allied conditions. 10th ed. Philadelphia: Lea & Febiger, 1985.

179. Jacobs MB: Eosinophilic fasciitis, reactive hepatitis, and splenomegaly. Arch Intern Med 145:162–163, 1985.

180. Hoffman R, Young N, Ershler WB, Major E, Gewirtz A: Diffuse fasciitis and aplastic anemia: a report of our cases revealing an unusual association between rheumatologic and hematologic disorders. Medicine 61:373–381, 1982.

181. Marinez Tello FJ, Navas-Palacios JJ, Ricoy JR, et al.: Pathology of a new syndrome caused by ingestion of adulterated oil in Spain. Virchows Arch A Pathol Anat Histopathol 397: 261–285, 1982.

182. Jaffe I, Kopelman R, Baird R, et al.: Eosinophilic fasciitis associated with the eosinophilia-myalgia syndrome. Am J Med 88:542–546, 1990.

183. Granter SR, Barnhill RL, Hewins ME, et al.: Identification of Borrelia burgdorferi in diffuse fasciitis with peripheral eosinophilia: Borrelial fasciitis. JAMA 272:1283–1285, 1994.

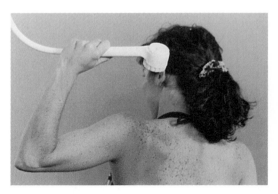

Figure 7.A. A hand-held shower allows heat to be applied to specific areas.

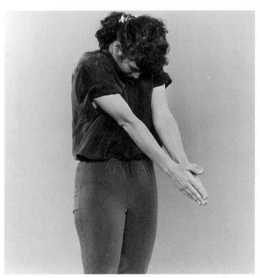

Figure 7.B. Lower Cervical/Upper Thoracic Stretch
Tuck chin into chest. Push arms forward and down. Hold 5–10 seconds and repeat. Stretch should be felt in the posterior neck and upper back.

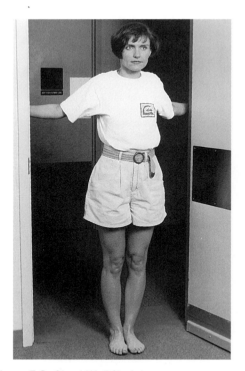

Figure 7.C. Chest Wall Stretch
With arms on door frame at shoulder level, step through door until stretch is felt across chest. Hold 10–30 seconds and repeat. *Use caution if patient has history of shoulder dislocation.* (Alternate method: Exercise 4.B, Corner Stretch.)

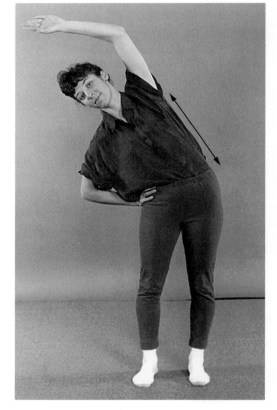

Figure 7.D. Lateral Body Stretch
Raise arm overhead and bend to the opposite side. Do not bend forward or backward. Hold 5–30 seconds and repeat. Stretch will be felt along body as indicated by *arrows*.

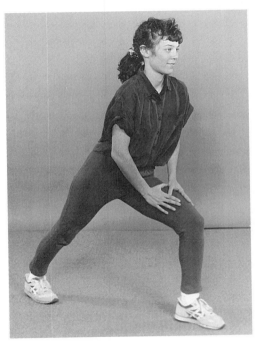

Figure 7.E. Lunge Stretch

Perform as illustrated. While performing this exercise, the neck and back should be in straight alignment and the back foot flat on the floor. Hold stretch 10–30 seconds. Stretch is felt in the back leg.

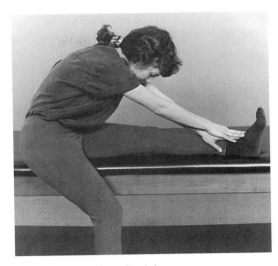

Figure 7.F. Hamstring Stretch

Sit with one leg/foot to the side of the bed. Bend forward, reaching the hands toward the foot. Hold 10–30 seconds. Stretch is felt in posterior trunk, thigh, and calf. (For an alternative method, see Exercise 5.L, Straight Leg Stretching).

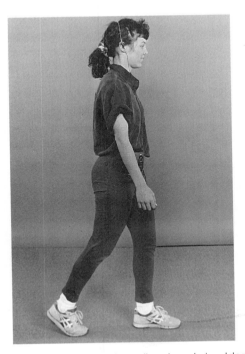

Figure 7.G. Correct posture aligns head, shoulders, and hips during gait and allows smooth transition of weight.

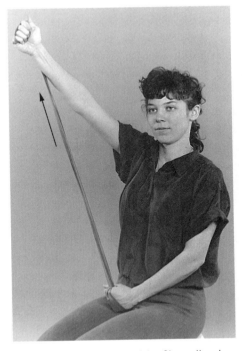

Figure 7.H. Theraband Shoulder Strengthening

Using one hand to stabilize the Theraband, the opposite arm can use its resistance to strengthen arm and shoulder girdle muscles during various movements—in this case, forward elevation at the shoulder.

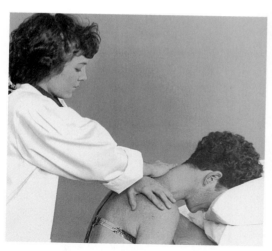

Figure 7.I. Myofascial release to upper trapezius muscles. This soft tissue mobilization technique can be taught to a support person by a qualified therapist.

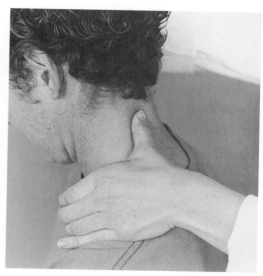

Figure 7.J. Ischemic pressure technique to a tender point provides pain relief.

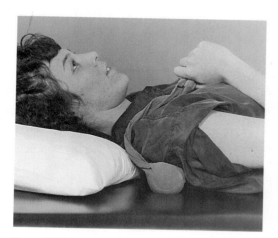

Figure 7.K. Tennis-ball trick. Self-pressure technique with a tennis ball in a stocking applied to a tender point.

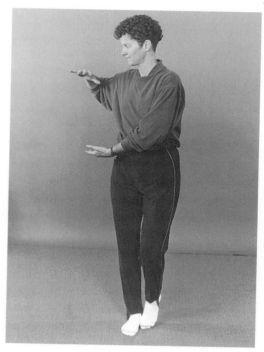

Figure 7.L. The slow sequential patterns of Tai Chi allow several benefits in fibromyalgia management, including relaxation, peace of mind, increased flexibility, improved endurance, and decreased pain.

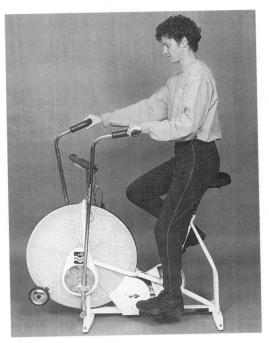

Figure 7.M. Aerobic exercise provides cardiovascular and positive neuroendocrine effects.

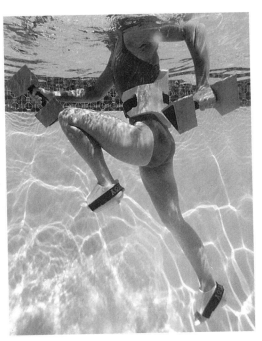

Figure 7.N. Aquatic Exercise

Aquatic exercise is well suited for many soft tissue conditions. The AquaJogger is an example of available flotation equipment. (See Appendix E for the source of this device.)

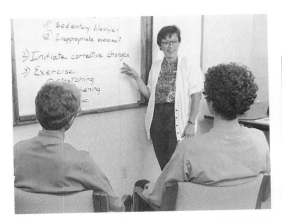

Figure 7.O. Patient education addresses many issues in self-management.

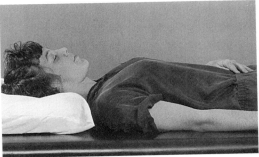

Figure 7.P. Relaxation is an important pain management technique. A variety of methods are available and can be demonstrated during patient education sessions.

8: Physical Interventions, Exercise, and Rehabilitation

BARBARA BANWELL AND PATRICIA HOEHING

BASIC CONCEPTS

Foundations and Interventions of Treatment

Physical interventions for systemic or regional soft tissues and musculoskeletal symptoms include the use of thermal (heat or cold), electrotherapeutic, ultrasound, and hydrotherapy modalities. Many types of exercise, posture and movement training, and a wide range of manual techniques such as massage, mobilization, and manipulation, are utilized by practitioners. These interventions can be applied in many settings, and many of them will have already been tried by patients as an intuitive "first aid" or "home remedy" approach before their first contact with a physician. It is quite common, for example, for people to apply heat or cold packs to sore muscles soon after the onset of discomfort or stiffness, or to soak in a warm tub to seek relief from joint pain. Changing position or taking a rest is a person's first reaction to postural fatigue, and stretching is a natural reaction to muscle spasm. However, other interventions are not first nature and require specific prescription and planning. Active exercise for low back pain is a good example of this situation, because most people in our society have become accustomed to the recommendation of rest and avoidance of strenuous activity for back problems.

The skill in using physical remedies for soft tissue disorders lies not so much in the choice of treatment components, but rather in judicial planning and staging of activities, active and creative exercise design, and motivating for long-term adherence to the program. Hadler provides excellent guidelines—"that physical interventions should be comfortable, that none are mandatory, and that nearly all are empirical. Benefits should clearly outweigh discomfort, inconvenience, stigmatization, or enforced disability" (1).

The foundations for practice use physical measures and exercise in soft tissue disorders; these are drawn from theory, tradition, belief, and research. Ideally, the choice of physical interventions in a treatment plan should be based on a research literature reflecting a body of knowledge that establishes a consensus for practice. However, Ottenbacher (2) notes that such consensus does not exist for every question of interest in the field of rehabilitation. He also describes shortcomings and difficulties in rehabilitation research that lead to the contradictory research literature and lack of statistical agreement. Ottenbacher notes in particular the problem of statistical invalidity in rehabilitation research because of small sample size and failure to establish the magnitude of treatment effect. He emphasizes, however, that many treatments may have important clinical effects even though they fail to achieve statistical significance in research studies. Therefore, it is necessary to distinguish between a treatment's statistical significance and effect and its clinical significance and effect; it is imperative that clinical, anecdotal, and empirical evidence not be entirely discounted as a basis for selection of physical intervention.

From another perspective, Spencer emphasizes that the "quantifiable is not all there is in rehabilitation. Counting or measuring is not sufficient as a way of understanding the resilience of patients or what inspires their despair or joy" (3). According to Spencer's model, treatment methods should be considered in light of three different dimensions: the overall context, the meaning of the treatment within that context, and the change that can be attributed to the treatment (3). In selecting or evaluating physical interventions or rehabilitation techniques, the practitioner might ask questions such as the following: In what context are the methods used? What is their meaning to the patient in that specific situation, environment, or cultural background? What types of changes are brought about by the use of these methods, and how important are they to the patient? In this light, foundations for the utilization of physical intervention and rehabilitation emerge from both the art and the science of rehabilitation and can offer many options and treatment strategies to complement pharmacologic intervention and provide the patient with self-management activities.

Current trends in health care economics mandate more specific and rigorous assessment of function and functional outcomes. Fortunately, the rehabilitation field has emphasized functional assessment during the past decade (4, 5). This volume consistently brings into focus the effect of rehabilitation upon functional status in soft tissue disorders and emphasizes a full spectrum of rehabilitation settings and activities including medical, community, and home based resources.

Patient Education

Patient education regarding soft tissue rheumatism management is crucial to successful prophylaxis, rehabilitation, and prevention of recurrence. This volume has emphasized the importance of thoroughly educating the patient about the problem, the purpose of and plan for management activities, and the expected outcomes of treatment. It is particularly important that the patient recognize and appreciate the time period expected for normal tissue healing and recovery so that continued pain after treatment has been initiated not be seen as treatment failure. The patient should understand the difference between healing and recovery. Healing is the body's natural process of restoring damaged tissues to normal or near-normal states. The process can occur with or

without intervention, but does not require effort on the part of the individual. Proper rest and nutrition, overall good health, and fitness can contribute to the healing process. Recovery, on the other hand, is the process in which persistent effort from the patient is applied toward getting well. It includes increases in strength, flexibility, coordination, and functional performance. In the recovery process, attention is focused on improvements even though symptoms may remain, and progress, effort, and functional return are emphasized.

Physicians and therapists should clarify the limited role and short-term benefits of passive treatments such as heat and cold packs or massage and encourage transition to more active, long-lasting treatment activities. Patients who understand the purpose and limitations of the physical management procedures will be more likely to comply with instructions and adhere to exercise schedules. A variety of patient education materials is available from specific organizations such as the Arthritis Foundation (6) and the Fibromyalgia Network (7) as well as from commercial sources. These materials will help the patient and family to understand various diseases, treatments, and related topics. Patient libraries can be assembled in treatment settings including materials such as these and complemented by individual information packets describing particular practices, resources, and philosophies. Patients should have ready access to these materials in community as well as medical libraries, treatment settings, or health fairs.

Self-Management and Home Programs

Many of the treatment activities aimed at soft tissue rheumatic problems can be carried out by the patient in the home or work setting. The goals of treatment must be related to restoration of function rather than comfort. Therapists must resist the temptation to provide only those services that result in patient comfort and gratitude, and choose instead those therapeutic activities that challenge and empower.

When exercises and home programs are taught to patients by nonprofessionals, teaching methods should be thorough and complete. Many patients are exposed to superficial teaching sessions in which no provision is made for follow-up, reassessment, modification, and revision. Any teaching activity requires good preparation and techniques, with appropriate materials, documentation, and follow-up procedures.

Efficiency and practicality should be considered in every component of the treatment program. For instance, adaptations to posture and movement patterns should be tailored to the home or work environment rather than to an ideal or esoteric model. The purchase of new equipment, aids, or furniture should be made only after appropriate trial periods, if possible. Carter provides an excellent and complete review of modifications and adaptations that can be made for the common musculoskeletal problems resulting from repetitive head or arm motions during computer work or from improper positioning of the video display terminal (8). Expensive physical modalities should be limited to short-term use and continued only if and when obvious benefit is obtained, with transition to less expensive home techniques as soon as possible. Particularly in the area of thermal (heat or cold) modalities, simple techniques such as a sock filled with dry rice and heated briefly in the microwave oven (see below), moist hot or cold packs, and ice or other items from the freezer should be used. The wise practitioner will have a variety of adaptive items available for trial and borrowing, and might consider furnishing the waiting room with samples of ergonomic items and sturdy posture-friendly furniture.

Treatment plans should have specific short-term and long-term goals, including competence in self-management and functional activities that are based in the home or work setting. Instruction in home activities should begin with the first treatment session and the patient should be aware that self-management is implicit in treatment progression. Many elements of the exercise program can be performed in a nonmedical setting such as the "Y," health clubs, community recreation facilities, or even the home basement gymnasium. Certified massage therapists can be located in most communities and can provide many of the massage techniques available in medical therapy departments. In addition, many massage therapists are willing to work with medical practitioners and therapists who have specific disease-related knowledge in order to better develop and adapt their techniques to specific client needs. Similarly, personal trainers can provide excellent guidance and encouragement for exercise clients who have clinical diagnoses, in collaboration with physicians or physical therapists. It may be very helpful for medically based practitioners to establish partnerships and collaborations with community-based counterparts and to maintain frequent and ongoing communication with these partners. Many of the treatment approaches to soft tissue rheumatism can be "de-medicalized" with thoughtful planning and use of community resources.

Because many soft tissue conditions are directly or indirectly attributed to injury, trauma, or other external force, some patients may take on a passive or dependent role in recovery, awaiting change in the external environment. Pain and decreased function may also bring about anger and frustration (see Chapter 9). When treatment activities such as exercise bring about increased discomfort or fatigue, the long-term goals of restoration to function are overshadowed by the short-term goals of pain relief. The short-term benefits of pain relief must be linked to self-management strategies for the long-term benefit.

Assessment Strategies

Comprehensive assessment of the patient with regional soft tissue problems has been addressed throughout this volume. The patient's history and report of symptoms and function provide initial guidance for the choice of assessment strategies. Additionally, the practitioner will observe certain functions as the patient performs them. For rheumatology rehabilitation management, certain physical tests, objective measurements, and descriptions are used. Strength and range of motion are tested, and individual body parts can be measured for girth or circumference. Pain is described with identification of pain points, and mapping the location of painful areas should be done with notation of the patient's response when pain is elicited. Certain patterns of joint laxity will identify patients with hypermobility syndrome, which may affect the choice of stretching and strengthening methods. The foot deserves special attention because of its relevance to posture and gait. Many assessment techniques are depicted throughout the chapters and text.

Assessment and evaluation provide the framework within which treatment planning and implementation occur. The therapist must balance the need for information against economic and patient-driven efficiency. Furthermore, data should be assembled in a format that will facilitate sequential recording and depict progress as it becomes apparent. With the current trend toward outcome-related data, the therapists must record more than simply the changes in ranges of motion, pain, and strength. Instead, documentation of reported and observed changes in abilities in daily function, difficulty in performance, and changes in levels of comfort or pain should be the primary focus and are crucial to measuring the effectiveness of care. However, *independence* in these areas may not be the only objective of treatment. Spencer (3) reminds us that the ability to *collaborate,* or seek, use, and accept help can be more valuable to clients than striving for absolute independence in function. She points out the bias toward a value on independence that is manifest in various assessment instruments rating independence rather than the ability to work *collaboratively with others.* The development in a patient's ability to seek and utilize appropriate assistance may contribute more to a meaningful encounter with a health care system than a rigid focus on functional independence.

Therapists are well advised to provide some form of treatment during the initial evaluation session, in order to assure the patient that some of their needs are being met. Instruction in some basic breathing and posture exercises (such as axial extension) and in the use of simple thermal modalities are excellent first session treatment activities. The assessment process may have caused the patient to experience anxiety, discomfort, or fatigue, and some active treatment can ease these problems.

Close communication between the referring physician and the therapist can and should streamline the assessment process. The use of ''faxed'' information or other telecommunica-tions with standardized evaluation formats, at least for the subjective component of the evaluation, can establish an efficient format for the flow of information from one source to another. Evaluation formats throughout this book provide suitable sources of information for the therapist to develop a treatment plan. Figure 8.1 is one format for a data sheet that records assessments appropriate to the rheumatology patient. It includes sections for recording data on range of motion, strength, tender points, foot disorders, spinal alignment and pain, joint status, and hypermobility. Some items on the hypermobility section are illustrated in Figure 8.A. Hypermobility is important to identify because of its proposed correlation with soft tissue disorders.

The formulation-of-problem statement, goals and objectives, and treatment activities with emphasis on functional performance issues will logically follow the history and assessment data. The incorporation of standardized functional status instruments with acceptable sensitivity to change will facilitate the accumulation of database and outcome material. Every patient assessment should reflect the therapists' appreciation of sequential data collection and the importance of internal consistency in the data. Sequential reports should indicate progress toward goals and objectives and revision of treatment plans.

Posture, defined as the carriage or position of the body during static and dynamic function, is a dimension that should be assessed in every evaluation. Many strategies for posture assessment have been used, such as grids, charts, photographs, and measures of specific curve. Again, it is important to document sequential changes in posture, highlighting such components as forward head position, shoulder on trunk position, kyphosis, lordosis, and scoliosis. Symmetry and position of landmarks such as scapulae, iliac crests, anterior superior iliac spines, and popliteal fossae should be described and followed. Overall alignment in static standing and sitting postures as well as observed postures during function should be described. Ability to sustain a particular posture over time is also a useful measurement. The ''Posture Score Sheet'' published by Reedco (P.O. Box 345, Auburn, NY 13621) is a conve-

ARTHRITIS ASSESSMENT

NAME _____ DATE _____

LEFT				RIGHT	
M.S.	Passive ROM			M.S.	Passive ROM
		SH	Flex		
			Ext		
			Abd		
			E.R.		
			I.R.		
			Traps-up		
			Traps-mid		
			Traps-low		
			Rhomboid		
			Lats		
		ELB	Flex		
			Ext		
			Sup		
			Pron		
		WR	Flex		
			Ext		
			U.D.		
			R.D.		
			Dominant		
			ABDOMS		
		HIP	Flex		
			Ext		
			Abd		
			E.R.		
			I.R.		
		KN	Flex		
			Ext		
		ANK	P.F.		
			D.F.		
			Inv.		
			Ev.		
			SUBTALAR		

POSTURE:

Cervical

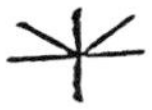

Thoracic

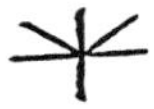

Lumbar

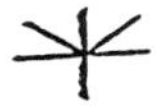

Active Joint Count:_____

Palpation Findings

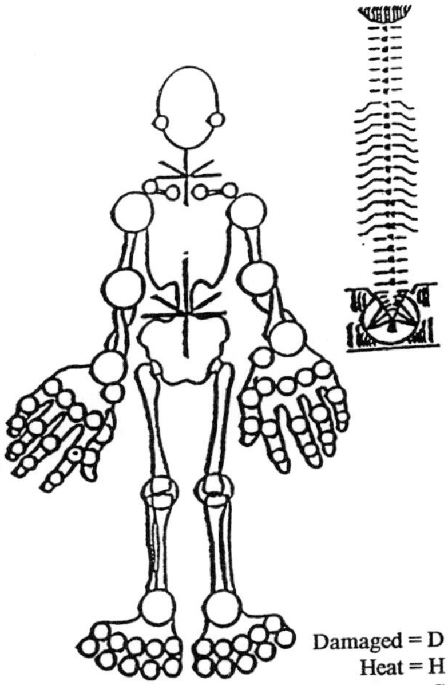

Damaged = D
Heat = H
Crepitus = C
Swelling = S
Effusion = ●
Tenderness/Stress Pain = ⊗

Fibromyalgia Tender Points

	R	L	R	L	
Occiput					Lat Epicondyle
L. Cervical					Med Epicondyle
Upper trap					Gluteal
Supraspinatus					Greater Trochanter
Paraspinals (T5)					Knees
2nd Rib					Forearm
Lat Pecs					Thumbnail
					Mid Foot

FEET	Pain		Valgus		Varus		Other: bunion, callus, sublux, crossed, hammer
	L	R	L	R	L	R	
Hindfoot							
Forefoot							
Hallux							
2nd							
3rd							
4th							
5th							

Special Tests _____

HYPERMOBILITY INDEX   PTS

1.	P DF 5th MP jts > 90°	1 pt R/L	_____
2.	P opp thumb/forearm	1 pt R/L	_____
3.	Hyperext elbows > 10°	1 pt R/L	_____
4.	Hyperext knees > 10°	1 pt R/L	_____
5.	Fwd flex trunk-palms touch floor	1 pt R/L	_____

TOTAL   _____

INDEX

Marked	= 5-9 pts
Mild	= 2-4 pts
Physiologic	= 0-2 pts

Therapist Signature

9/93 Forms#2:ARTHRIAS.PM5

Figure 8.1. The Rheumatology Data Sheet. (Adapted from the Physical Therapy Department, St. Lawrence Hospital, 2900 Hannah Blvd, East Lansing, MI 48840.)

nient recording form that provides a scoring method to document change in each area.

Treatment Progression

Progression of treatment activities is important in order to address the acute, moderate, resolving, and chronic phases of soft tissue problems.

Most patients with acute conditions will be receiving pharmacologic intervention, possibly by injection, that may produce immediate changes in their condition. Physicians who perform the injections often have a specific format for physical therapy activities, including treatment for the period immediately following injection, such as active and passive stretching with or without the use of vapocoolant spray or ice, massage, or manual therapy to increase range of motion. Progression of treatment after the acute stage will include modification of the program to meet specific needs. Treatment progresses to include movement retraining and strength, flexibility, and endurance activities when acute symptoms diminish. As the condition resolves, contact with the patient continues as necessary and possible for monitoring and reinforcement of treatment and teaching. The number of actual treatment sessions will vary according to individual situations.

Graded exercise progresses from (a) passive and assisted to active, (b) nonresistance to resisted, and (c) gross to fine movement. Exercises should be done in straight, rotational, and diagonal planes and should encompass specific activities of daily living (Fig. 8.B*a–d*) in order to achieve functional goals. Exercise activities can be varied and progressed by altering the amount of resistance offered, the arcs of motion performed, the number of repetitions performed, the total time in exercise performance, the speed of performance, and the complexity of movements involved. Weightbearing progresses from non-weightbearing to partial to full weightbearing with no support. Movement dysfunctions or improper patterns must be corrected before exercise can progress, or the dysfunctions will persist and be reinforced. Posture retraining is more than the admonition to ''straighten up, pull the head and shoulders back, and tuck in the stomach.'' Individual patterns of muscle ''firing'' must be identified

and corrected if necessary. For example, the lower trapezius muscles must function properly in order to retract the shoulders correctly. However, trapezius function may be limited and not well integrated into the entire process. The patient and therapist may have to start the retraining process in prone or even side-lying positions with guidance and some awareness of or facilitation to the lower trapezius in the shoulder retraction motion. Headley (9) emphasizes the importance of retraining in an orderly fashion.

Progress in rehabilitation activities should be recorded by means of functional scales that are adequately sensitive to clinical change. Selection of these scales is discussed by Deyo (10, 11).

PHYSICAL MODALITIES

Physical modalities employed to decrease pain should be presented in terms of their better preparing the patient to participate in conditioning or restorative activities rather than to preserve sedentary patterns. A 1993 review of physical interventions in the management of pain in arthritis included several soft tissue diagnoses such as frozen shoulder, shoulder periarthritis, epicondylalgia, muscle soreness, low back pain, and tendinitis. The review concluded that the results of studies of one or a combination of the physical intervention strategies were generally inconsistent. The studies were noted to be of varied methodology and design (12). Another review of the treatment of epicondylitis noted similar lack of evidence of the efficacy of physical measures (13). Certainly physical agents should be used only in combination with exercise and movement retraining, discontinued if positive effects are not apparent within a few treatment sessions, limited to 8–10 total treatments, and a transition to home techniques made as quickly as possible. In addition, the offending postures, movement patterns, or behaviors must be altered or eliminated.

Heat

Superficial heat in the form of heating pads, microwave heated packs, and moist compresses have been effective in providing temporary relief. The heat applications should be limited to 10–15 minutes. Here, even the most inexpensive materials can be highly effective and are to be recommended. For instance, 2 cups of dry rice in a white sock can be heated (1 minute, medium heat) in the microwave oven to provide a warm pack that conforms nicely to the body part and retains warmth for 8–10 minutes.

Cold

Cold applications should also be done as practically and cheaply as possible. Some suggested forms of cold application include ice cups, packets of frozen peas, and alcohol-water slush in a zip-lock plastic bag. Figure 8.C illustrates application of ice in a cup to the cervical and upper shoulder area. Cold applications should be applied for a time period sufficient to achieve analgesia, usually 4–6 minutes, with care always taken to prevent skin damage or frostbite. Michlovitz provides an excellent review of cryotherapy as a therapeutic agent (14).

Ultrasound

Ultrasound is frequently used with the goals of decreasing pain and promoting healing. Ultrasound therapy uses sound waves directed at specific tissues to achieve therapeutic (rather than diagnostic) goals. As the sound waves penetrate tissue, local temperature increases and tissue extensibility is altered. Treatment is targeted over the tissue lesion or area of pain. Ultrasound is applied directly to the skin over the target area with a coupling solution or through water as the body part is submerged. Treatment is frequently preceded by application of local superficial heat such as a hot pack, although research substantiating benefits in this procedure is not conclusive. Ultrasound is used for local tendinitis, bursitis, fasciitis, muscle pain or spasm, and is usually performed two or three times per week for 2- to 4-week series. Acute inflammation is a contraindication due to the focal increase in tissue temperature. Evidence from well-controlled studies is mixed and inconclusive regarding the effectiveness of ultrasound in relieving pain, contributing to overall functional outcomes, or reducing treatment time or cost (15–17).

Electrotherapeutic Modalities

Interferential current applications rely on techniques in which two different medium frequency currents are crossed or interposed to produce a comfortable frequency that will achieve a greater relief of pain. These electrotherapeutic modalities are costly and cannot easily be done in the home, and so they should be used judiciously. There is little evidence that they are of specific value. Microcurrent and phoresis have similar uses.

Biofeedback and surface electromyelography (EMG) are not treatment modalities, but are used in movement retraining, such as in upper quadrant posture and retraining and reactivating the parascapular mechanism. These modalities require therapist time, and it has not been clearly demonstrated that they are more effective than direct therapist intervention with sound teaching and guidance. Headley describes these measures in detail (9).

MANUAL TECHNIQUES

Manual techniques include soft tissue mobilizations such as massage, direct pressure (ischemic pressure or myotherapy), myofascial release, muscle energy techniques, and manual stretch to tender/trigger points. In addition, joint manipulation can be included in this category (18). These are treatment techniques in which the primary forces or effects are delivered by the practitioner's hands. For many therapists, manual techniques form the core of their approach to soft tissue problems. Physical, occupational, and massage therapists, osteopathic manipulative physicians, and chiropractors use many types of manual therapy for a wide range of conditions, not limited to muscle spasm. For instance, Anderson has used a comprehensive Australian approach to manual therapy in the treatment of one patient with complex problems related to de Quervain's tenosynovitis (19). Sucher describes the use of manual therapy in the treatment of carpal tunnel syndrome, tenosynovitis, and thoracic outlet syndrome (20–23).

Massage

Massage includes techniques of kneading, stroking, and rolling the muscles, skin, and other soft tissues (24). The practitioner's sense of touch is central to the massage technique, and tactile sensation is the avenue of communication between patient and practitioner. There are many general types of massage, including, for example, Swedish (kneading) and Shiatsu (Japanese finger pressure). Figure 8.D illustrates a massage practitioner using the supine position to treat the posterior cervical and upper thorax areas. Specific strokes include effleurage, petrissage, deep friction or cross-fiber massage, and tapotement. The primary massage professionals are physical therapists or certified massage therapists, and the number of skilled practitioners is growing. One source of information about massage is the *Massage Journal,* published by the American Massage Therapy Association (25). Deep friction massage (Fig. 8.E) is a specific technique used in local areas such as lateral epicondylitis and the iliotibial tract (26, 27) in which fibrosis is noted in the areas of pain or dysfunction. The availability of and access to massage therapy is increasing in many areas of health care as its beneficial effects are being recognized.

Direct Pressure Myotherapy

Direct pressure (ischemic pressure) as a means of deactivating tender or ''pain'' points is a technique extensively described by Prudden (28), Travell and Simons (29), and in Shiatsu. In this technique, progressively stronger and more painful pressure is applied to the tender point with the practitioner's finger or thumb, knuckle, or elbow. Generally, pressure is maintained 7–10 seconds and repeated four to five times per point, although techniques vary among practitioners. This pressure is theorized to blanch the compressed tissues, which then become hyperemic after compression is released. Patients can learn to apply this pressure independently by using their own hands, tennis balls, or other convenient surfaces. The

technique is reported to relieve painful or tender points and decrease pain. The practitioner locates the tender points to be treated by exploratory palpation, then systematically treats as indicated. Treatment is repeated as needed, with transition to self-applied technique when possible.

Myofascial Release

Myofascial release is a manual technique in which the practitioner mobilizes soft tissues, focusing on fascial planes as well as muscle tissue. The technique of myofascial release is illustrated in Figure 8.F.

Muscle Energy Technique

Muscle energy technique blends manual techniques with carefully guided muscle contractions to effect changes in alignment and muscle performance and to correct motion dysfunction.

Manual Stretch

Manual stretch for trigger points is a direct mechanical stretch to tissues that may be preceded by or accompanied by the use of a spray that chills the area (hence, ''stretch and spray''). Travell and Simons have described the technique in great detail and have been noted for its use (29).

Manipulation

The technique of manipulation involves passively moving the joint to the end of the functional range, but not to the limit of the anatomical range. There are two categories of manipulation: *long lever low impact* and *short lever high impact.* In the first, the practitioner uses the leverage of a long bone such as the femur to amplify the therapeutic force. This is a rather nonspecific technique and is used by chiropractors, physical therapists, osteopathic physicians, and orthopaedic specialists. The short lever high impact technique, used primarily by chiropractors and osteopathic physicians, is a more direct technique consisting of quick force directed at specific areas; in spinal manipulation the forces are directed at the selected transverse processes. Recent reviews of research reports concerning spinal manipulation indicate support for the efficacy of spinal manipulation for treatment of acute and subacute back pain, but not for chronic back disorders (30). Goodridge also describes its role in the treatment of shoulder dysfunctions (31).

Mobilization

Joint mobilization is similar to and often used interchangeably with joint manipulation, as described by Schoensee (32); both are techniques that use passive movement to restore normal motion to a joint. Soft tissue mobilization and massage are also frequently interchanged terms and refer to techniques of increasing the flexibility of soft tissues.

EXERCISE

There is now a growing body of data supporting the use of exercise in the management of soft tissue rheumatism, especially back pain. The good news is that exercise works! The bad news is that it has to be performed on a regular basis. Convincing people to exercise remains one of the great challenges in management. Even after the great strides of recent years in the popularization of exercise, health clubs, and recreation facilities, only about 40–50% of people get enough exercise to gain health benefits. Physicians who advise patients to exercise can be powerful motivators. Therapists can also set a good example and become involved in regular exercise at many levels.

Relaxation Exercise

Relaxation is essential in the management of soft tissue and back pain. The tendency to "tighten up" with pain creates the additional problems of postural alignment, pain perception, and muscle spasm. Good relaxation can reduce pain and improve comfort and muscle tone. Everyone should have a personal relaxation program. Some of the most popular types of relaxation techniques include the "contract and relax" technique (in which specific muscles are activated and relaxed), deep breathing, meditation, and guided imagery. Bensen provides an excellent discussion of the benefits of structured relaxation activities (33). Many relaxation audio tapes are available for instruction and guidance. These tapes are helpful when used during periods of stress or insomnia and are an excellent accompaniment to professional instruction. All these relaxation techniques provide solid strategies for "stress-busting" and can be selected according to individual preferences and circumstances.

Breathing Exercises

Breathing exercises are done to improve respiratory function and thereby vital capacity. These exercises serve to increase costal expansion laterally and posteriorly, to increase trunk movement in side-bending and rotation, and to improve the function and performance of the respiratory muscles. Proper breathing is an important component of relaxation alignment. Figure 8.G illustrates the technique of costal expansion performed on the therapeutic ball, to provide additional challenge to stability and control and facilitate the stretching motions.

The simple breathing instructions presented in Table 8.1 can be taught in the practitioner's office or waiting room. Persons with pain histories tend to "tense up" during strenuous exercise, limiting their breathing patterns and exercise durations. Proper breathing can increase the potential duration of an exercise session. The instructions presented in Table 8.2 for breathing during exercise can improve aerobic exercise breathing patterns.

One effective strategy to improve breathing is to instruct the exercising patient to measure exercise repetitions by a count of *breath cycles* rather than in seconds or repetitions. A sample instruction for quadriceps setting exercise would be: "Tighten the muscle in the front of your thigh and hold for *five breath cycles,* then relax"—rather than "hold 5 seconds and relax." This yoga technique seems to focus the patient on breathing and prevents breath-holding.

Movement Reeducation

Movement reeducation strategies such as the Feldenkrais Method (34) and the Alexander

TABLE 8.1 SIMPLE BREATHING INSTRUCTIONS

Try these simple breathing instructions with patients and provide a take-home copy of instructions. Place copies in the waiting room and encourage patients to try them as they sit. Place instructions on waiting room walls.

BASIC PREPARATION INSTRUCTIONS: "Sit comfortably erect, shoulders apart, not hunched together. Let your head fall forward slightly. Nod your brain to your heart. Close your eyes, relax your jaw, and focus your imagined vision down."

1. Increase and extend the time you spend exhaling. Alternate extended and normal breaths at first, then extend all exhalations.
2. Extend the time you spend inhaling until it matches the time you spend exhaling.
3. Focus totally on your breathing—the sound of it, the pace, the length, the feeling as the air enters and leaves the body.
4. As you breathe in, make the belly move out, so that the rib cage really expands. This will relax the diaphragm and allow the lungs to suck in the air deeply. Place the hands on the belly and feel the belly as you breathe.
5. Place the hands on the sides of the rib cage and feel the ribs move as you breathe. Focus attention on one hand as it moves in and out with the ribs.
6. Feel the rhythm of your breathing. Allow the breathing to slow, then to increase.

TABLE 8.2 EXERCISE BREATHING

Proper breathing during exercise is important to the aerobic program and can increase the duration of the aerobic exercise session. Provide these instructions to your exercising patients.

1. Warm up breathing as you warm up your muscles. Allow 5–10 minutes of gradual increase in workload before going all out. Do not go full blast at first.
2. Narrow the lips as you exhale. This will increase resistance to each expelled breath and reduce the tendency to hyperventilate.
3. Adjust exercise intensity so that you can carry on an occasional conversation as you work out. Just talk to yourself if you are alone.
4. Muscles should use oxygen at the same rate the lungs provide it so that you can exercise 20–30 minutes or more. Find your ideal rate of exercise breathing.

Techniques (35) are particularly suited to the management of soft tissue and back problems because of the emphasis on posture, relaxation, healthy breathing, and the gentle approach. These techniques emphasize efficiency of movement and elimination of unnecessary patterns. Feldenkrais is said to have been influenced by Alexander and adapted many techniques from his works. Therapists trained in the Alexander and Feldenkrais methods have undergone extensive training in movement study and offer a holistic approach to pain, posture, and kinesthetic awareness. Tai Chi is an Oriental movement education system that emphasizes relaxation and correct body alignment, as well as muscle lengthening activities to improve flexibility (36). Figure 8.H illustrates two Tai Chi movements, the squat and a rotation.

Posture and Alignment Training

Posture and alignment training is central to the management of soft tissue problems. The concept of "good posture" is frequently associated with directives to "stand straight," or "sit tall," or "be erect." In fact, being "straight" is simplistic and does not reflect the anatomical structure of spinal alignment, which consists of complex curves and relationships. A functional concept of good posture should be based upon efficiency of movement rather than static position or stature. Feldenkrais (33) states that the purpose of the skeleton is to counteract the force of gravity so that movements of the extremities can occur freely. "Good posture" is that in which minimal muscle action is used for skeletal support. Therefore, the functional concept implies that good posture is that in which efficient movement takes place on a skeleton that is properly aligned to support muscles. Postural problems are complex, because of the body's tendency to compensate for dysfunction and imbalance. For instance, the pattern of forward head and rounded shoulders will require compensatory patterns in the lumbar spine, pelvis, hips, and knees, often in multiple planes.

Accurate and comprehensive assessment of posture is the framework within which the retraining occurs, and should therefore comprise a major component of the evaluation process. Simple posture tips are frequently offered but may not completely address the identified posture problems and compensatory changes. Practitioners are cautioned to assess the impact of the posture retraining intervention on the entire body, and to seek comprehensive and long-range corrections.

Postural control relies on the ability of the trunk muscles to protect spine tissues from excessive motion or strain. These muscles must be able to co-contract and relax smoothly to meet functional needs. Therefore posture training must include strengthening, lengthening, relaxation, coordination, and skill development activities (37, 38).

One strategy to improve postural control is known as functional or lumbar stabilization. The overall goal of spinal stabilization is to improve the stabilizing mechanisms of the pelvis and lumbar spine in order to enhance function. Most stabilization programs begin with spine exercises done in the midrange positions and train the patient to recognize and control postures as they move away from the midline. The programs emphasize awareness of neutral spine positions and of actions necessary to control spine motions. The programs build strength and endurance in the spine muscles, enabling them to contract and protect the spine during functional activities of the extremities. Many stabilization programs utilize functional stabilization or a large ball exercise as a means of developing awareness and strength of pelvic motions (Fig. 8.I), and programs can be designed for either dry land or aquatic environments.

Stretching or Lengthening Techniques

Stretching and lengthening techniques are important in the management of soft tissue problems. Many stretching techniques are described throughout this book in individual chapters. These techniques emphasize mechanical stretching of soft tissue fibers and rely primarily on biomechanical forces. Another approach is to focus on lengthening techniques rather than tissue stretching. The lengthening techniques are favored over stretching as a more gentle approach, particularly in the case of fibromyalgia, where regular stretching or lengthening is a necessary component of the treatment program. The lengthening approach is slower, includes relaxation and breathing techniques, does not traumatize tissues, and allows for natural releases to occur. The Feldenkrais Method (34), the Alexander Techniques (35), and Tai Chi (36) (Fig. 8.H) are all movement systems that include lengthening strategies rather than biomechanical stretching.

Strengthening Techniques

Strengthening techniques are the core of posture restoration and functional activities. Studies indicate the presence of weakened muscles in the perpetuation of pain and the importance of strengthening exercise for recovery in neck (39–52), back (53–61), and patellofemoral pain (63–65) and in injuries related to manual handling tasks (66–68). The studies strongly suggest that strengthening activities are the most important component of management. The prophylactic value of strengthening is becoming more and more obvious, as studies in manual material handling tasks have shown (66–68).

Strengthening activities are possible in land and aquatic settings and can utilize a wide range of assistive devices such as weights, resistive bands, and mechanized resistive equipment. Figure 8.J illustrates lumbar strengthening done in the prone position over an exercise ball. In this position, broad range-of-motion exercises can be included in the strengthening exercises. Strengthening is essential in the complete rehabilitation of pain-producing disorder, but should be carefully staged to avoid exacerbation of pain. Individual strengthening activities are discussed in each chapter for specific diagnoses. The most important precaution is to correct dysfunctional movement patterns before strengthening activities take place, so that improper patterns are not reinforced.

Endurance or Aerobic Exercise

Endurance or aerobic exercise has many values and benefits, including cardiovascular and neurohormonal effects. Studies now indicate that even modest amounts of aerobic exercise (sustained exercise over time) have important preventive and therapeutic effects (69, 70). The challenge in soft tissue disorders is to develop aerobic programs that do not aggravate pain or compound existing motor dysfunction. For instance, patients with neck or back pain may not have adequate strength in muscles that provide spinal stability to support the extremities in prolonged exercise such as walking, cross-country skiing, or biking. Therefore, posture retraining and spinal stabilization exercises must accompany the aerobic program. This is particularly important for patients with chronic fibromyalgia in which trunk stability is compromised. The aerobic program for fibromyalgia must be preceded by posture and movement retraining as well as trunk strengthening. These fibromyalgia patients may increase their overall discomfort if endurance exercises are imposed upon patterns of poor posture due to trunk instability. Programs that include spinal stabilization can lay the foundation for more active and prolonged exercise.

Recreational Exercise

The need for a pleasurable, restorative form of exercise in daily life is unchallenged. Walking, swimming, dancing, and biking are but a few of the exercise options that bring a myriad of physical, psychological, and social benefits to the participant. The concept of recreation and exercise is basic to healthy lifestyles and should be promoted at every chance.

AQUATIC THERAPY AND EXERCISE

Aquatics is an ancient science with rich potential for therapy and rehabilitation of soft tissue rheumatism and back pain (71–73). The recent resurgence of interest is timely because aquatics activities can be performed in a wide variety of settings and can be transferred from medical to community and home settings. Aquatics can be a model for collaborative care involving numerous levels of professional training and specialty. The growing interest in aquatics is evidenced by the availability of new patient programs and continuing education opportunities for professionals. Aquatics is much more than "water aerobics"; in the following sections, principles of aquatics exercise will be discussed, various types of aquatics exercise and therapy will be compared, and specific techniques will be presented for treatment of some of the soft tissue disorders covered in this volume.

Aquatic Exercise Overview

Aquatics is a general term used to describe the full spectrum of water activities and includes topics such as pool/beach maintenance and management. Two terms important in rehabilitation are "aquatic exercise" and "aquatic therapy."

Aquatic exercise is any purposeful activity performed in an aquatic environment. Aquatic exercise includes calisthenics, aerobics, water walking, swimming, and sports activities. Aquatic exercise can be done for various purposes such as recreation, health enhancement, or rehabilitation. Aquatic exercise can also be done individually, in groups, or in an assisted/guided mode.

Aquatic therapy implies the use of aquatics principles and activities in the restorative or therapeutic process. Aquatic therapeutic movement is a goal-directed activity in water using the varied properties of water to achieve specific purposes. *Aquatic physical therapy* is defined by the Aquatics Section of the American Physical Therapy Association as "one-on-one therapy in the water utilizing the water's properties as the primary or adjunctive modality" (74). It is patient-focused, hands-on therapy, based on skilled assessment, evaluation, and treatment planning, and is directed at therapeutic goals. Aquatic therapy should be documented by therapists according to guidelines and criteria appropriate for any type of therapeutic exercise. Reimbursement from third-party payers is possible for aquatic therapy and therapeutic aquatic exercise if guidelines are followed and documentation is accurate and reflects activities aimed at specific goals with the desired progress documented (75). Guidelines for documentation are available in several recent publications of the Aquatics Section of the American Physical Therapy Association.

Aquatic exercise activities are many, varied, and imaginative. Several professional disciplines claim competency in various aspects of aquatic exercise, including physical and occupational therapists, athletic trainers, physical educators, exercise physiologists, and health educators. Although each of these professional disciplines includes basic instruction on aquatics as part of their educational curriculum, expertise in a breadth of practice is acquired by specialized training and certifications offered in continuing education programs. Aquatic therapists usually have a good knowledge of medical conditions and clinical applications of aquatics, whereas aquatics exercise professionals may be more attuned to the recreational/health-enhancing aspects of aquatic exercise and have more skills in leading groups, promoting adherence and the exercise habit, and utilizing community facilities. In many cases, the skills of various professionals overlap and are complementary. A full continuum of client-focused services is best attained through collaboration, communication, and partnership of the professionals and the patient/client.

One important advantage of the aquatic environment is that exercise can be finely and fully progressed with a minimum of equipment or position change. Extensive programs can be developed incorporating many types of activities to achieve varied goals. Exercise in water can make a major contribution to flexibility, strength, endurance, coordination, comfort, functional performance, and mood. By finely planning specific exercise activities and progression, the therapist can help the participant take full advantage of the water's resources. Aquatic exercise programs can be designed to address many problems in soft tissue disorders, from small areas such as the arm (e.g., in epicondylitis) to larger areas such as the back or lower extremities. General fitness training is nicely achieved for persons of all abilities through aquatics programs. The recent resurgence of interest in aquatics activities has benefited medical as well as health/fitness communities and interests, with many more pools available in small and large facilities. Many community pools such as schools, YMCA and YWCA, and fitness clubs are setting aside time for medical rehabilitation activities such as arthritis and back pain programs. Additionally, therapy departments are installing small pools for use by one or two patients at a time.

Organizations that promote aquatic exercise and therapy include the Aquatics Section of the American Physical Therapy Association (74), the Aquatics Exercise Association (76), and the Aquatic Rehabilitation & Therapy Institute (77).

Principles of Aquatics

The physical properties of water and its relationships to matter and force form the basis for therapeutic aquatics. Two important principles that are particularly important are *buoyancy* and *hydrostatic pressure*. A complete discussion of water and its principles and properties can be found in any good physics text. Incidentally, it is *physical* as in *physics,* not as in the physical body, from which physical therapy takes its name. Thus, all physical therapists should have gained basic knowledge of aquatic therapy in their core curriculum!

Buoyancy is the tendency of an object to float or rise when immersed in a fluid (78). The force of buoyancy is the upward thrust equal to the weight of water/fluid that a body displaces. The force of buoyancy experienced by a body or object is opposite to the force of gravity, which is the force pulling toward the center of the earth. Thus an object in water/fluid at rest is acted on by two opposing forces: (*a*) gravity pulling toward the earth and (*b*) buoyancy thrusting upward. Buoyancy counteracts gravity and thus enables the body to function in static or dynamic postures as if weight were reduced. Patients experience standing in water as if "weight had been lifted from my spine." Ambulating in water seems easier because "my body doesn't weigh as much," or "there's less weight on my knees and hips." The body stands straighter, limbs move easier and persons feel supported while immersed in water.

Low density items such as foam floats or rings can be attached to the body to increase buoyancy. Conversely, when distracting or stabilizing forces are desired, high density items such as lead diver's weights can be used.

Buoyancy is important for soft tissue disorders because it:

1. decreases forces on the spine (compression) and contributes to better alignment
2. decreases weight on the extremities as they move through the water
3. decreases the compressive forces on joints
4. decreases the weight of the shoulders and upper trunk on the pelvis, promoting more erect vertical posture
5. decreases the weight of the body on the hips and knees
6. decreases the weight of an extremity and allows more motion per unit of force supplied by muscle. For example, weak-

ened hip flexors may be inadequate to flex the hip on land and cause serious gait dysfunction. In the water, the force of buoyancy assists the hip/thigh as it is flexed and enables full flexing and normal gait pattern.

Hydrostatic pressure, the second important physical principle in aquatics, is the force exerted by a fluid upon the surfaces of immersed bodies at rest. Hydrostatic pressure is exerted equally at any given depth on all surface areas of an immersed object. Pressure is positively correlated to the depth of immersion and density of the liquid; the deeper the level of immersion, the greater the hydrostatic pressure experienced. Salt water exerts more hydrostatic pressure per unit of area because it is more dense that fresh water. Thus, salt water pools or the ocean comprise aquatic environments somewhat different from those of fresh water.

Hydrostatic pressure is exerted against the chest wall of a person partially or completely immersed in water, resisting chest expansion and making respiration more difficult. Persons with deceased vital capacity or weakness of respiratory muscles may experience unexpected fatigue as the demands of respiration are increased. The increased use of accessory muscles of respiration during water exercise can cause discomfort and fatigue of the neck and upper trunk and inability to maintain correct cervical and trunk alignment.

Hydrostatic pressure increases with depth of immersion; thus swelling is more effectively treated at greater depths. Edematous knees and ankles should be exercised as deeply as possible for at least part of a session. Other principles that are important to therapy in water include thermal properties, viscosity, and turbulence.

Aquatic exercise, whether for regional or generalized soft tissue problems, can be finely progressed by using the physical principles/properties of water. Exercise intensity and resistance can be varied according to the following factors:

1. the speed of motion through the water
2. the arc of motion through which the body part moves
3. the length of the lever arm moved
4. the eddy created
5. the streamline
6. inertia

The individual exercise patterns can be varied by using combinations of these principles in an almost limitless variety.

Specific Techniques

One-on-one aquatic therapy is accomplished with the therapist in the water with the patient. The therapist guides the patient through specific activities of exercise or movement. Two particular techniques are of importance in soft tissues disorders, the Bad Ragaz Ring Method (79, 80) and Watsu (81). In both of these techniques, the patient is supported/floated in the water with manual assistance (81) or with buoyant equipment such as foam collars or water-ski jackets (79, 80). The techniques are extremely useful for the acute back pain patient as well as for many other diagnoses. The techniques are unique to the water environment.

Bad Ragaz is named for the spa in Austria where it was developed. It involves use of "proprioceptive neuromuscular facilitation" (PNF) patterns in water exercise, accomplished by using the water as resistance rather than using the therapist's force. In Bad Ragaz, the therapist is the stable object around which various patterns are carried out (79, 80).

Watsu is a technique for relaxation and training in which Shiatsu (Japanese Finger Pressure) principles are used. The therapist in the water is in close contact with the patient during Watsu therapy (81).

General Considerations

There are disadvantages to pool therapy that must be considered realistically:

1. intensive therapist time and effort
2. limited tolerance and time in the water, regardless of physical conditioning
3. difficult and time-consuming patient preparation, including undressing, dressing, and drying the patient
4. possible need to assist the patient into the pool. The pool itself is a fragile environment and can be upset by an incontinent patient, a chemical error, plumbing problems, and so on, and repair and fixing

take time. Skin, cardiovascular, and respiratory concerns must be considered as well.

In general, for the enthusiastic therapist and willing patient, the advantages far outweigh the disadvantages. Some practitioners recommend transition from pool to land exercise as soon as possible. However, if the client is fond of water exercise and has an available water environment, there is no reason for exercise not to continue at least partially in water, as long as adequate weightbearing exercise is obtained.

BODY MECHANICS AND ERGONOMICS

Because so many diagnoses in soft tissue rheumatism are cumulative stress/strain-related, the importance of good body mechanics and appropriate ergonomics cannot be overemphasized. Improper movement patterns are responsible for many problems, and they must be recognized, analyzed, and addressed. Further change of offending patterns is of paramount importance. The therapist must work with the patient to assess obvious as well as not-so-obvious errors in body mechanics. Thorough activity evaluation will provide the necessary information—and it is often the least obvious habit that is the offending element! The professional research and literature of the ergonomics field are excellent resources for information regarding soft tissue disorders.

ADHERENCE AND PERFORMANCE ISSUES

As stated earlier, adherence to exercise programs is only about 40–50% for all types of exercise, recreational or therapeutic. Adherence to other components of the management plan is less well documented. Does the patient really use the warm pack, attend to posture, make the adaptations suggested for positioning? Are the exercises performed as instructed, or do patients make adaptations and changes as time goes on? Many exercises are not thoroughly taught at initial sessions and the patient's performance may be inadequate or incorrect. Misunderstandings about the purpose of various exercises, of the goals and objectives of the

program, or of the overall length of time that a program should be continued are common between exercisers and instructors. Referral to a physical or occupational therapist is appropriate for more complex or difficult exercise programs or when the patient is having difficulty following basic instruction. Consistent teaching and frequent follow-up form the basis for good exercise program performance.

Whether the exercise program is taught in the physician's office or therapy department, several guidelines can be helpful in correct performance and generating improved adherence. The suggestions listed in Table 8.3 can be helpful for programs that include physical measures and exercise.

SUMMARY

Physical measures and exercise interventions can and usually do make significant contributions to the management of soft tissue disorders and musculoskeletal pain. The art and science of their selection and application lies not so

TABLE 8.3 EXERCISE ADHERENCE AND PERFORMANCE TIPS

1. Provide clear teaching with
   a) consistent verbal instructions
   b) demonstration of techniques
   c) observation of exerciser's performance
   d) correction and reinforcement of technique
   e) clear printed picture directions in attractive, durable formats such as folders or booklets.
2. Develop a program that is reasonable and practical. Limit the total number of individual exercises to 10 or 12. Limit the total time of performance to 30 minutes plus an aerobic component.
3. Provide a method of recording performance of activities, immediate and delayed response, and any problems noted. Review these records on a regular basis and enter into the patient record if possible.
4. Provide reminders about exercise such as postcards, telephone calls, exercise posters.
5. Provide small visible rewards for successes such as pencils, gold stars, and key chains.
6. Let the patient know how strongly *you* feel about regular exercise and be a role model for healthy behaviors.
7. Provide clear guidelines about revising or altering programs according to responses, particularly increased pain following exercise. Take a marketing approach to exercise and health behaviors.

much in the choice of individual treatments as in development of appropriate and practical programs that will be effective in achieving functional outcomes and in fostering adherence to performance. Many aspects of the programs can be carried out in nonmedical settings with appropriate guidance from medical consultants and advisors.

REFERENCES

1. Hadler, NM: Arm pain in the work place. Bull Rheum Dis 42:6–8, 1993.
2. Ottenbacher KJ: Why rehabilitation research does not work (as well as we think it should). Arch Phys Med Rehabil 76:123–129, 1995.
3. Spencer JC: The usefulness of qualitative methods in rehabilitation: issues of meaning, of context, and of change. Arch Phys Med Rehabil 74:119–126, 1993.
4. Jette AM, Davis KD: A comparison of hospital-based and private outpatient physical therapy practices. Phys Ther 71:21–30, 1991.
5. Jette AM: Using health-related quality of life measures in physical therapy outcomes research. Phys Ther 73:528–537, 1993.
6. The Arthritis Foundation. Atlanta, GA 30309.
7. Fibromyalgia Network. Tucson, AZ 85751-1750.
8. Carter JB, Banister EW: Musculoskeletal problems in VDT work: a review. Ergonomics 37:1623–1648, 1994.
9. Headley B: Posture correction—begin with motor control re-training. Physical Therapy Forum 3:9–11, 1993.
10. Deyo RA, Centor RM: Assessing the responsiveness of functional scales to clinical change: an analogy to diagnostic test performance. J Chronic Dis 11:897–906, 1986.
11. Deyo RA: Measuring the functional status of patients with low back pain. Arch Phys Med Rehabil 69:1044–1053, 1988.
12. Minor MA, Sanford MK: Physical interventions in the management of pain in arthritis: an overview for research and practice. Arth Care Res 6:197–206, 1993.
13. Labelle H, Guibert R, Joncas J, Newman N, Fallaha M, Rivard CH: Lack of scientific evidence for the treatment of lateral epicondylitis of the elbow. An attempted meta-analysis. J Bone Joint Surg (Br) 74:646–651, 1992.
14. Michlovitz SL: Cryotherapy: the use of cold as a therapeutic agent. In: Michlovitz SL, ed.: Thermal agents in rehabilitation. Philadelphia: FA Davis, 1990:88–108.
15. Bearzy H: Clinical applications of ultrasonic energy in treatment of acute and chronic subacromial bursitis. Arch Phys Med Rehabil 34:228–231, 1953.
16. Downing DS, Weinstein A: Ultrasound therapy of subacromial bursitis: a double-blind trial. Phys Ther 66:194–199, 1986.
17. Crawford F, Snaith M: Therapeutic ultrasound as a treatment of plantar heel pain. (Abstract) Br J Rheumatol 34(Suppl I):42, 1995.
18. Farrell JP, Jensen GM: Manual therapy: a critical assessment of role in the profession of physical therapy. Phys Ther 72:843–852, 1992.
19. Anderson M, Tichenor J: A patient with de Quervain's tenosynovitis: a case report using an Australian approach to manual therapy. Phys Ther 74:314–325, 1994.
20. Sucher BM: Myofascial release of carpal tunnel syndrome. JAOA 93:92–101, 1993.
21. Sucher BM: Myofascial manipulative release of carpel tunnel syndrome: documentation with magnetic resonance imaging. JAOA 93:1273–1278, 1993.
22. Sucher BM: Palpatory diagnosis and manipulative management of carpal tunnel syndrome. JAOA 94:647–663, 1994.
23. Sucher BM, Heath D: Thoracic outlet syndrome: a myofascial variant. Part 3: Structural and postural considerations. JAOA 93:334–345, 1993.
24. Hofkosh JM: Classical massage. In: Basmajian JV, ed. Manipulation, traction, and massage. 3rd ed. Baltimore: Williams & Wilkins, 1985.
25. American Massage Therapy Association. Massage Therapy Journal.
26. Schwellnus MP, Mackintosh L, Mee J: Deep friction massage to the iliotibial band. Physiotherapy 78:564–568, 1992.
27. Steward B, Woodman R, Hurlburt D: Fabricating a splint for deep friction massage. JOSPT 21:172–175, 1995.
28. Prudden B: Pain erasure: the Bonnie Prudden way. New York: Ballantine Books, 1980.
29. Travell JG, Simons DG: Myofascial pain and dysfunction: the trigger point manual. Baltimore: Williams & Wilkins, 1983.
30. Shekelle PG: Spinal update: spinal manipulation. Spine 19:858–861, 1994.
31. Goodridge JP: Manipulation, exercise resolves shoulder dysfunctions. JAOA 93:426, 1993.
32. Schoensee SK, Jensen G, Nicholson G, Katholi C: The effect of mobilization on cervical headaches. JOSPT 21:184–196, 1995.
33. Bensen H: The relaxation response. New York: Morrow, 1975.
34. Feldenkrais M: Awareness through movement: health exercises for personal growth. New York: Harper & Row, 1977.
35. Brennan R: The Alexander technique. Rockport, MA: Element, 1991.
36. Crompton P: The Tai Chi workbook. Boston: Shambhala, 1987.

37. Jull GA, Richardson CA: Rehabilitation of active stabilization of the lumbar spine. In: Twomey LT, Taylor LT, eds. Physical therapy of the low back. 2nd ed. Edinburgh: Churchill Livingstone, 1994.

38. Dul J, Johnson GE, Shiavi R, Townsend MA: Muscular synergism. II: Minimum-fatigue criterion for load sharing between synergistic muscles. J Biomech 17:675–684, 1984.

39. Levoska S, Keinanen Kiukaaniemi S: Active or passive physiotherapy for occupational cervicobrachial disorders: a comparison of two treatment methods with a 1-year follow-up. Arch Phys Med Rehabil 74:425–430, 1993.

40. Martin GM, Corbin KB: Evaluation of conservative treatment for patients with cervical disc syndrome. Arch Phys Med Rehabil 35:87–92, 1954.

41. British Association of Physical Medicine: Pain in the neck and arm: a multicentre trial of the effects of physiotherapy. Br Med J 1:253–258, 1966.

42. Goldie I, Landquist A: Evaluation of the effects of different forms of physiotherapy in cervical pain. Scand J Rehabil Med 2:117–121, 1970.

43. Kvarnstrom S: Occurrence of musculoskeletal disorders in a manufacturing industry with special attention to occupational shoulder disorders. Scand J Rehabil Med (Suppl 8):1–114, 1983.

44. Bjelle A, Hagberg M, Michaelson G: Work-related shoulder-neck complaints in industry: a pilot study. Br J Rheumatol 26:365–369, 1987.

45. Kilbom A: Isometric strength and occupational muscle disorders. Eur J Appl Physiol 57:322–326, 1988.

46. Rundcrantz BL, Johnsson B, Moritz U, Roxendal G: Cervicobrachial disorder in dentists: a comparison between two kinds of physiotherapeutic interventions. Scand J Rehab Med 23:11–17, 1991.

47. Hidalgo JA, Genaidy AM, Huston R, Arantes J: Occupational biomechanics of the neck: a review and recommendations. J Hum Ergo Tokyo 21:165–181, 1992.

48. Tan JC, Nordin M: Role of physical therapy in the treatment of cervical disk disease. Orthop Clin North Am 23:435–449, 1992.

49. Berg HE, Gunnell B, Tesch PA: Dynamic neck strength training effect on pain and function. Arch Phys Med Rehabil 75:661–665, 1994.

50. Bovim G, Schrader H, Trond S: Neck pain in the general population. Spine 19:1307–1309, 1994.

51. Gogia PP, Sabbahi MA: Electromyographic analysis of neck muscle fatigue in patients with osteoarthritis of the cervical spine. Spine 19:502–506, 1994.

52. Ellenberg MR, Honet JC, Treanor WJ: Cervical radiculopathy. Arch Phys Med Rehabil 75:342–352, 1994.

53. Thomas LK, Hislop HJ, Waters RL: Physiological work performance in chronic low back disability: effects of a progressive activity program. Phys Ther 60:409–411, 1980.

54. Smidt G, Herring T, Amundsen L: Assessment of abdominal and back extensor function. Spine 8:211–219, 1983.

55. Biering-Sorensen F: Physical measures as risk indicators for low-back trouble over a one-year period. Spine 9:106–107, 1984.

56. Kohles S, Barnes D, Gatchel RJ, Mayer TG: Improved physical performance outcomes after functional restoration with chronic low back pain. Spine 15:1321–1324, 1990.

57. Mellin G, Harkapaa K, Hurri H, Jarvikoski A: A controlled study on the outcome of inpatient and outpatient treatment of low back pain. Part IV. Long term effects on physical measurements. Scand J Rehabil Med 22:189–194, 1990.

58. Mitchell RI, Carmen GM: Results of a multicenter trial using an intensive active exercise program for the treatment of acute soft tissue and back injuries. Spine 15:514–521, 1990.

59. Koes BW, Bouter LM, Beckerman H, et al.: Physiotherapy exercises and back pain: a blinded review. Br Med J 302:1572–1576, 1991.

60. Lindgren KA, Sihvonen T, Leino E, Pitkanen M, Manninen H: Exercise therapy effects on functional radiographic findings and segmental electromyographic activity in lumbar spine instability. Arch Phys Med Rehabil 74:933–939, 1993.

61. Moffroid MT, Haugh LD, Haig AJ: Endurance training of trunk extensor muscles. Phys Ther 73:3–10, 1993.

62. Brennan GP, Shultz B, Hood RS, Zahniser JC, Johnson SC, Gerber AH: The effects of aerobic exercise after lumbar microdiscectomy. Spine 19:735–739, 1994.

63. Doucette SA, Goble EM: The effect of exercise on patellar tracking in lateral patellar compression syndrome. Am J Sports Med 20:434–440, 1992.

64. Bockrath K, Wooden C, Worrell T, Ingersoll CD, Farr J: Effects of patella taping on patella position and perceived pain. Med Sci in Sports and Exercise 25:989–992, 1993.

65. Kannus P, Niittymaki S: Which factors predict outcome in the non-operative treatment of patellofemoral syndrome? A prospective follow-up study. Med Sci in Sports and Exercise 26:289–295, 1994.

66. Genaidy AM, Karwowski W, Guo L, Hidalgo J, Garbutt G: Physical training: a tool for increasing work tolerance limits of employees engaged in manual handling tasks. Ergonomics 35:1081–1102, 1992.

67. Guo L, Genaidy A, Warm J, Karwowski W, Hidalgo J: Effects of job-simulated flexibility and strength-flexibility training protocols on maintenance employees engaged in manual handling operations. Ergonomics 35:1103–1117, 1992.

68. Kroemer KHE: Personnel training for safer material handling. Ergonomics 35:1119–1134, 1992.

69. Burckhardt CS, Mannerkorpi K, Hedenberg L, Bjelle A: A randomized, controlled clinical trial of education and physical training for women

with fibromyalgia. J Rheumatol 21:714–720, 1994.

70. Nichols DS, Glenn TM: Effects of aerobic exercise on pain perception, affect, and level of disability in individuals with fibromyalgia. Phys Ther 74:327–332, 1994.

71. Rockel, I: Taking the waters: early spas in New Zealand. Wellington, New Zealand: Government Printing Office, 1986.

72. Cunningham J: Historical review of aquatics and physical therapy. Orthop Phys Ther Clin North Am 3:83–93, 1994.

73. Wynn KE: Lily ponds and warm springs, fortunate accidents: a brief history of aquatic physical therapy. PT Magazine 2:44–45, 1994.

74. APTA Aquatic Therapy Section: Statement of Purposes, Rationale, and Goals. Alexandria, VA: American Physical Therapy Association, 1993.

75. Charness AL: Outcomes measurement: interventions versus outcomes. Orthop Phys Ther Clin North Am 3:47–164, 1994.

76. Aquatic Exercise Association. Box 1609, Nokomis, FL 34274.

77. Aquatic Therapy & Rehabilitation Institute. Port Washington, WI 53074.

78. Skinner AT, Thomson AM, eds.: Duffield's exercise in water. 3rd ed. London: Bailliere-Tindall, 1983.

79. Boyle AM: The Bad Ragaz ring method. Physiotherapy 67:265–268, 1981.

80. Jamison L, Ogden D: Aquatic therapy using PNF patterns. Tucson: Therapy Skill Builders, 1994.

81. Dull H: Watsu—freeing the body in water. Middlefield, CA: Harbin Springs Publishers, 1993.

FIGURES

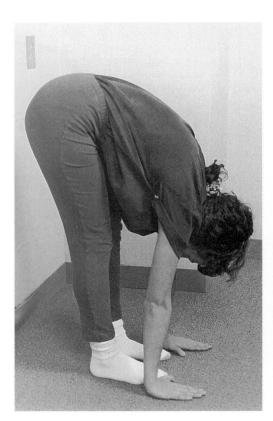

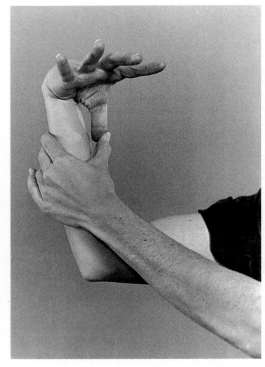

Figure 8.A. Hypermobility assessment positions. **8.A (a).** Palms flat on the floor with full standing lumbar flexion.

8.A (b). Thumb parallel to the forearm with full wrist flexion.

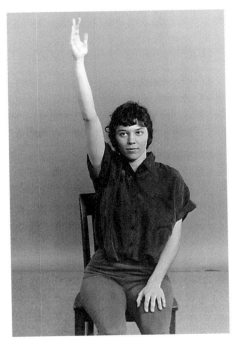

Figure 8.B. Four planes of shoulder exercise.
8.B (a). Forward flexion.

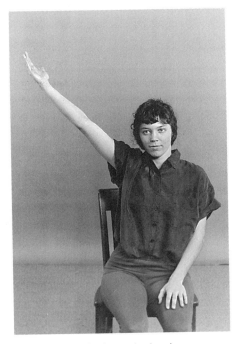

8.B (b). Diagonal flexion—single plane.

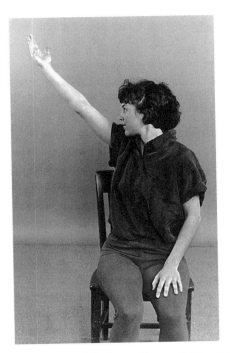

8.B (c). Diagonal flexion with rotation—combined planes.

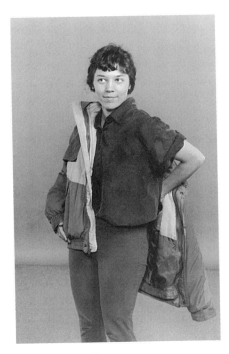

8.B (d). Functional plane.

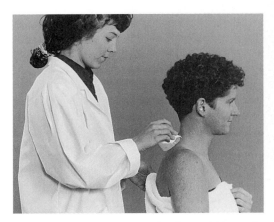

Figure 8.C. Ice application. The therapist is applying an ice cup to the lower cervical spine area.

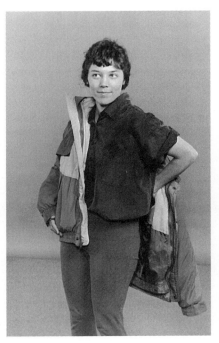

Figure 8.D. Supine massage position. The supine position provides the massage practitioner with excellent access to cervical and upper thoracic areas.

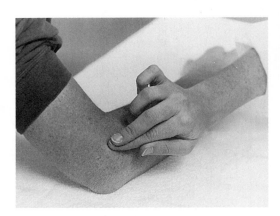

Figure 8.E. Deep friction massage. The therapist is applying deep friction (cross-fiber) massage to the area of the lateral epicondyle and extensor attachments.

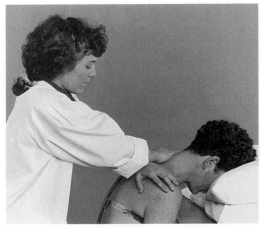

Figure 8.F. Myofascial release technique. The therapist is performing myofascial release technique to the upper posterior thorax.

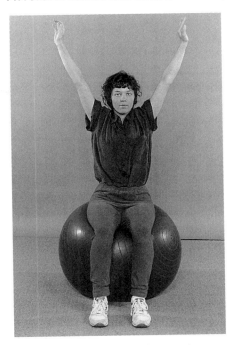

Figure 8.G. Breathing exercises such as costal expansion can be done on the therapeutic ball.

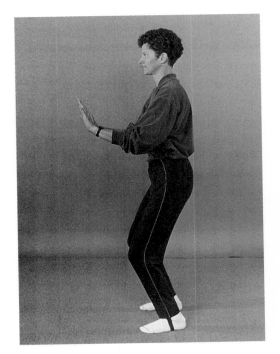

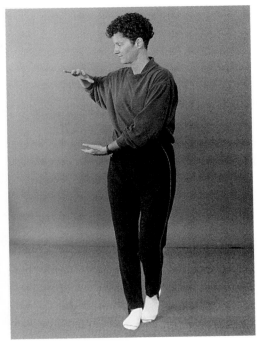

Figure 8.H. Tai Chi movements.
8.H (a). Tai Chi squat movement.

8.H (b). Tai Chi rotation movement.

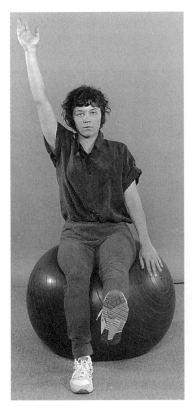

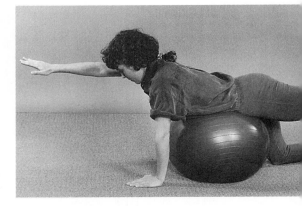

Figure 8.I. Lumbar stabilization techniques can be performed on the therapeutic ball to challenge stability and balance.
8.I (a). Combined hip and shoulder flexion, alternating sides.

8.I (b). Prone contralateral shoulder and hip extension.

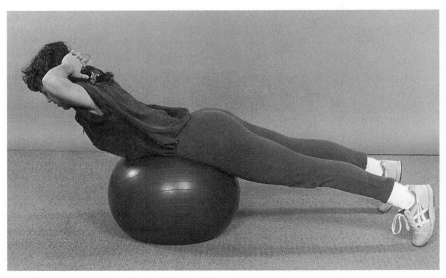

Figure 8.J. Lumbar extensor strengthening exercise performed from the prone position on the therapeutic ball.

9: Role of Nursing in the Management of Soft Tissue Rheumatic Disease

JANET E. JEFFREY

Soft tissue rheumatic diseases are nonarticular conditions that can have acute onset and are resolved with interventions. Soft tissue rheumatic diseases can also be chronic in nature and contribute to disability. For the purposes of this chapter, chronic pain is differentiated from acute pain simply on the basis of the length of time the pain has been experienced and not resolved with usual treatment—pain is chronic when not resolved within 6 months (1, 2). Managing the pain and prevention of further injury and/or exacerbation of illness requires a multimethod approach that, although best offered by an interdisciplinary health care team, is often only available from a physician, physical therapist, and/or nurse. The focus of this chapter is on the role of the nurse in the management of soft tissue rheumatic disease. Nurses are the health care professionals who are most directly responsible for the overall management of pain, given their direct contact with the patients who are experiencing pain (3). The term "management" is used here to include a more comprehensive approach than treatment alone. Management includes ongoing assessment, development of a comprehensive plan for intervention, guiding the implementation of the intervention strategies, and evaluating their effectiveness. These steps in managing soft tissue rheumatic disease form the organizing framework of this chapter. Although the emphasis of much of the chapter is on soft tissue rheumatic disease that involves chronic pain, nurses have an important role to play with acute problems both in primary care and occupational health. The role of the nurse in both acute and chronic problems is discussed.

IMPORTANCE OF THE TEAM APPROACH TO PATIENT CARE

In an ideal world of health care, patients with soft tissue rheumatic disease would receive health care from professionals who are expert in dealing with rheumatic diseases. There are clear advantages to a team approach to the care of patients with soft tissue rheumatic disease. First, assessment and treatment of the individual who has chronic pain requires a multidimensional approach that can best be accomplished using the expertise of professionals from different disciplines, because each brings a unique set of skills to the clinical situation (4, 5, 6). Second, a multidimensional approach to development of a treatment plan using expertise from health care team members may result in greater success (defined as a lower level of pain severity and lower levels of functional impairment and depression) because individual patients do not all respond equally well to all treatment strategies or to all persons offering treatment advice (5, 7, 8).

In the real world, adults have pain that may result from injury, repetitive strain, or systemic disease. Care is often sought from a family physician or general medical practitioner only when the pain does not go away with the use of usual home remedies. Referral to a treatment team or an individual specialist is not always feasible or possible. The use of an interdisciplinary health care team should be considered and is recommended when first-line approaches to the management of soft tissue disorders fail. However, emphasis should be placed on developing skills in individual prac-

TABLE 9.1 ROLE OF THE NURSE IN MANAGEMENT OF SOFT TISSUE RHEUMATIC DISEASE

Case manager or coordinator
Communicator, translator, interpreter
Facilitator
Advocate for the patient
Educator

titioners who are likely to diagnose and treat patients with soft tissue rheumatic disease. For example, in the study of one factory in which a nurse was employed, workers with work-related upper limb disorders continued to work or were able return to work (after some time off), and were unlikely to seek medical advice (9). A nurse in the work setting can not only help to prevent injury and disability, but can also learn the skills required to manage both acute and chronic work-related disorders. Family physicians or general practitioners are also often in a similar position when patients consult them for treatment of unresolved pain.

ROLE OF THE NURSE ON THE INTERDISCIPLINARY HEALTH CARE TEAM

Nurses work with other members of the health care team in acute or tertiary care settings. They do not prescribe medications (this is a role of the physician) or treatment modalities (role of physician and/or physical therapist). (Note: Nurses may have limited use of prescription if licensed to do so or when standing orders are provided.) However, they play a unique and important role in assisting patients with soft tissue rheumatic disease to manage their health problem (see Table 9.1). Nurses, with appropriate education, can diagnose minor acute soft tissue conditions (e.g., tendinitis, bursitis) as well as recommending what should be done early on (e.g., application of ice, use of nonprescription medications). Nurses also have an important role to play helping patients to manage chronic pain.

Given the changing roles of health care professionals, nurses are involved in the care of persons with soft tissue rheumatic disease in a variety of environmental settings, assuming a variety of specific roles, including: (a) occupational health specialist in work environments, such as in industrial or office settings; (b) nurse

at staff/student health centers, such as in a corporation or university; (c) primary care specialist in practice with physicians and other health care professionals, such as in a family physician or group practice; (d) staff nurse or manager in acute care or tertiary care center, such as a hospital; and (e) independent practitioner, such as a nurse practitioner in private practice.

Case Manager

Whether the interdisciplinary health care team is composed of many members or only of the patient (and his/her family), the physician, and the nurse, the primary role of the nurse on the team is similar—case manager or coordinator.

The role of the nurse as case manager or coordinator is more commonly understood in an acute or tertiary care setting. The goal of case management is the coordination of care throughout the episode of illness to achieve positive patient outcomes within a reasonable time frame using appropriate resources (10, 11, 12). A key component of this role in acute care is communication among members of the health care team (13, 14).

In the community setting, settings like those described above, the case management role of nurses is evolving. The health care consultant may be a physician, and the nurse may not have access to a team of any kind, depending on financial resources (including insurance and third-party payers). However, *communication remains central to coordination of care,* involving: (a) scheduling of consultation and diagnostic tests within reasonable yet practical time periods, (b) ensuring that findings from consultants and tests are compiled and communicated to those making recommendations about treatment (e.g., physician) and decisions about work status or required work-related change (e.g., employer, workers' compensation insurers), and (c) last, but not least, patients and their families.

Please remember that our patients are in foreign territory (complete with foreign language) when they deal with the health care system. Recovery and return to work are dependent, to a large extent, on the patients' and their families' understanding what is happening and what is expected of them. Given how much of the responsibility for "getting better"—reducing pain and improving functional ability—is up to the patients, it seems obvious that they (and their families) must be partners in the process of healing and recovery.

Integral to communication are translation/interpretation, facilitation, and education. To state the obvious, what patients are told by physicians, employers, and insurers often requires translation into a language that is understood by lay persons. Interpretation goes beyond translation of the language used by other professions: It requires a clear understanding of what is important to the patients and their families. Do not assume that patients with acute problems are the only ones who have a need for information; patients with chronic health problems may be equally poorly informed. As case manager, the nurse must function as a middle person between lay persons and health care professionals, so to speak.

The nurse must understand the perspectives of all. For example, if patients are told to take medications regularly but do not understand why "regularly" is important, or do not have the timing of taking the medication translated into a schedule that is practical for their lives, they are less likely to take the prescribed medication (and may be labeled "not compliant").

Facilitation and education cannot really be separated from interpretation, as they are part of what makes interpretation broader than translation. *Facilitation of communication* between patient and physician (14), employer, or insurer is essential to recovery and return to work. Patients are often given mixed messages or messages that are contradictory. For example, physicians instruct patients to take it easy for a period of time to see how they do, and employers use the end of this time period as a definitive date for return to work. Employers can also benefit from interpretation of medical reports into terms that apply in their context.

Education of patients and their families is also a key aspect of case management. Without knowledge, patients and their families cannot make informed decisions. A recent finding that the strongest correlate of negative mood for patients attending a pain clinic was lack of information (15) demonstrates the importance of keeping patients informed. Providing information should be more than telling facts. As

noted above, understanding the patients' situation as well as their prescribed treatment regimens will enable nurses to help patients and their families to follow the regimens in a manner that fits their lifestyle.

An example described in Chapter 7 provides an illustration. Prescription of amitriptyline or low dose tricyclics to help patients get to sleep and stay asleep requires tailoring of dose and the timing of taking the medication on the basis of individual response. The lowest dose should be tried for 2 weeks before increasing the dose in small amounts. Asking the patient to write the schedule on a calendar may be helpful to keep track of how much to take on each day. Many patients find that taking these medications at 10 PM or at bedtime leaves them feeling groggy or "hung over" in the morning, making it difficult to "get up and get moving." If this reaction occurs, the patient should try taking the medication earlier, up to as early as 5 to 6 PM, by moving the time back in 1-hour increments; writing the time it was taken on the calendar may again be a helpful way of keeping track and learning what time taking the medication results in the best effect and least side effects. Patients need to know that drinking extra coffee in the morning to "get going" is not the answer. Increasing caffeine intake only adds to difficulty sleeping. Finding the best dose and timing of medication taking, for most medications, requires persistence and knowledge. Asking patients to write time, dose taken, and response (including how well it works as well as side effects) on a daily basis will provide information for physicians for changing prescriptions or making recommendations about timing of medication taking. Instructing patients to take such records to their physicians provides helpful information and places less reliance on memory.

Finally, case managers may need to act as *advocates* for patients and their families. Depending on who employs the nurse, a clear understanding of who the nurse represents is essential. Although the nurse and patients may be employed by the same company, the nurse as case manager has an obligation to the employees/patients, as does the physician to whom the patients may be referred. The nurse in this situation can work for what is best for both employees and employers. The assumption must be made that employees want to return to work and that the employers want their employees to return to work. If employees believe that anything said to the nurse is reported to their employer, then the nurse will not be in a position to help employees any more than superficially.

Advocacy also requires the nurse to be aware of resources within the community. *Resources* refers to: (*a*) expert health care professionals and consultants (general practitioners, rheumatologists, orthopaedists, occupational and physical therapists, social workers, and psychologists); and (*b*) programs and services (e.g., assertiveness training, aquatics and exercise programs, support groups, self-help groups). Knowledge about resources must include cost and availability of the resource or service, including timing and flexibility of scheduling. For example, knowledge about a support group should include: (*a*) the fee to join the support group, (*b*) when (time and day of week) and how often the group meets, (*c*) the background of typical members—diverse or similar to that of the patient and his/her family, (*d*) who is contact for referral, and (*e*) the expertise of the group leader and the efficacy of the group. Note, however, that recommendation for a program, service, or consultant should only be provided if it is known to be expert and effective. Keeping up to date about the expertise and effectiveness of community programs and consultants requires frequent contact with the persons who administer and/or provide the program or service. An excellent way of learning how well a program or service works is to talk to individuals who have used it recently.

UNIVERSAL ASPECTS TO CONSIDER WITH SOFT TISSUE RHEUMATIC DISEASE

As previously noted in this book, pain is a common reason for visiting a physician (16). Chronic pain affects about 11% of the adult population at any given time (17). Determining the cause and treating this pain is not always a simple matter, as must be clear by now. The following aspects must be considered by any health care professional when dealing with pain and patients with soft tissue rheumatic disease, especially for patients who are experiencing pain that has not resolved spontaneously (which is why patients consult health care professionals).

Acute Pain: The Role of the Nurse

In a primary care or occupational health setting, nurses may be consulted by patients who have acute pain from soft tissue rheumatic disease. (Refer to the assessment techniques in previous chapters and to Appendix A.) The nurse should clearly differentiate localized soft tissue conditions from articular or systemic disease. Clear cases of minor localized conditions, such as tendinitis and bursitis, are within the scope of practice of appropriately trained nurses. History and physical examination to confirm such conditions forms the basis for diagnosis.

Prescription for the use of ice for acute inflammation, over-the-counter nonsteroidal antiinflammatory drugs (NSAIDs), and rest during acute phase is suggested (see the decision charts in preceding chapters). Once initial inflammation resolves, prescription of stretching and exercise using instruction sheets, as provided in many of the previous chapters, is recommended.

The role of the nurse in assessment, plan for treatment, education and direction regarding interventions, and evaluation of the outcomes of treatment is described in more detail later. The principles described apply to both acute and chronic conditions.

As noted in preceding chapters, local injections are recommended for many acute conditions. In some jurisdictions, nurses may be trained and certified to perform some injections, although in most cases physicians perform this procedure. The role of the nurse in practice with physicians is to assist with the procedure and teach patients how to care for injection sites (e.g., ice around the site immediately following injection, balancing rest and exercise once injections have reduced pain). When exercise is prescribed, follow the suggestions in previous chapters according to body region and generally in Chapter 8; that is, provide instruction, demonstrate the exercise, observe patients doing the exercise (return demonstration), and provide written instructions for each exercise.

Chronic Pain: A Multidimensional Experience

Chronic pain is a multidimensional, complex phenomenon that can affect every aspect of an individual's life (4, 14, 18, 19). The following dimensions must be considered: (a) physiological, (b) sensory, (c) affective, (d) cognitive, (e) behavioral, and (f) sociocultural (14).

The physiological dimension entails primarily the etiology of the pain and includes pain location, onset, and duration, whereas the sensory dimension focuses on how the pain feels to the patient and includes the intensity, quality, and pattern of the pain. These dimensions should be considered in taking the history from the patient (see Appendix A).

The affective dimension of chronic pain is based on the feelings experienced related to the pain. Pain affects and is affected by mood state, anxiety, fear, depression, and well-being (4). Ratings of overall pain are not a simple summation of sensory and affective ratings, but rather a mathematical additive function of both components, with anger, fear, and sadness accounting for the affective component (20). Anxiety can both enhance and inhibit coping with pain (21, 22).

A relationship clearly exists between depression and chronic pain, although there is no consensus about the nature of this relationship. The impact of pain on daily life and activities and feeling of life control may explain a resulting depression (23), while depression plays a role in the maintenance of chronic pain (24). The prevalence of depression for persons who have chronic pain is not age-specific; young and old alike experience both (23). Subjects with or without chronic pain who are depressed have been found consistently to report greater negative cognitive distortion than subjects with or without chronic pain who are not depressed (25, 26). Chronic pain patients in a spine program who were more depressed reported more negative traits in themselves (27). In other words, negative thinking contributes to depression and both have an impact on the management of chronic pain (28). What these findings really mean for clinicians is that depression and the report of depressive symptoms in the absence of major depression should not be ignored. The effectiveness of any intervention will depend on dealing with cognitions and depression while at the same time offering strategies to manage pain.

The cognitive dimension of chronic pain encompasses the meaning of pain to the patient and other related thought processes (4). Meaning is assigned to the pain in an attempt to understand the pain and its impact on the life of the individual experiencing the pain, as well as on the individual's family (29). Meaning is understood in the context of how one views the self, the attitudes and beliefs held by the individual and others, factors influencing pain, how pain has been treated in the past, and the type of coping skills and strategies used. Meaning and how meaning can be changed are important considerations when trying to understand the pain experience and to plan effective interventions.

The existence of pain contributes to pain-related behaviors, some of which are designed to decrease pain intensity, while others are indicators of the presence of pain (4, 29). These behaviors include communication and interpersonal interaction, physical activity, and interventions to reduce pain (e.g., taking medications). Learning effective behaviors or interventions is essential to reducing pain and learning to live with what cannot be eliminated. The subjective perception of a low level of control over pain accounts for a significant amount of the distress and disability that result from pain (30). Patients who have chronic pain have reported uncertainty about their ability to control pain (25, 26), and low levels of predictable control over their pain (31). Interventions that focus on acceptance of uncertainty and that increase perceived control over pain may increase the ability to manage chronic pain. The worst position for a person in pain to be in is one in which they believe that there is nothing that they can do about the pain. Setting goals that are attainable and reasonable is the key.

Finally, the sociocultural dimension of chronic pain focuses on the ethnocultural background of the individual, family and social life, work and home responsibilities, recreation and leisure, environmental factors, and social influences (4). Although sociocultural affiliation has been found to have a primary influence on the perception of and response to acute pain, only recently has this influence been studied in persons with chronic pain. A bio-cultural model has been found to be useful in explaining the complex factors that form the basis for perceptions about chronic pain (32). The age of the person with chronic pain has also only recently been considered because the focus of treatment and research has been on adults, but not on seniors or the elderly. Recently, characteristics of pain and treatment outcomes have been compared for younger and older adults. Although baseline measures were somewhat different between the two age groups, the comprehensive program (which included exercise and cognitive interventions) was equally effective when change in outcome measures was evaluated (33, 34). The same approach to pain management is effective for young and old alike.

Localized Versus Systemic Soft Tissue Rheumatic Disease

As previously emphasized in this book, soft tissue rheumatic disease may be localized or systemic. Localized diseases are often a result of injury or repetitive strain, whereas systemic diseases, although aggravated by some of the same factors as localized problems, are usually more problematic and difficult to treat. Persons with systemic disease, such as fibromyalgia, often have additional localized soft tissue problems that are difficult to resolve or manage—more difficult than for persons who have localized conditions without systemic disease. Assessment and treatment strategies for localized and systemic conditions are in some ways similar and the similarities are emphasized in the remaining sections of this chapter. For example, the role of difficulty in sleeping and of fatigue in myofascial pain and fibromyalgia is stronger than in localized soft tissue rheumatic disease (35, 36). Fatigue adds to the impact of pain and makes it more difficult to resume usual activities and a "normal" lifestyle. Strategies for management of fatigue are discussed later.

To emphasize a point made previously that cannot be stated too often, understanding the impact of home, work, and recreational activities on the condition—that is, understanding the factors that aid and that aggravate the condition—is essential to developing treatment strategies that will be successful. In fact, it may take as long to feel better as it took for the soft tissue problem to become significant. "Getting better" requires much effort for persons with chronic conditions. This effort is enhanced by the support of the health care professionals and the patient's family and coworkers.

The Role of Family

The role of the family—both the impact of individuals with acute or chronic pain on their families and the impact of the families on the individuals with pain—has received little scrutiny until recently. In the event of an acute illness the person who is ill assumes a "sick role," as it was named by Parsons (37). As there is a division of labor in all households, with family members performing different tasks, the division of labor in families who have a member who cannot complete usual tasks must be changed (38). Acute illness is accepted by and acceptable to the both the family and its member who must stop performing usual tasks because changes in roles and responsibilities are viewed as temporary. In the case of chronic health problems, however, this sick role is less clearly understood. The family is usually required to make permanent changes in how its members function—in the tasks performed and responsibilities assumed. Family members need to communicate openly and to discuss how changes can be made and how to manage additional tasks that may be required to manage the disease (e.g., exercise, transportation to medical or therapy appointments, rest) (38).

Two reviews of the literature on the impact of chronic pain on the family were reported in the early 1990s (39, 40). Factors that affect how individuals cope with their chronic pain are the same factors that are important to how the spouses of such persons cope with the situation (39). Spouses are at increased risk for emotional distress or depression (41, 42, 43), decreased satisfaction with their marriage (43), and health problems (42). How persons with the pain manage and cope has a greater influence on how their spouses cope than does the nature of the illness causing the pain, or its intensity (42, 43).

In recent qualitative studies, many areas of the lives of spouses were found to be adversely affected by their partners with chronic pains (44, 45). The social relationship of the marriage changed, including changes in partnership, sexual activity, contact with friends and relatives, and roles (46).

In the reciprocal relationships within a family, the response of the family to the member with chronic pain affects how the person with pain copes. Spouses have been found to reinforce the pain behaviors of their partners, and poor marital relationships may contribute to the pain (46). It is not uncommon for spouses to respond to negative cues and to attend selectively to their partners' pain and distress, thus reinforcing these behaviors (26, 39). Given the interrelationships between patients and their families, assessment of the impact of pain both on persons experiencing the pain and their families must be considered if interventions are to be effective. Family support is required for patients to recover.

In summary, knowledge about pain and its impact on life, the role of aggravating factors from the home and work environments on soft tissue rheumatic disease, and the inseparable role of physiological and psychological factors (7, 45, 47–49) on the complex multidimensionality of pain are important in assessing and treating adults who have pain from soft tissue rheumatic disease. The decision charts in this book provide excellent guidelines for practitioners, especially nurses in independent practice. Consultation of appropriate specialists must always be considered, as well as what role the nurse has in conjunction with other health care professionals. As previously emphasized, knowledge of expert community resources and consultants is an essential role of the case manager.

ASSESSMENT OF PATIENTS WITH SOFT TISSUE RHEUMATIC DISEASE

Nurses who work in conjunction with family physicians or general practitioners in a generalist role should be prepared to conduct an assess-

TABLE 9.2 NURSING ASSESSMENT OF PATIENTS WITH CHRONIC PAIN

I. History and physical examination if not already performed by a physician.

II. Supplemental assessment:
   a) factors that influence pain at home, work, and play
      i) factors that aggravate pain
      ii) factors that alleviate pain
   b) strategies used to manage pain in the past
      i) strategies that helped
      ii) strategies that did not help
   c) meaning and impact of pain to the individual and family
   d) role of others (family, friends, coworkers)

III. Consider:
   a) injury and repetitive strain versus systemic disease
   b) person in context with the environment— at home, work, and play
   c) values related to pain and illness

ment that supplements that of the medical history and physical examination and to participate in the development of a treatment plan in collaboration with both physicians and patients (including their families). In an occupational health setting, the nurse may have a more independent role to play and be the first-line health care professional consulted by the patient. In this role, the nurse may conduct history and physical examinations or may be required to refer the patients for medical examination and diagnostic tests according to a protocol established with employers. Table 9.2 presents a summary of assessment measures (see also Appendix A and suggested procedures described in previous chapters).

The nurse should focus assessment on the nonphysiological dimensions of pain, assuming that the history and physical examination focus on the physiological dimension, whether performed by physician or nurse. The focus of this section is on supplemental assessment to the history and physical examination.

Although physical assessment of the patient in pain is similar whether the pain is acute or chronic, the approach to both history taking and supplemental assessment requires a different approach for chronic pain. The impact of chronic pain has similarities and differences based on the etiology of the pain as well as on what body part is involved (15). Therefore, assessment of all dimensions of chronic pain is essential to understanding the experience fully and being able to recommend appropriate interventions. The following areas for assessment are suggested.

First, the cognitive dimension of chronic pain—the meaning of pain and other related thought processes—forms the basis for pain-related behaviors. Asking what the pain means to persons with pain is as simple as asking what it is like to live with their pain. Second, the nurse needs to be aware of sociocultural influences on pain. More specifically, nurses, who are usually young to middle-aged, middle class Caucasians, need to be aware of their assumptions about persons from different cultural groups and ages from theirs. Beliefs and values about pain are diverse and they influence response to treatment. Try to be open to what patients and their families say that may be different from your own experiences.

Start with a general question and follow it with more specific questions to clarify responses or help individuals expand on ideas or thoughts. Four sets of questions (summarized in Table 9.3) follow with the rationale for the questions. Many of these questions are appropriate for patients who are experiencing acute or chronic pain, although the fourth set is most appropriate to chronic pain experiences.

1. Description of Pain. Describe your pain. What words would you use to describe your pain? Where is your pain—point to the place. How bad is your pain right now—what number would you give in on a 0 to 10 scale when 0 means no pain and 10 means worst pain? How long have you had this pain? What other problems or symptoms are you having?

Description of the pain and other symptoms places the physiological problems experienced on the table for discussion. A clear description of symptoms that are bothersome provides the baseline from which to define goals to be accomplished on the way to living a life that is acceptable even with chronic pain. Tools that can be used to help patients describe their pain include: (*a*) marking on a diagram of the body the areas that experience pain (*b*) rating scales for pain intensity (e.g., the 0–10 rating), and (*c*) questionnaires that provide choices of word descriptors of pain (e.g., the McGill Pain Questionnaire). Understanding what is experienced by the patient is important: Individual differ-

TABLE 9.3 QUESTIONS TO ASK PATIENT AND FAMILY

1. Describe your pain.
   What words would you use to describe your pain? Where is your pain—point to the place. How bad is your pain right now—what number would you give it on a 0 to 10 scale when 0 means no pain and 10 means worst pain? How long have you had this pain? What other problems/symptoms are you having?

2. What affects your pain?
   What makes your pain worse? What changes your pain? What improves your pain? What activities make your pain worse (e.g., work, hobby)? What activities reduce your pain (e.g., work, hobby)?

3. What have you done to manage this pain in the past?
   What has worked? What has not worked? How has this pain been treated in the past? What has worked? What has not worked? How much control do you have over the pain? What gives you more control? Ask the same question about symptoms other than pain.

4. How have other people reacted to your pain?
   Your family? Your friends? Your coworkers? What do other people do that helps your pain? What do other people do that makes your pain worse? Think about family, friends, and coworkers. How has your condition (pain) influenced your relationships? With your husband/wife? Your family? Your friends? Your coworkers?

ences in pain severity between patients are more striking than among groups of patients with different medical diagnoses (14, 50).

Pain may not be the only symptoms experienced. Living with pain is an exhausting experience. Not only do people who have pain become physically tired as a result of the pain, but also those who have fibromyalgia experience fatigue that is in part a result of nonrestorative sleep. Fatigue adds to the impact of pain and makes it more difficult to resume usual activities and a ''normal'' lifestyle (35, 36, 51). For patients who describe being tired, ask about sleep habits, what interferes with sleep, caffeine intake, and what promotes sleep (see the section below on interventions related to fatigue). Clarify other symptoms (e.g., numbness, tingling) if not previously reported in the history or physical examination.

2. Factors That Influence Pain. What factors or things affect your pain? What makes your pain worse? What changes your pain?

What improves your pain? What activities make your pain worse (e.g., work, hobby)? What activities reduce your pain (e.g., work, hobby)?

As noted in Appendix B, many activities can aggravate symptoms and pain. Aggravating factors contribute to pain not only when the injury is from repetitive use or strain, but also when the condition is more generalized (e.g., fibromyalgia). Focus on persons in their environments (e.g., work, home, and recreation), and be certain to talk with the patient about activities at home and play (e.g., hobbies, social activities). It may be something that the patient does not do often that exacerbates pain and/or other symptoms. Think about body positions (e.g., standing, reaching). Ask about differences in pain during the day and at night; pain during rest differentiates diagnoses (52). Consider how stress (psychological) and tension (physiological) influence pain. Be specific—ask if stopping an activity that aggravates symptoms stops them temporarily or does the activity need to be avoided to reduce pain/symptoms. Finally, ask how typical daily activities are performed. What activities are performed and how they are performed provides information about how the patient handles everyday life (53).

The use of a journal or diary is a strategy than can be used both for assessment and as an intervention. Some patients are not sure what makes their pain or symptoms worse or better, just that they feel better at some times than at others, or have good and bad days. Ask patients to rate the intensity of their pain and to describe it hourly, along with what they were thinking and/or doing at the time, for 1 week. The detailed information should provide insights for both nurse and patient about factors that contribute to pain as well as the role of family and friends. The second strategy, although more time-consuming, is to ask patients to tell their stories. Active listening validates their experiences and feelings (54). (See the format suggested by McCaffery and Beebe on page 30 of their text [14].)

3. Management of Pain in the Past. What have you done to manage this pain in the past? What has worked? What has not worked? How has this pain been treated in the past? What has worked? What has not worked? How much control do you have over the pain? What gives you more control? Ask the same question about symptoms other than pain.

Experience with acute and chronic pain in the past may be predictive of the ability to deal with pain in the present. If an exacerbation has been relieved with specific strategies in the past, patients may be more willing to believe that the same or similar strategies will work in the present. On the other hand, if patients experienced little or no relief of symptoms from interventions tried previously, they may be skeptical about trying anything new. What patients know about rehabilitation influences how they feel about the pain and what is happening (15). Given the diversity that exists in people, it is likely that some strategies will be more effective than others in managing chronic pain. Knowing what interventions have been effective or helpful in the past, and which ones did not work, is essential information when developing a treatment plan.

Remember to consider the affective dimension of chronic pain. Pain affects and is affected by mood state, anxiety, fear, depression, and sense of well-being (4, 55). Evaluation of affect is an important component of assessment, although some of the symptoms of depression or dysphoria are common to persons who have pain (e.g., difficulty sleeping). A questionnaire like the Center for Epidemiological Studies Depression Scale (CES-D) (56) can be used to determine the likelihood of depression or to screen for depression, but should not replace skilled clinical assessment. The score on the CES-D that indicates possible depression has recently been determined to be 19 for persons who have chronic pain (57), and not 16 as traditionally used in the general population; thus scores greater than 19 indicate possible depression and scores less than 19 are ''normal.'' If major depression is suspected, rather than dysphoria or sadness, consider referral to a psychologist for confirmation and/or treatment. Medical intervention may be required.

Given that the strongest correlate of negative mood for patients attending a pain clinic was lack of information, followed by lack of sleep, unemployment, and fear of the future (15), what the patient knows about his condition or pain should also be assessed. Education about what is happening and what to expect should be based on what the patient and his/her family know, so a baseline assessment is helpful.

Beliefs about pain and its management can facilitate healing and treatment, but may also interfere with recovery if beliefs interfere with willingness to provide complete information about the pain experience (58). Beliefs are grounded in cultural norms and may be influenced by age and gender. Such beliefs need to be incorporated into the assessment so that, if necessary, some beliefs can be dispelled so that treatment can be effective (58).

Worry and anxiety contribute to functional limitations and ability to work (59). Although most people want to be well and free from pain, there are secondary gains to having a chronic soft tissue rheumatic disease. Secondary gain is not the same as malingering. Malingering— lying about the presence of pain—is relatively uncommon (14). As discussed earlier, assuming a chronic sick role may excuse an individual from certain duties and responsibilities in the family. At times, dependency on others for assistance is perceived as requisite to keeping the family together. External roles are also affected (e.g., employment [60], friendship). Negative secondary gains include disability, whereas positive secondary gains for persons who have pain and diagnosed disease include reasons to avoid tasks and actions (14). Understanding the gains and losses that result from living with pain provides important clues to developing a treatment plan that will be effective.

4. *The Reaction of Others to the Patients' Pain.* How have other people reacted to your pain? Your family? Your friends? Your coworkers? What do other people do that helps your pain? What do other people do that makes your pain worse? Think about family, friends, and coworkers. How has your condition (pain) influenced your relationships? With your husband/wife? Your family? Your friends? Your coworkers?

Being in pain influences relationships with others, even if the person in pain lives alone. Understanding individuals' perceptions about how their health problem and pain have changed relationships with family and friends and the reactions experienced from others is essential to being able to help patients set goals. For example, the goal of getting out of the house more often is not possible if the patient perceives that this activity places an unacceptable burden on family to arrange their schedules to provide transportation. With the patients' permission, over time, talking with spouses and other family members may be helpful in helping patients and their families make plans and set goals together.

Return to work for patients who are employed is usually set as a realistic goal unless the work involves tasks that aggravate the rheumatic disease and cannot be modified. In a recent study, persons who lived alone, were not actively involved in treatment plan, and/ or experienced long periods of disability without support from the immediate family were found to be more likely never to return to work (61). Nurses should consider strategies to involve the patients in their care and assess their family support system to identify strategies that could be used to strengthen support provided to patients.

PLAN FOR CARE OF INDIVIDUALS WITH SOFT TISSUE RHEUMATIC DISEASE

Serious, acute problems stemming from soft tissue rheumatic disease should be referred for medical evaluation and not treated by the nurse without consultation. Use the decision charts in other chapters of this book to distinguish true emergencies from urgent or acute situations and take the appropriate action. As noted previously, acute problems that are not serious are within the scope of practice of the nurse with appropriate training. Many of the interventions described later in this chapter can be appropriately prescribed by nurses.

The plan for the care of individuals with soft tissue rheumatic disease should be based on data collected during assessment by all health care professionals involved in the assessment (see Table 9.4). In addition, as suggested above, the use of a journal or diary to keep track of pain and other symptoms, activities, actions taken and their impact on pain/symptoms, provides excellent data about aggravating factors and the impact on pain by others. This information is also helpful in determining the most appropriate referral. For example, descriptions

TABLE 9.4 PLAN FOR CARE OF THE INDIVIDUAL WITH CHRONIC PAIN FROM SOFT TISSUE RHEUMATIC DISEASE

Diagnosis of the syndrome or cause of pain in collaboration or referral with a physician

Referral to physician for medical management (e.g., local injections, prescription of medications, further referral for physical therapy or to medical specialist)

Consider and prioritize what is important to the patient and his/her family when developing treatment plan

Set goals with the patient and/or the family

Develop plan for multidimensional approach to treatment (see Table 9.5)

Communicate treatment plan to patient, family, health care professionals, and employer (if appropriate)

---

of sadness and depression may suggest referral to a psychologist or social worker; descriptions of pain worsening following altercations with an adolescent child may indicate that family should be asked to become involved in the development of the treatment plan and/or to meet with a counselor. Remember, learning about the patient and his/her family will take time and cannot happen in one meeting.

The plan for care is usually developed by the nurse and patient in conjunction with advice and direction from other health care professionals. The prescribing of medications and therapeutic modalities is done by physicians and physical therapists, except in the case of standing orders or of jurisdictions in which others may prescribe (e.g., nurse practitioners). Strategies to educate patients about all of these aspects of the treatment plan are important and are discussed in the next section.

Setting realistic, achievable goals with patients and their families is vital to successful response to treatment. The goal of being pain-free may not be reasonable, but reducing pain so that patients can rest or sleep may be reasonable. These goals must be agreed upon: Goals set by the health care professional are rarely met if their achievement is dependent on compliance with a treatment plan that is not clear or does not make sense to the patient. Patients are more likely to ''stick with'' a program of exercise, rest, medications, and so on, if they have been involved to some extent in the development of the overall treatment plan. The opportunity for choice is a key to success and is addressed more fully below.

As discussed previously, the interrelationship between physiological and psychological factors cannot be overstated. Return to work is often a goal set by health care professionals on the basis of the physical findings. Yet, research supports the complex nature of this outcome and indicates physiological factors to be poor predictors of return to work (62, 63).

Finally, consider what is important to the patients and what the health care team or consultants suggest. Coordinate communication among patients, families, and other health care team members. Make sure that information is provided to those who require it. And remember that the patient is a member of the team.

INTERVENTIONS FOR INDIVIDUALS WITH SOFT TISSUE RHEUMATIC DISEASE

Researchers at the University of Washington have concluded that the majority of patients with chronic pain can learn to function normally despite the presence of pain and depressive symptoms (64). Identification of factors that contribute to adaptation for each individual is integral to successful adaptation.

Strategies to manage a soft tissue rheumatic disease depend in part on the nature of the disease. Rather than to focus on specific diseases and their treatment, which are well reviewed in other chapters in this book, the focus of interventions for the nurse is on generic strategies that can be applied to a general practice setting.

Traditional Strategies to Manage Chronic Pain

Traditional strategies to manage chronic pain include: (a) medications, (b) use of heat and cold, (c) splinting and footwear, (d) exercise, (e) surgery, and (f) removal of aggravating factors. Each of these interventions has been described in previous chapters, so comments here are limited to specific directions and references, and to the role the nurse has as case manager—that is, coordination of care, communication, translation/interpretation, facilitation, and education. To restate the obvious, what patients need to understand fully is how

TABLE 9.5 INTERVENTION STRATEGIES FOR TREATMENT OF CHRONIC PAIN FROM SOFT TISSUE RHEUMATIC DISEASE

Assist in setting goals that are reasonable to attain

Translate instructions from health care professionals, employers, and other parties into understandable language

Involve family and others as agreed by patient

Educate regarding safe and effective use of medications

Educate regarding safe and effective practice of exercise

Educate regarding identification and elimination of aggravating factors, modification of how activities are performed

Educate regarding prevention of further injury or exacerbation of systemic disease

Educate regarding methods to reduce or manage pain:
- use of ice, heat
- resting regularly during activity
- wearing splints and proper footwear
- relaxation and stress management (e.g., guided imagery)
- cognitive strategies

Provide information about community programs and resources (e.g., support groups, stress management courses)

---

to implement treatments and interventions. ''Noncompliance'' is often an issue of poor understanding of what is expected and the consequences of action or inaction. Patients require support and education to carry out a treatment plan as prescribed, as well as directions that translate it into their language and lifestyle. Education about pain and strategies to manage it are both essential (65), as is information about the rheumatic condition and what it means to their lives and lifestyle both in the short and the long term. A general plan for care is summarized in Table 9.5.

MEDICATIONS

Record the name of the medication, dosage, and date started as part of documenting medication use and effectiveness. Ask patients to transcribe this information to a medication calendar or diary; the actual time pills are taken and the effectiveness and side effects can be recorded daily. Make sure that patients have information from the pharmacy about safe and effective practices for taking each medication (e.g., which to take with meals or on a full stomach) (66).

Translate when to take medications into a timetable that fits the lives of patients. For

example, if the patient is working night shifts, change the timing of taking medications to nighttime while at work and not daytime when sleeping; and medications might be taken at the same time as meals or other events that are usually on the same schedule. When patients are taking several prescription and over-the-counter medications, review all medications to check for any that may potentiate or interfere with the pharmacokinetics of another. Consultation with a local pharmacist is recommended.

The timing of taking medications is also an important issue. Analgesics should be taken on a regular basis, and not when the pain has become too bad to handle. Taking acetaminophen (extra strength—500 mg) prior to completing activities that produce pain may reduce the level of pain experienced. If an aggravating activity cannot be avoided, take the analgesics at least 30 minutes before starting the activity and every 3 to 4 hours. Instruct patients that waiting until pain is severe will result in less effective relief from analgesic medication. The example of amitriptyline discussed earlier is another illustration of the effects of the timing of medications. Consultation with drug handbooks and clinicians with expertise in the effective taking of medications is recommended (an excellent reference is text by McCaffery and Beebe [14]).

As noted above, medications include more than prescription medicines. Over-the-counter remedies for pain relief, such as acetaminophen and topical preparations, are commonly taken. Ointments and gels can be purchased over the counter to produce heat or cold. Review cautions and contraindications with patients (e.g., not to use a topical preparation with acetylsalicylic acid to produce heat and simultaneously to use a heating pad; or not to use topical preparations on skin with a rash or scratches).

USE OF HEAT AND COLD

There is no standardized recommendation for use of heat versus cold for soft tissue rheumatic disease, except to use cold during early stages of injury or inflammation rather than heat. Like the effectiveness of medication, response to all therapeutic modalities in terms of pain management is individualized. Heat and cold can be used interchangeably and one is often pre-

TABLE 9.6 RESULTS OF USING HEAT VERSUS COLD

Heat	Cold
Comforting and relaxing	Counter-irritant for pain
Vasodilation	Vasoconstriction
Reduces muscle spasm	Reduction in muscle spasticity and tone
Reduces pain	Increases pain threshold

ferred over the other by individual patients (14, 67) (Table 9.6). Use of heat and cold are contraindicated for patients with tissues with poor vascular supply (67) and in persons with decreased sensation or ability to respond when they feel too hot or cold (68). Caution applies to both modalities. Do not place the source of heat or cold directly on the skin; wrap the source in a dry cloth or thin towel. (See text by McCaffery and Beebe for patient instructions and information [14].)

In general, inflammation is treated with cold, and stiffness and muscle spasm not accompanied by inflammation are treated with heat, although, as noted above, some patients find heat preferable to cold for inflammation. Heat is applied via convection (changes in environmental temperatures), conduction (direct contact with a warm substance), or radiation (e.g., sunshine) (68). Heat is commonly applied with hot packs (by physical therapists) or a hot water bottle at home. In addition, heating pads that provide dry electrical heat may be used. Heat is contraindicated after trauma and during the acute stages of an injury (14, 68). Heat should be applied for no longer than 20 minutes. The skin should be examined every 2 minutes for the first few applications to ensure that skin is not being damaged.

Cold is applied using bags of ice, frozen gel, and cold packs. Although application of ice using a wet cloth next to the skin results in the greatest reduction in skin temperature, the use of dry cloth is recommended for comfort (68). Maximum cooling occurs in the first 3 minutes and is accompanied by a sensation of cold. Local numbness occurs usually in 5 to 12 minutes, followed by reflex vasodilation of deep tissue at 12 to 15 minutes. Cold should be applied for a minimum of 15 to 20 minutes per session, but not longer than 30 minutes. On first application, skin should be observed every 2 minutes for hives indicating an allergy

to cold (68). Contraindications for use of cold in addition to those listed above are muscle spasm secondary to skeletal or neurological pathology, itching, or following surgery (14).

SPLINTING AND FOOTWEAR

When symptoms are exacerbated by specific movements that cannot be avoided, the wearing of splints to support the limb during the activity can be as helpful as proper footwear in reducing strain. Consultation with an occupational therapist may be required for custom splinting and orthoses. However, items such as over-the-counter wrist supports or running shoes with good support may suffice for many patients. Review of the assessment of what makes pain worse and what improves it will facilitate the identification of any need for support.

EXERCISE AND POSTURE

Correct posture and body mechanics during activities at home and at work are essential to healthy musculoskeletal structures. Exercises to strengthen muscles and improve flexibility also have uncontested benefit and are typically a key part of a multidimensional treatment plan (see below). Review Chapter 8 for specific instructions about exercise. Nurses should teach exercises as prescribed in earlier chapters by demonstrating the exercise while reviewing written instructions, followed by having the patient return to demonstrate the exercise(s). Providing patients with written instructions is recommended. Illustrations in this text can be photocopied for use by patients.

PLANNING FOR SURGERY

Surgery may be an option for some patients. They need to be prepared for what to expect with surgery and recovery as well as what to expect without surgery. The most helpful approach may be to have the patient ask questions of the surgeon or to talk to other patients who have had similar procedures. The nurse's role in surgical care is not within the scope of this text.

REMOVAL OF AGGRAVATING FACTORS

As emphasized throughout this book, identification of factors that aggravate the soft tissue rheumatic disease is an important part of assessment, and strategies to reduce these factors are integral to recovery. Modifying how some activities are performed is as important as avoiding certain other activities. Please refer to Appendix B for common aggravating factors and solutions. General guidelines to consider include the following:

1. Take a break from performing the same activity by stopping the activity every 20 minutes for 5 minutes, stretching and changing body position. Take a break every half hour when driving long distances, getting out of the car to stretch. Try to vary your activities rather than doing one thing for a long period of time.

2. When performing any activity, think about how to do it without straining. For example, when getting something from a high shelf, use a step stool rather than to reach over your head; work at a table or other surface that is positioned so that you can sit comfortably with arms supported.

3. Learn how to lie, sit, and stand in positions that are both comfortable and correct.

4. Learn how to move and lift things and to perform activities using proper body mechanics. Talk to a safety officer or occupational health specialist at work, or an occupational therapist for non–work-related activities.

5. Think before you do. Plan how you are going to do any task. Look for the simplest way to do things. Do tasks when you are at your best—well rested, not overtired, and calm, not angry.

6. Pace yourself and learn your limits. It is smart to stop before aggravating symptoms; it does not make sense to push to get something done and pay for it later. Doing any one activity for too long will make you feel worse. Do an activity for a short period of time, such as 5 minutes, then rest. If you feel no worse for the attempt, add 5 minutes next time. Find the amount you can do without aggravating symptoms and learn to respect your limits.

IMPROVING SLEEP AND REDUCING FATIGUE

As most of us have come to realize, ''getting a good night's sleep'' is essential for health and well-being. Given the relationship between pain and sleep, interventions that improve sleep reduce pain, and decreasing pain intensity improves sleep (52). As simple as this sounds, neither may be easy. Timing the taking of medication for optimum effectiveness and use of heat to relax are strategies to consider to reduce pain. Body position or alignment also contributes to comfort and can reduce pain. The use of pillows for neck support and under the knees (lying on back) or between the knees (lying on side) should be suggested. Low doses of tricyclic antidepressants or serotonin reuptake inhibitors are helpful for some patients (66). As previously discussed, finding the optimum dose and timing of these medications requires patience and persistence.

Activities prior to going to bed to sleep should be reviewed. Discuss with the patient the avoidance of activities that stimulate the body physically or psychologically:

1. Do not exercise in the evening. Avoiding strenuous exercise does not mean avoiding stretching or sexual activity (if evening is a time that you are physically comfortable and wish to engage in sexual activities). In fact, orgasm releases endorphin in the brain, a natural pain reducer.

2. Consider the use of touch or massage for relaxation and not just for sexual stimulation. Touch can also be comforting.

3. Do not watch shows on television or read material that is upsetting or worrying. Try catching up on the news earlier in the day.

The phrase *sleep hygiene* is used to describe the usual routines followed by someone getting ready to go to sleep (e.g., changing out of daytime clothes, brushing teeth) (69, 70). These routines get people physically and psychologically ready for bed. Also related to sleep hygiene is how adults traditionally view the bedroom and bed as being for sleep or sexual activity. When adults have chronic pain they may spend more time in bed and in the bedroom but not sleeping. They may change out of daytime clothes earlier in the day. With change in routines and abandonment of long-standing habits, our brains do not get the message that it is time for sleep. The following advice applies:

1. Spend time in the bedroom only for sleep or sexual activity. Watch television and read in another room.
2. Follow usual routines prior to going to bed (e.g., brushing teeth, changing out of daytime clothes). Change from work clothes into comfortable clothes, but not the clothing you sleep in (until bedtime). Change into clothing you sleep in prior going to bed.
3. Avoid caffeine after 4 PM (coffee, tea, chocolate, medications that have caffeine—check the labels of over-the-counter pain or cold medicines. If possible remove caffeine from your diet. Try a snack of warm milk at bedtime.
4. Try to settle down for the night at the same time. When you feel drowsy, position yourself comfortably in bed. Make sure the bedroom is a comfortable temperature and the lights are turned off or down low. If you are not asleep in 15 minutes, get up and go to another room. Read something light but do not watch television. When you feel drowsy return to bed. Repeat until you fall asleep. Get up when you usually do—do not sleep in to compensate. You are trying to retrain good sleep habits.
5. Get up at the same time every day, even on weekends. Once you are back to a routine of sleeping well so that you get up feeling like you have slept, you may wish to test the occasional staying up late and sleeping in.
6. Try to avoid naps during the day and do not return to bed to rest if you are having trouble sleeping at night. If you are tired, sit in a comfortable chair or lean back in a reclining armchair or on a sofa/couch/chesterfield. Rest is important and should not be confused with sleep. All activities should be followed by rest. If you lie down during the day, do so for no more than 30 minutes at a time. Dreaming during daytime naps is a clear indication that you are not getting enough sleep at night.

Multidimensional Approach to Managing Chronic Pain

What should be obvious is that managing chronic pain that results from soft tissue rheu-matic disease takes time, persistence, and a multidimensional approach. Unlike some acute conditions, this pain will not disappear with the taking of pills or the performance of a few exercises. All of the above and more may be required by the persons with the health problem as well as family members to reach a point where the patient can say ''I am better'' (but not ''all better'').

The role of the nurse is to help the patient and family to identify strategies that seem reasonable on the basis of systematic assessment, and to develop methods of evaluating the effectiveness of strategies or combinations of strategies for managing pain and other symptoms. All of the interventions described above may be used in combination. As previously suggested, keeping a journal or diary to keep track of strategies that were used and their impact, as well as how patients feel on a day-to-day basis, can be used to evaluate treatment outcomes (14).

Do not underestimate the value of belief in a strategy, even if it seems of little benefit. Although health care professionals have an obligation to protect patients from practices that may be harmful or of no benefit (but are often expensive), they also have a responsibility to be informed of options open to their patients. Belief in the effectiveness of recommended interventions will result in their being more effective. If a patient follows directions given by a health care professional, some benefit may be achieved; but if the patient believes that a strategy or combination of strategies will work, the benefit will be greater.

Given that no one strategy will work for all patients, the problem-solving approach to treatment is recommended: systematic trial and evaluation of strategies. Keep in mind that patients and health care professionals view aspects of treatment differently. For example, patients value information more than physicians (71). Note, too, that listening to patients is highly underrated.

Assessment and treatment (as well as its outcomes) are complex. Researchers have been unable to predict who will respond best to what treatment plan, but have suggested that some people will get better no matter what is done. Others respond best to specific interventions, and some will not get better no matter what is done. The hope is that the latter group is small. In one study, the best predictors of variance in outcome measures are the initial level of the measures, but they accounted for only 30% of the variance in outcomes (72).

The remainder of this section is devoted to strategies that are a part of a multidimensional approach to the management of pain, especially chronic pain.

RELAXATION

The goal of relaxation is to facilitate the reduction of physiological tension in muscles and other structures and to promote psychological calming or unwinding. Relaxation breaks the cycle of the effect of stress on the body (67). People cannot relax on command; they require guidance. (McCaffery and Beebe's text is recommended for patient instruction sheets and information about all of the following strategies [14].)

There are many methods that promote relaxation: (a) sensory or movement interventions—biofeedback, progressive muscle relaxation, music, and massage or touch, and (b) cognitive interventions, which are strategies of the mind—meditation, guided imagery, and sensory information (68). All of these methods have been found to be effective strategies to promote relaxation for some persons some of the time (8, 67, 73), but like exercise, they must be practiced daily. Just as muscles become weak without use and training is reversed by a few weeks of inactivity, the results of any of these methods are lost without regular practice. Health care professionals should provide patients with a selection of strategies from which to choose. Some patients prefer the exclusive use of one strategy, and others find that the use of several methods enhances relaxation.

Biofeedback was used in early work exclusively to reduce heart rate and blood pressure levels. As a technique that provides patients with immediate and continuous signals about body function, biofeedback provides patients with opportunities to become aware of body functions that are not usually consciously experienced. As biofeedback is a method of teaching the relationship between anxiety or stress and body function, patients learn to recognize actions that relax and those that do not. For

more information about this technique, please refer to the more detailed references (e.g., Snyder [68]; Brown [74]).

Progressive muscle relaxation has been practiced for centuries as a part of meditation. In this century, the procedure has been used to teach relaxation to reduce pain (e.g,. women in labor, persons with chronic pain). The technique can be self-taught, but it is easier to learn if another person provides verbal direction. Alternatively, books and audiotapes can be found in the health sections of most large bookstores. Directions ask patients to focus on specific muscle groups and to tense or tighten them for 5 seconds and then to relax them. Then patients are asked to focus on the relaxed muscles (68). This process is repeated in a systematic pattern from upper to lower body.

The use of *music* to treat illness was reported more than 4000 years ago by the Egyptians (68). Five elements are important: frequency (pitch), intensity (volume), tone color, interval (that which is the melody and harmony), and duration (that which creates rhythm and tempo). The type of music is in part personal preference, although most often classical music is preferred and has been found to reduce both pain and anxiety (68). Listening to music for 20 to 30 minutes with the same frequency during the day that other methods are used (e.g., ice) is suggested. Music used several times a day is as effective as using ice several times a day; once a day is not enough.

Massage, touch, and distraction are strategies that involve others and not just the individual who wishes to relax. Although the first two methods require training for maximal effectiveness, gentle touch and basic skills can be taught by a health care professional in a few minutes. Distraction is an important strategy to review with patients and their families (14, 72). Just as children can be distracted from doing something that parents wish them to stop doing by involving them in other activities, spouses and other family members can provide distraction for persons who are in pain. Activity, reading, play, singing, listening to music, and humor are all methods of distraction (3). Promoting laughter, doing quiet activities at home, and talking can all distract patients from dwelling on their pain. Health care professionals should promote creativity and discourage behaviors that promote pain behaviors. For families in which support is not available, consider referral for marital or family counseling (39, 40, 46). Do not assume that the chronic pain problem predates family difficulties.

Laughter is an adjunct to relaxation and should not be discounted. However, what is humorous differs among individuals. The relevant body of literature concentrates on the impact of laughter and music on patients with cancer pain, but the messages apply equally to all persons who have pain and discomfort. Mental outlook is half of the battle.

It is beyond the scope of this book to describe these interventions, but many texts are available that address the subject in detail.

COGNITIVE INTERVENTIONS

Cognitive interventions are those which use thought or thinking processes to reduce pain and other symptoms. In lay terms, these techniques use mind over matter, or use the mind to control pain and other symptoms. These techniques are not any more effective in alleviating symptoms than others described above, but they can be as helpful as traditional strategies in reducing symptoms. By promoting relaxation and reducing stress, depression, fear, anxiety, and pain are often reduced (19). Cognitive interventions include: (*a*) guided imagery, (*b*) meditation, (*c*) contracting, (*d*) reminiscence, (*e*) decisional control, and (*f*) sensory information. The first three are presented here, as they have the strongest scientific basis for practice.

Guided imagery is used for many purposes, from helping athletes to focus on winning the competition, to helping patients reduce pain or other symptoms by focusing on images or pictures in which they are not having pain or other symptoms. It has been used effectively in conjunction with other pain-management techniques to reduce both acute and chronic pain (3). Imagery can be fostered first at a subtle, conversational level by the use of specific phrases by health care professionals (e.g., floating, melting, dissolving, releasing, healing, letting go, less and less) (14). More direct instruction is required to assist patients to visualize, in their mind's eye, pictures that have visual, auditory, olfactory, and/or tactile qualities (68). Instruction sheets for health care profes-

sionals to direct imagery themselves or to teach family members to direct imagery can be found in the McCaffery and Beebe's text (14). Commercial audiotapes are also available for individuals who wish to use imagery as a technique on their own.

Meditation has been used as a cognitive strategy in many cultures for many centuries. It is an exercise that requires patients to focus their attention and awareness on a single object (68). The steps followed, although varied, usually involve progressive relaxation and deep breathing. There are many sources of information about meditation to be found in libraries or bookstores.

The use of *contracting* or *contracts* is common in some areas of practice (e.g., behavior modification). Development and signing of contracts is suggested for use with patients who do not clearly understand the required steps or who do not take responsibility for getting better. This strategy may be helpful when patients who have acute problems are not responding to treatment and they are suspected of failing to follow prescribed regimens of exercise or other treatments, as well as for patients with chronic problems who are not taking an active role in their recovery. A contract, simply stated, is a document that outlines what both parties, health care professional and patient, can expect of each other, as well as rewards and sanctions when expectations are not met. The agreement formalizes the responsibility patients have for their recovery. However, a description of the roles of both parties is essential because the contract is not just for what the patient is to do; it also covers the health care professional's obligations.

COGNITIVE-BEHAVIORAL INTERVENTION PROGRAMS

Cognitive-behavioral interventions are usually part of a program of treatment or rehabilitation for persons who have chronic pain that has not resolved in 6 months with usual medical interventions (e.g., local injections, medications). Although cognitive therapy can be provided by trained professionals as a specific treatment and has been evaluated as a single therapy (75–79), it has usually been part of a more comprehensive approach to pain management (1, 3, 19, 80). Participation in such programs on an outpatient basis usually involves attending a 2-hour meeting with other patients once a week, as well as "homework" (activities to perform independently at home). Many programs formally include family in the group sessions of the program (75, 77). The chapter "Expressing" in McKay, Davis, and Fanning's *Messages: The Communication Book* (81) is recommended by Turner et al. (77), and Sternbach's *Mastering Pain: A Twelve-Step Program for Coping with Chronic Pain* (82) is recommended by Nielson et al. (75).

These programs usually include physiological as well as cognitive and behavioral interventions. Medication regimens are reviewed and simplified as much as possible before starting such a program. Physiological interventions include: (*a*) physical reconditioning through a program that gradually proceeds from stretching to strengthening, aerobic fitness, and endurance (19, 75–78); (*b*) breaking down activities and exercise into components to be mastered one at a time and setting goals relative to personal tolerance (75, 76); and (*c*) activity pacing to enhance pain tolerance (75). Visual presentation of progress (e.g., graphs or charts of gains) is an effective strategy to highlight the impact of "sticking with a program" (19).

The goals of cognitive-behavioral interventions are: (*a*) to combat demoralization, (*b*) to enhance outcome efficacy, (*c*) to foster self-efficacy, (*d*) to break up automatic maladaptive patterns, (*e*) to acquire skills, and (*f*) to facilitate maintenance of effective coping strategies (83).

Cognitive-behavioral components of a comprehensive program usually include: (*a*) education about how to use cognitive techniques to reconceptualize the pain experience to gain control over thoughts, feelings, and behavior (e.g., cognitive reappraisal, reducing distortions) (19, 75–78, 80); (*b*) education about medication and physical strategies to reduce pain (80); (*c*) relaxation using the strategies described above (3, 19, 75, 77–79, 80); (*d*) learning new coping strategies and rehearsal of these strategies (e.g., role playing) (75–78, 80); (*e*) scheduling of pleasant activity to shift focus away from self (80); and (*f*) contracting (19, 76, 77).

Although cognitive-behavioral programs are designed for persons who have chronic pain, their effectiveness is far from universal. Cognitive-behavioral interventions work about as well as any other interventions. They work best in combination with the other interventions described above, and they work best for persons who have a desire to recover and who do not have psychiatric problems. Screening potential participants for clinical depression, mood disorder, and involvement in litigation is recommended by many clinicians (75, 84).

INVOLVEMENT OF FAMILY

As noted above, in the case of chronic pain, families of patients enrolled in cognitive-behavioral programs are often involved in learning how to live with chronic pain. Families play a role in distraction and supporting behaviors that do not focus on pain. In the case of acute pain, family should be equally involved. Patients and their families need to know what has happened and what to do to manage acute pain and recovery. Temporary change in household responsibilities may be anticipated by most family members. However, families may benefit from learning how to help patients manage pain (e.g., using ice or heat, distraction) and to identify and avoid aggravating factors. In other words, any information that benefits patients benefits their families.

Health care professionals should be aware of the resources available within their community, including: (*a*) expert health care professionals and consultants (general practitioners, rheumatologists, occupational and physical therapists, social workers, and psychologists); and (*b*) programs and services (e.g., assertiveness training, aquatics and exercise programs, support groups, self-help groups). Knowledge about resources should include the cost, availability, and scheduling of the resource or service (see section on advocacy in the section "Case Manager" above). A program, service, or consultant should only be recommended if it is known to be expert and effective. Frequent contact should be maintained with those who administer and/or provide the program or service, in order to keep up-to-date with both their methods and their expertise and effectiveness. Note that the self-help groups for specific diseases (e.g., the Fibromyalgia Support Group) are often valuable to patients and their families; contact the Arthritis Society or Foundation (or related national or local organization) for more information.

MIND OVER MATTER

As much as cognitive-behavioral strategies are designed to strengthen the impact of mind over matter or body, other practices used by persons who have chronic pain are effective. Although some of these methods have received very little study, they should not be underestimated (54). The value of faith and spirituality as well as prayer has not been clearly established, but they are important strategies for some persons when used in conjunction with the methods described above (54, 72). Health care professionals should not encourage specific practices, but rather should support those that provide specific patients and their families with strength and support. The belief that one has not been given more to deal with than can be managed is reassuring for many.

PREVENTION

Prevention is part of treatment—both prevention of exacerbation of the soft tissue rheumatic disease and prevention of repetitive strain injuries. Although little research has been conducted in the industrial sector, physical training of a nature specific to the tasks required at work has been found to prevent injury (85) and to reduce claims for compensation (86). Like the contribution of smoking to illness, poor muscle tone, strength, and flexibility predispose workers to injury (both at work and at home). Back schools also contribute both to the prevention of injury and to returning to work after injury (87, 88).

Both the work and home environments should be examined for factors that contribute to injury or aggravate the soft tissue rheumatic disease, whether acute or chronic. The time spent working at a specific activity should be limited. Stretching and exercise breaks should be taken at work and at home. It is less expensive to use strategies that reduce the incidence of injury than to compensate workers for inability to work. It is also less expensive to families to have all members contributing to its function than for one member to have a chronic health problem. Appropriate attention to acute conditions is likely to result in their resolution rather than in their becoming chronic problems.

EVALUATION OF INTERVENTIONS WITH INDIVIDUALS WITH SOFT TISSUE RHEUMATIC DISEASE

The role of the nurse is to help the patient and family to identify strategies that seem reasonable based on the completed assessment, and to evaluate the effectiveness of a strategy or combination of strategies to managing the condition. This evaluation is required to determine whether the interventions are working, from the patient's perspective, and if they are not, to inform the patient and other health care team members as required so that the treatment plan can be revised . . . and so the cycle continues. Prediction of outcomes, even from comprehensive pain treatment centers, is neither guaranteed nor easy (73, 89).

As in a good mystery, it takes time to identify all of the possibilities (assessment) and to test different solutions (strategies or interventions). Establishing open communication with patients so that they may talk freely about what works and what does not, and so that they know that their health care professionals believe them, places value on their experiences and their partnership in the team. The goal of all team members is to help the patients learn to do what needs to be done, to change what can be changed, and to live with what cannot be changed.

REFERENCES

1. Burckhardt CS: Chronic pain. Nurs Clin North Am 25:863–870, 1990.
2. Emmelkamp PMG, van Oppen R: Cognitive interventions in behavioral medicine. Psychother Psychosom 59:116–130, 1993.
3. Mobily PR, Herr KA, Kelley LS: Cognitive-behavioral techniques to reduce pain: a validation study. Int J Nurs Stud 30:537–548, 1993.
4. McGuire DB: Comprehensive and multidimensional assessment and measurement of pain. J Pain Symptom Manage 7:312–319, 1992.
5. Klapow JC, Slater MA, Patterson TL, Doctor JN, Atkinson JH, Garfin SR: An empirical evaluation of multidimensional clinical outcome in chronic low back pain patients. Pain 55:107–118, 1993.
6. Simon, JM: A multidisciplinary approach to chronic pain. Rehabil Nurs 14(1):23–28, 1989.
7. Jensen MP, Turner JA, Romano JM: Correlates of improvement in multidisciplinary treatment of chronic pain. J Consult Clin Psychol 62:172–179, 1994.
8. Flor H, Birbaumer N: Comparison of the efficacy of electromyographic biofeedback, cognitive-behavioral therapy, and conservative medical interventions in the treatment of chronic musculoskeletal pain. J Consult Clin Psychol 61: 653–658, 1993.
9. Helliwell PS, Mumford DB, Smeathers JE, Wright V: Work related upper limb disorder: the relationship between pain, cumulative load, disability, and psychological factors. Ann Rheum Dis 51: 1325–1329, 1992.
10. Hampton DC: Implementing a managed care framework through care maps. JONA 23(5): 21–27, 1993.
11. Etheredge ML, ed.: Collaborative care: nursing case management. Chicago: American Hospital Publishing Inc., 1989.
12. DeZell AV, Comeau E, Zander K: Nursing case management: managed care via the nursing case management model. In: Scherubel JC, Shaffer FA, eds. Patients and purse strings II. New York: National League for Nursing, 1988.
13. Mosher C, Cronk P, Kidd A: Upgrading practice with critical pathways. Am J Nurs 92(1): 41–44, 1992.
14. McCaffery M, Beebe, A: Pain: clinical manual for nursing practice. St. Louis: Mosby, 1989.
15. Sofaer B, Walker J: Mood assessment in chronic pain patients. Disability & Rehabil 16(1): 35–38, 1994.
16. Bowman JM: The meaning of chronic low back pain. AAOHN J 39:381–384, 1991.
17. Merskey H: "Foreword." In: RD France, Krishnan KRR, eds. Chronic pain. Washington, DC: American Psychiatric Press, 1988:xvii.
18. Bowman JM: Experiencing the chronic pain phenomenon: a study. Rehabil Nurs 19(2):91–95, 1994.
19. Slater MA, Good AB: Behavioral management of chronic pain. Holistic Nurs Pract 6(1): 66–75, 1991.
20. Fernandez E, Milburn, TW: Sensory and affective predictors of overall pain and emotions associated with affective pain. Clin J Pain 10:3–9, 1994.
21. McCracken LM, Gross RT: Does anxiety affect coping with chronic pain? Clin J Pain 9:253–259, 1993.
22. Hafjistavropoulos HD, Craig KD: Acute and chronic low back pain: cognitive, affective, and behavioral dimensions. J Consult Clin Psychol 62:341–349, 1994.
23. Herr KA, Mobily PR, Smith, C: Depression and the experience of chronic back pain: a study of related variables and age differences. Clin J Pain 9:104–114, 1993.
24. Herr KA, Mobily PR: Geriatric mental health: chronic pain and depression. J Psychosoc Nurs 30(9):7–12, 1992.
25. Smith TW, O'Keefe JL, Christensen AJ: Cognitive distortion and depression in chronic pain: association with diagnosed disorders. J Consult Clin Psychol 62:195–198, 1994.
26. Jeffrey JE, Nielson W, McCain GA: Cognitive factors as mediators between disease activity and adjustment to rheumatic disease: comparison of rheumatoid arthritis and fibromyalgia. Unpublished research report, 1993.
27. Holzberg AD, Robinson ME, Geisser ME: The relationship of cognitive distortion to depression in chronic pain: the role of ambiguity and desirability in self-rating. Clin J Pain 9:202–206, 1993.
28. Gaston-Johansson F, Gustafsson M, Felldin R, Sanne H: A comparative study of feelings, attitudes, and behaviors of patients with fibromyalgia and rheumatoid arthritis. Soc Sci Med 31: 941–947, 1990.
29. Davis GC: Measurement of the chronic pain experience: development of an instrument. Res Nurs Health 12:221–227, 1989.
30. Wells N: Perceived control over pain: relation to distress and disability. Res Nurs Health 17: 295–302, 1994.
31. Toomey TC, Mann JD, Abashian SW, Carnrike CLM, Hernandez JT: Pain locus of control scores in chronic pain patients and medical clinical patients with and without pain. Clin J Pain 9:242–247, 1993.
32. Bates MS, Edwards WT, Anderson KO: Ethno-cultural influences on variation in chronic pain perception. Pain 52:101–112, 1993.
33. Cutler RB, Fishbain DA, Rosomoff RS, Rosomoff HL: Outcomes in treatment of pain in geriatric and younger age groups. Arch Phys Med Rehabil 75:457–464, 1994.
34. Sorkin BA, Rudy TE, Hanlon RB, Turk DC, Steig RL: Chronic pain in old and young patients: dif-

ferences appear less important than similarities. J Gerontol 45:64–68, 1990.

35. Boissevain MD, McCain GA: Toward an integrated understanding of fibromyalgia syndrome. I. Medical and pathophysiological aspects. Pain 45:227–238, 1991.

36. Anch AM, Lue FA, MacLean AW, Moldofsky H: Sleep physiology and psychological aspects of the fibrositis (fibromyalgia) syndrome. Can J Psychol 45:179–184, 1991.

37. Parsons T: The sick role: definitions of health and illness in the light of American values and social structure. In: Jaco EG, ed. Patients, physicians, and illness. New York: The Free Press, 1979:120–144.

38. Strauss AL, Corbin J, Fagerhaugh S, Glaser BG, Maines D, Suczek B, Wiener C: Chronic illness and the quality of life. St. Louis: Mosby, 1984.

39. Schwartz L, Slater MA: The impact of chronic pain on the spouse: research and clinical implications. Holistic Nurs Pract 6(1):9–16, 1991.

40. Snelling J: The role of the family in relation to chronic pain: review of the literature. J Adv Nurs 15:771–776, 1990.

41. Schwartz L, Slater MA, Birchler GR, Atkinson JH: Depression in spouses of chronic pain patients: the role of patient pain and anger, and marital satisfaction. Pain 44:61–67, 1991.

42. Flor H, Turk DC, Scholz OB: The impact of chronic pain on the spouse: marital, emotional, and physical consequences. J Psychosom Med 31:63–71, 1987.

43. Ahern KD, Adamns AE, Follick MJ: Emotional and marital disturbance in spouse of chronic low back pain patients. Clin J Pain 1:69–74, 1985.

44. Subramanian K: The multidimensional impact of chronic pain on the spouse: a pilot study. Social Work in Health Care 15(3):47–52, 1991.

45. Sullivan MD, Turner JA, Romano J: Chronic pain in primary care: identification and management of psychosocial factors. J Fam Pract 32:193–198, 1991.

46. Snelling J: The effect of chronic pain on the family unit. J Adv Nurs 19:543–551, 1994.

47. Melzack R: Pain: past, present, and future. Can J Exp Psychol 47:615–629, 1993.

48. Deyo RA, Tsui-Wu YJ: Functional disability due to back pain. Arthritis Rheum 30:1247–1253, 1987.

49. Julkunen J, Hurri H, Kankainen J: Psychological factors in the treatment of chronic low back pain. Psychother Psychosom 50:173–181, 1988.

50. Hawley DJ, Wolfe F: Pain, disability, and pain/disability relationships in seven rheumatic disorders: a study of 1522 patients. J Rheumatol 18:1552–1557, 1991.

51. Spencer B: Fibromyalgia: fighting back. Toronto: LRH Publications, 1992.

52. Hart FD, Taylor RT, Huskisson EC: Pain at night. Lancet 1(7652):881–884, 1970.

53. Henriksson C, Gundmark I, Bengtsson A, Ek A: Living with fibromyalgia: consequences for everyday life. Clin J Pain 8:138–144, 1992.

54. Howell SL: Natural/alternative health care practices used by women with chronic pain: findings from a grounded theory research study. Nurse Practitioner Forum 5(2):98–105, 1994.

55. Goldenberg DL: An overview of psychologic studies in fibromyalgia. J Rheumatol 16 (Suppl 19):12–14, 1989.

56. Radloff LS: The CES-D scale: a self-report depression scale for research in the general population. Appl Psychol Measure 1:385–393, 1977.

57. Turk DC, Okifuji A: Detecting depression in chronic pain patients: adequacy of self-reports. Behav Res Ther 32:6–16, 1994.

58. Hofland SL: Elder beliefs: blocks to pain management. J Gerontol Nurs 18(6):19–24, June 1992.

59. Robbins JM, Kirmayer LJ, Kapusta MA: Illness worry and disability in fibromyalgia syndrome. Int J Psychiatry in Med 20:49–63, 1990.

60. Lusk SL: Low back pain. AAOHN J 41: 450–455, 1993.

61. Parascandola JM: A behavioral approach to determining the prognosis in patients with lumbosacral radiculopathy. Rehabil Nurs 18:314–320, 1993.

62. Gallagher RW, Rauh V, Haugh LD, Milhous R, Callas PW, Langelier R, McClallen JM, Frymoyer J: Determinants of return-to-work among low back pain patients. Pain 39:55–67, 1989.

63. Härkäpää K: Psychological factors as predictors for early retirement in patients with chronic low back pain. J Psychosom Res 36:553–559, 1992.

64. Jensen MP, Turner JA, Romano JM, Karoly P: Coping with chronic pain: a critical review of the literature. Pain 47:249–283, 1991.

65. Chase JA: Outpatient management of low back pain. Orthop Nurs 11(1):11–20, 1992.

66. Dean BZ, Williams FH, King JC, Goddard MJ: Pain rehabilitation. 4. Therapeutic options in pain management. Arch Phys Med Rehabil 75: S21–S30, 1994.

67. Owens MK, Ehrenreich D: Literature review on non-pharmacologic methods of the treatment of chronic pain. Holistic Nurs Pract 6(1):24–31, 1991.

68. Snyder M: Independent nursing interventions. New York: John Wiley & Sons, 1985.

69. Catalano EM: Getting to sleep. Oakland, CA: New Harbinger Publications, 1990.

70. Lacks, P: Behavioral treatment for persistent insomnia. New York: Pergamon Press, 1987.

71. Potts MK, Silverman SL: The importance of aspects of treatment for fibromyalgia (fibrositis): differences between patient and physician views. Arth Care Res 3:11–18, 1990.

72. Smith IW, Airey S, Salmond SW: Nontechnologic strategies for coping with chronic low back pain. Orthop Nurs 9(4):26–34, 1990.

73. Cutler RB, Fishbain DA, Yu Y, Rosomoff RS, Rosomoff HL: Prediction of pain center treatment outcome for geriatric chronic pain patients. Clin J Pain 10:10–17, 1994.

74. Brown B: Stress and the art of biofeedback. New York: Bantam Books, 1977.

75. Nielson WR, Walker C, McCain GA: Cognitive behavioral treatment of fibromyalgia syndrome: preliminary findings. J Rheumatol 19:98–103, 1992.

76. Williams AC, Nicholas MK, Richardson PH, et al.: Evaluation of a cognitive behavioural programme for rehabilitating patients with chronic pain. Br J Gen Pract 43:513–518, 1993.

77. Turner JA, Clancy S, McQuade KJ, Cardenas DD: Effectiveness of behavioral therapy for chronic low back pain: a component analysis. J Consult Clin Psychol 58:573–579, 1990.

78. Jensen IB, Nygren A, Lundin A: Cognitive-behavioural treatment for workers with chronic spinal pain: a matched and controlled cohort study in Sweden. Occup Environ Med 51:145–151, 1994.

79. Bradley LA: Cognitive-behavioral therapy for primary fibromyalgia. J Rheumatol 16(Suppl 19):131–136, 1989.

80. Basler HD: Group treatment for pain and discomfort. Patient Educ Counsel 20:167–175, 1993.

81. McKay M, Davis M, Fanning P: Messages: the communication book. Oakland, CA: New Harbinger Publications, 1983 (Chapter ''Expressing'').

82. Sternbach RA: Mastering pain: a twelve-step program for coping with chronic pain. New York: Putnam, 1987.

83. Turk DC, Rudy TE: A cognitive-behavioral perspective on chronic pain: beyond the scalpel and syringe. In: Tollison CD, ed. Handbook of chronic pain management. Baltimore: Williams & Wilkins, 1988:222–236.

84. Richardson IH, Richardson PH, Williams ACC, Featherstone J, Harding VR: The effects of a cognitive-behavioural pain management programme on the quality of work and employment status of severely impaired chronic pain patients. Disability & Rehabil 16:26–34, 1994.

85. Genaidy AM, Karwowksi W, Guo L, Hidalgo J, Garbutt G: Physical training: a tool for increasing work tolerance limits of employees engaged in manual handling tasks. Ergonomics 35:1081–1102, 1992.

86. Shi L: A cost-benefit analysis of a California county's back injury prevention program. Publ Health Rep 108:204–221, 1993.

87. Varslott JM, Orozemann A, van Son AM, van Akkerveeken PF: The cost-effectiveness of a back school program in industry: a longitudinal controlled field study. Spine 17:22–27, 1992.

88. Hellsing AL, Linton SL, Kaivemark M: A prospective study of patients with acute back and neck pain in Sweden. Phys Ther 74:116–128, 1994.

89. Barnes D, Smith, D, Gatchel RJ, Mayer TG: Psychosocioeconomic predictors of treatment success/failure in chronic low-back pain patients. Spine 14:427–430, 1989.

THE RHEUMATOLOGIC HISTORY AND PHYSICAL EXAMINATION

The art of the rheumatologic history and physical examination is so important to cost-effective medical care that this review of the processes involved, though brief, is provided. All skilled practitioners develop personal methods of history-taking that work well for them. We assume that our readers come from a variety of health care professions with individual approaches and hope that this review will address some of their specific interests.

Differential Diagnosis of Rheumatic Disease

First, decide whether the presenting problem is regional or systemic, inflammatory or noninflammatory, or a combination of these categories. Is the presenting problem a component of a more systemic disorder? Inflammatory disorders should be suspected when joints appear red, hot, or swollen or if the patient reports morning stiffness or gelling in the joints of more than 30 minutes' duration. Fever, weight loss, and fatigue also indicate systemic disorders. Table A.1 lists the important features that distinguish noninflammatory from inflammatory rheumatic disease.

When the disorder appears to be inflammatory, a differential diagnosis may be based upon the number of joints involved. Table A.2 summarizes the major diagnostic considerations if the presentation is a single swollen joint (monarticular), which at times is the most difficult task for a rheumatologist. Table A.3 summarizes the differential diagnosis if the presentation consists of four or fewer swollen joints (pauciarticular onset), often occuring in an asymmetric pattern. Table A.4 summarizes the differential diagnosis when onset consists of a mostly symmetrical polyarthritis affecting more than four joints (hands and feet are considered as one joint each for counting purposes).

Noninflammatory rheumatic diseases include osteoarthritis (osteoarthrosis), osteoporosis, and nonarticular rheumatism. Nonarticular soft tissue rheumatic disorders include myofascial pain, bursitis and tendinitis, structural disorders, nerve entrapment disorders, and the generalized disorders including fibromyalgia and the hypermobility syndrome. Table A.1 summarizes the features that distinguish these from the inflammatory or systemic rheumatic diseases.

Osteoarthritis is often a coincidental accompaniment to a nonarticular rheumatic pain disorder. Whereas osteoarthritis would cause pain during use or weightbearing, a superimposed nonarticular disorder such as bursitis would cause pain both during movement and at rest. Pain after rest that is worse than pain during

TABLE A.1 FEATURES OF INFLAMMATORY AND NONINFLAMMATORY RHEUMATIC DISORDERS

Inflammatory Rheumatic Diseases	Noninflammatory Disorders
Pain during movement	Pain after rest
Palpable joint swelling	Swelling is sensation only
Abnormal laboratory test results	All laboratory tests normal
Aggravating factors possible	Aggravating factors likely
Diagnosis based on clinical examination and test results	Diagnosis based on physical examination maneuvers and outcome

From Sheon RP: Nonarticular rheumatism and nerve entrapment disorders. Resident and Staff Physician 35(12):65–70, 1989.

TABLE A.2 DIFFERENTIAL DIAGNOSIS OF MONOARTICULAR ARTHRITIS

Noninflammatory	Inflammatory	Infectious
Trauma/osteoarthritis	Rheumatoid monoarthritis	Acute (bacterial, viral)
Internal derangements	Gout/pseudogout	Chronic (tuberculosis, fungal)
Osteonecrosis	Juvenile monoarthritis	AIDS-associated
Reflex sympathetic dystrophy	Spondyloarthropathy	
Hemarthrosis		
Neuropathic/Charcot		
arthropathy		
Paget's disease		
Joint tumors		
Pigmented villonodular synovitis		

TABLE A.3 DIFFERENTIAL DIAGNOSIS OF PAUCIARTICULAR POLYARTHRITIS (FOUR OR FEWER JOINTS)

Spondyloarthropathies (HLA-B27 positive)
Reactive Arthritis
    Reiter's syndrome
    Psoriatic arthritis
    Acute rheumatic fever
    Enteric arthropathies
Metabolic and crystal-induced arthropathies
Paraneoplastic syndromes
Septic arthritis
    AIDS-related arthritis
    Parvovirus
    Lyme disease arthritis
Seronegative rheumatoid arthritis

movement is likely to be due to an extraarticular soft tissue disorder.

Syndrome Analysis: The Rheumatic History and Physical Examination

Most connective tissue diseases lack any single diagnostic feature. The examiner must know the elements of each disease or syndrome and elicit those features during the examination. The history-taking will vary with the mode of presentation and age of the patient, but should quickly assess critical features that may suggest serious underlying disease requiring prompt workup. Table A.5 presents a list of critical features for rheumatic disease, and Table A.6 provides a checklist for features important in a rheumatic history and physical examination. Look for critical features early and quickly.

For example, when the patient reports swelling, is the swelling visible/measurable or only a sensation? The timing, duration, and location of stiffness or gelling will help to differentiate inflammatory disease from noninflammatory disease or gout. Gout seldom causes stiffness.

Make certain that stiffness is in true joint areas, not "all over," and not episodic. Inflammatory rheumatic disease often begins with prolonged morning stiffness that occurs daily and in true joint locations. The stiffness of osteoarthritis often occurs in involved joints after periods of inactivity such as sitting in one position. However, fibromyalgia and Parkinson's disease can cause "all over" stiffness after inactivity.

Constitutional features of fever, chills, sweats, weight loss, and decreased endurance indicate urgent diagnosis and treatment. Chills are rarely present in connective tissue diseases unless there is accompanying infection.

Weakness is a common complaint but must be objectively quantified and distinguished from fatigue. Is there specific muscle weakness or generalized loss of strength? Can the patient arise unassisted from a chair, lift the head from bed, raise the arms above the head, and arise from a squat position? Does the weakness vary according to time of day? What functions of daily living are affected?

Attributes of pain, as determined by history, can follow the PQRST questioning:

Provocative factors: head position, coughing, straining, emotion

Quality: burning, aching, throbbing, continuous, superficial

Region: location of pain

Severity: on a scale from none to terrible

Timing: duration and periodicity

If the onset of the problem followed trauma, elicit information regarding the extent and nature of the trauma (e.g., whether the car was totalled, or if the patient was physically assaulted), presence of abrasions, lacerations, or fractures at the time of injury, and availability of radiographs. Is litigation pending? Has

TABLE A.4 DIFFERENTIAL DIAGNOSIS OF POLYARTICULAR ARTHRITIS (SIX OR MORE JOINTS)

Rheumatoid Diseases	*Hematologic*	*Infectious*
Seronegative RA	Leukemia	Endocarditis
Seropositive RA	Hemochromatosis	Lyme disease
Sjögren's syndrome	*Metabolic*	Parvovirus B 19
Felty's syndrome	Polyarticular gout	Rocky Mountain spotted fever
Other Connective Tissue	Pseudogout	*Miscellaneous*
Diseases	Dialysis arthropathy	Serum sickness
Systemic lupus erythematosus		Henoch-Schönlein purpura
Mixed connective tissue		Enteric arthropathy
disease		Paraneoplastic syndrome
Adult Still's disease		Sarcoidosis
Reactive Arthritis		
Acute rheumatic fever		
Reiter's syndrome		
Psoriatic arthritis		
Spondylarthritis		

TABLE A.5 CRITICAL FEATURES FOR RHEUMATIC DISEASES

Fever, chills, sweats
Weight loss
Pain localized to a single site, and worsening
Skin color change
Bruits or diminished pulse
Asymmetric weakness
Neurologic deficit

Potentially Serious Findings

Lymphadenopathy
Raynaud's phenomenon
Joint swelling and tenderness
Limitation of spinal or joint movement
Any unexplained laboratory abnormality

the patient been able to perform the usual daily routine at work or at home? Specify the disabilities (e.g., cannot dress, grasp, climb). Had the patient suffered prior injuries as well?

To determine how the patient has been affected by the condition, include a *misery index*:

"If you were so bad that you could not get out of bed, and if that is like being in the bottom of a pit; and being restored to perfect is like being out of the pit; and if there are 100 steps down into the bottom of the pit, with step number one being terrible, where is your level of misery this week?" This version of a pain scale can discriminate irrational pain concern or alert you to search more closely for evidence of critical disease. A visual pain scale can also be helpful. (See Table I.5.)

It is not rare for patients to have overlapping features, such as the pain of a nonarticular rheumatic disorder laid upon an inflammatory rheumatic disease or osteoarthritis.

Physical Examination

Physical examination should be done with the patient's spine and extremities exposed. You may wish to advise females to bring shorts and a halter to the initial visit.

Begin with assessment of static and dynamic posture and alignment. Look for structural abnormalities and asymmetries. Facial asymmetry (see Figure I.2) can suggest temporomandibular joint pain and dysfunction with resulting neck pain and headache; or it may be associated with other skeletal deformities such as a short leg and scoliosis. Observe the patient arising from a chair; have patient walk away and then toward you; note gait, leg alignment or torsion, and balance and trunk/spine mobility. Measure true leg length from the anterior superior iliac spine to the medial malleolus at the ankle.

Palpate for joint tenderness and swelling. Swelling can be determined by palpating small joints with the examiner's two index fingers used at the sides of the joint. Is the synovium normal, palpable, or boggy thick (like soft dough)? Always examine the feet; sometimes they are deformed by a previous unrecognized attack of rheumatoid arthritis. Assess the feet for signs of abnormal weightbearing and other deformities.

Trigger points and tender points should be searched for when pain and symptoms occur beyond the joint boundary. Refer to Anatomic

TABLE A.6 HISTORY AND PHYSICAL EXAMINATION CHECKLIST

HISTORY

Current Illness:	Onset, pattern of spread Swelling: duration, timing; is swelling visible? *Chills, fever, rash *Weight loss/gain? Stiffness: duration, location Results of medications tried	*Review of Systems:*	Skin rashes; psoriasis Raynaud's phenomenon Sun sensitivity & rash *Alopecia Jaw/fist clenching Headache, convulsions *Jaw claudication Depression, stressful event
Family History:	Inflammatory bowel diseases Other rheumatic diseases Migraine headaches Joint laxity		Dryness of eyes and mouth Stomatitis *Pleuropericarditis Dyspnea, cough, wheeze

Social:	Stairs at home; location of
	   bathrooms
	Activity level: managing
	   daily activities, work,
	   recreation
	Tick exposure
	Smoking/drinking
			*Edema, discoloration of
			   limbs
			Dysphagia, acid reflux
			Liver diseases, peptic
			   ulcers
			Change in bowel habit
			Kidney stones, hematuria

Past History:	Allergies/operations Current medical diseases Past medical diseases		Dysuria, frequency Nocturia, balanitis Genital discharge Cervicitis
Current Rx:	Prescription and nonprescription drugs		Paresthesias, weakness

PHYSICAL FINDINGS

General:	Vital signs
	Appearance, movement
	Body symmetry, limb length
	Flexibility, strength
			Pulses; range of motion,
			   active and passive;
			   muscle symmetry

Skin:	Hair loss; rashes, psoriasis
	*Nailfold infarctions; leg
	   ulcers
		Joints:	Crepitus, tenderness,
			   deformity
			Synovitis: bogginess
			Joint effusions

HEENT:	Temporal arteries palpable?
	Conjunctiva, mucous
	   membranes
	Dentition, fundoscopy
		Spine:	Periarticular tenderness/
			   inflammation
			Appearance, bending and
			   extending effect on pain

Neck:	Thyroid abnormalities; pulses, bruits	*Neurologic:*	Appearance, reflexes Pathologic reflexes Gait, ability to arise
Cardiac/ pulmonary:	Rubs, murmurs, wheezes Chest expanse		unassisted
Abdomen:	Organs, masses, bruit	*Function:*	Rise from chair, arms over head, put on coat,

Extremities:	Deformity, color,
	   temperature
			grasp, write, button,
			   unbutton, feed self, drink

*May be a critical finding.

Plates XIV and XV for common trigger point locations, and refer to Chapter 7 for the pattern of tender points in fibromyalgia. Palpation should approximate 4 kg pressure or enough pressure to induce blanching of the palpating finger's nail bed. You can use the anterior thigh and the styloid process as control points. Palpation of the trigger point will often reproduce the distant pain and paresthesia. Palpation of tender points will elicit expressions of pain from the patient.

Assessment of the range of joint and spinal movement should be part of the examination. More complete general examination will depend upon the history and age at presentation.

The examination should be completed with the neurologic examination, principally noting motor nerve function. A pelvic or rectal examination is performed depending upon the age and presentation. Figure 8.1 may be used to record findings.

SUGGESTED READING

1. Sheon RP: Rheumatic disorders. In: Kahn MG, ed. Medical diagnosis and therapy. Philadelphia: Lea & Febiger, 1994 (Chapter 30).

2. Shmerling RH, Fuchs HA, Lorish CD, et al.: Guidelines for the initial evaluation of the adult patient with acute musculoskeletal symptoms. Arthritis Rheum 39, 1996, in press.

APPENDIX B: Joint Protection Guide for Rheumatic Disorders

ROBERT P. SHEON AND PATTY M. ORR

Joint protection should be introduced to every patient with a musculoskeletal disorder in order to prevent recurrent sprains and strains added to inflammation and degeneration (1). Conservative care includes preventive care, and joint protection is a fundamental way to provide preventive joint care.

It is recognized in the joint protection guide that we participate in a wide variety of activities today and are not limited by age or sex. Octogenarians are playing tennis, women now participate in virtually all manual labor activities, and everyone works at maintaining their strength and endurance as well as maintaining their property (cleaning, mowing, gardening, and so on). Thus our joints are going through more varied activity than ever before, and joint protection has become increasingly important.

Joint protection has the following aims:
- To prevent disability
- To enhance performance
- To supplement function with adaptive aids, and when necessary, to learn to perform tasks in different ways

The principles of joint protection are:
1. To respect pain (signals patient to moderate or avoid activity)
2. To balance work and rest
3. To maintain strength and range of motion
4. To reduce musculoskeletal effort
5. To simplify work
6. To avoid positions inducing deformity
7. To use stronger, larger joints whenever possible
8. To avoid staying in one position for too long

These are derived from the simple, practical application of proper body mechanics, posture, and positioning of joints. Joint protection reduces local joint stress and preserves joint integrity.

Aggravating factors are those habits and activities that can initiate and/or perpetuate soft tissue rheumatic pain and disability. Whenever pain persists beyond the expected duration for a given problem such as bursitis or tendinitis, the clinician should consider a perpetuating aggravating factor as detailed in the Joint Protection Guide. Delving into the patient's routine at work, at home, and in sports is the starting point. Personality assessment may also be important. The patient who is a compulsive worker with the attitude, "I'm going to finish this job if it kills me," must learn to respect the pain signals, to recognize potentially self-destructive behavior, and to let reason prevail. Telling a patient not to do a task may not be as helpful as guiding the patient to perform the task in a manner that puts less stress on joints.

The joint protection guide is provided as an aid for identifying aggravating factors and applicable corrective measures.

Joint Protection Guide for Rheumatic Disorders

GENERAL MEASURES

Use each joint in its most stable anatomical and functional plane.

Prevent rotational forces that stretch joint ligaments excessively.

Maintain good posture and alignment.

Stop a task if it causes pain.

Arrange rest breaks to interrupt repetitive tasks. Alternate repetitive hand movements from one hand to the other.

Perform stretching exercises between tasks.

Alternate sitting and standing positions.

Exercise at midday, when possible, or right after work.

Alternate heavy jobs with lighter jobs.

Carry heavy objects with the weight distributed over many of the strongest joints and the largest muscle groups.

Push rather than pull an object in order to move it. Use the hips and larger joints when pushing.

Perform strengthening exercises when work requires increased strength.

Adjust the work station to fit your task. For example, the height of a work surface can be changed with an adjustable chair.

Desks that provide adjustable levels are ideal. The desk should be at a height that supports the elbows next to the body. Use a gas lift or easily height-adjustable chair. Extensive reading and writing should be done at an angle with a tilted desk top.

Maximize control of the work environment to minimize emotional stress.

Maintain ideal body weight without excess fat.

Avoid high risk behavior.

When injuries occur, apply RICE techniques:
Rest the injury
Ice initial stages of inflammation
Compression bandage
Elevate the injured limb

Injuries are more likely if muscles are fatigued; avoid strenuous activity when fatigued.

Build tolerance and strength by gradually increasing duration and intensity of training. Use a qualified trainer.

Detect malalignment in the young athlete with a preparticipation evaluation.

Design training programs for youths according to skeletal maturity and degree of conditioning and preparedness.

Adult training is necessary for fitness and flexibility, including aerobic and strengthening exercises.

Use a warm-up routine before playing sports that includes neck, trunk, upper limb, hamstring, groin, and Achilles stretching.

Prevent imbalances of muscle strength by careful training.

Always use the proper equipment and safety gear for a particular sport.

Prevent repetitive overactivity; stop or switch to another activity.

Avoid contact sports that have repetitive impulsive loading such as ice hockey and football if risk behavior has been prevalent.

Head and Neck

GENERAL

Avoid sitting or standing for more than 30 minutes. It can induce more neck strain than lifting heavy objects.

Take frequent breaks during tasks in which the body does not move (e.g., knitting). Include tasks that allow the body greater movement (e.g., sweeping).

Align the head, neck, and trunk during rest and activities.

Avoid stressful head positions (e.g., lying on a sofa with the head propped up; falling asleep in a chair and allowing the head to drop forward; using more than one thin pillow).

Align the entire trunk, chest, and head on a slanted wedge or a very large pillow if you must watch television or read in a reclining position.

If required to sleep with the head high, elevate the entire mattress or the head of the bed.

Sleep on the side or the back, keeping the arms below chest level.

Clenching the jaw can cause muscle spasms in the neck; use relaxation techniques or a bite spacer.

Store heavy items that are used daily no higher than shoulder height and no lower than knee height.

Use a step stool when lifting heavy items from shelves higher than the shoulders.

Avoid the "birdwatcher's neck" (jutting the head forward as if watching birds through field glasses) (also called video display terminal or VDT neck).

Be conscious of stressful head positions when concentrating, when driving, or when tense.

Use headsets or a speaker phone for prolonged or frequent telephone calls.

Place a computer screen at eye level and use a ''draft holder'' to place work at eye level next to the screen.

Use an adjustable chair and vary the height of the seat frequently during prolonged sitting.

Maintain the proper hand-to-eye work or reading distance of 16 inches.

Position the body and work materials in such a way that the neck remains straight during activities.

SPORTS

Use plastic goggles or eyeglasses with plastic lenses.

Wear a safety helmet when cycling.

Vary swim strokes and head position during swimming and water exercise. When diving, be certain that pools are of proper depth.

Shoulder

Prevent cumulative movement disorders by frequently interrupting repetitive tasks such as washing windows, vacuuming, and working on an assembly line. Keep the elbow close to the body. Change the angle of shoulder motion when possible.

Sleep with the arms below the level of the chest.

If using crutches, adjust them properly to 2 inches (about 5 cm) below axillae; carry weight on ribs and hands, not under the arms. A forearm cane may be preferred.

Rise from a chair by pushing off with thigh muscles, not the hands.

Take frequent breaks when working with the arms overhead.

To grasp an object at your side or that is behind you, turn your body and face the object.

To reach a car seat belt, use the far arm and hand across the front of the body.

A swivel or wheeled chair may be useful when tasks done from a seated position are in various locations.

When driving, keep the hands below the 3 o'clock and 9 o'clock positions on the wheel. If possible, use a steering wheel that tilts.

SPORTS

Swimming: Strengthen and maintain shoulder muscles with proper exercises.

Tennis: Learn proper overhead and stroke technique.

Avoid tendinitis and impingement. Respect pain; avoid overuse; use frequent rest breaks. Relax your grip between strokes.

Maintain shoulder strength through exercise; be aware of proper posture and positioning of joints.

Cycling: Avoid falling onto an outstretched arm; learn to fall by pulling your arm in and rolling onto your shoulder.

Golf: To avoid golf shoulder injuries, perform conditioning exercises year-round. Learn proper swing and impact.

Elbow/Forearm

Avoid pressure and impact to the elbow.

When sitting, do not contact any firm surface with the elbow.

In moving out of bed, use the abdominal muscles to help roll over.

When changing body position, do not push off with the elbow against a hard surface.

Use elbow pads for protection.

Use relaxation techniques focused on the hands and arms to protect the forearm muscles.

Recognize and avoid repetitive hand clenching or excessively hard gripping. For nocturnal hand clenching, wear stretch gloves with the seams to the outside.

Avoid forced gripping or twisting.

Use kitchen aids such as jar openers, enlarged grips on utensils, or power tools.

Take periodic breaks and alternate tasks during manual activities.

Use a light and two-handed grip when shaking hands repeatedly.

Avoid prolonged use of tools requiring twist/force motions.

Hold tools with a relaxed grip. Use foam/plastic pipe insulation (sold at hardware stores) on tool handles.

Take frequent short breaks.

Do not lean directly on elbows; stabilize with the forearms.

Change to a better work position or use elbow pads.

SPORTS

Use proper grip and play techniques with golf clubs, racquets, bats, or other pieces of sports equipment. For grip problems, consult a pro.

Use elbow protective equipment (hockey, roller-blading, skating).

Use stretch, strengthening, and relaxation exercises to condition the tissues that surround the elbow.

Hand/Wrist

Avoid cumulative movement patterns.

Interrupt repetitive tasks (e.g., typing, peeling vegetables, knitting, playing cards) by short breaks.

Rest the hands flat and open rather than tight-fisted.

Pad the handles on utensils, tools, and the steering wheel with pipe insulation.

Use the stronger, larger joints, especially the shoulders.

Use the palms and forearms to carry heavy objects.

Push, slide, or roll objects instead of lifting them.

Use pencil grips and pad the stapler.

Keep the hands off chairs when arising.

Be aware of hand clenching and wear stretch gloves to bed when nocturnal hand clenching is recognized.

Interrupt lengthy writing sessions by stopping for 1 to 2 minutes every 10 minutes.

Use relaxed grip on tools.

Enlarge the handles of work tools—2¼-inch diameter is optimum for most people.

Texturize handle surfaces to provide an easy hold with less grip.

Bend and straighten (wiggle) your fingers and wrist often.

Wear stretch gloves while driving and at night if hand clenching is a habit.

Grasp objects with the hand and all fingers. Use both hands as much as possible when lifting heavy objects.

Use real tools, not the thumbs, to pinch and push in your daily job activities. Use pliers for hard-to-remove velcro fasteners.

Power tools (screwdriver, drill) are often preferable and easier to use than manual tools.

Avoid uncomfortable hand positions.

Keep hand and wrist extended for work activities. Adapt tools with handles designed so that the wrist is straight.

Use a wrist rest while working on a keyboard.

Use an appropriate tool to hit or move objects.

Fit the handles of vibrating tools with shock absorbers or rubber, or wear gloves with gel inserts.

If joints are painful, wear an appropriate splint for rest and activity.

Consult an occupational therapist about work-induced problems, splinting, and modifying or adapting tools and equipment.

SPORTS

For racquet sports or golf, use proper grip size. Relax the grip until just before ball impact.

For grip problems, consult a pro.

Use proper grip and play techniques with golf clubs, racquets, and other sports equipment.

Use a bowling ball with five finger holes. Bevel edges of the finger holes.

Golfers with arthritis should try using cushion grips and the baseball grip style (no interlocking fingers).

Chest

Posture: practice good body alignment, especially during reading, writing, keyboarding, and sewing. The head, neck, and shoulders should be supported by the trunk and in line with it.

Use good breathing patterns to maintain chest wall flexibility.

Smoking-induced cough aggravates chest wall pain. *STOP SMOKING.*

Sleeping with the arms overhead can pinch nerves, thus causing chest wall pain. Sleep with the arms below chest level, not overhead.

When working with the arms overhead (e.g., painting a ceiling), place the body strategically so as to work upward and forward. Perform shoulder strengthening and spine extension exercises.

SPORTS

Improper weight lifting techniques can cause chest wall muscle strain. Use supervised conditioning and warm-up procedures.

Use appropriate protective equipment during sports activities.

Low Back

Strengthen and use the abdominal muscles that support the back.

Attain and maintain ideal weight.

Avoid prolonged periods of sitting or standing.

Wear supportive cushion-soled shoes when standing or walking on concrete surfaces.

Use proper rest and sleep positions.

Perform trunk and hamstring flexibility exercises regularly.

To release a "locked back," lie on the back and elevate the legs to the 90/90 position (see Exercise 5.A). Rest the lower legs on a chair or piano stool.

Turn the body while moving the feet in alignment so that the toes point in the direction you are facing.

To move objects at your side, rotate the entire body by moving the feet.

To lift large or heavy objects, move the object to the chest, lift it with the arms, and use the thigh muscles for strength. Hold the object close and centered in front of you.

When lifting children or pets, be prepared for sudden shifts of weight. Do not carry a child on your side. Carry the child Indian or Oriental style on your back, or use a front or back harness pack.

For a sore "tailbone," protect the point of tenderness at the tip of the coccyx. Sit on a foam cushion 3 inches thick and the size of the seat cushion. Cut a 3-inch circle out of the cushion center for pressure relief. Place the cushion under the tailbone whenever seated or doing exercises on the floor.

Sleep side-lying with the legs slightly bent and a pillow between the knees, or back-lying with the knees and feet elevated with a cushion or pillow.

Do not sleep on the stomach. Place a tennis ball in a pocket sewn onto the front of a tee shirt so that the pressure will awaken you if you roll onto the stomach.

A leg length discrepancy more than 0.5 inches may be the cause of back pain. Try a corrective insert to raise the shorter leg, and determine if pain is improved.

Avoid prolonged sitting. Use active sitting techniques such as "wiggling the pelvis" and rocking to activate and relax the pelvic muscles.

Break up seated tasks like desk work and card games by standing and moving around for 2 minutes every 15 minutes or so.

Use cruise control when driving long distances.

Do not carry a large wallet in a back pocket. Check for pressure placed on the pelvic bones by a wallet, tight belt, or constricting jeans that can squeeze nerves in the pelvis or groin.

Always bend at the knees, not at the waist.

When lifting an object, bend the knees, keeping the back straight. Use the palms of both hands or the forearm, rather than one hand to pick up and carry an object.

Do a regular strengthening and lengthening program for abdominal and back muscles.

Use a step stool to reach overhead objects.

When standing for prolonged periods, place one foot on a higher surface (stool, brick, phone book) for a while and then alternate.

SPORTS

Do trunk stretching and leg stretching warm-up exercises before the sport activity.

Knee

Strengthen the thigh muscles (quadriceps/hamstrings) to protect the knee.

If stair climbing causes or increases knee pain, limit the activity and strengthen the thigh muscles until the pain subsides.

Knee pain can be caused by foot disorders: evaluate the entire lower leg when investigating knee pain.

Avoid deep knee bending—use reacher tools for assistance.

During prolonged sitting, straighten the knees or stand up at least every 30 minutes to relieve pressure and stretch tight muscles.

Short, brisk walks will increase leg circulation and exercise muscles.

Buy shoes with proper heels and check them often for signs of wear.

Use the thigh muscles to rise from a chair—it provides good exercise.

Use a mechanic's or milker's stool when working on the floor or on the ground. Sit with the legs apart and reach forward to perform tasks such as gardening or scrubbing floors.

If you must work on hands and knees, use protective knee pads.

Consider raised or container gardening to reduce stress and effort.

Stationary biking provides safe, low-impact exercise. Adjust the seat height so that the knees are slightly bent at the low point of the down-stroke and no more than 90 degrees flexed on the up-stroke. Increase resistance gradually.

Perform a regular stretching program for the muscles of the upper and lower leg.

Tight muscles can contribute to knee problems.

SPORTS

Treat knee injuries promptly with RICE techniques. If pain and instability persist, seek medical attention.

Adjust bicycle seats as described above.

Engage in exercise and sports activities on a regular basis rather than occasional weekend participation. Include warm-up and cool-down activities as well as appropriate stretching in your routine.

Modify or avoid knee-twisting dance steps or exercises.

Ankle and Foot

Choose footwear with comfort, support, and utility in mind.

Do not wear shoes that cause pain or fatigue. Get professional advice when necessary.

Loose-jointed persons should be especially careful to protect the ankles and feet. Sprains and strains can increase instability.

Orthoses can provide needed support and positioning assistance. Consult an experienced professional regarding the choice of an orthosis, whether having it custom-made or obtaining it over-the-counter.

Maintain appropriate weight to reduce stress on feet and ankles.

Running shoes, walking shoes, or aerobics shoes are more supportive and comfortable to the flexible or arthritic foot.

Use a metatarsal pad or bar to relieve pressure or pain at the forefoot.

If you must stand or walk on concrete (even if it is carpeted), select shoes with shock-absorbing soles.

Treat ankle sprains promptly with RICE techniques. Seek medical advice if swelling and pain do not subside.

SPORTS

Use footwear that is especially designed for the sport you are playing.

Run on dirt or track surfaces—avoid running
on concrete or asphalt.

REFERENCES

1. Sheon, RP: A joint protection guide for nonarticular rheumatism. Postgrad Med 77(5):331–337, 1985.
2. Melvin JL: Joint protection and energy conservation. In: Melvin JL, ed. Rheumatic disease in the adult and child: occupational therapy and rehabilitation. 3rd ed. Philadelphia: FA Davis, 1989.
3. Anderson, JA: Arthrosis and its relation to work. Scand J Work Environ Health 10:429–433, 1984.
4. Bergenudd H, Nilsson B: Knee pain in middle age and its relationship to occupational work load and psychosocial factors. Clin Orthop Rel Res 245:210–215, 1989.
5. Dalton SE: Overuse injuries in adolescent athletes. Sports Med 13(1):58–70, 1992.
6. Radin EL: The effects of repetitive loading on cartilage: advice to athletes to protect their joints. Acta Orthop Belg 49:225–232, 1989.
7. Isani A: Prevention and treatment of ligamentous sports injuries to the hand. Sports Med 9(1):48–61, 1990.
8. Martis B: Health effects of recreational running in women. Sports Med 11(1):20–51, 1991.
9. Sheon RP: Peripheral nerve entrapment, occupation-related syndromes, and sports injuries. Current Science 4:219–225, 1992.

APPENDIX C: Intralesional Soft Tissue Injection

INTRALESIONAL SOFT TISSUE INJECTION RATIONALE

Over two decades of experience in the use of local anesthetics or corticosteroid suspensions for soft tissue injection have established both its safety and its effectiveness in therapy (1). Orthopaedists, who for many years feared the injurious effects of the steroid on tendon strength, now increasingly accept this form of therapy (2). In one survey of 233 orthopaedists in 1989, 96% were found to use intralesional injections (3). Long-term follow-up of corticosteroid injections for tenosynovitis has conclusively shown it to be safe (4, 5). Corticosteroid and/or local anesthetic injections at intervals of 6 to 12 weeks into myofascial pain (trigger) points (over a 10-year period) were not found to be associated with any long-term deleterious effects (6).

Very few blinded, placebo-controlled studies of this treatment have been conducted, and these tend to suffer from too few subjects, from design problems, or a lack of objective outcome parameters. When the subject of injections of fibromyalgia points was raised at a forum in San Francisco in 1989, some of the participants suggested that corticosteroid and local anesthetic intralesional injections were of no value. Others in attendance thought otherwise, with many claims of significant benefit. In our experience, two-thirds of our patients have significant benefit, with less tightness and pain, and are more likely to perform and benefit from aerobic exercise. Also, for those patients who do respond, future immobilizing flare-ups can be quickly restored to self-control maintenance with an injection and at small cost.

Throughout the chapters in this text, mostly anecdotal reports are referenced. For the past decade, we have tried to design a random study with placebo control for regional pain disorders but have not yet been able to develop satisfactory objective criteria for diagnosis or outcome. We encourage others to try!

Namba et al. investigated the deleterious effect of intraarticular corticosteroid (triamcinolone) in ankle joints of rabbits after distal tibial fractures; no effect on tibial torsion strength was found, but stiffness was reduced 66%, suggesting that steroid injections probably do not detract from positive outcome following fracture (7).

In this era of concern for cost containment, soft tissue injection is recognized for its value in reducing the need for more complex, prolonged medical measures and for surgical intervention (8–10).

The use of intralesional corticosteroids and local anesthetic agents for tendinitis and myofascial disorders as well as for nerve entrapment involving the shoulder, elbow, hip, knee, and foot has been widely reported. The importance of careful localization of the site of involvement before injection has been pointed out. A number of studies report superior results with a variety of agents, and none has been found to be superior. Often, the operator's experience and technique are more important to outcome than which agent is used. Failure of benefit has been attributed to a variety of factors including higher levels of perceived pain, prolonged duration, unemployment, lower coping ability, and use of analgesic medications (11).

Local injection for myofascial pain is preferred by many nonphysiatrists, whereas physiatrists tend to utilize physical therapy modalities. Interestingly, trigger points and acupuncture points are at similar locations (12). The controversy surrounding trigger points is discussed in Chapter 1. Cost comparison between various treatment regimens has not been reported. Functional restoration often occurs promptly when the soft tissue problem is amenable to an intralesional injection.

Fifty years ago, Janel Travell popularized the use of procaine for trigger point injection (13). Dry needling of the points has also been advocated (14, 15) but requires multiple sessions (average is eight treatments) (14). In a study comparing repeated injections of saline solution with injections of mepivacaine hydrochloride for myofascial pain, more pain relief occurred after the first injection in the saline solution group. The subsequent injections resulted in similar pain relief with either saline or mepivacaine, lasting 1.5 to 4.5 hours (16). In another double-blind crossover trial, bupivacaine and etidocaine were found to be superior to saline solution and dry needling (17).

Of interest is Janssens's study of the treatment of lame dogs as a model of myofascial pain disorder, using needling and the injection of trigger points with local anesthetic agents. Despite previous failure with the customary treatment, 34 of 48 dogs recovered with an average of three treatments (18).

INTRALESIONAL SOFT TISSUE INJECTION TECHNIQUE

The technique of soft tissue injection has been presented in each chapter of this text. We recommend combining a corticosteroid with a local anesthetic in most cases. *We do not recommend use of epinephrine.* Some package inserts accompanying the corticosteroid agents suggest that other agents should not be mixed with them; in our experience, untoward reactions have not occurred when local anesthetics are mixed in the same syringe with the corticosteroid suspension. The addition of the local anesthetic has the advantage of providing immediate symptomatic relief as well as of diluting the steroid preparation, allowing a more diffuse distribution of the drug with less hazard of local tissue atrophy. In addition, the methylprednisolone and local anesthetic mixture flocculates in the syringe, providing prolonged local contact before absorption. The total amount of local anesthetic administered to the patient should be kept to less than 6 to 8 mL if possible. Local postinjection pain is alleviated with the application of ice. Tables C.1 and C.2 list local anesthetics and corticosteroids, respectively, in current use.

Studies documenting the safety and efficacy of local soft tissue injections with a crystalline corticosteroid and local anesthetic agent have been reviewed in each chapter of this text. In our experience, a single pain (trigger) point injection using a mixture of a corticosteroid and a short-acting local anesthetic, along with joint protection advice and the other points in management as detailed in this book, will usually eliminate the pain (trigger) point and the pain indefinitely (fibromyalgia excepted). Costly additional physical therapy is rarely needed. At least 80% of our patients respond to this regimen. The hazards and frequency of injection must be considered in each case as well, and are detailed below.

Hollander reported on the safety of local soft tissue and joint injection therapy in over 100,000 injections in 4,000 patients (19). The incidence of infection was less than 1 per 16,000 injections. Others report 3000 or more injections per year (Mayo Clinic) with no untoward reaction (20, 21). In the past 20 years we, too, have performed thousands of soft tissue injections with few complications.

Although *tendon rupture* following local steroid injection may occur, this complication is infrequent if injections are made around the tendon rather than directly into it and if overexertion is avoided for a week or longer. Most research supports the finding that harmful effects of corticosteroids on tendons generally result from use of massive corticosteroid doses (22–25). In one study, rabbits' Achilles tendons were partially transected and then injected with 0.3 mg/kg triamcinolone acetonide at 2, 8, 14, and 20 days, and compared to controls that were injected with equal volumes of normal saline solution. The saline-treated animals had a greater final tendon weight, 66% more adhesions, and superior mechanical properties of failure load, strain, and energy to failure as compared to the steroid-injected animals (24). A more recent study confirmed these observations (23). Thus, repeated administration of local steroids should be performed with caution and in the lowest possible dose for palliation of tendon injuries (24).

In other studies comparing soluble versus relatively insoluble steroid preparations injected into musculotendinous junctions of rabbits, which were then examined up to 30

TABLE C.1 LOCAL ANESTHETICS IN CURRENT USE

Anesthetic Agents	Concentrations Available	Duration of Action (minutes)
Procaine hydrochloride (Novocaine)	1–2 mg/mL	50
Lidocaine hydrochloride (Xylocaine)	10–15–20 mg/mL	100
Chloroprocaine hydrochloride (Nesacaine)	10–20 mg/mL	60
Mepivacaine hydrochloride (Carbocaine, Polocaine)	10–20 mg/mL	100
Bupivacaine hydrochloride (Marcaine, Sensorcaine)	2.5–5 mg/mL	175
Etidocaine hydrochloride (Duranest)	2.5–5–10 mg/mL	200

Modified from Covino BG, Vassallo HG: Local anesthetics: Mechanisms of action and clinical use. New York: Grune & Stratton, 1976.

TABLE C.2 CORTICOSTEROIDS IN CURRENT USE

Corticosteroid	Concentrations Available	Dose Range
Prednisolone tebutate (Hydeltra TBA)	20 mg/mL	5–15 mg
Betamethasone acetate and betamethasone sodium phosphate (Celestone Soluspan)	6 mg/mL	1.5–3 mg
Methylprednisolone acetate (Depo-Medrol)	20–40–80 mg/mL	10–20 mg
Triamcinolone acetonide or diacetate (Aristocort)	10–25–40 mg/mL	5–15 mg
Triamcinolone hexacetonide (Aristospan)	5–20 mg/mL	5–20 mg
Dexamethasone acetate suspension (Decadron-LA)	8 mg/mL	0.8–3.2 mg

days later, findings revealed that the insoluble corticosteroids were associated with more local inflammation and calcium deposits than seen with the soluble steroids; however, when these agents were mixed with lidocaine, no calcium deposits developed (25). When physiologic doses of steroids are injected directly into rabbit tendons, the injury had nearly returned to normal after 2 weeks. Experimental studies of corticosteroid injections into rabbit tendons using usual therapeutic doses revealed disorganization of collagen and a 35% loss of tendon strength; this healed within 14 days. Athletes who receive intralesional steroid injections are therefore urged to rest the involved limb for at least 2 weeks (23).

Corticosteroid injections into the region of the Achilles tendon should never be performed, since tendon rupture at this site is a disastrous complication. Patellar tendon rup-

ture following a corticosteroid injection is a distinct hazard in athletes (26). Bowstring deformity of a digit following corticosteroid injections for flexor tenosynovitis has been described but is rare (27).

The use of local anesthetics without corticosteroids has been advocated by some; however, this requires more frequent injections (28–30) and is less often effective in subacute or chronic disorders. Longer-acting local anesthetic agents, such as bupivacaine and etidocaine, may prove more effective and improve injection technique (31). However, bupivacaine, in particular, is cardiotoxic (32); sudden death has occurred during administration. We have seen one cardiac arrest occur with bupivacaine used for stellate ganglion block. The myotoxicity of bupivacaine, demonstrated by magnetic resonance imaging, was found to persist for up to 10 days (33).

The addition of a corticosteroid suspension to a local anesthetic is recommended for the following reasons:

1. Benefit is often longer-lasting and in most cases one injection suffices.
2. The safety of infrequent injections has been established over time.
3. More frequent injections (generally required when a local anesthetic is used alone) increase the risk of inadvertent intravascular instillation of the anesthetic.
4. The incidence and intensity of reactions to local anesthetics are proportional to the number of sites injected as well as the volume and total dosage utilized at any one time.
5. In the treatment of entrapment neuropathies, tendinitis, tenosynovitis, or bursitis, the local anesthetic–corticosteroid injection results in such predictable benefit that diagnosis is assisted by the results of injection.

Moreover, a local anesthetic–corticosteroid injection facilitates an exercise and physical therapy regimen. It is one of the few regional analgesic-antiinflammatory techniques that are suitable for everyday practice and requires little special training (28).

Indications

Soft tissue injection is indicated (*a*) in traumatic, inflammatory, or degenerative processes of the musculoskeletal system, especially when associated with local tenderness or trigger points (21, 28); (*b*) to assist in confirming the diagnosis of bursitis, tendinitis, and entrapment neuropathies; and (*c*) in certain periarticular soft tissue conditions that can lead to limitation of motion; in these situations, injection is helpful in providing a more rapid resumption of active range of motion, thus preventing more serious sequelae (20).

Epidural steroid injections for the treatment of lumbar disc disease and lumbar spinal stenosis are recommended for consideration when profound disability occurs. In one study of spinal stenosis patients, pain relief occurred in 11 of 25 patients. The relief persisted for 4 to 16 months (34). However, in a controlled study of patients with chronic back pain and sciatica, epidural steroids were compared with procaine alone; no difference was noted (35). But simple deep paravertebral muscle and presacral/sacroiliac injections using a No. 22 needle 2.0–3.5 inches long will also provide relief in those patients with tight, tender muscles, at much less expense.

Contraindications

Hypersensitivity to any anesthetic preparation is rare but can occur (36). Dermal allergy is less common with lidocaine and its derivatives (36). Soft tissue injection is obviously contraindicated in the vicinity of infections. A relative contraindication is an extremely apprehensive or neurotic patient (28). Injections into tendon areas are contraindicated in anyone who tends to overuse these structures as they may result in tendon rupture (37).

Hazards

A corticosteroid agent for soft tissue injection should be used with some caution in patients who have had a recent peptic ulcer or brittle diabetes, or who are using anticoagulants. The diabetic who is taking insulin may be advised to use a sliding scale of increased insulin dosage for 1 or 2 days following the injection based upon the result of fractional urine sugar or blood sugar determinations. Aggravation of the diabetic state is rarely a problem. Application of local compression following soft tissue injection prevents significant hematomas in most patients receiving anticoagulants. An *active* peptic ulcer is a relative contraindication to a local corticosteroid injection unless a small dose is used. Local injections with corticosteroids should also be used with caution, if at all, in patients with recent thromboembolic disease, pneumonia, or active systemic infection (28). Introducing infection with local injection has become remarkably rare since the introduction of disposable needles and syringes (19).

Certain hazards are related to the specific site of injection. A *pneumothorax* may result when soft tissue injections are made into the chest or trapezius region (35). Intravascular injection or *hematoma formation* is a risk following injection of the popliteal, antecubital, or groin regions. *Reflex sympathetic dystrophy* and nerve injury with paralysis may follow inadvertent injection of a neurovascular bundle, but these are rare complications.

The use of these agents may be associated with specific pharmacologic or hypersensitivity reactions as described below.

LOCAL ANESTHETICS

Accidental intravenous introduction of the local anesthetic agent may result in central nervous system or cardiovascular reactions. These effects may depend on the blood levels of the agents, which in turn depend upon the site of the injections, the number of sites injected, and the dose. A linear relationship exists between number of reactions and the total dose of the local anesthetic (36).

Central nervous system effects include lightheadedness, dizziness, visual or auditory (tinnitus) complaints, slurred speech, muscle twitching, or muscle tremors, particularly about the face (36). Cardiovascular effects include prolongation of the conduction time with resultant bradycardia, and stimulation of vascular smooth muscle contractions. Another rare hazard of local anesthetics is anaphylaxis (36). More severe reactions following intravenous injection include clonic and tonic convulsions, shallow respirations, diminished blood pressure and pulse rate, and finally, cardiorespiratory collapse. These reactions may begin 5 to 15 minutes or even several hours following the injections (28). Serious hypersensitivity or toxic reactions are more likely to occur when large amounts of local anesthetic are used for soft tissue injection therapy.

The clinician should have an airway tube, oxygen, intravenous diazepam, short-acting parenteral barbiturates, phenylephrine, epinephrine, and rapid-acting intravenous corticosteroids available for emergency use (28, 36).

More common than these serious reactions is the more immediate vasovagal reaction seen in patients with vasomotor instability. The vasovagal reaction occurs within seconds following the injection. The patient becomes pale, sweaty, and lightheaded, and may faint. The pulse rate is slow but blood pressure remains normal. A crushable ampule of ammonia is helpful for use in such patients. Often, the reaction occurs in patients who are dehydrated. If the patient is seen long after the last meal or when fasting, we provide 8 oz water before the injection.

Focal muscle injury, proportional to the potency and duration of action of the local anesthetic agent, has been reported and was usually reversible (36). We have not had that experience with lidocaine hydrochloride or procaine hydrochloride. Localized nerve damage has not been seen following use of a local anesthetic agent unless the injection is inadvertently made into a nerve.

CORTICOSTEROIDS

Systemic toxicity from local injections of corticosteroids is infrequent when the interval before subsequent injections is longer than 6 weeks and the number of injections is less than eight per year (38). Adrenal suppression may occur but is usually transient (39). Local complications include infections, which of course are rare if the clinician uses disposable equipment and careful aseptic techniques (38). Although infection is a rare complication, the patient should report any postinjection development of pain, redness, or swelling (28). Local cutaneous atrophy or depigmentation may occur (28, 40); the atrophy usually resolves but may require weeks or months to regress. A postinjection ''flare'' or local crystal reaction occurs in 1 to 2% of patients receiving steroid injections, and is ameliorated with ice packs (41). When triamcinolone preparations are used for injection in women, menstrual irregularity, breast tenderness, and skin flushing can occur.

Corticosteroids used for local injections should be the repository preparation in suspension (28). We generally use the dose ranges indicated in Table C.2 for any given injection site, depending on the size of the area and the total number of sites to be injected (1). Although we prefer to use procaine hydrochloride or lidocaine hydrochloride in a 1% solution and methylprednisolone acetate or triamcinolone acetonide, the preparations' cost and availability as well as personal experience will assist each clinician in choosing the most suitable agents. The addition of epinephrine to the local anesthetic is not recommended.

Other agents are under investigation for soft tissue injection. Diclofenac has been reported to be helpful in myofascial pain (42), and antioxidants are under investigation.

Technique

Tables C.3 and C.4 summarize some of the details of injection technique. Prior to injection, the point of maximum tenderness should be located by palpation. Then the clinician can use the open end of the needle container cover to indent and mark the trigger point location (RI Finkel, personal communication, 1973) or the back of blunt end of a ballpoint pen. Strict skin sterilization is essential. If iodine-containing material is to be used, a history of iodine sensitivity should be sought prior to skin preparation. Injections should be made with appropriate sterile precautions. Gloves are recommended to protect the patient and the physician. Raising a skin wheal before deep injection has not been essential since the introduction of disposable needles that are sharp and without barbs. A vapocoolant spray such as ethyl chloride may provide surface anesthesia if desired.

A ½-inch No. 25, No. 26, or No. 27 dermal needle is most appropriate for a "trigger finger" tendon injection. A 1-inch No. 22 or No. 23 needle is used for carpal tunnel injection. In myofascial pain disorders, the needle point may be used as a probe to reproduce the patient's pain. A 4-inch No. 20 spinal needle may be necessary for injecting the piriformis muscle, the trochanteric bursa, or the low back region.

TABLE C.3 SOFT TISSUE INJECTION—HELPFUL POINTS ON TECHNIQUE

1. Mark site of injection with circular end of needle container cover or ballpoint pen
2. Prepare a sterile field; use gloves or sterile technique
3. Use the shortest needle that will reach the lesion
4. For injecting tender points, use the needle as a probe
5. For injecting tendon sheaths, insert the needle parallel to the tendon
6. At site of nerve entrapment, wait a moment after needle is inserted; be certain the needle has not penetrated a nerve or vessel
7. Use 1 or 2% local anesthetic *without epinephrine*

From Sheon RP: Non-articular rheumatism and nerve entrapment syndromes. In: Roth SH, ed. Rheumatic therapeutics. New York: McGraw-Hill, 1985.

TABLE C.4 SOFT TISSUE INJECTION TECHNIQUE

Injection Site	Needle Size (No.)	Needle Length (inches)	Local Anesthetic (mL)	Crystalline Steroid (mg)	Comments
Temporomandibular joint	23–27	1/2–1	0.5	5–20	Have mouth open
Cervical TP	23–27	1/2–1	0.5–1.0	5–10	Use needle as a probe
Trapezius or scapular TP	23–27	1/2–1	0.5–1.0	10–20	
Shoulder tendons	23–27	1/2–1	1.0–2.0	10–20	Watch for twitch response
Epicondyle (humerus)	23–27	1/2–1	1.0	10–20	Inject tender spot and tendon
Carpal tunnel	23–27	1/2–1	1.0	10–20	Inject radial side of palmaris longus
Hand tendons	23–27	1/2–1	0.25	10–20	Distal to tendon nodule
Chest or thorax TP	23–27	1/2–1	1.0	10–20	Inject intercostal nerve also
Erector spinae TP	20–22	1–3.5	1.0–2.0	10–20	Determine if needle site
Gluteus TP	20–22	1–3.5	1.0	10–20	reproduces sciatica, if present
Trochanteric bursitis	20–22	1–3.5	1.0–3.0	20–40	Use needle as probe for TP
Fascia lata fasciitis	20–22	1–2	0.5–1.0	10–20	May have 6–12 sites along fascia
Knee and foreleg	20–22	1–2	1.0	10–20	Avoid peroneal nerve
Tarsal tunnel	23–27	1/2–1	1.0	10–20	Avoid nerve and vessels
Plantar fascia	23–27	1/2–1	0.5	10–20	Locate at least 3 sites
Intermetatarsal bursitis	23–27	1/2–1	0.5	5–10	Just proximal to web of toes

Note: TP = trigger point or tender point.
From Sheon RP: Non-articular rheumatism and nerve entrapment syndromes. In: Roth SH, ed. Rheumatic therapeutics. New York: McGraw-Hill, 1985.

Pitfalls to Injection Therapy

These injections are not solvents for hypertrophic or degenerated tissue (28). The injection must be part of a comprehensive program for soft tissue rheumatic pain as described throughout this text. Among the pitfalls leading to failure are the following (28):

1. A wrong diagnosis or incorrect localization of the soft tissue rheumatic pain site
2. Advanced or irreversible changes
3. Uncorrected contributory factors such as poor body mechanics, or systemic factors that are unrecognized or untreated
4. Multiple lesions that are unrecognized
5. Refractoriness to local anesthetics if used alone
6. Treatment of subjective complaints without findings
7. Persons who are hypersensitive or who have low pain thresholds

If infection is suspected, local injection therapy should not be used until infection has been excluded. A previous mild crystal reaction or a vasovagal reaction is not an absolute contraindication to future reinjection.

Frequency of Injections. How often and how many times a soft tissue lesion should be injected requires the use of common sense. Disorders known to be occasionally stubborn in their response, such as a carpal tunnel syndrome or a thickened olecranon bursitis, may best be treated by surgery rather than by many repeated local injections.

Repeated need for injection of the same site should raise the possibility of continued strain or aggravation. Review of work, hobby, sport, or homemaking activity should be undertaken. In general, more than three corticosteroid-anesthetic injections over 6 months into the same site should be avoided.

REFERENCES

1. Moskowitz RW: Clinical Rheumatology. 2nd Ed. Philadelphia: Lea & Febiger, 1982.
2. Zuckerman JD, Meislin RJ, Rothberg M: Injections for joint and soft tissue disorders: when and how to use them. Geriatrics 45(4):45–55, 1990.
3. Hill JJ Jr, Trapp RG, Colliver JA: Survey on the use of corticosteroid injections by orthopaedists. Contemp Orthop 18(1):39–45, 1989.
4. Fauno P, Andersen HJ, Simonsen O: A long-term follow-up of the effect of repeated corticosteroid injections for stenosing tenosynovitis. J Hand Surg (Br) 14:242–243, 1989.
5. Marks MR, Ganther SF: Efficacy of cortisone injection in treatment of trigger fingers and thumbs. J Hand Surg (Am) 14:722–727, 1989.
6. Bourne IHJ: The treatment of pain with local injections. Practitioner 227:1877–1883, 1983.
7. Namba RS, Kabo JM, Dorey FJ, et al.: Intra-articular corticosteroid reduces joint stiffness after an experimental periarticular fracture. J Hand Surg 17A:1148–1153, 1992.
8. Alexander SJ: Cost containment in carpal tunnel syndrome. Arthritis Rheum 22:1415–1416, 1979.
9. Clark DD, Ricker JH, MacCollum MS: The efficacy of local steroid injection in the treatment of stenosing tenovaginitis. Plast Reconstr Surg 51:179–180, 1973.
10. Janecki CJ: Extra-articular steroid injection for hand and wrist disorders. Postgrad Med 68: 173–181, 1980.
11. Hopwood MB, Abram SE: Factors associated with failure of trigger point injections. Clin J Pain 10:227–234, 1994.
12. Melzak R, Stillwell DM, Fox EJ: Trigger points and acupuncture points for pain: correlations and implications. Pain 3:3–23, 1977.
13. Travell J: Conferences on therapy: management of pain due to muscle spasm. New York State J Med 45:2085–2097, 1945.
14. Lewit K: The needle effect in the relief of myofascial pain. Pain 6:83–90, 1979.
15. Gunn CC, Milbrandt WE, Little AS, Mason KE: Dry needling of muscle motor points for chronic low-back pain. Spine 5:279–291, 1980.
16. Frost FA, Jessen B, Siggard-Anderson J: A control, double-blind comparison of mepivacaine injection versus saline injection for myofascial pain. Lancet 1:499–501, 1980.
17. Hameroff SR, Crago BR, Blitt CD, et al.: Comparison of bupivacaine, etidocaine, and saline for trigger-point therapy. Anesthesia Analgesia 60:752–755, 1981.
18. Janssens LA: Trigger points in 48 dogs with myofascial pain syndromes. Veterin Surg 20: 274–278, 1991.
19. Hollander JL, Jessar RA, Brown EM: Intra-synovial corticosteroid therapy: a decade of use. Bull Rheum Dis 11:239–240, 1961.
20. Fitzgerald RH: Intrasynovial injection of steroids: uses and abuses. Mayo Clin Proc 51:655–659, 1959.

21. Finder JG, Post M: Local injection therapy for rheumatic diseases. JAMA 172:2021–2030, 1960.

22. Kennedy JC, Willis RB: The effects of local steroid injections on tendons: a biomechanical and microscopic correlative study. Am J Sports Med 4:11–21, 1976.

23. McWhorter JW, Francis RS, Heckmann RA: Influence of local steroid injections on traumatized tendon properties. Am J Sports Med 19:435–439, 1991.

24. Kapetanos G: The effect of the local corticosteroids on the healing and biomechanical properties of the partially injured tendon. Clin Orthop Res 163:170–179, 1982.

25. Trapp RG, Hill JJ, Su C, Mody N: Effects of injectable corticosteroids on extra-articular soft tissues of the extremities. (Abstract #D56) Arthritis Rheum 28(4) [Suppl], 1985.

26. Ismail AM, Balakrishman R, Rajakumar MK. Rupture of patellar ligament after steroid infiltration. J Bone Joint Surg 51B:503–505, 1969.

27. Gottlieb NL, Riskin WG: Complications of local corticosteroid injections. JAMA 243:1547–1548, 1980.

28. Steinbrocker O, Neustadt DH: Aspiration and injection therapy in musculoskeletal disorders. New York: Harper & Row, 1972.

29. Swezey RL, Weiner SR: Rehabilitation medicine and arthritis. In: McCarty DJ, ed. Arthritis and allied conditions. 10th ed. Philadelphia: Lea & Febiger, 1985.

30. Brown BR: Myofascial and musculoskeletal pain. Inst Anesthiol Clin 21:139–151, 1983.

31. Brown BB: Diagnosis and therapy of common myofascial syndromes. JAMA 239:646–648, 1978.

32. Adverse reactions with bupivacaine. Health Human Services Bull, p. 23, 1983.

33. Newman RJ, Radda GK: The myotoxicity of bupivacaine: a 31P NMR investigation. Br J Pharm 79:395–399, 1983.

34. Hozman R, Eisenberg G, McLaughlin D, Arnold W: Epidural steroid injection (ESI) in the treatment of lumbar spinal stenosis (SS). (Abstract #93) Arthritis Rheum 27(4) [Suppl], 1984.

35. Cuckler JM, Bernini PA, Wiesel SW, et al.: The use of epidural steroids in the treatment of lumbar radicular pain. J Bone Joint Surg 67A:63–66, 1985.

36. Covino BG, Vassallo HG: Local anesthetics: mechanisms of action and clinical use. New York: Grune & Stratton, 1976.

37. Sweetnam R: Corticosteroid arthropathy and tendon rupture. J Bone Joint Surg 1:397–398, 1969.

38. Hollander JL: Arthrocentesis technique and intrasynovial therapy. In: McCarty DJ, ed. Arthritis and allied conditions. 10th ed. Philadelphia: Lea & Febiger, 1985.

39. Reeback JS, Chakraborty J, English J, et al.: Plasma steroid levels after intra-articular injection of prednisolone acetate in patients with rheumatoid arthritis. Ann Rheum Dis 39:22–24, 1980.

40. Cassidy JT, Bole GG: Cutaneous atrophy secondary to intra-articular corticosteroid administration. Ann Intern Med 65:1008–1018, 1966.

41. McCarty DJ, Hogan JM: Inflammatory reaction after intrasynovial injection of microcrystalline adrenocorticosteroid esters. Arthritis Rheum 7:359–367, 1964.

42. Frost A: Diclofenac versus lidocaine as injection therapy in myofascial pain. Scand J Rheumatol 15:153–156, 1986.

APPENDIX D: Coding for Your Services

Soft tissue pain or functional impairment may be a visit of low or moderate intensity. However, you may upcode when you teach the patient exercises and/or provide joint protection and energy conservation advice. Furthermore, your medical assistant may use the 99211 code (for brief encounters, not necessarily with the physician), if the assistant provides this information on another day. If the condition is layered over an existing connective tissue disease, similar upcoding should reflect the time spent in that counseling in addition to the care rendered for the connective tissue disease.

If you perform a procedure and provide evaluation and additional management, be sure to add the -25 modifier. This informs the insurer that additional evaluation and management time was provided at the time of the intralesional injection.

If you perform a bilateral joint procedure, then the treatment code should be preceded by a -50 modifier. This informs the insurer that a bilateral procedure was performed and usually the second procedure is reimbursed at a lesser fee. In general, we do not recommend counting the individual locations that are injected beyond three. Thus, for performing tender point injections at eight locations we would charge for three. If the treatment is rendered as a soft tissue problem, then the 20550 code is used; the -50 modifier is not used with the 20550 code.

You may also add a charge for the ingredients injected. Some examples are:

Lidocaine	J2000
Methylprednisolone	J1030
Triamcinolone	J3301

Obviously, these codes pertain only to insurers in the U.S.

Some soft tissue ICD-9 CM (International Classification of Diseases of the World Health Organization Code Manual) diagnosis codes are presented in Table D.1.

Coding for your services must be done correctly the first time. Make certain that the modifier -25 is included when you provide additional examination or management care in order to receive payment for both the office call and the procedure.

TABLE D.1 SOFT TISSUE ICD-9 CM CODES

Head and Neck

723.4	Cervical neuritis
353.0	Thoracic outlet syndrome
723.1	Myofascial pain, cervical
524.6	TMJ syndrome

Upper Limb

719.41	Myofascial pain, shoulder
726.0	Frozen shoulder
726.1	Bursitis/Tendinitis, shoulder
726.11	Calcific bursitis, shoulder
726.12	Bicipital tenosynovitis
719.42	Myofascial pain, elbow
726.32	Tennis elbow
726.33	Olecranon bursitis
719.43	Myofascial pain, wrist
719.44	Hand pain
352.0	Carpal tunnel syndrome
727.04	de Quervain's tenosynovitis
727.05	Wrist/Hand tendinitis
727.03	Trigger finger

Chest Region

733.6	Tietze's syndrome
733.99	Costochondritis
786.5	Chest pain

Lumbar/Pelvis Region

724.02	Lumbar spinal stenosis
724.2	Myofascial pain, low back
847.2	Lumbar strain
724.6	Sacroiliac pain
724.3	Sciatica
724.4	Lumbar radiculopathy
724.5	Back pain

Lower Limb

719.45	Hip or thigh pain
726.5	Trochanteric bursitis
717.9	Internal derangement, knee
719.46	Pain, knee
726.64	Patellar tendinitis
726.6	Knee bursitis
727.51	Baker's cyst
726.61	Pes anserine bursitis
726.65	Prepatellar bursitis
719.46	Pain, lower leg
719.47	Pain, ankle
353.5	Tarsal tunnel syndrome
727.3	Heel bursitis
728.71	Plantar fasciitis
728.79	Nodular fasciitis
726.7	Metatarsalgia
719.47	Foot pain

Generalized Disorders

729.0	Fibromyalgia
719.49	Myofascial pain, multiple sites
780.7	Fatigue
718.89	Hypermobility syndrome

Unspecified Region

729.5	Pain in limb
726.9	Tendinitis, unspecified
729.1	Myalgia, unspecified
729.4	Fasciitis, unspecified

APPENDIX E: Sources for Illustrated Equipment

1. Jackson Cervipillo
   Designed by Dr. Ruth Jackson
   Assistant Professor of Orthopedic Surgery
   University of Texas, Dallas

   Manufactured by Tru-Trac for
   Sunrise Medical Guardian
   Arieta, CA 91331

2. The Original McKenzie Cervical Roll
   OPTP Orthopedic Physical
   Therapy Products
   P.O. Box 47009
   Minneapolis, MN 55447
   (612) 553-0452

3. The Cervical Roll
   Saunders Therapy Products
   Chaska, MN 55318

4. The Wal-Pil-O
   Roloke Co.
   5760 Hannum Avenue
   Culver City, CA 90230
   (213) 649-1807

5. Matey Reaching Aid
   P.O. Box 12
   Pequannock, NJ 07440-1993

6. Posey Footguard
   J.T. Posey Co.
   Arcadia, CA 91006

7. Aircast Pneumatic Armband
   Aircast Inc.
   Summit, NJ 07901
   (800) 526-8785
   (908) 273-6349

8. Handeze Therapeutic Craft Gloves
   Berroco
   Uxbridge, MA 01569

9. Over-Door Traction
   Duro-Med Industries, Inc.
   Hackensack, NJ 07602

10. "Carex" Hand-Held Shower Spray
    Model 765000
    Division of Acorn Development Cos., Inc.
    Newark, NJ 07114

11. X-Depth Shoes
    P.W. Minor
    P.O. Box 678
    Batavia, NY 14021-0678

12. Running Shoes — New Balance
    New Balance Athletic Shoe, Inc.
    Boston, MA 02134

13. Walking Shoe — Rockport
    The Rockport Co.
    220 Donald J. Lynch Blvd.
    P.O. Box 30
    Marlboro, MA 01752

14. The AquaJogger: Approved for insurance
    payment as a Stabilization aid for hydro-
    therapy programs. The CPT code is Aqua-
    Jogger 99070.
    Sports Science International
    P.O. Box 1453
    Eugene, OR 97440
    (800) 922-9544

15. Theraband
    The Hygenic Corp.
    1245 Home Avenue
    Akron, OH 44310
    (800) 321-2135
    Fax: (216) 633-9359

INDEX

Page numbers followed by "f" refer to figures, those followed by "t" refer to tables.